NURSING INTERVENTIONS

Essential Nursing Treatments

Second Edition

NURSING
INTERVENTIONS
Essential Nursing Treatments

GLORIA M. BULECHEK, RN, PhD

College of Nursing
University of Iowa
Iowa City, Iowa

JOANNE C. McCLOSKEY, RN, PhD

College of Nursing
University of Iowa
Iowa City, Iowa

W. B. SAUNDERS COMPANY
Harcourt Brace Jovanovich, Inc.

Philadelphia / London / Toronto / Montreal / Sydney / Tokyo

W.B. SAUNDERS COMPANY
Harcourt Brace Jovanovich, Inc.

The Curtis Center
Independence Square West
Philadelphia, Pennsylvania 19106

Library of Congress Cataloging-in-Publication Data	
Nursing interventions : essential nursing treatments / [editors], Gloria M. Bulechek, Joanne C. McCloskey. --2nd ed.	
p. cm.	
Includes bibliographical references and index.	
ISBN 0-7216-3802-3	
1. Nursing. 2. Nursing diagnosis. 3. Nurse and patient.	
I. Bulechek, Gloria M. II. McCloskey, Joanne Comi.	
[DNLM: 1. Acute Disease--nursing. 2. Health Promotion--nurses instruction. 3. Nurse-Patient Relations. 4. Nursing Process.	
5. Self Care--nurses' instruction. 6. Therapeutics--nurses instruction. WY 100 N973]	
RT48.N8835 1992	
610.73--dc20	
DNLM/DLC	
for Library of Congress	91-37725
	CIP

Editor: Thomas Eoyang

NURSING INTERVENTIONS
Essential Nursing Treatments . . . . .ISBN   0-7216-3802-3

Printed in Mexico.

Last digit is the print number: 9   8   7   6   5   4   3   2

CONTRIBUTORS

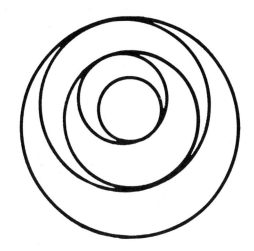

LAURIE L. ACKERMAN, MA, RN, CNRN
Clinical Nurse Specialist, Neuroscience Nursing Division, University of Iowa Hospitals and
Clinics, Iowa City, Iowa
Secondary Brain Injury Reduction

JANET DAVIDSON ALLAN, PhD, RN, FAAN
Associate Professor, School of Nursing, University of Texas at Austin, Austin, Texas
Exercise Program

MICHELE A. ALPEN, BSN, RN, CCRN
Nurse Clinician, Critical Care, University of Iowa Hospitals and Clinics, Iowa City, Iowa
Ventilatory Support

GAIL ARDERY, PhD, RN
Patient Care Coordinator, Iowa City Hospice, Iowa City, Iowa
Terminal Care

LINDA JO BANKS, MS, MA, RN, CS
Clinical Specialist in Medical-Surgical Nursing, Mercy Hospital Medical Center, Des
Moines, Iowa
Counseling

NANCY BERGSTROM, PhD, RN, FAAN
Professor, College of Nursing, University of Nebraska Medical Center, Omaha, Nebraska
Pressure Reduction

SUSAN BOEHM, PhD, RN, FAAN
Associate Professor, and Arthur F. Thurnau Professor, School of Nursing, University of Michigan, Ann Arbor, Michigan
Patient Contracting

BARBARA J. BRADEN, PhD, RN
Professor, School of Nursing, Creighton University, Omaha, Nebraska
Pressure Reduction

JERRI BRYANT, MPH, RN, CIC
Nurse Epidemiologist, Cleveland Clinic Foundation, Cleveland, Ohio
Infection Control

KATHLEEN C. BUCKWALTER, PhD, RN, FAAN
Professor, College of Nursing, University of Iowa, and Associate Director, Office of Nursing Research and Development, University of Iowa Hospitals and Clinics, Iowa City, Iowa
Confusion Management

GLORIA M. BULECHEK, PhD, RN
Associate Professor, College of Nursing, University of Iowa, Iowa City, Iowa
Nursing Diagnoses, Interventions, and Outcomes; Future Directions

MARTHA A. CARPENTER, PhD, RN
Assistant Professor, College of Nursing, University of Iowa, Iowa City, Iowa
Support Groups

KATHLEEN CASTIGLIA, MSN, RN
Critical Care Educator, Desert Samaritan Medical Center, Mesa, Arizona
Hemodynamic Regulation

NORMA J. CHRISTMAN, PhD, RN, FAAN
Associate Professor, College of Nursing, and Department of Behavioral Science, College of Medicine, University of Kentucky, Lexington, Kentucky
Concrete Objective Information

FELISSA L. COHEN, PhD, RN, FAAN
Professor and Head, Department of Medical-Surgical Nursing, and Director, Center for Narcolepsy Research, College of Nursing, University of Illinois at Chicago, Chicago, Illinois
Sleep Promotion

JANET K. CRIST, MA, RN
Owner/Counselor, Weight & Wellness Management, and Adjunct Instructor, University of Iowa, College of Nursing, Iowa City, Iowa
Weight Management

SANDRA CUMMINGS, MSN, RN, CS
Program Director, Jackson Brook Institute, South Portland, Maine
Group Psychotherapy

JEANETTE M. DALY, PhD Candidate, MS, RN
Director of Nursing, Oaknoll Retirement Residence, Iowa City, Iowa
Discharge Planning

CYNTHIA M. DOUGHERTY, PhD, RN
Postdoctoral Fellow, School of Nursing, University of Washington, and Cardiac Rehabilitation Coordinator, Swedish Hospital Medical Center, Seattle, Washington
Surveillance

NANCY J. EVANS, MSN, RN, CNSN
Clinical Specialist in Nutrition Support, Hospital of the University of Pennsylvania, University of Pennsylvania, Philadelphia, Pennsylvania
Feeding

MARGERY O. FEARING, MA, RN
Clinical Nursing Specialist, University of Iowa Hospitals and Clinics, Iowa City, Iowa
Dialysis Therapy

DIANE L. GARDNER, PhD, RN
Assistant Professor, College of Nursing, University of Iowa, Iowa City, Iowa
Presence

MEG GULANICK, PhD, RN
Clinical Nurse Specialist/Program Director Cardiac Rehabilitation, Humana Hospital—Michael Reese Hospital and Medical Center, Chicago, Illinois
Shock Management

DIANE BRONKEMA HAMILTON, PhD, RN
Assistant Professor, College of Nursing, Medical University of South Carolina, Charleston, South Carolina
Reminiscence Therapy

MARY ANDERSON HARDY, PhD, RN
Associate Professor, College of Nursing, University of Iowa, Iowa City, Iowa
Dry Skin Care

LAURA K. HART, PhD, RN
Associate Professor, College of Nursing, University of Iowa, Iowa City, Iowa
Dialysis Therapy

ADA JACOX, PhD, RN, FAAN
Professor and Independence Foundation Chair in Health Policy, Johns Hopkins University, School of Nursing, Baltimore, Maryland
Pain Control

GERRY A. JONES, MA, RN, CCRN
Clinical Nurse Specialist, University of Iowa Hospitals and Clinics, Iowa City, Iowa
Airway Management

KATHLEEN C. KELLY, PhD, RN
Assistant Professor, College of Nursing, University of Iowa, Iowa City, Iowa
Discharge Planning

CAROLYN K. KINNEY, PhD, RN
Assistant Professor, School of Nursing, University of Texas at Austin, Austin, Texas
Support Groups

KARIN T. KIRCHHOFF, PhD, RN, FAAN
Professor, College of Nursing and Director of Nursing Research, University Hospital, University of Utah, Salt Lake City, Utah
Concrete Objective Information

JANE S. KNIPPER, MA, RN
Clinical Instructor and Lecturer, College of Nursing, University of Iowa, and Staff Nurse and Staff Educator, University of Iowa Hospitals and Clinics, Iowa City, Iowa
Ventilatory Support

ROBERT J. KUS, PhD, RN
Associate Professor, College of Nursing, University of Iowa, Iowa City, Iowa
Crisis Intervention; Art Therapy

LINDA J. LEWICKI, MSN, RN
Nurse Researcher, Cleveland Clinic Foundation, and Program Coordinator, Medicare Clinic Pilot Project, Cleveland, Ohio
Infection Control

DEBRA J. LIVINGSTON, MS, RN
Clinical Nurse Specialist, Psychiatric Nursing, University of Iowa Hospitals and Clinics, Iowa City, Iowa
Truth Telling

JENNIFER M. LOEPER, MS, RN
Clinical Nurse Educator, Abbott-Northwestern Hospital, Minneapolis, Minnesota
Positioning

MERIDEAN L. MAAS, PhD, RN, FAAN
Associate Professor and Chair, Organizations and Systems, College of Nursing, University of Iowa, Iowa City, Iowa
Intermittent Catheterization

ELEANOR McCLELLAND, PhD, RN
Associate Professor and Associate Dean, Undergraduate Studies, College of Nursing, University of Iowa, Iowa City, Iowa
Discharge Planning

JOANNE COMI McCLOSKEY, PhD, RN, FAAN
Professor, College of Nursing, University of Iowa, and Adjunct Associate Director of Nursing, University of Iowa Hospitals and Clinics, Iowa City, Iowa
Nursing Diagnoses, Interventions, and Outcomes; Future Directions

AUDREY M. McLANE, PhD, RN
Professor Emerita, Marquette University, Milwaukee, Wisconsin
Bowel Management

RUTH E. McSHANE, PhD, RN
Assistant Professor, University of Wisconsin–Milwaukee, Milwaukee, Wisconsin
Bowel Management

REBECCA MANNETTER, PhD, RN
Therapist, Eastern Iowa Psychiatric Services, Cedar Rapids, Iowa
Support Groups

MICHELE S. MAVES, MSN, RN
Quality Assurance Director, Gastrointestinal Associates, Knoxville, Tennessee
Mutual Goal Setting

THÉRÈSE CONNELL MEEHAN, PhD, RN
Honorary Associate Lecturer, Department of Nursing Studies, Massey University, Palmerston North, New Zealand, and Staff Nurse, Northland Base Hospital and Nurse Researcher, Whangarei Area, Northland Area Health Board, Northland, New Zealand
Therapeutic Touch

SHARON L. MERRITT, EdD, RN
Assistant Professor, Department of Medical-Surgical Nursing, and Assistant Director, Center for Narcolepsy Research, College of Nursing, University of Illinois at Chicago, Chicago, Illinois
Sleep Promotion

MARY ANN MILLER, BLS, RN, CARN
Nurse Clinician and Art Specialist, University of Iowa Chemical Dependency Center, University of Iowa Hospitals and Clinics, and Clinical Instructor, College of Nursing, University of Iowa, Iowa City, Iowa
Art Therapy

LORRAINE C. MION, MSN, RN
Assistant Professor, School of Nursing, Yale University, New Haven, and Gerontological Clinical Nurse Specialist, Yale-New Haven Hospital, New Haven, Connecticut
Environmental Structuring

PAMELA H. MITCHELL, PhD, RN, FAAN, ARNP, CNRN
Professor, Department of Physiological Nursing, University of Washington, Seattle, Washington
Secondary Brain Injury Reduction

NANCY K. MYERS, RN
Nurse Clinician, Iowa Veterans Home, Marshalltown, Iowa
Intermittent Catheterization

MARSHA G. OAKLEY, MSN, RN
Research Assistant, College of Nursing, University of Kentucky, Lexington, Kentucky
Concrete Objective Information

KATHLEEN A. O'CONNELL, PhD, RN
Associate Professor, School of Nursing, University of Kansas, Kansas City, Kansas
Smoking Cessation

ALICE S. POYSS, PhD, RN
Assistant Professor, College of Nursing, Villanova University, Villanova, Pennsylvania
Fluid Therapy

MARLA PRIZANT-WESTON, MN, RN, CCRN
Critical Care Clinical Nurse Specialist, Desert Samaritan Medical Center, Mesa, Arizona
Hemodynamic Regulation

BARBARA K. REDMAN, PhD, RN, FAAN
Executive Director, American Nurses' Association, Washington, DC
Patient Teaching

CAROL RUBACK, MSN, RN, CCRN
Clinical Nurse Specialist, Critical Care, Copley Memorial Hospital, Aurora, Illinois
Shock Management

SHARON SCANDRETT-HIBDON, PhD, RN, AAMFT
Associate Professor, College of Nursing, University of Tennessee, Memphis, Tennessee
Cognitive Reappraisal; Relaxation Training

JANET P. SPECHT, MA, RN, C
Director of Nursing, Iowa Veterans Home, Marshalltown, Iowa
Intermittent Catheterization

JACQUELINE M. STOLLEY, MA, RN, C
Gerontological Clinical Nurse Specialist, Mercy Hospital, Davenport, Iowa
Confusion Management

BETTY PATTERSON TARSITANO, PhD, RN
Health Services Assessment RN, Elmhurst Memorial Home, Elmhurst, Illinois
Structured Preoperative Teaching

SUE ANN THOMAS, PhD, RN
Ellicot City, Maryland
Patient Teaching

MARITA G. TITLER, MA, RN
Clinical Nurse Specialist, University of Iowa Hospitals and Clinics, Iowa City, Iowa
Airway Management

CATHERINE A. TRACEY, MS, RN, CRRN
Vice-President, Patient Care Services, Northeast Rehabilitation Hospital, Salem, New Hampshire
Hygiene Assistance

SUSAN UECKER, MSN, RN, PCN
Director, Nursing Support Services, St. Luke's Episcopal Hospital, Houston, Texas
Relaxation Training

WENDY L. WATSON, PhD, RN
Associate Professor, Education Coordinator — Family Nursing Unit, University of Calgary, Calgary, Alberta, Canada
Family Therapy

ELIZABETH A. WEITZEL, MA, RN
Consultant, R.B. Weitzel Co., Inc., Marshalltown, Iowa
Medication Management

VERONICA WIELAND, MA, RN, CS
Psychotherapist, Mid-Eastern Iowa Community Mental Health Center, Iowa City, Iowa
Group Psychotherapy

JAMES Z. WILBERDING, MA, RN
Clinical Nurse Specialist, Bone Marrow Transplant Unit, Veterans Administration Medical Center, Seattle, Washington
Values Clarification

SALLY WILLETT, BS, RN, C
Nurse Clinician, Iowa Veterans Home, Marshalltown, Iowa
Intermittent Catheterization

CASSANDRA B. WILLIAMSON, MA, RN, CS
Clinical Nurse Specialist, Psychiatric-Mental Health Nursing, Oxford, Ohio
Truth Telling

PREFACE

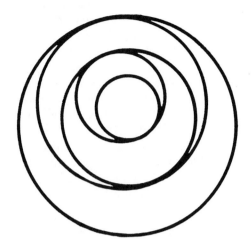

In 1985 we published the first edition of this book. It included 26 chapters each on a different nursing intervention. It was a pioneering work developed to fill a void. Up until this time, little attention had been paid to the conceptualization and identification of nursing interventions. While nurses had done treatments for patients for decades, the idea of discussing nursing interventions as concepts was new. Our text and another that year were the first to focus on independent nursing interventions.

Much has happened in nursing and health care since the first edition. With the increase in computerization, the need to contain costs, and the emphasis on establishing quality of care, there is recognition among nursing leaders and policy makers that we need to document and evaluate the effects of nursing care. In order to do that, we need to systematically label and define those things that nurses do so that nursing care can be included in information system databases; we need to understand the research base for our current interventions in order to study and add to our body of practice knowledge; and we need to develop a common language about our care that can be used to better educate our new members and can communicate with the language of other health care providers.

New features of the second edition

The second edition of the book has several new features.

1. It has been expanded from 26 to 45 chapters. Seventeen of the chapters are on interventions that were included in the first edition. These were updated by previous authors or have new authors. The remaining 28 chapters are new to this edition. Regretfully, we had to leave out some interventions which were included in the first edition in order to make space for the new ones. The choice of what to include was difficult but it was based on our estimation of frequency of use by clinicians (for example, Culture Brokerage, Role Supplementation, and Music Therapy from the first edition are important and helpful interventions, but they are not used as frequently as others) and elimination of redundancies (for example,

in the first edition we had three chapters on Counseling, Nutritional Counseling, and Sexual Counseling while in this one we only have Counseling).

2. The first edition had chapters organized in four sections: Stress Management, Lifestyle Alteration, Acute-Care Management, and Communication. This edition is organized in five sections: Self-Care Assistance; Acute-Care Management; Life-Style Alteration; Health Promotion; and Life Support. The overviews to each section highlight the material in each of the chapters and can be used to select individual chapters for reading.

All of the chapters in the Self-Care Assistance section are new. The interventions included here are the basics of nursing care, for example, Hygiene Assistance, Feeding, Positioning, and Sleep Promotion. While nurses have always done this care, in the past there has been little conceptualization and research about some of these interventions. The section on Acute-Care Management has been expanded. In this edition it includes both psychosocial (for example, Crisis Intervention and Presence) and physiological (for example, Fluid Therapy and Infection Control) interventions that are commonly used by hospital nurses. Discharge Planning concludes this section as it is chiefly used by hospital nurses to help patients adjust to care needs after discharge. The section of Life-Style Alteration includes 6 chapters that were updated from the first edition and five new chapters. The chapters in this section (for example, Values Clarification and Family Therapy) are used most often by nurses who work with patients and families needing to establish and reach new life goals. The section on Health Promotion is an expansion of the section in the previous edition that was called Stress Management. Chapters in this section include both physical (for example, Smoking Cessation and Weight Reduction) and mental (for example, Relaxation Training and Contracting) interventions to improve the health status of the patient. The final section on Life Support is new. Only one chapter in this section (Surveillance) was included in the first edition; all of the rest are new. The chapters in this section demonstrate the essential life saving role of nurses who work in critical care areas.

3. The selection of chapters and sections are based on our expanded definition of nursing interventions. In the first edition we defined a nursing intervention as "an autonomous action based on scientific rationale that is executed to benefit the client in a predicted way related to the nursing diagnosis and the stated goals." Since then we have revised our thinking and our definition: "A nursing intervention is any direct care treatment that a nurse performs on behalf of a client which includes nurse-initiated treatments, physician-initiated treatments, and performance of daily essential functions. These are at the conceptual level and require a series of actions or activities to carry them out." The revised definition captures both the autonomous and collaborative roles of the nurse. A nursing intervention is the action of the nurse in response to either a nursing diagnosis, a physician diagnosis and order, or the patient who may simply need some help with something that does not require a diagnosis. As we continue to work on the conceptualization of nursing interventions, we anticipate that this definition will continue to be refined.

4. The introductory chapter has been rewritten to reflect the inclusiveness of the new definition. The chapter also has new sections on nursing outcomes and on clinical decision making. We believe that the term "nursing process" is now obsolete and that we should now talk about nursing content (diagnoses, interventions and outcomes) and clinical decision making (the process of choosing these and making relationships).

5. The chapters are more clinically useful than in the first edition. While each of the authors was asked to cover the research base for the intervention, they were

instructed for this edition to define in a clinical protocol what it is one does to carry out the intervention. The book as a whole thus has more clinical application than the first edition, without sacrificing the overview of research. Case studies included in nearly all chapters also illustrate the use of the content.

Who should use this book

The book is useful for several audiences. While the book was chiefly written with graduate students in mind, it should be useful in both undergraduate and graduate programs. The book can be used as the text in graduate courses that focus on interventions. It can be a supplementary text in a theory course when an instructor desires to provide illustrations of nursing's developing theory. It also can be used as a supplement to undergraduate clinical textbooks. Some undergraduate programs may want to choose this as a text that can be used across the curriculum in several courses. In this case the interventions in the section on Self-Care Assistance would be included in the foundation course, those in Acute-Care Management in the course that focused on acute hospital care, those in the Life-Style Alteration section in the course on chronic illness, those in the Health Promotion section in the course on wellness, and those in the Life Support section would be covered when the student had critical care content and experience. The book could be particularly useful in RN-to-BSN programs, where nurses can approach familiar activities from a conceptual perspective, having already been exposed to them through basic education and clinical practice. As in the past, clinical specialists will also find the book helpful to document their treatments, and researchers developing studies in any of these areas will find the content here an excellent starting point.

The growth in nursing knowledge

All of the contributors made enormous efforts to define and clarify the interventions. Synthesizing the literature and their practical experience, they have made explicit what has previously been implicit. As the movement to define and articulate the treatments that nurses perform grows, this book has expanded. In a few more years it will be impossible to hold all of the nursing interventions in one text. Several of the chapters in this edition will become books in themselves in order to develop the intervention labels in particular specialty areas. We are excited about the book's contribution to the growth in nursing knowledge. We look forward to the response from the professional community.

Gloria M. Bulechek
Joanne Comi McCloskey

ACKNOWLEDGMENTS

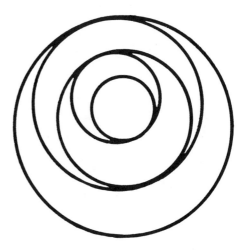

The success of this book is a result of the combined efforts of many people.

We thank the contributors who have synthesized large amounts of literature and applied excellent conceptual skills to define their interventions. In many chapters they have made explicit what has previously been implicit.

We thank the readers and users of the book for your continued support. We were able to publish this second edition because you found the first helpful.

We thank our colleagues at Iowa who are engaged with us in an effort to define a taxonomy of nursing interventions. This book has benefited from our continuing dialogue with them.

In addition, we thank several individuals. Our editor, Thomas Eoyang and his assistant, Terri Fortiner, at Saunders have provided timely and helpful comments. We particularly appreciate Tom's continued support of this book and his recognition and appreciation of its contribution to the knowledge base of nursing. We also thank Jennifer Clougherty, Sue Templin, and Kara Logsden, all members of the staff at the College of Nursing at Iowa, who provided administrative and secretarial support for the book. They helped keep us on time and made it possible for busy people to complete this project.

CONTENTS

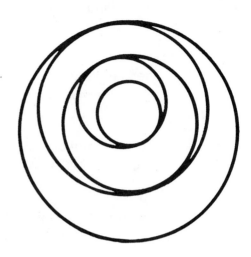

NURSING DIAGNOSES, INTERVENTIONS, AND OUTCOMES

GLORIA M. BULECHEK
JOANNE C. McCLOSKEY

The key to an autonomous profession is a clearly defined base of knowledge. Certainly nursing will continue to use knowledge from other disciplines, but it must define what it is that nurses do and whether what they do makes a difference. In the late 1960s, the nursing process movement—a systematic problem-solving methodology used to describe the process of delivering patient care—initiated work in this area. More recently, it is being recognized that there are also products resulting from the nursing process movement; these are the concepts that have evolved to describe nursing diagnoses, interventions, and outcomes. These concepts are providing the building blocks for a base of knowledge that is uniquely nursing.

This chapter sets forth an overview of diagnoses, interventions, and outcomes to provide a framework for the forty-four intervention chapters that follow.

PAST PERSPECTIVES

Past perspectives focus on the definition and use of the nursing process, a description of the nurse thinking. In a sense, the nursing process was an offshoot of earlier attempts to define nursing. Although nurses have been licensed in the United States since 1903, it was not until 1938, when the first mandatory nursing practice act was passed in New York, that there was a recognized need to define nursing. Until 1938, all acts were permissive, allowing unlicensed persons to practice as long as they did not use the title registered nurse. Although the laws were called nurse practice acts, none of those written before 1938 included a definition of nursing in terms of practice. Rather, a registered nurse was someone who had completed an acceptable nursing program and passed an exam; the emphasis was thus placed on the educational process. With a mandatory act that made it illegal for an unlicensed person to practice nursing, it became necessary in 1938 to define nursing. Nevertheless, attempts at definition have been frustrated by the sheer size of the profession, its diversity in educational preparation, and its work demands.

If it is impossible to say what nursing is, perhaps at least what a nurse does can be described. In 1955, Lydia Hall suggested that the quality of nursing care be judged on a continuum from bad to good by whether the nurse did nursing at the patient, to the patient, for the patient, or with the patient. In 1961, Ida Jean Orlando addressed the interpersonal aspects of the client-nurse relationships. Five years later, Lois Knowles stated that a nurse's success as a practitioner depends on mastery of the 5 Ds (discover, delve, decide, do, and discriminate). The attempts of these and other nurses to describe nursing were important because they put into words the intellectual activity of the nurse, previously labeled as intuitive.

In 1967, faculty at the school of nursing at the Catholic University of America in Washington, D.C., identified four phases of the process — assessment, planning, implementation, and evaluation — which were popularized in Yura and Walsh's book, *The Nursing Process: Assessing, Planning, Implementing and Evaluating* (3d ed.) According to Yura and Walsh, "The nursing process is an orderly, systematic manner of determining the client's problems, making plans to solve them, initiating the plan or assigning others to implement it, and evaluating the extent to which the plan was effective in resolving the problems identified" (p. 20). In Yura and Walsh's steps, assessment begins with the nursing history and ends with the nursing diagnosis, planning includes goal setting and writing the care plan, implementation is the nurse's carrying out the nursing actions called for in her care plan, and evaluation is a rethinking of the diagnosis and treatment in terms of the patient's response. For many years, the popularity of these steps overshadowed other available alternatives. With the advent of nursing diagnosis, a four-step model was replaced by a five-step model, with the most popular steps being assessment, diagnosis, plan, intervention, and evaluation.

The nursing process, then, is a problem-solving systematic approach to care delivery that describes the intellectual activity of the nurse. It connects what a nurse does with why she does it; the nursing process requires actions based on judgment (Gordon 1982). The nursing process standardizes nursing care while providing individual service. Most nurses, however, continue to advocate individual care planning while using a process that encourages group care planning modified for an individual when necessary. A passage from Henry Mintzberg on the professional bureaucracy explains the situation: "The professional has two basic tasks: (1) to categorize the client's need in terms of a contingency, which indicates which standard program to use, a task known as diagnosis and (2) to apply or execute that program. [This categorization] allows the professional to move through the world without making continuing decisions at every moment" (Mintzberg 1979, p. 352).

As examples of the professional, Mintzberg cites the psychiatrist who examines a patient, declares him to be manic-depressive, and thus initiates psychotherapy, and the professor who, finding 100 students registered in the course, executes a lecture program, but facing 20 students instead runs the class as a seminar. Similarly, a professional nurse using the nursing process recognizes such problems as anxiety, pain, and knowledge deficit and has a precise and tested repertoire of skills designed to treat each of these problems. "A professional nurse, while cognizant of individual differences, seeks to identify nursing interventions and patient outcomes that are applicable to identifiable groups of patients" (CURN Project 1981, p. xiv).

Professional nursing practice is the diagnosis and treatment of health problems within the scope of nursing. But what is the scope of nursing? What problems do or should nurses diagnose? What treatments do or should nurses use? What treatments work for what diagnoses? The chapters in this book are a continuing attempt to outline nursing treatments and to relate them to nursing diagnoses. The term *interventions* denotes these nursing treatments.

TABLE 1.   ANA'S MAJOR CATEGORIES OF HUMAN RESPONSES

Self-care limitations
Impaired functioning in areas such as rest, sleep, ventilation circulation, activity, nutrition, elimination, skin, and sexuality
Pain and discomfort
Emotional problems related to illness and treatment, life-threatening events, or daily life experiences, such as anxiety, loss, loneliness, and grief
Distortion of symbolic functions, reflected in interpersonal and intellectual processes, such as hallucinations
Deficiencies in decision making and ability to make personal choices
Self-image changes required by health status
Dysfunctional perceptual orientations to health
Strains related to life processes, such as birth, growth and development, and death
Problematic affiliative relationships

Source: American Nurses' Association. 1980. *Nursing: A social policy statement.* Kansas City: Author.

NURSING DIAGNOSES

The profession's acceptance of making nursing diagnoses came in 1980 when the American Nurses' Association (ANA) published *Nursing: A Social Policy Statement,* which stated that "nursing is the diagnosis and treatment of human responses to actual or potential health problems" (p. 9). The major categories of human responses delineated by ANA appear in Table 1.

A comparison of the ANA's model practice acts of 1955 and 1980 (Table 2) demonstrates the profession's acceptance of diagnosis as an integral part of the nurse's role. In 1955, the act specifically precluded acts of diagnosis, while in 1980, the act acknowledged that nurses diagnose and treat.

The North American Nursing Diagnosis Association (NANDA) has taken the lead in developing the standardized language for the human responses that nurses treat. This group was formed in the early 1970s as the National Conference Group for the Classification of Nursing Diagnoses at St. Louis University. Through a series of invitational conferences, the group began the work of identifying nursing diagnoses (Gebbie and Lavin 1975; Gebbie 1975; Kim and Moritz 1982; Kim, McFarland, and McLane 1984). In work sessions, the participants developed, reviewed, and grouped diagnoses based on their expertise and experience. By

TABLE 2.   ANA'S MODEL PRACTICE ACTS, 1955 AND 1980

1955 Act
"The practice of professional nursing means the performance for compensation of any act in the observation, care and counsel of the ill, injured, or infirm, or in the maintenance of health or prevention of illness of others, or in the supervision and teaching of other personnel, or the administration of medications and treatments prescribed by a licensed physician or dentist; requiring substantial specialized judgement and skill and based on knowledge and application of the principles of biological, physical and social sciences. The foregoing shall *not* [emphasis added] be deemed to include acts of diagnosis or prescription of therapeutic or corrective measures." (Kelly, 1974, p. 1314)

1980 Act
"The practice of nursing means the performance for compensation of professional services requiring substantial knowledge of the biological, physical, behavioral, psychological, and sociological sciences and nursing theory as the basis for assessment, diagnosis, planning, intervention, and evaluation in the promotion and maintenance of health; the case finding and management of illness, injury or infirmity; the restoration of optimum function; or the achievement of a dignified death." (ANA, 1980b)

1982, they had produced an alphabetical list of fifty nursing diagnoses accepted for clinical testing. There was a great deal of discussion about a conceptual framework that would provide a classification schemata for the diagnoses, and a group of nurse theorists assisted with analyzing the various levels of abstractions in the list and proposed various ways of clustering the diagnoses.

In 1985, a taxonomy committee was appointed. This was the first conference open to all nurses and the first held under the bylaws of the new organization, the North American Nursing Diagnosis Association (Hurley 1986). At the next conference, the taxonomy committee proposed Taxonomy I based on nine human response patterns: Exchanging, Communicating, Relating, Valuing, Choosing, Moving, Perceiving, Knowing, and Feeling. The membership endorsed Taxonomy I for development and testing and approved 21 new diagnoses (McLane 1987). Guidelines for classification were developed to incorporate new diagnoses as they evolved. New diagnoses were accepted at the eighth conference (Carroll-Johnson 1989) and the ninth conference (Carroll-Johnson 1991). The most recent version of the taxonomy is Taxonomy I Revised 1990, which lists 99 nursing diagnoses approved for clinical testing. After several years of liaison activity between NANDA and ANA, ANA endorsed NANDA's work on the classification of nursing diagnoses as the official nursing diagnosis taxonomy (Warren and Hoskins 1990).

Although the profession has accepted the making of a diagnosis as part of a nurse's role and developed Taxonomy I, there continues to be debate about the nature of a nursing diagnosis. The NANDA struggle with operationalizing a definition is recounted by Mills (1991). At the ninth conference, the following definition was accepted after floor debate and revision: "A nursing diagnosis is a clinical judgement about individual, family or community responses to actual or potential health problems/life processes. Nursing diagnoses provide the basis for selection of nursing interventions to achieve outcomes for which the nurse is accountable" (Carroll-Johnson 1990, p. 50).

Miers (1991) concluded that the first sentence of the definition is conceptual; it describes the meaning of the term. The second sentence of the definition is contextual; it describes the relationship of nursing diagnosis to nursing process. Miers applied rules and principles of definition in analyzing this definition and recommended areas for clarification.

Developing the definition has been so difficult because the definition is predicated on the scope of nursing. Should nursing diagnoses guide both independent and interdependent aspects of nursing care? Gordon (1987) has taken the position that nursing diagnoses should be used only if independent interventions are needed. Carpenito (1987) also recommends use of nursing diagnoses to guide independent interventions but suggests the use of collaborative problems to guide interdependent interventions. In viewing health status, nursing has a tradition of holism that takes into account the physiologic, psychologic, sociologic, cultural, and spiritual aspects of health. This focus makes it difficult to divide nursing care into independent and interdependent realms.

Two issues have had recurrent debate in regard to the nature of nursing diagnosis. First, there has been continuing controversy surrounding the use of physiology and pathophysiology in the nursing diagnostic process. Should physiological labels be included in the taxonomy? Can nurses collect the data to determine such diagnoses, or are the needed laboratory tests physician controlled? Is the use of protocols autonomous practice? Kim (1984) and Cassmeyer (1989) present convincing arguments that nursing needs to reemphasize the biologic sciences in the diagnostic process. The primary concern for nurses in critical care and many chronic care situations are alterations in the physiological aspects of health. Two sections of this book, Section 1, "Self-Care Assistance," and Section 5, "Life Support," include several interventions for physiological nursing diagnoses. There is need for more physiological diagnoses to direct some of these interventions.

The second issue concerns how the wellness perspective of nursing can be incorporated in the nursing diagnosis movement. Should wellness labels be represented in the taxonomy? The problem orientation has dominated the nursing diagnosis development. Yet nursing claims health promotion as a philosophic basis for practice. Popkess-Vawter (1991) reviews literature supporting wellness nursing diagnosis and advocates their incorporation in the taxonomy. We reaffirm our previous statement (Bulechek and McCloskey 1989) that wellness diagnoses are not necessary. We believe that nurses work to enhance client strengths through interventions to treat actual diagnoses or in redirection of risk factors for potential diagnoses. In our view, most of the examples of wellness diagnoses (e.g., increased activity tolerance, effective airway clearance, effective breast feeding, health-seeking behaviors) are outcome statements, not diagnostic nomenclature.

The question, What is a nursing diagnosis? will continue to be revisited. In our own words, a nursing diagnosis is the identification of a patient's problem that the nurse can treat. Some diagnoses are both nursing and medical. Some patients have many nursing diagnoses, some only one or two, and some none at all. Nursing diagnoses change more frequently than medical diagnoses, and some patients with no nursing diagnoses one day may have several a few days later as a result of medical intervention. Nursing diagnoses are more fluid, varying, and episodic than medical diagnoses (ANA 1980a).

In order to classify and standardize nursing diagnoses and treatments, it is necessary to accompany a diagnosis with the signs, symptoms, and etiology that led to the making of it. Several formats exist for stating a nursing diagnosis: PES (Problem-Etiology-Signs/Symptoms) format, related to format, supporting data format, and POR (Problem-Oriented Record) format. Examples of diagnoses made in each format are in Table 3. The basic elements of each format are the diagnosis (problem), its etiology (cause), and its characteristics (signs and symptoms). Whatever the format, supporting data (etiology and characteristics) are important because they give clues as to how to treat the problem. This will not always be necessary; at some point in the future, a nursing diagnosis will mean, just as a medical diagnosis does now, a precise set of signs and symptoms and etiology, which will call for certain treatments. NANDA is striving to move in this direction by requiring all new diagnosis submissions to include a label, a definition, a list of etiologies, and a list of defining characteristics.

NURSING INTERVENTIONS

Multiple terms are used to label the treatment portion of the nursing process, including *action, activity, intervention, treatment, therapeutics, order,* and *implementation*. There is overlap in the literature between what constitutes intervention versus assessment and evaluation. The following are typical of treatments listed in current textbooks: "measure intake and output;" "measure central venous pressure;" "help patient with personal hygiene;" "watch for signs and symptoms of infection;" "have patient turn, cough, and deep breathe." Are these assessment, treatment, or evaluation activities? These examples show that interventions are viewed as discrete actions with little conceptualization of how the actions fit together. The result is wordy, lengthy care plans that are difficult to use.

TABLE 3. NURSING DIAGNOSIS EXPRESSED IN FOUR DIFFERENT FORMATS

PES format
Problem: Impaired Reality Testing (Acute)
Etiology: Psychosis
Signs and symptoms
1. Impaired perception
2. Impaired attention span
3. Impaired decision making (Bruce 1979)

Related to format
Anxiety related to impending surgery as characterized by verbalization.
Knowledge deficit related to diabetes as characterized by inability to give self insulin, inadequate diet, and poor hygiene.

Supporting data format
Knowledge deficit
Supporting data: Newly diagnosed diabetic. Does not know how to give daily insulin injections. Daily intake list for past week reveals diet not followed, although instruction by dietitian 7/1. Overweight. Poor hygiene practices. Believes diabetes will go away in a few years.

POR format (Problem-Oriented Record)
S. Believes diabetes will go away in few years. Says does not know how to give daily insulin.
O. Newly diagnosed diabetic. Daily intake for past week reveals does not follow diet although was instructed by dietitian 7/1.
Weight 180. Ht./wt. chart puts desirable weight at 144. Nails dirty and large toenails ingrown.
A. Knowledge deficit related to diabetes.
P. List above diagnosis as problem 3 on patient's problem list.
Teach patient and wife about diabetes, complications, and insulin.
Stress need for foot care, diet and urine testing. Referral to visiting nurse for postdischarge evaluation.

Nurses perform many activities to benefit clients. The focus of concern with nursing intervention is nurse behavior: those activities that nurses do to assist client status or behavior to move toward a desired outcome. This differs from nursing diagnosis and nursing outcome, where the focus of concern is client behavior (McCloskey et al. 1990). Our research team at the University of Iowa has identified seven types of nurse activities (Table 4). All are done by the nurse to benefit the client; but are they all nursing interventions? We have incorporated three of the seven types of activities in our expanded definition of a nursing intervention:

> A nursing intervention is any direct care treatment that a nurse performs on behalf of a client. These treatments include nurse-initiated treatments resulting from nursing diagnoses, physician-initiated treatments resulting from medical diagnoses, and performance of the daily essential functions for the client who cannot do these. (Bulechek and McCloskey 1989, p. 25)

The core of nursing interventions should be the nurse-initiated treatments, and the first edition of this book included only interventions of this type. However, any

TABLE 4. SEVEN TYPES OF NURSING ACTIVITIES

1. Assessment activities to make a nursing diagnosis
2. Assessment activities to gather information for a physician to make a medical diagnosis
3. Nurse-initiated treatments in response to nursing diagnoses
4. Physician-initiated treatments in response to medical diagnoses
5. Daily essential function activities that may not relate to either medical or nursing diagnoses but are done by the nurse for clients who cannot do these for themselves
6. Activities to evaluate the effects of nursing and medical treatments
7. Administrative and indirect care activities that support the delivery of care

Source: Adapted from Bulechek and McCloskey (1989).

listing of nursing interventions (for example, for a computerized care planning system) must also include physician-initiated treatments and perhaps the daily essential function activities. The activities in categories 1 and 2 in Table 4 are assessment (prediagnosis) rather than intervention (postdiagnosis) functions. Category 6 also includes assessment activities, but these are done for purposes of evaluation, not diagnosis. Evaluation activities are best identified when a classification of patient outcomes is articulated. Category 7, administrative and indirect care activities, would not be included in a listing of direct care activities. The identification of indirect nursing actions, however, may be needed to assist with a determination of nursing costs.

The first edition of this book and Snyder's *Independent Nursing Interventions*, both published in 1985, were the first to propose nursing interventions as symbolic concepts that require a series of actions for implementation. Acceptance of the conceptual approach in nursing was a prerequisite to the nursing diagnosis movement. "A concept expresses an abstraction formed by generalization from particulars" (Kerlinger 1973, p. 28). A diagnosis requires that the nurse assess the client and identify the etiology and characteristics of a problem (the particulars). Naming the problem (generalization) completes the process of conceptualization. This book moves the conceptual approach to interventions forward. Each chapter develops one intervention at the conceptual level.

Several research teams are working to clarify the intervention concepts for nursing through classification and taxonomy construction. The Iowa research team, formed in 1987, is composed of 11 investigators from the College of Nursing and the Department of Nursing at the University of Iowa Hospitals and Clinics. Several graduate students and three consultants also assist with the project. The project, Classification of Nursing Interventions, was funded in 1990 (NIH, National Center for Nursing Research, Grant NR02079-02) to construct and validate a taxonomy of nursing interventions. The research is addressing two questions: (1) What are the interventions that nurses use? (2) How are nursing interventions related and classified? The steps to answer these questions and construct the taxonomy are ongoing in two phases:

Phase 1

   1.   Identification and resolution of the conceptual and methodological issues involved in the development of the taxonomy.
   2.   Generation of an initial list of interventions.
   3.   Refinement of the intervention list and defining activities.

Phase 2

   4.   Arrangement of the intervention list in an initial taxonomic structure and articulation of the rules and principles governing the structure.
   5.   Validation of the intervention labels, defining activities, and taxonomy.

The result of Phase 1, recently completed, is an alphabetical classification of approximately 340 intervention labels, each with a definition and set of related activities that describe the behaviors of the nurse who implements the intervention (Iowa Intervention Project, in press). Phase 2 of the work, which is ongoing, is organizing the labels into a conceptual framework with clearly articulated rules and principles. The final product will be a standardized language that can be coded for computer and reimbursement utilization to describe the treatments provided by nurses and to be used in a nursing data set for evaluating the effectiveness of nursing care.

Additional work in the area of classification of nursing interventions has been reported. Saba and colleagues (1991) have developed a taxonomy for home health care. This project, conducted at Georgetown University School of Nursing, developed a method for classifying home health Medicare patients in order to predict resource requirements and measure outcomes. The classification was developed from textual descriptions taken from patient records. A series of keyword sorts by computer produced 200 unique nursing services. Grobe (1990), at the University of Texas at Austin, is using informatics analysis methods to examine nursing terms. Natural language is being used to develop a lexicon (a vocabulary) and a taxonomy of nursing intervention statements. Grobe emphasizes the importance of designing automated systems with the capability of language-based analysis. Brooten's research team at the University of Pennsylvania School of Nursing has published a taxonomic classification of nursing interventions for the transitional follow-up care of low birthweight infants (Cohen et al. 1991). The data were from a study that tested a model of early hospital discharge with transition care by master's-degree-prepared nurses (Brooten et al. 1986). The interventions employed by the nurse specialists were classified according to the Taxonomy of Ambulatory Care Nursing (Verran 1981). The approaches taken by Saba, Grobe, and Brooten differ, but collectively they point to the significance of such work.

Selection of a Nursing Intervention

The selection of a nursing intervention depends on several factors. We have identified six: (1) the desired patient outcome, (2) the characteristics of the nursing diagnosis, (3) the research base associated with the intervention, (4) the feasibility of successfully implementing the intervention, (5) the acceptability of the intervention to the client, and (6) the capability of the nurse.

Desired Patient Outcome

The primary consideration in selecting a nursing intervention is to identify one that will facilitate the client to move toward one or more desired outcomes. This action has traditionally been referred to as the planning portion of the nursing process. It involves a number of steps, including the establishment of client goals with client input as appropriate, the development of outcome criteria that will serve as a measure of successful nursing intervention, and the establishment of priorities among multiple goals. Outcomes describe behaviors, responses, and feelings of the client in response to the care provided. Outcomes are discussed more fully in the next section.

Characteristics of the Nursing Diagnosis

The selection of a nursing intervention also depends upon the characteristics of the nursing diagnosis. The intent is to direct the intervention toward altering the etiological factors associated with the diagnosis. If the etiology is correctly identified during the nursing assessment and if the intervention is successful in altering the etiology, the client's status can be expected to improve. Improvement can be measured by a change in the signs and symptoms associated with the diagnosis.

The case study presented in Table 5 illustrates a nursing diagnosis in which the intervention is directed at altering the etiological factors. Anything that can be done to simplify the therapeutic regimen will help this client. For example, he could monitor his blood glucose with an autolet and chemstrips and eliminate the

TABLE 5. CASE STUDY 1

T.K. is a 22-year-old male who has been diabetic for four years. He sought admission to his local hospital because of right upper quadrant abdominal pain. The following signs and symptoms were found on admission:

T—98.5	Glucose—450
P—120	Urine—4+
R—24	pH—7.13
BP—128/80	

The medical diagnoses were diabetic ketoacidosis and possible cholelithiasis. Surgery was recommended. T.K. requested a second opinion and was transferred to a university medical center.

Nursing assessment revealed that T.K. is a high school dropout who works as a baker from 3 A.M. until noon. He eats breakfast at a local café around 9 A.M. and takes his insulin at that time. The employer is aware of his diabetes, but T.K. states that he has been let go from previous jobs when the employer found out about his diabetes. He earns $4.50 per hour, lives alone, and has difficulty affording living expenses, proper food, insulin, and medical bills. He does not have health insurance and is reluctant to ask his parents for assistance. T. K. stated that he requested transfer to the university hospital in hope that the state would pay his medical expenses and also because he thought his diabetes should be brought into control before surgery.

T. K. was able to discuss diabetes and his treatment regime accurately. He scored very high on a paper-and-pencil test concerning diet. However, T. K. stated that for the past year, he has not followed his diet or tested his urine. He related that he found it very repulsive to save and test his urine. He does take his insulin daily, increasing it when he plans to party with his friends. He checks his feet daily. Because of his work schedule, he has erratic sleeping, eating, and exercise patterns. He states that he is depressed much of the time, and when he is depressed, he binges on sweets. He also states that he will probably not follow his regimen after discharge.

Nursing Diagnosis: Noncompliance

Etiology: 1. Complex therapeutic regimen
2. Inadequate financial resources
3. Inadequate coping
4. Stigma due to illness

Signs and Symptoms: 1. Lab values that indicated ketoacidosis upon admission
2. Knowledgeable about therapeutic regime but complies with only some aspects of treatment plan
3. States that he will probably not comply after discharge

---

need for urine testing. He is in desperate need of skills that will qualify him for a job with better pay, daytime hours, and insurance benefits. A referral to job training resources should be considered. This client needs to make many changes in his life-style to cope with his illness more adequately. Changes in diet, sleep, and exercise patterns are indicated. He needs assistance in ways that will be socially acceptable to him and his friends. The following nursing interventions could be considered for implementation in this case: Counseling (Chapter 22), Patient Contracting (Chapter 33), Cognitive Reappraisal (Chapter 35), and Patient Teaching (Chapter 24). The ultimate choice depends on the desires of the client and the capability of the nurse.

Although the prognosis of successfully treating a nursing diagnosis is better if the etiological factors can be changed, this is not always possible. Sometimes the etiology cannot be altered, and it is necessary instead to treat the signs and symptoms. In such instances, it may be possible to achieve the desirable outcome criteria for a finite period of time.

The case study contained in Table 6 illustrates a nursing diagnosis in which the nursing intervention must be directed toward the signs and symptoms because it is not possible to eliminate the etiology. The client desires to continue the chemotherapy as recommended. Nursing intervention must focus on helping her cope with the nausea and vomiting. The client has already identified that exercise helps her. The nurse could reinforce the client's use of this intervention, do an exercise

TABLE 6.   CASE STUDY 2

M.J. is a 63-year-old female admitted to the surgical oncology clinic for chemotherapy following a left-sided, modified mastectomy. Her surgical incision is well healed, and she denies any pain. Her chemotherapy regime is a combination of two oral and one intravenous drugs, which will be administered on a rotating basis for two years. She consented to participate in a national drug study being conducted at the university medical center where she is receiving care and where she is employed as a unit clerk. She plans to keep her job while receiving chemotherapy and retire at age 65. M.J. is divorced and has two grown sons, whom she sees on a regular basis. Both M.J.'s mother and sister died subsequent to breast cancer. A close friend died within the past year from malignant melanoma. This friend experienced nausea and vomiting throughout her chemotherapy, resulting in anorexia and cachexia.

When asked about coping strategies, M.J. reports, "My stomach is sensitive in stressful situations, and I sometimes feel nauseated. I'm afraid I will be as sick as my friend was on chemotherapy." She reports that exercise is an effective way to relieve her anxiety and walks to and from work.

By the end of the first week, M.J. reports severe nausea and episodes of vomiting. She is able to tolerate some of her meals but has no appetite for candy or bananas, which are her favorite foods. She states, "Today it makes me sick just to walk in this place. I think it is the smell."

Nursing Diagnosis: Altered Nutrition: Less Than Body Requirements

Etiology: 1. Chemotherapy
2. Negative past experience with chemotherapy through friend's experience
3. History of nausea and vomiting in stressful situations

Signs & Symptoms: 1. Persistent nausea and 10 episodes of vomiting over past 24 hours
2. Gastric hypomotility on auscultation
3. Sensitivity to olfactory stimuli in treatment area
4. No appetite for favorite foods

assessment, and develop an Exercise Program (Chapter 32). Relaxation Training (Chapter 34) is another possible intervention for helping this client control her stress-related symptoms. Help will be needed to assist her in maintaining an adequate intake. Feeding (Chapter 3) and Fluid Therapy (Chapter 18) may be considered. Sound decisions about collaborative nursing practice are also important in reducing the incidence of nausea and vomiting. Medication Management (Chapter 16) is an intervention related to the following types of questions: What is the best time of day to administer the chemotherapy? When should prn antiemetics be given? Can the clinic environment be altered to minimize odor and waiting?

Nurses also treat clients with potential health problems—clients who display known risk factors that are predictive of future development of a health problem. NANDA has identified several such diagnoses and has included the phrase "potential for" in the diagnostic label. In these diagnoses, the risk factors are viewed as the etiology; the preventive intervention is aimed at altering or eliminating the risk factors. Examples of interventions include Exercise Program (Chapter 32), Patient Teaching (Chapter 24), Smoking Cessation (Chapter 36), and Weight Management (Chapter 37).

Research Base

A third consideration when selecting an intervention is the research base associated with it. Since the early 1960s, the profession has been working to produce clinical research that will give direction to nursing practice. Dumas and Leonard's (1963) classic study on preoperative preparation demonstrated that it is possible to test nursing interventions in the natural setting. Subsequently, many clinical studies have been produced by faculty, graduate students, and clinical specialists. The results of these studies have been slow to appear in practice for many reasons, which have been well described by other authors (Jacox 1974; Aydelotte 1976; Martinson 1976; Smoyak 1976).

In the mid-1970s, the Michigan Nurses' Association undertook a statewide federally funded project to bridge the gap between research and practice. The Conduct and Utilization of Research in Nursing Project (CURN Project) developed and tested a model to facilitate the use of scientific nursing knowledge in clinical practice settings. Three categories of criteria were established for selecting research that was sufficiently developed to merit utilization in practice (Haller, Reynolds, and Horsley 1979). The first category pertained to evaluation of the research base of the studies and included criteria on replication, scientific merit, and risk; the second dealt with relevance to practice and included criteria on clinical significance, nursing control, feasibility, and cost; and the third dealt with potential for clinical evaluation by clinicians. Through application of these criteria, the CURN Project developed and field-tested 10 research-based practice protocols:

1. Structured preoperative teaching
2. Lactose-free diet
3. Sensory information: Distress reduction
4. Sensory information: Recovery rate
5. Nonsterile intermittent urinary catheterization
6. Prevention of catheter-associated urinary tract infections
7. Intravenous cannula change regimen
8. Prevention of decubiti by means of small shifts of body weight
9. Mutual goal setting
10. Deliberative nursing: Pain reduction

More recently Brett (1987) has identified 14 innovations ready for implementation in clinical practice. She found that the majority of nurses in her samples were aware of the innovations but that use of the innovation had no relationship to hospital policies or procedures concerning the research findings. Subsequently Brett (1989a) found that in small hospitals, a higher level of integration was related to increased nurse innovation adoption, while in large hospitals, the reverse occurred. Goode and colleagues (1987) have reported on the implementation of research-based practice in a rural, community hospital. With the leadership of a master's-degree-prepared nurse administrator, staff nurses learned to critique research, identify a research base, and translate the findings into clinical innovations. This project resulted in an award-winning video, *Using Research in Clinical Nursing Practice* (Goode 1989). A second video, *Research Utilization: A Process of Organizational Change* (Goode 1990), emphasizes that research-based practice requires organizational commitment and support when nurses work in groups in bureaucratic settings. The videos are excellent resources for nurses and agencies who are attempting to establish research-based practice. Another source of help in implementing research findings is Stetler (1989), who has described a teaching strategy designed to assist nurses in integrating research use into daily practice.

The research base associated with specific nursing interventions varies widely. Pressure Reduction (Chapter 7) and Structured Preoperative Teaching (Chapter 12) have had extensive amounts of research, which is providing direction for practitioners. Other interventions, such as Presence (Chapter 14) and Truth Telling (Chapter 11), are still at the concept development stage and have had little empirical testing. Still other interventions, such as Relaxation Training (Chapter 34) and Support Groups (Chapter 26), have been widely utilized but need more testing with specific nursing diagnoses. More work, such as the CURN Project and the Goode work, is needed to help transfer research findings into practice.

Feasibility

Many factors contribute to concerns about feasibility when selecting a nursing intervention. Most patients have several nursing diagnoses, and the order or priority in which to treat them must be decided. There may also be several medical diagnoses and other health professionals in addition to the nurse working with the client. Therefore, it is necessary to think about the total plan of care for the client. Consideration must be given to interaction of the nursing interventions with treatments being provided by other health professionals. Such interactions may be either beneficial or detrimental for the client. A concerted effort by everyone involved is needed to achieve a successful client outcome; at times the health team must establish a priority ranking of treatments to avoid overwhelming the client.

Cost and time are other feasibility concerns. Will there be third-party reimbursement for the treatment? Is there a critical path associated with a diagnosis-related group? Will the intervention be conducted in the hospital, clinic, or home? Can both the client and the nurse give the amount of time required for the intervention? Today's consumers expect quality health care but are also concerned about the cost.

Acceptability to Client

Each client comes for health care with a perception of the problem and a notion of what should be done about it. Whatever the nurse assesses, diagnoses, and treats will be interpreted by the client within his or her own frame of reference. The treatment plan must be congruent with the client's reality, or it is doomed to failure. If the nurse has established rapport during the assessment, the client should be ready to participate in selecting outcomes. Whenever possible, it is important for the client to participate in goal formulation and deciding goal priority. The nurse is frequently able to recommend a choice of nursing interventions to assist in reaching the outcome. For each intervention, the client should be given information about the conduct of the intervention and how he or she is expected to participate to help make an informed choice. The client's values, beliefs, and culture must also be considered when selecting a nursing intervention.

Capability of the Nurse

To implement an intervention successfully, a nurse must have knowledge of the scientific rationale for the intervention, the necessary psychomotor and interpersonal skills, and the ability to function within the setting to utilize health care resources effectively. All nurses are not alike. Each has unique knowledge with skills developed through education and experience. It is important for each nurse to differentiate the clients and nursing diagnoses she or he can treat from those that should be referred to other nurses or other health professionals.

OUTCOMES

Patient outcomes, which should be specified before an intervention is chosen, serve as the criteria against which to judge the success of a nursing intervention.

Outcomes describe behaviors, responses, and feelings of the patient in response to the care provided.

Many variables influence outcomes: the interventions prescribed by the health care providers, the health care providers themselves, the environment in which care is received, the patient's own motivation and genetic structure, and the patient's significant others. The task for nursing is to define which patient outcomes are sensitive to nursing care, that is, to identify for each patient the expected and attainable results of nursing care.

Defining patient outcomes is the newest initiative of the federal government. In December 1989, the Agency for Health Care Policy and Research (AHCPR) was established to enhance the quality, appropriateness, and effectiveness of health care services and to improve access to that care (AHCPR, September 1990). The agency's Medical Treatment Effectiveness Program (MEDTEP) is charged with examining the effects of variations in health care practices on patient outcomes. As part of this program, practice guidelines are being formulated with the help of the professional community. They will "convert science-based knowledge into clinical action in a form accessible to practitioners, thus enabling professional judgment to inform the health care provider of preferred treatment; clarify health care choices and their consequences for the patient; and link quality assurance and cost effectiveness to health care management" (AHCPR, February 1990, p. 1). An advisory panel of nurses to AHCPR concluded that the purpose of guidelines "is to guide practice by providing linkages among diagnoses, treatments, and outcomes, and by describing the alternatives available for each patient" (AHCPR, February 1990). The government is concerned about the high cost of health care, and this newest approach to lower costs seeks to determine whether the most expensive treatment is always warranted or even effective.

In order to evaluate guidelines or interventions, however, one needs to identify and measure the desired patient outcomes. This has led to further interest in outcome measurement and classification. As part of its mandate to develop a research agenda for outcomes and effectiveness research, the AHCPR, in cooperation with the Health Care Financing Administration (HCFA), sponsored in April 1991 a conference mandated by Congress to develop agendas for future research in 10 different areas of outcomes and effectiveness research. That there is much need for standardization of language in this area and that instruments need to be validated has been determined.

AHCPR's efforts are paralleled in nursing by efforts by the National Center for Nursing Research (NCNR) and the ANA. A major nursing initiative on outcomes research was initiated by the NCNR in May 1990 when it convened an expert planning group to discuss strategies concerning patient outcomes and nursing research. This group coined the term "nurse-sensitive outcomes," meaning those patient outcomes that are sensitive to nursing intervention. A follow-up state-of-the-science of nurse-sensitive patient outcomes research occurred in fall of 1991.

One major issue in developing a classification of outcomes is the level of measurement. As we are doing with diagnoses and interventions, we need to develop outcome variables as concepts with measures at several levels — that is, measures that can be used across different populations and settings so that we can compare population- and setting-specific measures to provide the detailed information necessary to improve care.

Measurement of outcomes for particular patients or patient groups needs to be done in relationship to the nursing diagnoses. For example, dialysis patients often have nursing diagnoses of Ineffective Individual Coping, Fear, Powerlessness, and Self-Esteem Disturbance. Interventions directed toward altering the etiologies of the diagnoses might be Cognitive Reappraisal (Chapter 35), Counseling (Chapter 22), Concrete Objective Information (Chapter 10), or Crisis Intervention (Chapter 13). An outcome measure to assess the effectiveness of the interventions and to document whether the diagnoses are resolved, elevated, or controlled could be the Hemodialysis Stressor Scale (Baldree, Murphy, and Powers 1982), specifically for dialysis patients, or the Jalowiec Coping Scale (Jalowiec and Powers 1980), which could be compared to other patients with Ineffective Individual Coping (Moorhead 1990).

Pinkley (1991) urges choosing outcomes that will be measured at the macro level — that is, in the context of all the nursing diagnoses, not just those aimed at alleviating the etiology of one diagnosis. According to Pinkley, the choosing of outcomes should be directed at optimizing health, as well as alleviating problems.

To date, there is no common classification in the area of outcomes. Two types of classification are in existence: the change in status type and the content type (Table 7). We believe that over the course of the next several years, a common classification of patient outcomes will emerge. These variables and their common measures will be used by a variety of health providers to determine the quality of care. Nursing needs to take an active part in this effort so that outcomes that are sensitive to nursing care are part of the classification.

CURRENT PERSPECTIVES

Organized nursing has come to recognize that classifications of nursing knowledge are essential in making explicit the nature of nursing. The value of nursing care cannot be universally recognized until we have standardized databases that provide ongoing evaluation of nursing's effectiveness. Consensus is emerging that standardized language is needed in the areas of diagnoses, interventions, and outcomes (ANA 1989; Bulechek and McCloskey 1990). Five purposes for classification systems of nursing practice are overviewed:

Purpose 1: To link knowledge about diagnoses, treatments, and outcomes.

The widespread use of NANDA's nursing diagnosis language by health care practitioners and agencies has increased awareness of the needs for similar standardized classifications in the areas of interventions and outcomes. Practice guidelines are needed to help practitioners determine which of several courses of action are best given a particular set of circumstances — that is, to determine what interventions, based on research, are most effective for patients with a particular diagnosis or set of diagnoses. We need to define the standardized language in the areas of interventions and outcomes, improve and expand the NANDA terminology in the area of diagnoses, and then use this language in information systems to determine the linkages among the variables. When we have standardized documentation by nurses about the diagnoses of their patients, the treatments they performed, and the resulting patient outcomes, we will be able to determine the best interventions for a given population.

Purpose 2: To facilitate the development of nursing and health care information systems.

In 1983, at a conference in nursing information systems, it was pointed out that although nurses spend much of their time documenting their care, this documentation has not been systematically organized to advance nursing knowledge, to develop nursing practice, or to improve patient care (Study Group on Nursing Information Systems 1983). In 1984, Zielstroff asserted that the major impediment

TABLE 7. CLASSIFICATIONS OF PATIENT OUTCOMES

Status Classifications
Nursing Management Minimum Data Set (Werley and Lang 1988)
- Resolved
- Not Resolved
- Referred for Continuing Care (e.g., referral or transfer)

Direction of Change (McCormick 1991)
- Improvement
- Stabilization
- Deterioration
- Death

Content Classifications
Starfield (1974)
- Resilience (resilient, vulnerable)
- Achievement (achieving, not achieving)
- Disease (not detectable, asymptomatic, temporary, permanent)
- Satisfaction (satisfied, dissatisfied)
- Comfort (comfortable, uncomfortable)
- Activity (functional, disabled)
- Longevity (normal life expectancy, dead)

Donabedian (1980, cited by Hodges and Icenhour 1990)
- Physical health status
- Mental health status
- Social and physical function
- Health attitudes/knowledge/behavior
- Utilization of professional health resources
- Patient's Perception of quality care

Mayers (1983)
- Patient verbalization regarding what he or she knows, understands, or feels
- Patient behavior pattern relating to a specific situation
- Patient signs or symptoms related to the disease process
- Patient management of the environment

Visiting Nurse Association of Omaha (1986)
- Knowledge — the ability of the client to remember and interpret information (poor – excellent)
- Behavior — the observable responses, actions, or activities of the client fitting the occasion or purpose (poor – excellent)
- Status — the condition of the client in relation to objective and subjective defining characteristics (poor – excellent)

Brett (1989)
- Patient satisfaction
- Patient knowledge or understanding of disease or treatment
- Functional health status
- Clinical health status
- Psychoemotional health status
- Perceptions of patients, family, nurses, physicians
- Disposition of patients
- Negative results — complications
- Discharge readiness of the patient
- Patient compliance
- Appearance of the patient

Medical Outcomes Study (Tarlov et al. 1989)
- Clinical end points: Symptoms and signs, laboratory values, death
- Functional status: Physical, mental, social, role
- General well-being: Health perceptions, energy/fatigue, pain, life satisfaction
- Satisfaction with care: Access, convenience, financial coverage, quality, general

McCormick's Outcomes in Hospitalized Patients (1991)
- Admission assessment within 24 – 48 hours
- All diagnosis and treatment orders fulfilled
- Discharged in safe physical, emotional, and mental health
- No abnormal diagnostic findings left unattended
- Normal fluid hydration
- Continent (urinating and defecating appropriately)
- Mobile, steady gait without threat of falls
- Without drug interactions
- Comfort achieved to the extent possible
- Without decubitus ulcers and oral mucosal membrane ulcers
- Capable of bathing, toileting, feeding, and dressing self
- No nosocomial infection
- No purulent or blood drainage from wounds
- Patient understands home treatment plan and was satisfied with care given by nursing staff

to the development of computerized nursing information systems is the deficiencies in nursing's knowledge base:

> Those who work in the design and development of nursing information systems constantly bemoan the fact that there are so few clinical problems in nursing for which the etiology, symptoms, treatments, and expected outcomes are known. There are no known probability estimates for prevalence or incidence of common nursing problems; or for relating symptoms to diagnosis, or treatment to outcome. Indeed, there is neither a standard terminology nor a widely accepted format for data gathering. It is impossible to derive hard and fast rules for computer assistance in decision making with such an ill-defined data base. (p. 9)

At a January 1988 Conference on Research Priorities in Nursing Science, the NCNR identified as a high priority the development of nursing information systems (Hinshaw 1988). In order to achieve this goal, the need for standardized data sets that document nursing care across settings and the need for a taxonomy to classify nursing treatments in a standard language were recognized.

Purpose 3: To facilitate the teaching of decision making to nursing students.

Clinical judgment has been defined as the use of knowledge in making one or more of several kinds of decisions: the decision of which observations to be made in a particular situation, the decision of what the observed data mean with the recognition of patterns, and the selection of actions to be taken on behalf of the patient (Tanner 1987). There are two important aspects of clinical judgment: the knowledge used for the judgment and the thinking process used by the nurse in making the judgment (Tanner 1989).

Currently, we teach students from medical-surgical and specialty textbooks, based mostly on medical knowledge; from nursing process books, based mostly on untested nursing theory; and from audiocassettes, films, and skills manuals, based mostly on tradition (McCloskey 1988). Students practice technical skills in a laboratory before they try them with patients, but they have little opportunity to practice the more difficult decision-making skills. Some help is available in case study books and some computer patient simulations, and increasing numbers of texts are based on nursing diagnoses. We believe that nursing diagnoses and interventions textbooks based on tested theory eventually will replace medical-surgical, pediatric, psychologic, and other textbooks, and more films and audiocassettes demonstrating nursing interventions will be available. We envision that the analysis of actual client data will assist in the instruction of clinical decision making.

Purpose 4: To help determine the costs of services provided by nurses.

In the past decade, there have been multiple efforts reported in the literature to "cost out" nursing. Most of the studies had small sample sizes, were conducted in one institution, and used patient classification systems without much regard to their validity and reliability (McCloskey, Gardner and Johnson 1987). The wide variety and nonstandardization of patient classification systems is, in fact, a key reason for the difficulty of obtaining large data sets for comparison of nursing costs. The determination of costs based on interventions performed would be a great improvement but would require a standardized list of interventions.

Indeed, reimbursement to nurses is a key issue in the reduction of health care costs. Physicians bill for their services based on the codes in the *Physician's Current Procedural Terminology* (CPT) manual published by the American Medical Association (1986). Griffith, Thomas, and Griffith (1991) have shown that nurses often perform some of the procedures for which physicians are paid; however, there is no uniform mechanism other than the CPT that can be used for reimbursement to nurses.

Purpose 5: To articulate with the classification systems of other health care providers.

The federal government, insurance companies, and the medical community have been collecting standardized health information for a number of years to direct reimbursement, guide research priorities, and develop health policy. Several health data sets have been developed under the auspice of the National Committee on Vital and Health Statistics, including the Uniform Hospital Discharge Data Set (UHDDS), the Ambulatory Medical Care Minimum Data Set, and the Longterm Health Care Minimum Data Set. Included variables are patient-identifying information, provider information, medical diagnoses, and procedures. The major systems for classification of the variables are the *International Classification of Diseases* (ICD), the *Current Procedural Terminology* (CPT), *The Diagnostic and Statistical Manual of Mental Disorders* (DSM), the *Systematized Nomenclature of Pathology* (SNOP), and the *Systematized Nomenclature of Medicine* (SNOMED). These classifications are overviewed by Gebbie (1989).

These data sets and coding classifications, however, are not representative of nursing practice. The nursing community is recognizing the need to have nursing variables included in these and other data sets. Harriet Werley and colleagues have published extensively on the need for a unified Nursing Minimum Data Set (NMDS) that would be collected systematically in all agencies (Werley, Lang, and Westlake 1986; Werley and Lang 1988; Devine and Werley 1988). The nursing care variables identified for inclusion in the NMDS are diagnoses, interventions, outcomes and acuity. In 1989 the ANA and NANDA began work to put forward to the World Health Organization a proposal to include NANDA's list of nursing diagnoses in the tenth edition of the *International Classification of Diseases* (Fitzpatrick, Kerr, Saba, Hoskins, Hurley, Mills, Rottkamp, Warren, and Carpenito 1989). If accepted, this would be the first inclusion of nursing content in a major health care coding system.

In summary, the existing data sets and classification systems do not include nursing. As a result, nursing is invisible in its impact on patient care or health care costs. We need classifications of nursing practice that include diagnoses, interventions, and outcomes. As classifications develop, the research base for nursing practice will grow. The 44 chapters in this book document the growing research in the area of nursing treatments. These interventions are nursing's essential treatments and the core of any classification system of nursing interventions. The chapter authors have taken nursing a step closer to a unique body of knowledge.

REFERENCES

Agency for Health Care Policy and Research (AHCPR). 1990. Purpose and programs, Washington, D.C.: USDHHS PHS Agency for Health Care Policy and Research, February.

AHCPR Program Note. 1990. Nursing advisory panel for guideline development: Summary, Washington, D.C.: USDHHS PHS, September.

American Medical Association. 1986. *Physicians' current procedural terminology* (4th ed.). Chicago.

American Nurses' Association. 1989. *Classification systems for describing nursing practice: Working papers.* Publication NP-74. Kansas City: American Nurses' Association.

American Nurses' Association. 1980a. *Nursing: A social policy statement.* Kansas City: American Nurses' Association.

American Nurses' Association. 1980b. *The Nursing Practice Act: Suggested state legislation.* Kansas City: American Nurses' Association.

Aydelotte, M.K. 1976. Nursing research in clinical settings: Problems and issues. *Reflections* 2:3–6.

Baldree, K.S., Murphy, S.D., and Powers, M.J. 1982, Stress identification and coping patterns in patients on hemodialysis. *Nursing Research* 31(2):107–112.

Brett, J.L. 1989a. Organizational integrative mechanisms and adoption of innovations by nurses. *Nursing Research* 38(2):105–110.

Brett, J.L. 1989b. Outcome indicators of quality care. In B. Henry, C. Arndt, M. diVincente, and A. Marriner-Tomey (eds.), *Dimensions of nursing administration: Theory, research, education, practice*, pp. 353–369. Boston: Blackwell.

Brett, J.L. 1987. Use of nursing practice research findings. *Nursing Research* 36(6):344–349.

Brooten, D., Kumar, S., Brown, L., Butts, P., Finkler, S., Bakewell-Sachs, S., Gibbons, A., and Delivoria-Papadopoulos, M. 1986. A randomized trial of early hospital discharge and home follow-up of very low birthweight infants. *New England Journal of Medicine* 315:934–939.

Bruce, J. 1979. Implementation of nursing diagnoses: A nursing administrator's perspective. *Nursing Clinics of North America* 14(3):509–515.

Bulechek, G.M., and McCloskey, J.C. (eds.). 1985. *Nursing interventions: Treatments for nursing diagnoses*. Philadelphia: W. B. Saunders.

Bulechek, G.M., and McCloskey, J.C. 1989. Nursing interventions: Treatments for potential nursing diagnoses. In R.M. Carroll-Johnson (ed.), *Classification of nursing diagnoses*, pp. 23–30. Philadelphia: J.B. Lippincott.

Bulechek, G.M., and McCloskey, J.C. 1990. Nursing intervention taxonomy development. In J.C. McCloskey and H.K. Grace (eds.), *Current issues in nursing* (3d ed.), pp. 23–28. St. Louis: C.V. Mosby.

Carpenito, L.J. 1987. *Nursing diagnosis: Process and application* (2d ed.). Philadelphia: J.B. Lippincott.

Carroll-Johnson, R.M. (ed.). 1989. *Classification of nursing diagnoses: Proceedings of the Eighth Conference*. Philadelphia: J.B. Lippincott.

Carroll-Johnson, R.M. 1990. Reflections on the Ninth Biennial Conference. *Nursing Diagnosis* 1:50.

Carroll-Johnson, R.M. (ed.). 1991. *Classification of nursing diagnoses: Proceedings of the Ninth Conference*. Philadelphia: J.B. Lippincott.

Cassmeyer, V.L. 1989. Using physiology and pathophysiology in the nursing diagnostic process. *Journal of Advanced Medical Surgical Nursing* 1(3):1–10.

Cohen, S.M., Arnold, L., Brown, L., and Brooten, D. 1991. Taxonomic classification of transitional follow-up care nursing interventions with low birthweight infants. *Clinical Nurse Specialists* 5(1):31–36.

CURN Project. 1981. *Distress reduction through sensory preparation*. New York: Grune and Stratton.

Devine, E.C., and Werley, H.H. 1988. Test of the nursing minimum data set: Availability of data and reliability. *Research in Nursing and Health* 11(3):97–104.

Donabedian, A. 1978. The quality of medical care. *Inquiry* 200(4344):856.

Dumas, R.G., and Leonard, R.C. 1963. The effect of nursing on the incidence of post operative vomiting. *Nursing Research* 12:12–15.

Fitzpatrick, J.J., Kerr, M.E., Saba, V.K., Hoskins, L.M., Hurley, M.E., Mills, W.C., Rottkamp, B.C., Warren, J.J., and Carpenito, L.J. 1989. Translating nursing diagnosis into ICD code. *American Journal of Nursing* 89(12):493–495.

Gebbie, K.M. 1975. *Classification of nursing diagnoses: Proceedings of the Second National Conference*. St. Louis: Clearinghouse for Nursing Diagnosis.

Gebbie, K.M. 1989. Major classification systems in health care and their use. In Staff, *Classification systems for describing nursing practice: Working papers*, pp. 48–49. Kansas City: American Nurses' Association.

Gebbie, K.M., and Lavin, M.A. (eds.). 1975. *Classification of nursing diagnoses: Proceedings of the First National Conference*. St. Louis: C.V. Mosby Company.

Goode, C. (Producer). 1989. *Using research in clinical nursing practice* (videotape). Ida Grove, Iowa: Horn Video Productions.

Goode, C. (Producer). 1990. *Research utilization: A process of organizational change* (videotape). Ida Grove, Iowa: Horn Video Productions.

Goode, C.M., Lovett, M., Hayes, J., and Butcher, L. 1987. Use of research based knowledge in clinical practice. *Journal of Nursing Administration* 17(12):11–18.

Gordon, M. 1982. *Nursing diagnosis: Process and application*. New York: McGraw-Hill.

Gordon, M. 1987. *Nursing diagnosis: Process and application* (2d ed.). New York: McGraw-Hill.

Griffith, H.M., Thomas, N., and Griffith, L. 1991. MDs bill for these routine nursing tasks. *American Journal of Nursing* 91(1):22–25.

Grobe, S.J. 1990. Nursing intervention lexicon and taxonomy study: Language and classification methods. *Advances in Nursing Science* 13(2):22–33.

Hall, L.E. 1955. Quality of nursing care. Address at Meeting of Department of Baccalaureate and Higher Degree Programs of the New Jersey League for Nursing. *Public Health Nursing* (New Jersey State Department of Health).

Haller, K.B., Reynolds, M.A., and Horsley, J.A. 1979. Developing research based innovation protocols: Process, criteria and issues. *Research in Nursing and Health*, 2:45–51.

Hinshaw, A.S. 1988. The new national center for nursing research: Patient care research programs. *Applied Nursing Research* 1(1):2–4.

Hodges, L.C., and Icenhour, M.L. 1990. Measuring the quality of nursing care. In J. C. McCloskey and H.K. Grace (eds.), *Current issues in nursing* (3d ed.), pp. 242–248. St Louis: C.V. Mosby Company.

Hurley, M. (ed.). 1986. *Classification of nursing diagnoses: Proceedings of the Sixth National Conference.* St. Louis: C.V. Mosby Company.

Iowa Intervention Project. Forthcoming. Nursing Intervention Classification (NIC). St. Louis: Mosby Year Book.

Jacox, A. 1974. Nursing research and the clinician. *Nursing Outlook* 22:382.

Jalowiec, A., and Powers, M.J. 1980. Stress and coping in hypertensive and emergency room patients. *Nursing Research* 30(1):10–14.

Kelly, L.Y. 1974. Nursing practice acts. *American Journal of Nursing* 23(1):4–13.

Kerlinger, F.N. 1973. *Foundations of behavioral research.* New York: Holt, Rinehart & Winston.

Kim, M.J. 1984. Physiologic nursing diagnosis: Its role and place in nursing taxonomy. In J.M. Kim, G.K. McFarland, and A.M. McLane (eds.), *Classification of nursing diagnoses: Proceedings of the Fifth National Conference.* St. Louis: C.V. Mosby Company.

Kim, M.J., McFarland, G.K., and McLane, A.M. (eds.). 1984. *Classification of nursing diagnoses: Proceedings of the Fifth National Conference.* St. Louis: C.V. Mosby Company.

Kim, M., and Moritz, D.A. 1982. *Classification of nursing diagnoses: Proceedings of the Third and Fourth National Conferences.* New York: McGraw-Hill.

Knowles, L.N. 1967. Decision making in nursing—A necessity for doing. *ANA Clinical Sessions, 1966.* New York: Appleton-Century-Crofts.

McCloskey, J.C. 1988. The nursing minimum data set: Benefits and implications for nurse educators. *Perspectives in Nursing 1987–1989.* National League for Nursing Pub. No. 41-2199.

McCloskey, J.C., Bulechek, G.M., Cohen, M.Z., Craft, M.J., Crossley, J.D., Denehy, J.A., Glick, O.J., Kruckeberg, T., Maas, M., Prophet, C.M., and Tripp-Reimer, T. 1990. Classification of nursing interventions. *Journal of Professional Nursing* 6(3):151–157.

McCloskey, J.C., Gardner, D., and Johnson, M. 1987. Costing out nursing services: An annotated bibliography. *Nursing Economics* 5(5):245–253.

McCormick, K.A. 1991. Future data needs for quality of care monitoring, DRG considerations, reimbursement and outcome measurement. *Image* 23(1):29–32.

McLane, A.M. (ed.). 1987. *Classification of nursing diagnoses: Proceedings of the Seventh National Conference.* St. Louis: C.V. Mosby Company.

Martinson, I.M. 1976. Nursing research: Obstacles and challenges. *Image* 8(1):3–5.

Mayers, M.G. 1983. *A systematic approach to the nursing care plan* (3d ed.). New York: Appleton-Century-Crofts.

Miers, Linda J. 1991. NANDA's definition of nursing diagnosis: A plea for conceptual clarity. *Nursing Diagnosis* 2(1):9–18.

Mills, W.C. 1991. Nursing diagnosis: The importance of a definition. *Nursing Diagnosis* 2(1):3–8.

Mintzberg, H. 1979. *The structure of organizations.* Englewood Cliffs, N.J.: Prentice-Hall.

Moorhead, S. 1990. Example from a paper written for a doctoral nursing administration class, University of Iowa, Iowa City.

North American Nursing Diagnosis Association. 1990. *Taxonomy I Revised 1990: With official nursing diagnoses.* St. Louis: North American Nursing Diagnosis Association.

Orlando, I.J. 1961. *The dynamic nurse-patient relationship.* New York: Putnam's.

Pinkley, C.L. 1991. Exploring NANDA's definition of nursing diagnosis: Linking diagnostic judgments with the selection of outcomes and interventions. *Nursing Diagnosis* 2(1):26–32.

Popkess-Vawter, S. 1991. Wellness nursing diagnoses: To be or not to be? *Nursing Diagnoses* 2(1):19–25.

Saba, V.K., O'Hare, P.A., Zuckerman, A.E., Boondas, J., Levine, E., and Oatway, D.M. 1991. A nursing intervention taxonomy for home health care. *Nursing and Health Care* 12(6):296–299.

Smoyak, S.A. 1976. Is practice responding to research? *American Journal of Nursing* 76:1146–1150.

Snyder, M. 1985. *Independent nursing interventions.* New York: John Wiley.

Starfield, B. 1974. Measurement of outcome: A proposed scheme. *Milbank Memorial Fund Quarterly* 52(Winter):39–50.

Stetler, C.B. 1989. A strategy for teaching research use. *Nurse Educator* 12(3):17–20.

Study Group on Nursing Information Systems. 1983. Special report. Computerized nursing information systems: An urgent need. *Research in Nursing and Health* 6:101–105.

Tanner, C.A. 1987. Teaching clinical judgement. In J.J. Fitzpatrick and R.L. Taunton (eds.), *Annual review of nursing research,* vol. 5. New York: Springer.

Tanner, C.A. 1989. Research needs and priorities related to clinical decision making in nursing. Unpublished paper commissioned by National Center for Nursing Research, August.

Tarlov, A.R., Ware, J.E., Greenfield, S., Nelson, E.C., Perrin, E., and Zubkoff, M. 1989. The medical outcomes study: An application of methods for monitoring the results of medical care. *Journal of the American Medical Association* 262(7):925–930.

Verran, J. 1981. Delineation of ambulatory care nursing practice. *Journal of Ambulatory Care Management* 4:1–13.

Visiting Nurse Association of Omaha. 1986. Client management information system for community health nursing agencies. US DHHS, PHS, NTIS Accession No. HRP-0907023.

Warren, J.J., and Hoskins, L.M. 1990. The development of NANDA's nursing diagnosis taxonomy. *Nursing Diagnosis* 1(4):162–168.

Werley, H.H., and Lang, N.M. (eds.). 1988. *Identification of the nursing minimum data set.* New York: Springer Publishing Company.

Werley, H.H., Lang, N.M., and Westlake, S.K. 1986. The nursing minimum data set conference: Executive summary. *Journal of Professional Nursing* 2:117–224.

Yura, J., and Walsh, M.B. 1978. *The nursing process: Assessing, planning, implementing, evaluating* (3d ed.), New York: Appleton-Century-Crofts.

Zielstroff, R.D. 1984. Why aren't there more significant automated nursing information systems? *Journal of Nursing Administration* 14(1):7–10.

SECTION I

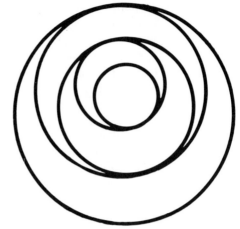

SELF-CARE ASSISTANCE

Overview: The Basics of Nursing Care

GLORIA M. BULECHEK
JOANNE C. McCLOSKEY

The basics of nursing care include those activities necessary for normal life function. Usually people do these for themselves, but when illness or disability prevents this, the tasks fall to the nurse or the family. The interventions in this section are those usually taught in the first course in a nursing curriculum. They help the patient with self-care activities, and although they are basic, they are most important to the person in need. Sometimes we take these interventions for granted; for being so basic, there is surprisingly little research on some of them.

In Chapter 1, Catherine A. Tracey discusses the important intervention of Hygiene Assistance, composed of multiple cleansing activities related to the skin, mouth, ears, eyes, hair, and other body parts. In the future, it may be desirable to identify other, more discrete, interventions, such as Bathing, Mouth Care, Hair Care, and Eye Care, with their related activities. In this chapter, however, all of these related activities are treated together as the intervention of Hygiene Assistance. Tracey relates the research, most of it on bathing, and describes the intervention as applicable to a number of nursing diagnoses. Two case studies illustrate the importance of this intervention that should be part of the expertise of all nurses.

In Chapter 2, on Dry Skin Care, Mary Anderson Hardy outlines the components of another important intervention. Dry skin, accompanied by itching, burning, and scaling, is a special problem for the elderly, for people who engage in frequent hand washing, such as nurses, and for those who undergo radiation therapy. Hardy reviews and organizes the vast literature on this topic. She proposes and outlines

21

the components of a new nursing diagnosis: Impaired Skin Integrity: Dry Skin. Although multiple descriptive studies have been done on the topic, only four have tested interventions for dry skin. Based on her own research and that of others, Hardy discusses the pros and cons of each component of the intervention: soaps, bathing frequency, bathing mode, length of bath/shower, occlusive agent, and humidity. Two case studies illustrate the use of the intervention. This is a comprehensive chapter that delineates the parameters of this often-needed but little-understood intervention.

Food is a basic need of everyone, and feeding those who cannot do this for themselves is not as simple as it sounds. In Chapter 3, Feeding, Nancy J. Evans discusses the components of feeding and the clinical implications of malnutrition. The ultimate goal of feeding is to provide adequate nutrients to prevent malnutrition. A secondary goal is to restore the patient's independence in this basic self-care area. Evans outlines several high-risk situations that may indicate a feeding problem: people with neuromuscular problems, those with cognitive deficits, and those with sensory perceptual deficits. A good deal of nursing time is spent helping people eat, and research shows that eating problems create much anxiety for caregivers. The author discusses multiple strategies that a nurse needs to use to feed a patient successfully. Although feeding is a basic and, at times, simple nursing intervention, nurses must have a "strong theoretical knowledge base regarding the physiological and psychological components of nutrient intake."

The basics also include assisting with urine and bowel elimination. Chapter 4 by Janet P. Specht, Meridean L. Maas, Sally Willett, and Nancy Myers, discusses the intervention, Intermittent Catheterization. The authors review the strong research base for this intervention and make a convincing case that it should be used more often by nurses. They discuss the pros and cons of sterile versus clean technique and recommend the clean procedure, which has the advantages of flexibility, convenience, and low cost. Two case studies illustrate the use of the intervention for the nursing diagnoses of overflow incontinence, reflex incontinence, urge incontinence, and iatrogenic incontinence. The procedures for nurse catheterization of a male and a female patient and for teaching self-catheterization are included. Incontinence is a major problem for many people. The intervention of Intermittent Catheterization has demonstrated value to prevent incontinent episodes, reduce urinary infections, and regain bladder tone.

Nurses frequently encounter bowel incontinence. Audrey M. McLane and Ruth E. McShane define Bowel Management as a "progressive program of elimination designed to regulate and control bowel incontinence." In Chapter 5, they review the mechanisms underlying normal elimination and bowel dysfunction and discuss three types of neurogenic bowel: uninhibited, reflex, and autonomous. Other components of a bowel management program are also discussed: diet, physical activity, pelvic floor exercise, medications, digital stimulation, toileting regime, caretaker instructions, and the use of flow sheets. The protocol for the intervention includes first identifying the components to be used as these relate to specific goals. Two case studies illustrate how to choose and implement the components. The authors conclude that the paucity of research in this important area is a cause for concern. Their chapter, in addition to being a practical guide, provides the basis for future research in this area.

Chapter 6 on Positioning by Jennifer Loeper focuses on the intervention as a proactive response to the hazards of immobility. In particular, it addresses the patient who has suffered a neurological insult to the central nervous system. The goal of positioning is to reduce muscle spasticity. Two nursing diagnoses are identified: Impaired Physical Mobility and Potential for Physiologic Injury. Based on a review of the physiology of movement and the developmental sequence of motor activity, the author provides an overview of the nursing activities for several types of positioning: supine bed positioning, positioning on the unaffected side, positioning on the affected side, prone positioning and wheelchair positioning. The chapter concludes with a case study illustrating the application of the content.

Nurses change patients' position frequently to reduce pressure, which might cause skin sores. In Chapter 7 on Pressure Reduction, Barbara J. Braden and Nancy Bergstrom review the many factors that lead to pressure sore development and provide a conceptual model of these factors. The chapter also features two tools: the Braden Scale for assessing pressure sore risk and the Bergstrom Skin Assessment Tool for assessing stages of pressure sore development. The research base and appropriate use of various intervention strategies are discussed. Strategies include frequent repositioning, the use of pillows or wedges, protective devices for bony prominences, monitoring the elevation of the head of the bed, use of lifting devices, and special mattresses and beds. The choice of strategies depends on the goal of the intervention and the level of risk. Three case studies demonstrate the use of the Braden Scale to determine the level of risk and the choice of intervention strategies.

Sleep problems affect many individuals, both well and ill. In preparation for the discussion of the intervention of Sleep Promotion, Felissa L. Cohen and Sharon L. Merritt provide an overview in Chapter 8 of the sleep-wake cycle and types of sleep disorders. They cover the assessment areas a nurse needs to be familiar with to make a diagnosis of Sleep Pattern Disturbance. The authors discuss three sleep promotion interventions: Sleep Promotion: Hygiene Measures, Sleep Promotion: Environmental Alterations, and Sleep Promotion: Drug Therapy. A case study illustrates the thorough assessment and intervention measures that are necessary for a successful outcome to this troublesome problem.

The last chapter in the section, by Jacqueline M. Stolley and Kathleen C. Buckwalter on Confusion Management, focuses on the treatment of chronic confusion in institutionalized clients. Although many conditions can cause a chronic state of confusion, the most common is Alzheimer's disease. The authors first delineate the stages of Alzheimer's disease and the associated behavioral states and losses. They give detailed suggestions for implementing the intervention in regard to seven areas: maximizing safe functioning, giving unconditional positive regard, determining limits of activity, listening, modifying the environment, providing physical care, and facilitating caregiver/family support. The intervention is aimed at maximizing the strengths and minimizing the losses of chronically confused patients, who have multiple needs and present a major challenge to caregivers. The chapter helps to sort out this complex picture.

The nine chapters in this section outline the basic interventions that all nurses do regularly. These encompass the areas of hygiene, skin care, feeding, elimination, positioning, sleep enhancement, and memory loss. Depending on the research base and the nature of the intervention, some authors have taken a broad approach, while others have a narrower focus. Assisting with self-care is an important and fundamental part of nursing. The implementation of these interventions based on knowledge of the individual patient, the disease process, and the particular environment will do much to increase the well-being of the individuals and their family, as well as prevent additional complications. While nurses have long done these basic self-care interventions, there has been little systematic study and documentation of the effects of the care provided. The chapters in this section provide a strong basis for future work in this important area.

1

HYGIENE ASSISTANCE

CATHERINE A. TRACEY

Every nurse should keep this fact constantly in mind, — for, if she allow her sick to remain unwashed, or their clothing to remain on them after being saturated with perspiration or other excretion, she is interfering injuriously with the natural processes of health just as effectually as if she were to give the patient a dose of slow poison by the mouth. Poisoning by the skin is no less certain than poisoning by the mouth — only it is slower in its operation.

Florence Nightingale

Activities provided by nurses to assist individuals with personal hygiene have generally been considered fundamental to nursing. Nightingale (1970) emphasizes the importance of these activities, especially in efforts to reduce infection. Many beginning nursing textbooks contain instructions on techniques to use during hygiene. As health care continues to become more technologically complex, nurses could devalue the activities associated with bathing or give them lower priority. Even now, in some settings, the bath is carried out by the least skilled care provider. Nevertheless, assisting with hygiene is truly a hallmark of the nursing profession, and when it is carried out with knowledge and skill, it yields not only the expected outcome of cleanliness but also a comprehensive assessment of any individual's physical and psychosocial status. Assisting with bathing is also an excellent opportunity for communication, education, and demonstration of a caring approach through physical contact.

DESCRIPTION OF THE INTERVENTION

Personal hygiene encompasses many activities. Bathing is the activity whereby an individual satisfies a need for personal cleanliness (Webster 1988). Meeting that need can include any or all of the following activities: cleansing the body, including the perineum, the eyes, ears, nose, and mouth; oral hygiene, including teeth brushing, flossing, cleaning dentures, and general cleansing of the oral cavity; washing and combing hair; shaving the face or body parts; and care of nails. This set of activities encompasses a broad range, and in the future it may be desirable to define multiple, more discrete interventions in this area. For now, the activities are grouped together under the broad intervention of Hygiene Assistance.

REVIEW OF RESEARCH

Research-based literature supports the complexity of personal hygiene assistance. Most of the research is on bathing; other aspects of hygiene assistance have not been researched. Variables studied include nursing rituals, patients' and nurses' opinions about the hygiene activity of bathing, physiological and psychological response to bathing, and the influence of cognition on bathing ability.

Wolf utilized the definition of a ritual "as a patterned, symbolic action that refers to the goals and values of a social group" (1988, p. 60) in studying nurses working on a medical unit of a large, urban American hospital. In a descriptive analysis, a number of rituals were identified, including the bath and other aseptic practices. Observations of nurses working on all shifts over a 12-month period identified a number of bath practices and beliefs. The bath was utilized for cleansing, assessing skin and the patient's general condition, and teaching and conversing with patients. Avoidance of giving baths was considered a violation of patient and family wishes. The timing of bathing activities gave structure and organization to the work of each shift, and nurse satisfaction was attained when baths were completed.

Webster (1988) studied nurses' and patients' opinions about bathing through a researcher-developed questionnaire and found a variety of discrepancies between nurses' and patients' feelings about bathing. The most significant difference was the importance each group placed on bathing. Patients in a large British acute care facility indicated that nurses have far more important duties than bathing patients, whereas nurses held the opposite opinion. Patients indicated that they are clearly less embarrassed about being bathed by nurses than nurses think they are. Additionally, nurses in this study seemed to be inaccurate in judging patient satisfaction with bathing. Although the study had a small sample, these three items suggest that nurses should validate patients' opinions about bathing.

In two separate studies, Wagnild examined bathing processes in a geriatric long-term-care setting (1985) and the number and nature of personal care complaints made to the Texas Department of Health over two years (1986). Data from the Department of Health revealed that 49 intermediate and skilled nursing facilities in 14 randomly selected counties had 853 complaints over the two study years. Of that total, 340 (40%) were classified as personal care complaints. Bathing and personal hygiene accounted for 27% of the complaints, respect and consideration, 19%, incontinence care, 8%, and decubitus care, 5%. Other areas of complaint involved safety, feeding care, and comfort.

In the follow-up study, Wagnild (1985) observed 42 nursing home residents and 20 nurse aides during the bathing process. In the eight study settings, all personal hygiene was carried out by nurse aides. Observations in the study noted how the resident was addressed by the nurse aide, procedural and nonprocedural touch during the bath, eye contact of the nurse aide, conversation, and nurse aide self-introduction. Twenty-nine (69%) residents received nonprocedural touch. There was only procedural conversation or no conversation preceding or during 21 (50%) of the observed interactions. The researcher noted that none of the aides introduced themselves to the resident receiving the care, and yet only 15% of the residents knew the name of the aide who assisted them with bathing. Residents' memory deficits could have played a role in this finding. Of the 42 baths observed, only 6 were given privately. The remaining 36 baths (86%) were given in the company of at least one other nurse aide and a resident. All residents in the survey indicated they were satisfied with the bath they received. Interpretation of the residents' satisfaction is unclear. The researcher postulated that it may be related to residents' comfort with the routine of bathing or perhaps their acquiescence to the researcher's question.

In two studies, the physiological impact of personal hygiene was examined. Parsons (1985) studied the effects of three hygiene activities on the cerebrovascular status of severe closed-head-injured persons. Nineteen subjects were assessed during mouth care, bathing, and indwelling catheter care. Heart rate, mean arterial blood pressure, mean intracranial pressure, and cerebral perfusion pressures were recorded at baseline, peak nursing activity, and 1 minute recovery times. All subjects had a Glasgow Coma Scale score of less than 6. All three of the hygiene activities produced significant mean increases in the four physiological variables when compared with baseline measurements. The findings were not considered clinically significant because the hygiene activities were considered to cause safe, transient increases in the four physiological measures. This study suggests that these selected hygiene activities can be performed safely with closed-head-injured persons whose resting mean intracranial pressures are less than 20 mm Hg without compromising cerebral blood flow.

The second study used bathing as the independent variable in 12 subjects with uncomplicated myocardial infarctions. Johnson (1981) used a 12-lead electrocardiogram (ECG), blood pressure, cardiac auscultation, and oxygen consumption (Vo_2) as the dependent variables in determining responses to bathing in this population. Physiologic data revealed that a shower (standing) demanded greater Vo_2 than either tub or bed bath. "Hemodynamic response [peak systolic blood pressure $\times$ heart rate (PRP)] was greater for showering when compared to bed bathing but not tub bathing" (p. 668). Heart rate contributed more to this finding. Analysis of ECGs revealed that a greater number of changes occurred after showering than after tub or bed bathing. Four of the five subjects with ECG changes had inferior infarctions. No angina was noted during any of the bathing activities. The researchers suggested that responses to showering may be caused by subclinical left ventricular dysfunction, alterations in peripheral circulation, and/or medications that may cause hemodynamic changes related to position. Limitations of the study include the absence of matched normal controls and cardiac catheterization data.

In a study comparing the effects of two bathing techniques on anxiety, Barsevick (1982) utilized the State-Trait Anxiety Inventory (STAI), the Palmar Sweat Index (PSI), and the Behavioral Cues Index (BCI). The study techniques were the conventional bed bath — a method using a basin of water and a sponging technique — and a towel bath — a method of bathing a patient in bed using a body-sized towel soaked in water with an antiseptic solution and lubricant; the towel is placed over the entire body and the skin is massaged and cleansed through the towel (see Wright, 1990). The study sample contained two groups: patients receiving an invasive procedure and patients with unrelieved pain. Subjects in each diagnostic group were randomly assigned to the towel bath or conventional bath groups. Two research assistants, both registered nurses, participated in the study; one collected the data, and the other administered the bath. The anxiety measures were administered prebath, immediately postbath, and 1 hour postbath.

Prebath data for all groups showed no significant differences. In postbath measures, the PSI and BCI yielded nonsignificant data. Overall, the STAI was the most useful measure of anxiety in this study population. The results of the study indicated that bathing in general reduced anxiety. No significant differences were observed between the two techniques in the unrelieved pain group. Within the invasive procedure group, the STAI scores were significantly lower in the towel bath group than the conventional bath group. In controlling for age and sex, no significant differences between groups were noted.

Among other activities of daily living, the ability of cognitively impaired stroke patients to carry out personal hygiene was studied by Carter (1988). The treatment group in this study received cognitive skills retraining for visual scanning, visual-spatial perception, and time judgment. The control group participated in other therapy treatment programs with the treatment group but did not receive the retraining. Stroke patients who received cognitive skills retraining showed significant improvement in personal hygiene activities, including bathing and toileting, as measured by the Barthel Index (Mahoney and Barthel 1965). This research indicates to nurses the importance of consultation and referral to occupational therapy for evaluation and treatment of individuals with cognitive impairments. Then nurse and therapist can collaborate for the best functional outcome.

REVIEW OF RELATED LITERATURE

Nonresearch-based literature generally focuses on descriptions of techniques used to carry out personal hygiene. An excellent example of a less commonly practiced technique was described by Wright (1990). This article describes the steps in giving a towel bath and the response of a group of patients to this technique compared to a conventional bath. Logistical concerns of equipment, cleansing products, and laundering were also discussed.

Potter and Perry (1989) comprehensively reviewed all hygienic practices, including a chapter on personal hygiene that reviewed methods and issues. One issue they discussed, elaborated in Brink (1976), concerns the cultural influence on hygiene practices. For example, in some cultures, bathing is a social activity, whereas in others, it is a private function. Both sources urge practitioners to determine individual values, desires, and practices before establishing a plan of care. Cleansing oneself is an individual practice, and rote or standard techniques and schedules may prove to be nontherapeutic.

ASSOCIATED NURSING DIAGNOSES

A number of nursing diagnoses are directly and indirectly related to personal hygiene assistance. The most salient is Bathing/Hygiene Self-Care Deficit. In addition to assessing an individual's ability to carry out hygiene, the nurse can use the time and the activities carried out during hygiene assistance to assess and carry out many other related interventions. The associated diagnoses, listed under their assigned human response pattern, follow:

Exchanging
Impaired Skin Integrity
Impaired Tissue Integrity
Altered Oral Mucous Membrane
Altered Tissue Perfusion
Altered Nutrition: Less Than Body Requirements
Potential for Infection
Potential Disuse Syndrome
Potential Altered Body Temperature
Ineffective Thermoregulation
Bowel Incontinence
Urinary Incontinence

Choosing
Ineffective Coping
Impaired Adjustment

Moving
Impaired Physical Mobility
Activity Intolerance
Altered Health Maintenance

Perceiving
Sensory-Perceptual Deficit
Powerlessness
Body Image Disturbance
Unilateral Neglect

Knowing
Knowledge Deficit

Feeling
Pain
Anxiety
Fear

PERSONAL HYGIENE ASSISTANCE: AN INTRODUCTION TO THE PATIENT

Nurses work in a variety of settings where hygiene activities are performed, from nursing homes and critical care units to homes. The time a nurse spends in these activities is often their only time alone with a patient. Taking advantage of this time can allow the nurse to establish a rapport with a patient and accomplish many other activities.

Patient values must be considered first. Each individual learns or adopts values about hygiene based on family, culture, religion, and other factors. In addition, hygiene is an activity with many personal preferences and idiosyncrasies. If the setting puts limitations on honoring personal preferences, these should be explained to the patient. Clean hair, filed and cleaned nails, or a shave can contribute to a client's sense of well-being. For some individuals, being bathed or having certain body parts washed is uncomfortable. The nurse's sensitivity is critical.

Nurses must be careful about projecting their own values onto the patient. For example, there are varying cultural attitudes toward using deodorants, other perfumed hygiene products, and cosmetics. Assessment and acknowledgment of these values must precede any activity.

Moving

Before carrying out hygiene activities, the nurse first assesses the patient's level of independence. Necessary adaptive equipment should be sought to maximize independence. Many items exist to aid those physically impaired individuals in hygiene activities. An occupational therapist can be helpful in identifying and acquiring appropriate equipment — shower chairs, tub benches, grab bars, long-handled sponges, and other items. A quadriplegic with no voluntary movement of any extremity can safely be showered in a padded shower chair, generally considered as providing a thorough and satisfying bath. Simple adaptations like a regular chair placed in front of the bathroom sink can allow an individual with low activity tolerance to complete self-bathing. The nurse must also carefully evaluate an individual's response to these activities, ensuring that the client is paced to maintain vital sign parameters.

In the case of a bedfast patient, the nurse also assesses self-care ability even if the individual is only able to carry out washing the face or mouth care. Especially in hospital settings, patients can regress to a level of dependence not consistent with their abilities. Some expect that the nurse should do certain things for them because they believe that is the nurse's role. In this situation, the nurse should explain to the patient the importance of self-care in the gradual process of recovery and the nurse's role in facilitating that process.

The method selected for bathing the bedfast patient who has a high level of dependence is contingent on a number of variables: available equipment, his or her preference, time available, and equipment associated with treatment. For example, it may be appropriate to use the towel bath technique for a post–cerebrovascular accident patient on an acute neurology unit but would not be useful in a post–myocardial infarction patient client in critical care with an arterial line, peripheral intravenous lines, and cardiac monitoring leads. The towel bath technique (Wright, 1990) is an excellent option and has been shown to reduce anxiety. In the absence of the recommended body-sized towel, a bath blanket could be substituted.

Bathing is an excellent time to encourage the immobilized patient to perform self-range of joint motion (ROJM) exercises. If the patient is unable, the nurse should put the major joints through complete ROJM to prevent contractures. Severe joint contractures can lead to decreased function and difficulty in accessing an area of the body. For example, a severe contracture of the shoulder can limit access to bathing the axilla, putting this area at risk for infection and/or skin rashes and breakdown. Early consultation with physical and occupational therapy can assist the nurse in collaborating on contracture prevention.

Exchanging

Many physiologic conditions should be assessed during hygiene. Beginning practitioners need time to master the task of bathing before they can include the array of other activities associated with this intervention. Skilled, experienced nurses can accomplish much during the bath.

A number of conditions affect an individual's ability to regulate body temperature. For example, a warm bath in a warm room could elevate the temperature of an individual with a brain infarct or injury. Generally, water temperature is recommended to be 43°C to 46°C or 110°F to 115°F (Potter 1989). Adjustments to this recommendation may need to be made for certain patients with Ineffective Thermoregulation.

While cleansing the skin, hair, nails, eyes, ears, nose, mouth, and perianal area, the nurse can assess the condition of these areas. The skin should be slightly moist and of a color consistent with the race or ethnicity of the client. In light-skinned clients, signs of pressure appear pink or red, whereas in dark-skinned clients, pressure areas appear darker. The nurse should pay particular attention to the skin over bony prominences because these areas are at the greatest risk for breakdown from pressure. Care should be taken in the selection of products to cleanse the skin. Heavy use of soap without lubrication can cause or worsen skin dryness. Antiseptic solutions and lubricants will adequately cleanse and moisten the skin. Care should also be taken in the strength of the motion of cleansing the skin. Especially in the elderly, skin can be extremely fragile and can tear during the process of bathing.

Potential for Infection is a diagnosis that should be kept in mind during hygiene assistance. Any breaks in the skin or mucous membranes leave the patient at risk for infection. Prevention is best, but early detection and treatment of skin breaks or rashes can minimize the risk of infection. The diagnoses of Bowel and Urinary Incontinence put an individual at even greater risk for skin breakdown and infection. Again, prevention will always better serve the patients, but early treatment may be more realistic in some populations. Particular care should be taken in treating skin that has been in frequent contact with fecal material. Repeated cleansing with soap and water can be more injurious than the incontinence. Suggestions for treatment of skin exposed to diarrhea are found in Case Study 2 in this chapter. Incontinence is often accompanied by immobility or the diagnosis of Potential Disuse Syndrome. The combination of immobility and incontinence is serious, requiring nursing diligence to prevent or treat skin breakdown.

Cleansing other body parts requires special considerations. The eyes are subject to both dryness and infection. Eye lubricants should be used for patients whose blink is reduced, resulting in inadequate tearing. Care should also be taken to use a separate or clean cloth when cleaning the eyes so as not to contaminate the eyes from other body parts. Excess nasal secretions could impair breathing; therefore it may be necessary to remove the secretions. The ears also may need cleansing of excess secretions. Nurses should not use and should instruct patients not to use sharp instruments in the ears. In addition, only the outer ear should be cleaned.

Medications or irrigations may be necessary for cleansing wax from the inner canals of the ear.

Hygiene of the oral cavity can present some unique challenges to the nurse. When patients are unable to meet their own oral care needs, the nurse needs to provide care to teeth, dentures, gums, and the mucous membranes of the oral cavity. Two important areas in the hygiene of the mouth are management of food and altered oral mucous membrane. Patients with swallowing problems may leave or pocket food in the mouth. Food can cause deterioration of the oral membrane and could occlude the airway. Careful examination of the mouth is necessary. A number of conditions can contribute to changes in the oral mucosa, including dehydration, poor-fitting dentures, radiation and chemotherapy, braces, endotracheal tubes, malnutrition, infection, decreased salivation or lack of it, and medications. Frequent examination of all areas of the mouth can identify problems early.

Choosing

Lack of attention to hygiene can be one of the first signs of Ineffective Coping or Impaired Adjustment. Vegetative signs of depression also include lack of interest and attention to personal appearance. In addition to the interdisciplinary treatment of the psychological condition, the nurse may need to contract with the patient to complete agreed-upon hygiene measures. The contract should allow for the patient's increasing involvement in all activities as mental status improves.

Perceiving

Similar to coping and adjustment, Powerlessness and Body Image Disturbance can affect a patient's ability and motivation to carry out hygiene. Involving him or her in parts of hygiene can be the beginning steps to treatment of the problem. In the case of an amputee, for example, the nurse can demonstrate the proper care of the skin over the stump and slowly involve the patient in that care. Using the time to discuss the patient's feelings about the change in body image can also assist in the adjustment and resulting self-care of the affected body part.

A Sensory-Perceptual Deficit is important to assess and consider in carrying out hygiene. Neurological impairments resulting in the inability to sense texture or temperature can have implications for hygiene. Also in some of the conditions, a hypersensitive state exists, causing the touch of certain areas to be uncomfortable. An inability to sense temperature can be a safety issue in regulating the heat of water for bathing or showering. The nurse should ensure the proper water temperature and, if appropriate, teach the patient the same process. The diagnosis, Unilateral Neglect, also requires that the nurse instruct and reinforce attention to the affected side of the stroke client: Consultation with an occupational therapist for cognitive skills retraining may be necessary or helpful (Carter 1988). Nurse and therapist co-treatment of this diagnosis will lead to a more positive outcome.

Knowing

In certain client populations, basic instruction in hygiene may be necessary. Age, poverty, neglect, and psychological state may all contribute to a Knowledge Deficit regarding hygiene. In many other conditions, the nurse may be involved in reeducation and adaptation of hygiene measures following illness or change in functional status. For example, a postpartum mother may need instruction on special perineal care following an episiotomy.

Feeling

Anxiety or Fear can inhibit patients from participating in hygiene at the level of their ability. Like other psychological conditions, treatment of the cause of anxiety or fear can improve participation in hygiene. Pain can also be prohibitive in self-care or the hygiene activities of the nurse. Pharmacological and nonpharmacological interventions to reduce or eliminate pain prior to any activity can allow necessary hygiene to be done. Bathing should also be considered as an option to reduce pain. Submersion of the body or a body part in water can relax muscles and reduce anxiety and pain.

CASE STUDIES

Case Study 1

Patrick is a 16-year-old black male who sustained a gunshot wound, resulting in paraplegia (no voluntary movement below the waist). The day following his admission to a rehabilitation setting, Pam, his primary nurse, begins to explain some of the precautions she will be taking to protect his body below the level of his injury. While bathing Patrick's lower extremities, Pam instructs Patrick on the need to protect his heels from skin breakdown due to his lack of any sensation below the waist. When she questions him on his understanding of this material, Patrick closes his eyes and does not respond. He also refuses to participate in any self-bathing of his upper body although he is able to do so. Patrick states that he will wash when he obtains his own toiletries the next day.

Having received his own supplies the following day, Patrick proceeds to spend over an hour washing his upper body, brushing and flossing his teeth, combing and applying gel to his hair, and applying deodorant and powder. After this lengthy process, Pam checks on his progress to find his upper body well cared for and his lower body untouched. He explained, "That's your job!" Pam is able to convince him that he could wash his thighs, which he barely touched.

Over the course of the next week, Pam is able to get Patrick out of bed into a padded shower chair that rolls into a large, private shower room. Gradually she instructs him in the use of a long-handled sponge to reach his feet, back, and buttocks. On the third time in the shower, after struggling to reach the soap he dropped on the floor, Patrick begins to cry. Pam urges him to express his feelings about his new disability and the new ways he needs to care for his body. Pam continues to use the shower time to urge Patrick to discuss his feelings, as well as reinforce her instruction about his new self-care responsibilities.

Case Study 2

Mrs. V, an 87-year-old white female, had been a nursing home patient for two weeks following a large right cerebrovascular accident. On several of her daughter Sue's visits, Mrs. V is found to have been incontinent of stool. Sue speaks with a staff member about her concerns but is not pleased with the response. She decides to move her mother to her own home, where she cares for Mrs. V herself. She refuses the nursing home's suggestion for a visiting nurse referral.

In addition to Mrs. V's total dependence in all self-care, she has an indwelling catheter for urinary drainage and a gastrostomy tube for nutritional feedings. The nursing home staff instructed Sue in all aspects of her mother's care. After a week at home, Mrs. V develops diarrhea, with four or five episodes a day. In addition, Mrs. V chokes when Sue tries to clean her mouth. Sue is diligent in cleaning Mrs. V's skin after each incontinence, but it worsens with each episode. Finally, the skin over the buttocks is so reddened it begins to bleed. Sue calls the local Visiting Nurse Association (VNA) and asks for assistance.

On her initial visit, the VNA nurse discovers that Sue has substituted a different tube feeding. The VNA nurse believes that this has caused the diarrhea. She instructs Sue to use the previously established feeding, starting at half-strength and working up to full strength over the next several days. The VNA nurse also instructs Sue to give an antidiarrhea medication for one day to try to reduce the episodes. In treatment of the skin, the nurse suggests Sue eliminate the use of soap and water and substitute a non–water based skin wash, gently applied with a soft cloth. Once the skin is clean, a protective medicated ointment is applied as a barrier. After two days, the diarrhea is completely resolved, and after a week, Mrs. V's skin is essentially healed.

The nurse continues to visit Mrs. V while instructing Sue in various techniques to keep her mother clean. She also obtains a portable suction machine to prevent Mrs. V from choking on mouthwash. Although the work is extremely time-consuming, Sue prefers caring for her mother and is more sure of herself with the support of the VNA nurse.

SUMMARY

Florence Nightingale emphasized the fundamental purpose of hygiene to "keep the pores of the skin free from all obstructing excretions" and to remove "noxious matter from the system as rapidly as possible" (1970, p. 53). This purpose remains unchanged today. In addition, hygiene assistance serves many other functions, including the opportunity to assess the condition of skin, hair, nails, and mucosa. It provides an opportunity to educate, communicate, and develop a caring relationship while reducing anxiety and pain and improving the patient's sense of well-being. Advanced nursing practice allows for all or any combination of these activities to be carried out simultaneously. In striving for excellence, the nurse will maximize the therapeutic value of hygiene.

REFERENCES

Barsevick, A., and Llewellyn, J. 1982. A comparison of the anxiety-reducing potential of two techniques of bathing. *Nursing Research* 31(1):22–27.

Brink, P. (ed.) 1976. *Transcultural nursing: A book of readings.* Englewood Cliffs, NJ: Prentice-Hall.

Carpenito, L.J. 1987. *Nursing diagnosis: Application to clinical practice.* Philadelphia: J.B. Lippincott Co.

Carter, L.T., et al. 1988. The relationship of cognitive skills performance to activities of daily living in stroke patients. *The American Journal of Occupational Therapy* 42(7):449–455.

Johnson, B.L., Watt, E.W., and Fletcher, G.F. 1981. Oxygen consumption and hemodynamic and electrocardiographic responses to bathing in recent post-myocardial infarction patients. *Heart & Lung* 10(4):666–671.

Nightingale, F. 1970. *Notes on nursing.* London: Brandon/Systems Press, Inc.

North American Nursing Diagnosis Association. 1989. *Taxonomy I: Revised.* St. Louis, MO.

Parsons, L.C., Smith Peard, A.L., and Page, M.C. 1985. The effects of hygiene interventions on the cerebrovascular status of severe closed head injured persons. *Research in Nursing and Health* 85(8):173–181.

Potter, P.A., and Perry, A.G. 1989. *Fundamentals of nursing: Concepts, process and practice.* St. Louis: C.V. Mosby Co.

Tracey, C.A. 1989. Etiologies of the nursing diagnosis of self-care deficit. In Carroll-Johnson, R.M. (ed.). *Classification of nursing diagnosis: Proceedings of the eighth conference* (pp 349–351). Philadelphia: J.B. Lippincott Co.

Wagnild, G., and Manning, R.W. 1985. Convey respect during bathing procedures. *Journal of Gerontological Nursing* 11(12):6–10.

Wagnild, G. 1986. Personal-care complaints: A descriptive study. *The Journal of Long-Term Care Administration* 86(3):27–29.

Webster, R., et al. 1988. Patients' and nurses' opinions about bathing. *Nursing Times* 84(37):54–57.

Wolf, Z.R. 1988. Nursing rituals. *The Canadian Journal of Nursing Research* 20(3):59–69.

Wolf, Z.R. 1986. Nurses' work: the sacred and the profane. *Holistic Nursing Practice* 1(1):29–35.

Wright, L., 1990. Bathing by towel. *Nursing Times* 86(4):36–39.

2

DRY SKIN CARE

MARY ANDERSON HARDY

Even before Florence Nightingale, bathing was known to be more than a hygienic practice. Writing in *Notes on Nursing*, Nightingale recognized that a little water and a rough towel to rub away dirt was all that was needed to keep clean but that

> washing . . . with a large quantity of water has quite other effects than those of mere cleanliness. The skin absorbs the water and becomes softer and more perspirable. To wash with soap and soft water is, therefore, desirable from other points of view than that of cleanliness. (Nightingale 1946)

The intervention outlined in this chapter is a bathing treatment for dry skin. The goal of treatment for dry skin (xerosis)—to maintain hydration of the epidermis—can be achieved by increasing the water content of the skin or retarding transepidermal water loss.

Water, not lipids, is most responsible for the pliability of and resistance to cracking of skin (Dotz and Berman 1984): "Skin is dry not because it lacks grease or skin oils, but because it lacks water. All therapeutic efforts are aimed at replacing water in the skin and in the immediate environment" (Arndt 1983). Humectants, such as glycerin and propylene glycol, draw moisture from the air into the stratum corneum. But, in environments with low humidity, these agents do not increase the water content of the skin significantly. Water, absorbed by the skin through bathing, hydrates the skin but is rapidly lost to the atmosphere and has minimal long-term effects. Therefore, therapy for dry skin emphasizes the use of occlusive topical agents, such as petrolatum, lanolin, and mineral oil, to prevent moisture loss from the skin (Parent 1985); the "greasier," the better, suggests Gilchrest (1986).

The intervention of Dry Skin Care is based on a consensus of dermatological and gerontological nursing literature. It is composed of the following activities:

1. Use a superfatted soap for cleansing.
2. Maintain a water temperature of 90°F to 105°F.
3. Immerse the patient in a tub up to the chest while pouring water over body parts not immersed or shower with a continuous spray over all body parts for 10 minutes.
4. Pat the skin dry with a cotton towel rather than by rubbing.
5. Maintain a humid environment.
6. Apply an emollient over all body parts as an occlusive.
7. Use linen that has been thoroughly rinsed of detergent and without antistatic.
8. Wear cotton clothing.

RELATED LITERATURE: GENERAL AND RESEARCH

Skin, the largest organ of the body, makes up about 15% of the total body weight. It has many valuable functions: it protects internal organs, guards against foreign substances, provides tactile perception, helps regulate temperature, stores fats, and discharges electrolytes and water. Skin consists of three anatomically distinct layers: the epidermis, the dermis, and the subcutaneous tissue.

The epidermis consists of the horny outer layer known as the stratum corneum and comprises mostly closely packed dead cells that are being continually brushed off by clothing and washing. These cells are constantly replaced by the bottom, living basal layer. It takes approximately 26 days for cells from this layer to migrate up to the stratum corneum and be completely replaced in the young and double that in elderly patients. About 20% of an adult's protein requirements are needed for this purpose.

Immediately after birth, an infant's skin has a mean pH of 6.34; within 4 days after birth, the pH declines to about 4.95. An acid skin surface with a pH lower than 5.0 has bactericidal quality. As the infant's skin pH decreases after birth, the acid mantle is formed from the epidermis, sweat, superficial fat, metabolic products, and external substances such as amniotic fluid, microorganisms, and cosmetics (Kuller, Lund, and Tobin 1983).

The lower levels of the epidermis contain melanocytes whose function is to produce melanin or pigment and keratin-forming cells, which cornify the outer layer of the epidermis. The number of active melanocytes diminishes with aging, thus reducing the skin's protective function against ultraviolet light.

The dermis lies directly under the epidermis and is 2 mm to 4 mm thick at birth. It is a closely woven layer of fibrous protein, collagen, and elastin fibers. It contains many nerves and a rich supply of blood vessels that nourish the skin cells and act as carriers of the sensations of heat, touch, pressure, and pain from the skin to the brain. Hair originates from deep in the dermis. With aging, the dermis becomes thinner and less pliable, and the number of blood vessels decreases, which in turn decreases the number of hair bulbs and sweat glands. The surface area between the dermis and epidermis decreases with aging, secondary to flattening of the derm-epidermal junction. This narrowing between the two skin components can lead to decreased transfer of substances, including nutrients, and can increase the potential for skin tears.

The major component of the subcutaneous layer is fatty connective tissue. The subcutaneous fat functions as a heat insulator, shock absorber, and calorie storage area. Accumulation of fat occurs predominantly during the last trimester of gestation. Sebaceous glands are found in both the dermis and subcutaneous layer. These are well developed and potentially functional at birth but in fact have only minimal function until puberty. Sweat glands are also found in the dermis and subcutaneous layer and are affected directly by external environmental temperature. Sweat gland maturation occurs between 21 and 33 days of life in premature infants and at about 5 days in term infants. Poor sweat production in premature infants is due to sweat gland immaturity. Adult skin function in any child, however, is not achieved until the second or third year of life.

Epidemiology of Dry Skin

Dry skin, or xerosis, with its accompanying itching, burning, scaling, and social isolation, is a problem for 59% to 75% of the elderly (Eliopoulos 1988; Frantz and Kinney 1986; Parent 1985; Tindall and Smith 1963). Of aging skin problems, pruritus is most common (Herman and Gilchrest 1989), and xerosis is responsible for up to 85% of this. Whether water loss increases in the elderly or the absolute amount of water embedded in the stratum corneum decreases — or neither — is unknown, but clinically the result is rough, dry, scaly, and sometimes fissured skin. This condition worsens during the winter months, when sharply reduced environmental temperature and humidity are compounded by the use of central heating.

In a survey of skin problems and skin care regimens among 68 noninstitutionalized volunteers aged 50 to 91 years (average 74 years), the most prevalent complaint was pruritus (29%); 61% acknowledged a history of dry skin, and on physical examination 85% had xerosis (Beauregard and Gilchrest 1987). Thus, there was no association between the objective finding of xerosis and the patient complaint. Men and women (71% and 87%, respectively) presented with dry skin despite the fact that many fewer men than women (29% versus 63%) acknowledged the existence of this condition, even on direct questioning. In the majority of cases, subjects treated their skin problems without consulting a physician, although these approaches were infrequently helpful. A moisturizer was used regularly by 79% of the subjects with a diagnosis of xerosis and by 88% of those subjects with a history of dry skin. However, the rate of regular moisturizer use was 80% and 65%, respectively, among those subjects lacking xerosis on physical examination or by history, thus complicating interpretation of this finding (Beauregard and Gilchrest 1987).

The frequent hand washing and resulting dry and cracked skin found in nursing personnel warranted attention from Seitz and Newman (1988). Season, age, geographic locale, frequency of hand washing, and work area were the major variables analyzed for their effects on skin dryness. The conclusion of the study was that winter season, northern locale, and age over 30 were the most significant factors contributing to skin dryness. Nurses over 30 years of age most susceptible to dry, chapped hands lived in a northern climate and were high-frequency washers (more than three times an hour). The authors suggested further study of the requisite number of hand washings to prevent nosocomial infection and the use of products that would be therapeutic but also prophylactic against drying skin.

Because radiation increases the mitotic production of basal cells and upsets the balance between basal cell production and surface cell destruction, dryness, pruritus, and redness often occur during radiation therapy (Hassey 1987). Thought to be related to a decrease in the function of the sweat glands and sebaceous glands, dryness and pruritus present about the third week of radiation treatment at an accumulated radiation dose of 3000 to 3500 cGy (Hassey 1987). The immunosuppressed patient is counseled to maintain a skin condition that prevents the entry of bacteria by using oils and avoiding drying the skin (Crow 1983).

Research Literature

The overwhelming conclusion from the literature is that dry skin can be treated by adding moisture through bathing, preventing moisture loss through the use of a mild, superfatted soap for cleansing, maintaining a controlled environment, and applying an emollient that will prevent rapid evaporation (Anderson 1971; Arndt 1983; Atkins 1977; Fitzsimmons 1983; Gilchrest 1986; Hogstel 1983). There is little agreement, however, on brand of soap, frequency of bathing, use of shower or tub, type of occlusive agent, or desired environmental humidity. Although there is agreement that water should be tepid and that laundry should be treated without starch or antistatic agents in drying, there is little research base supporting any of these multiple treatment choices (Boisits 1986; Cornell 1986; Epstein 1983;

Fenske 1982; Fitzsimmons 1983; Gaul and Underwood 1951; Hogstel 1983; Parent 1985; Parth and Kapke 1983; Pearson and Kotthof 1979; Walther and Harber 1984; Weiner, Belser, Giudice, Kanat, Kaplan, Kauth, and Stone 1983).

Four studies testing interventions for dry skin have been reported. Spoor (1958) analyzed the effects of a water-dispersable oil as an additive for the bath in the treatment of patients with "dry, itchy, scaly, lichenified skin" (p. 3299) and reported successful therapeutic effect and personal acceptance in 10 of 12 subjects. Weiner et al. (1973) used a nationwide sample of 153 persons over the age of 50 and reported limited success in the treatment of dry skin with a topical moisturizing and lubricating lotion. Brown, Boosinger, Black, Gaspar, and Sather (1982) tested the use of 10-minute water soaks followed by mineral oil application for the treatment of skin dryness of the feet in 31 long-term-care residents. An analysis of the treatment, which was introduced three times per week for 2 weeks, resulted in significant ($p < .01$) improvement in the skin condition of the feet.

The fourth study, by Hardy (1990a), reported the results of a pilot study designed to improve measurement and treatment of dry skin in the elderly. The sample consisted of 15 institutionalized elders with a mean age of 70 years. The Skin Condition Data Form (SCDF), developed by Frantz and Kinney (1986), was administered every 2 weeks, making nine data collection points: three pretest, three during intervention, and three postintervention. No effort was made to control the time of the day of assessment, the bathing and skin treatments in the pre- and postintervention periods, the amount of mineral oil, or whether a bath or shower was used. Six weeks was determined as sufficient for testing the effectiveness of the intervention because the normal cell moves from the basilar level to the epidermis in about 4 weeks, and skin changes in the elderly may take up to 2 weeks to be manifested (Fenske 1982). MANOVA was used to analyze the repeated measures of total skin dryness and the four individual dimensions of skin dryness (redness, scaling, cracking, and flaking). Significant differences were found over time on total skin dryness and on redness, scaling, and flaking. Cracking did not change significantly over time, perhaps because this dimension was difficult to assess or did not contribute significantly to dryness scores. The expected pattern of dryness — decreasing during the intervention and returning to baseline postintervention — was reflected in all of the mean scores except on redness, which peaked during the last 2 weeks of the intervention period. This may have been because redness is not a valid variable of skin dryness, that one or more aspects of the intervention was responsible for increasing redness, or that skin takes on a pinker color as it becomes less dry. The limitations of small sample size and moderate interrater reliability on the SCDF must be weighed against the fact that the dry skin of the 15 residents in the study did follow the pattern expected following intervention.

INTERVENTION TOOLS

Although extensive work exists on the history and assessment of the integument (Delancey and North 1983; Hannigan 1978; Hogstel 1983; Malkiewicz 1981; Pearson and Kotthof 1979: Urosevich 1981), the research base for measurement of dry skin is limited to two instruments: the Skin Condition Data Form (SCDF) and the Black and Gaspar Foot Assessment Tool. The SCDF was used to gather information from 76 subjects over the age of 65 on bathing and skin treatment practices and factors believed to contribute to dry skin. In addition to questions pertaining to practices and etiologic factors, the SCDF measures skin condition by redness, scaling, fissuring, rash, excoriation, greasy appearance, and thickening. One check is made each time a sign occurs on any of the 11 areas of the body rated, making the range of possible scores from 0 to 77 (Frantz and Kinney 1986).

Brown and co-workers (1982) used the Black and Gaspar Foot Assessment Tool to evaluate the effectiveness of an intervention for treating elderly persons with dry feet. The Black and Gaspar instrument measures skin condition on a scale of 1 (oily) to 7 (very dry) for dorsal and plantar surfaces of the foot. No psychometric properties were reported for either instrument.

Hardy (1990a) reported testing a modified SCDF. Observed skin condition was contained to four concepts of the dryness construct (redness, flaking, scaling, and cracking); the observation was expanded to 22 areas of the body, and the rating was changed to a 4-point scale, ranging from absent (0) to severe (3). This made the range of possible scores from 0 to 66 (Figure 2 – 1). Content validity and interrater reliability of the SCDF were assessed as part of the pilot study (Hardy 1990a). Content validity was based on literature and expert review. Interrater reliability using percentage agreement among raters was 87%, 63%, and 68%, respectively, on history, current skin practices, and observed dryness. The fact that the mean score for the three preintervention dryness scores was 18.4 for this known group (subjects with dry skin) provided preliminary evidence of the construct validity of the instrument.

Three instruments recently described by Blichman and Serup (1988) hold some hope for more objective and perhaps more reliable measures of skin dryness in the future. The Skicon-100, the Coreomter CM 420 hydrometers, and the Servo Med EPI evaporimeter all measure electrical conductance, capacitance, and transepidermal water loss. Water is an effective electrical transmitter, and dry skin is directly related to the water content of the skin. These biomedical instruments may be useful in measuring skin dryness and, thus, the effectiveness of interventions designed to treat dry skin.

ASSOCIATED NURSING DIAGNOSES AND CLIENT GROUPS

A review of the nursing literature on skin care reveals that a wide variety of clients are affected by dry skin: the elderly (Eliopoulos 1988; Frantz and Kinney 1986; Herman and Gilchrest 1989; Parent 1985; Tindall and Smith 1963), nursing staff who do a lot of hand washing (Seitz and Newman 1988), patients undergoing radiation therapy (Crow 1983; Hassey 1987), and premature infants in isolettes for an extended length of time (Kuller, Lund, and Tobin 1983).

Diagnosis

No diagnostic label for dry skin is included in the North American Nursing Diagnosis Association Taxonomy I (Revised) (1989). However, Hardy (1990a, 1990b) has provided considerable support for the addition of a diagnostic label: Impaired Skin Integrity: Dry Skin.

Signs and Symptoms

Dry skin is usually said to be primarily on the extremities, although the trunk and face may be affected (Arndt 1983; Parent 1985). Symptoms include roughness, flaking, scaling, chapping, pruritus, and, in severe cases, inflammation, fissuring,

Body Site		redness	scaling	cracking	flaking
Face					
Neck					
Upper arms-	anterior				
	posterior				
	lateral				
Forearms-	anterior				
	posterior				
	lateral				
Hands-	dorsal				
Trunk-	anterior				
	posterior				
	lateral				
Thighs-	anterior				
	posterior				
	lateral				
Lower leg-	anterior				
	posterior				
	lateral				
Feet-	dorsal				
	plantar				
	heels				
	between toes				

Enter a number in each box: 0 = absent
1 = mild
2 = moderate
3 = severe

FIGURE 2–1. Skin Appearance Observations (Skin Condition Data Form)

and erythema of the affected areas (Arndt 1983; Dotz and Berman 1984; Parent 1985). Gilchrest (1986) described xerosis as pruritic, inflamed, scaly, and chapped. The modified SCDF used by Hardy (1990a) captures data about the degree of pruritus as well as direct observation of the signs of dry skin for which there is consensus in the literature. Hardy reports the following operational definitions for the signs of dry skin:

1.   Redness: Inflammation varying from pink to bright red in the area of xerosis.

2. Flaking: Dandrufflike flakes that appear when the fingers are lightly rubbed over skin surface.

3. Scaling: Fishlike scales on the skin's surface that are easily rubbed off of skin surface with fingers.

4. Cracking: Parched appearance of skin that resembles dry earth.

Although there seems to be some consensus on the signs and symptoms of dry skin, research to isolate valid defining characteristics and incorporate these into valid instruments is needed. To this end, Hardy is replicating the pilot study in a larger study of 300 community living as well as institutionalized subjects over age 60 with dry skin.

Etiologies

The literature suggests several etiologies, including maturational, environmental, and pathological. It has long been thought that age-related decrease in sebum production, which allows increased loss of water from the skin surface and decreased hydration of the stratum corneum from underlying tissues, is responsible for the prevalence of dry skin among the elderly. Yet Frantz and Kinney (1986) found no significant relationship between skin dryness and nutritional or hydration status, medical history, sebum content in the skin, or diuretic regime, all factors purported to contribute to dry skin. Some of these factors, like hypothyroidism, diabetes, malignancies, hepatic or renal diseases, psychoneuroses, or medications, are amenable only to medical treatment (Dotz and Berman 1984; Parent 1985) and must be ruled out in cases of severe pruritus or xerosis (Atkins 1977; Shelley and Shelley 1982; Walther and Harber 1984). Other hypothesized contributing factors are amenable to nursing intervention: frequency of bathing and use of soap (Gioella and Bevil, 1985; Parent 1985; Walther and Harber 1984), excessive perspiration (Cornell 1986), dehydration and vitamin A deficiency (Hogstel 1983; Parent 1985), smoking (Fitzsimmons 1983), stress (Atkins 1977), lack of humidity (Fenske 1982; Hogstel 1983), and exposure to the sun (Arndt 1983; Parth and Kapke 1983). Skin is also drier in the winter months when forced-air heating systems and cold winds accelerate the loss of skin moisture. Many variables, such as the condition and chemical content of water, as well as kinds of skin lotions and diet, have not yet been discussed. Although the small sample size in the Hardy (1990a) pilot study precluded analysis of many of these variables because of insufficient cell sizes, the only significant variable for skin dryness was use of soap prior to the treatment protocol. Research is needed to test the multiple factors that have been identified and those still to be discovered.

My belief is that attention to the condition and treatment of skin will increase in nursing practice. The fact that the International Association of Enterostomal Therapy is discussing a change in its name to reflect a function that encompasses skin care in general rather than the narrower stoma care (President's Message 1990) coupled with the rich literature addressing this area of nursing practice are welcome evidence.

PROTOCOL

The overwhelming conclusion of the literature is that dry skin can be treated. The measures suggested have as a common objective the addition of moisture through bathing. The loss of moisture is prevented through the use of a mild, superfatted soap for cleansing, maintenance of a controlled environment, and active retention of the moisture by application of an emollient that will prevent rapid evaporation (Anderson 1971; Arndt 1983; Atkins 1977; Fitzsimmons 1983; Hogstel 1983). There is little agreement, however, on the brand of soap, the frequency of bathing, shower or tub, the occlusive agent, or the desired environmental humidity.

Soaps

Soaps are used for removing dirt and grease; their degreasing and oil-dissolving properties, however, may make skin dry after the early and middle stages of life (Shelley and Shelley 1982). A mild, nonirritating soap has a decreased detergent content but also a decreased cleansing ability. Superfatted soaps, on the other hand, attack the problem of reducing dehydration by providing an excess of emollient material, which results in a thick film of oil being deposited on the skin surface (Dotz and Berman 1984). The consensus is that nonperfumed superfatted soaps that do not contain hexachlorophine are most effective in treating dry skin in the elderly. The specific brands are Basis, Dove, Tone, Caress (Arndt 1984; Walther and Harber 1984), Neutrogena, and Emulave (Parth and Hapke 1983). Many of these soaps are also suggested for newborns: Lowila, Aveeno, Basis, Neutrogena, Purpose, and Oilatum (Tobin 1984a). Only Dove has been reported as being tested in a laboratory study and was found to be less "irritating" than only soaps (Frosch and Kligman 1979).

Tobin (1984a) suggests water-only baths be given between soap baths for newborns. Beauregard and Gilchrest (1987) found in a study of the bathing practices of older adults, that 6% claimed use of only water while the others used conventional soap, liquid soap, or cold cream. The efficacy of the choice of soap or no soap may be important because one of the findings in Hardy's pilot study of a bathing treatment for dry skin in the elderly was that subjects with dry skin who reported using no soap prior to the intervention had lower preintervention dryness scores throughout the pilot study (1990a).

Bathing Frequency

There is little consensus in the literature about the frequency of bathing. Tobin (1984b) suggested a soap bath once to twice weekly for newborns because of the need to maintain an acid pH (acid mantle) for its bactericidal quality. Hogstel (1983) suggested a partial bath daily and a complete bath two to three times a week for an elderly individual. Shelley and Shelley (1982), in contrast, suggested one short, cool shower per week for any older individual suffering from itching due to dry skin. Arndt (1983) suggested that an adult with dry skin bathe once every 1 to 2 days. Epstein (1983) suggests, however, that there is no reason for those with dry skin to cut down on bathing unless they bathe more than once a day. This suggestion is consistent with the theory that one element of effective treatment for dry skin is superhydration. Age may be an important factor to consider in prescribing bathing frequency; Beauregard and Gilchrest (1987) reported that subjects aged younger than 80 years had a tendency to bathe somewhat more frequently (6.1 versus 5.4 baths or showers per week).

Bathing Mode

A bed bath or partial bath is suggested by Walther and Harber (1984) for treatment of dry skin. This suggestion has not been tested, however, and is intuitively contradictive to the theory that water absorption must be maximized in dry skin treatments. Although Spoor (1958) and Brown et al. (1982) reported successful treatment with soaking baths, total immersion may not always be practical. Hardy reported that many subjects in a pilot study of the effects of a bathing treatment for dry skin (1990a) did not tub bathe due to limited mobility, and often nursing units lacked adequate transfer and bathing equipment that would promote tub bathing. Hardy also reported that the efficacy of bathing versus showering was unclear and that one dermatologist wrote that showering was as effective as bathing (Epstein 1983).

Because many hospitalized and nursing home elderly are showered, showering was incorporated in Hardy's intervention protocol (1990a). Incorporating both modes of bathing in treatment research is important because the differing effects of each are unknown, the clinical feasibility of nursing intervention must be a consideration, and the elderly report using both bathing modes. In a study of 68 noninstitutionalized subjects aged 50 to 91 years, subjects aged younger than 78 years used both the tub and the shower frequently, while subjects aged 80 years and older often exclusively used either the tub (38%) or shower (21%). Whether this was due to available bathroom facilities, physical limitations, or simple preference was not ascertained. Only 2% of those aged younger than 80 years required assistance in bathing or showering, and 17% of the independently living subjects aged 80 years or older required assistance.

Mode of bathing is not only a question for the frail elderly. In a study in Sweden designed to compare the effects of washing and bathing on umbilical infection rates, comfort as indicated by crying, and body temperature, 618 babies were either immersed in a tub filled with 37°C water and washed by hand or washed using a washcloth without soap. All other care was the same for both groups. Infection rates did not differ significantly; however, babies were significantly more comfortable with the tub bath ($p < .001$), and heat loss was significantly lower in the tub-bathed group ($p < .001$) (Hylen et al. 1983).

Although no research reports the rationale nurses use in making bathing mode treatment choices, safety, time, and the medical regimen are often major considerations, whether the nurse is in an assistive role or counseling a client on bathing choices. For instance, nurses working with demented elderly make this choice based on prevention of catastrophic reactions often brought on not only by the bath but by transportation to the tub or shower room. The effects of two treatment choices often made by nurses — a bed bath versus shower — have been reported. Lindell and Olsson (1990) reported that in a study comparing personal hygiene between 28 elderly women in a long-term-care setting and 35 healthy home-living elderly women, the institutionalized women were most often bathed in bed, while the home-living women showered. Second, 89% of the institutionalized women had vulvovaginal signs and symptoms, which the authors attributed to inadequate rinsing of soap following bed baths, as compared to 20% of the home-living women who complained most often of vaginal pruritus.

Length of Bath/Shower

Pearson and Kotthof (1979) suggest a soaking or submerging for 10 minutes to 15 minutes. Brown et al. (1982) reported significant improvement in the condition of dry feet after 2 weeks of 10-minute soaking treatments three times per week in the elderly. Hardy replicated the 10-minute soak in designing a pilot study to test the effects of a bathing protocol on dry skin and reported significant improvement in the dry skin of 15 institutionalized elders (1990a).

Occlusive Agent

An oil base is consistently suggested as the primary ingredient or factor in the agent of choice following a bath while the skin is still wet and water will be trapped (Arndt 1983; Dotz and Berman 1984; Shelley and Shelley 1982). Occlusive agents lubricate the skin surface and make the skin feel smoother and less dry. This improves the greasy feeling, and once the water has been trapped, the oily film remaining on the skin is generally sufficient to retard transepidermal water loss. Keratin softening agents, such as urea, lactic acid, and allantoin, may be added to dry skin products to soften the skin and improve its appearance. They do not affect the water content of the skin and should be used in conjunction with occluding agents.

In a study by Brown et al. (1982), mineral oil was used because of its cost and ability to hold water. Pearson and Kotthof (1979) suggest petrolatum, Eucerin (water in oil), or vegetable oil and note that some debate exists about the efficacy of lanolin and mineral oil, the former because it may sensitize skin (Parent, 1985) and the latter because it may act as a drying agent. Epstein (1983) suggested using mineral oil or petrolatum because a vegetable oil may leave an odor. Arndt (1983) also suggests that the elderly "may be best able to tolerate" petrolatum as an occlusive agent but additionally mentions commercial brands such as Keri, Nivea, Aquaphor, and Eucerin. Mineral oil, petrolatum, and lanolin are noted as effective agents, but because of the greasy feeling, petrolatum may result in less compliance than the oil-in-water or water-in-oil preparations (Dotz and Berman 1984; Parent 1985). Cornell (1986, p. 33) suggested that the best occlusive agent to use following a bath and throughout the day for the treatment of dry skin in the elderly is a compound of equal parts water and "one of the greasier over the counter products." Weiner et al. (1973) used Dermo-Pedic Foot Lotion, a lotion containing "ethoxylated" lanolin in an aqueous base, and Allantoin. Spoor (1958) tested the effects of a water-dispersable bath oil, Sardo. Since, then, however, the argument has been made that bath oil may be hazardous to safety and that oil becomes suspended rather than absorbed (Epstein 1983; Parth and Kapke 1983). Boisits (1986) reported that in a clinical trial of occlusive agents at a relative humidity of 20%, there was a 98% reduction in moisture loss with petrolatum, an 83% reduction with lanolin, and a 31% reduction with mineral oil. Other less commonly used products tested by Cheeseborough-Ponds resulted in reductions ranging from 59% with avocado oil to −19% with anhydrous glycerine.

Lanolin is more expensive than either mineral oil or petrolatum, and baby oil (fragranced mineral oil) is less expensive than mineral oil. Because of its economical nature and its effectiveness reported in the literature and because it has been tested empirically by Brown et al. (1982), I consider mineral oil the agent of choice. Petrolatum, although potentially very effective as an occlusive agent, may be unappealing to patients concerned with staining clothing. The nurse and patient must evaluate the effectiveness and desirability of products, and research to test the effects of these agents is needed. Since lubricants make surfaces slippery and can easily cause a fall, caution should be used when applying a skin lubricant (Parent 1985).

In addition to being used after bathing, emollients should be applied during the day as necessary to maintain the skin in a moist, supple condition. Creams and ointments are generally more effective than lotions, and gels should be avoided because their alcohol content causes drying. Moisturizers with added ingredients such as scents, deodorants, anesthetics, and colorings should be avoided because they can cause sensitivity reactions in damaged skin. If pruritus is severe or does not respond to lubricants, topical corticosteroids or oral antihistamines may be used; however, topical steroids can increase skin atrophy in the elderly, and antihistamines cause drowsiness and can alter mental status. These agents should be used only for a limited time period, if at all (Parent 1985). For lubrication, all perfumed lotions should be avoided in newborns (Tobin 1984a).

Humidity

Although the maintenance of sufficient environmental humidity is suggested by nearly all persons addressing the subject of dry skin, some variance in the ideal level is observed. Dry skin is common at humidities of less than 30% and uncommon at humidities over 60%. The majority of authors state that humidity should be maintained at over 60% in order for treatments for dry skin to be effective (Gaul and Underwood 1951; Hogstel 1983). The fact that Hogstel (1983) found humidities ranging from 25% to 40% in one nursing home suggests that institutions need to address this factor if dry skin is to be avoided. Room temperature, because it is directly related to humidity, should also be considered. Room temperature should be kept as low as is comfortable because the dry heat associated with winter contributes to further drying (Arndt 1983).

A tool used to measure humidity, a hygrometer, will aid in determining the need for intervention in increasing environmental humidity. In private homes, the use of humidifiers or pans of water on radiators or, where possible, humidifiers installed in forced-air systems will increase humidity (Arndt 1983; Walther and Harber 1984). In institutional settings, central environmental controls may have such humidifying elements and may require adjustment. In other cases, such equipment may need to be added.

Although there is agreement that water should be tepid, that rough clothing should be avoided (Arndt 1983; Shelley and Shelley 1982), that vigorous drying should be avoided (Parent 1985), and that laundry should be treated without starch or antistatic agents in drying, there is little research base supporting any of these multiple treatment choices (Boisits 1986; Cornell 1986; Epstein 1983; Fenske 1982; Fitzsimmons 1983; Gaul and Underwood 1951; Hogstel 1983; Parent 1985; Parth and Kapke, 1983; Pearson and Kotthof 1979; Walther and Harber 1984; Weiner et al. 1973).

Water Temperature

Tepid rather than hot water should be used (Hogstel 1983). The consensus is that water between 90°F and 105°F be used (Arndt 1983; Dotz and Berman 1984; Fitzsimmons 1983; Parth and Kapke 1983; Pearson and Kotthof 1979). This is consistent with the 105°F safety valve regulation for water temperature required in most long-term-care facilities.

CASE STUDIES

Case Study 1

Ms. J is a 50-year-old active professional woman. Her health is generally good, with no chronic illnesses and no positive history of hospitalization except for the birth of one child. She is on no medications except for occasional analgesic for headaches or muscle aches following workouts. Ms. J has a nutritionally balanced diet and an adequate intake of water (approximately six glasses daily). She experiences dry skin, especially flaking and itching, particularly on her lower anterior legs, her posterior forearms, and her face. The dryness on her arms and legs is exacerbated during the winter, but she experiences the dryness on her face throughout the year. She prefers long, hot showers or baths every morning and following each workout at a local spa. Thus, Ms. J showers approximately 10 times per week and sometimes has a long bath for relaxation. She lives in a cold climate, and although she attempts to keep the temperature of her home low, the temperature of her office is impossible to control and is always too warm. Her home furnace has no humidifier, but she does keep a room humidifier in the family room. Her bathing routine includes a deodorant soap, hot water, and brisk drying. She wears nylon hose daily.

Upon consultation with a clinic nurse during a routine physical exam, Ms. J discusses her dry skin and is assessed as having a score of 6 on the SCDF (moderate dryness in three body sites). She mutually agrees with the nurse to increase her intake of water to 8 glasses per day and to change her bathing routine to include a 10-minute tub bath or shower daily with a water temperature of 105°F (she purchased a bath thermometer), using Dove soap, patting dry following the bath, applying mineral oil immediately while her body is still wet, and wearing cotton stockings or hose. It is agreed that the protocol should be followed for 6 weeks before any evaluation of the outcome is attempted.

Within 1 week, Ms. J notes a decrease in the itching and flaking she usually experiences, and within 6 weeks, she feels much improved as long as she continues with the protocol. Upon a return visit to see the clinic nurse, Ms. J has a score of 1 on the SCDF (mild dryness on lower legs). Because she sometimes attempts a hot bath and experiences some dryness, Ms. J realizes that the protocol has to be maintained to be effective.

Case Study 2

Mr. K is a 75-year-old man who has been in a nursing home for 5 years. He was admitted following a stroke that severely affected his left side. He is taking methyldopa 250 mg daily and Diazide 2 caps every morning, along with 40 mEq of potassium. Sebulex shampoo has been prescribed for several months because of an itchy, scaly scalp. His anterior lower legs, posterior forearms, face, and scalp are dry. Following his twice-weekly baths without soap, Aquaphilic is applied. Further applications are made between baths if itching persists. Mr. K's skin is moderately flaky and scaly, giving him a score of 12 on the SCDF. No seasonal differences have been observed by his primary nurse. Although he has been treated with Sebulex and Aquaphilic, little improvement has been observed. Potential for Impaired Skin Integrity because of limited mobility and itching has been treated with application of Aquaphilic between bathing and frequent position changes.

The environmental humidity of the unit is about 40% at all times. Mr. K eats a balanced diet, although he tires easily when eating and often does not eat all that is served in his 2400 calorie, 2g to 4g sodium diet. His fluid intake has decreased to less than 200 cc per day during the past year because of losses in functional abilities, increasing episodes of impaired alertness, and choking. He has been hospitalized for dehydration at least once in the past 10 months, and during that time his weight dropped steadily from 158 to 150 pounds. Mr. K's primary nurse discusses the problem and her concern with Mr. K and tells him she would like to consult another primary nurse in the facility whose specialty is skin care.

While observing Mr. K, the two nurses and Mr. K decide to change his bath routine to include a soaking bath in the whirlpool using Dove soap, water between 90°F and 105°F, and a mineral oil application while still wet; to wear cotton clothing; and to increase his daily fluid intake to 3000 cc and substitute mineral oil applications for Aquaphilic.

The most difficult element of the prescription for treating the dry skin is the fluid intake, but within 2 weeks, an improvement is observable, and within 6 weeks Mr. K's SCDF score decreases to 1 (mild dryness persisted on his lower legs).

SUMMARY

Dry skin is a problem among nurses and in many populations with which nurses work. Dry Skin Care is an intervention designed to treat dry skin. It is based on the consensus found in the dermatology and nursing literature on treatment for dry skin and on the findings of a pilot study (Hardy 1990a). The intervention includes the following:

1. Use a superfatted soap for cleansing.
2. Maintain a water temperature of 90°F to 105°F.
3. Immerse the patient in a tub up to the chest while pouring water over body parts not immersed or shower with a continuous spray over all body parts for 10 minutes.
4. Pat the skin dry with a cotton towel rather than by rubbing.
5. Maintain a humid environment.
6. Apply an emollient over all body parts as an occlusive.
7. Use linen that has been thoroughly rinsed of detergent and without anti-static.
8. Wear cotton clothing.

REFERENCES

Anderson, H.C. 1971. Newton's Geriatric Nursing. St. Louis: Mosby.

Arndt, K.A. 1983. *Manual of dermatologic therapeutics.* Boston: Little, Brown.

Atkins, J. 1977, March. Care of the hair and scalp. *Nursing Mirror.* 45–48.

Beauregard, S., and Gilchrest, B. 1987. A survey of skin problems and skin care regimens in the elderly. *Archives of Dermatology* 123:1638–1643.

Blichmann, C.W. and Serrup, J. 1988. *Acta Derm Venercol* (Stockholm). 68:284–290.

Boarini, J., Bryant, R., and Irrgang, S. 1986. Fistual management. *Seminars in Oncology Nursing* 2(2):287–292.

Boisits, E.K. 1986, May. The evaluation of moisturizing products. *Cosmetics and Toiletries,* 31–39.

Broadwell, D. 1987. Peristomal skin integrity. *Nursing Clinics of North America* 22(2):321–332.

Brown, M., Boosinger, J., Black, J., Gaspar, R., and Sather, L. 1982. Nursing innovation for dry skin care of the feet in the elderly. *Journal of Gerontological Nursing* 8(7):393–395.

Bryant, R. 1988. Saving the skin from tape injuries. *American Journal of Nursing* 88(2):189–191.

Cornell, R.C. 1986. Aging and the skin. *Geriatric Medicine* 5(1):26–33.

Crow, S. 1983. Nursing care of the immunosuppressed patient. *Infection Control.* 4(6):465–467.

Delancy, V., and North, C. 1983. Skin assessment. *Topics in Clinical Nursing* 4:5–10.

Dotz, W., and Berman, B. 1984, August. Aids that preserve hydration and mitigate its loss. *Consultant,* 46–62.

Eliopoulos, C. 1988. *Gerontological nursing.* 2d ed. Philadelphia: J.B. Lippincott.

Epstein, E. 1983. *Common skin disorders.* 2d ed. Oradell, N.J.: Medical Economics Books.

Fenske, N.A. 1982, January. Problems of aging skin. *Consultant,* 287–300.

Fitzsimmons, V.M. 1983. The aging integument: A sensitive and complex system. *Topics in Clinical Nursing* 4(6):32–38.

Fowler, E. 1986. Skin care for older adults. *Journal of Gerontological Nursing* 11(11):34.

Frantz, R.A., and Kinney, C.N. 1986. Variables associated with skin dryness in the elderly. *Nursing Research* 35(2):98–100.

Frosch, P.J., and Kligman, A.M. 1979. The soap chamber test: A new method for assessing the irritants of soaps. *Journal of the American Academy of Dermatology.* 1(1),35 – 41.

Gaul, L.E. and Underwood, G.B. (1951). Relation of dew point and barometric pressure to chapping of normal skin. *Journal of Investigative Dermatology* 19:9 – 19.

Gilchrest, B.A. 1986. Skin diseases in the elderly. In E. Calkins, P.L. Davis, and A.B. Fords (eds.), *The practice of geriatrics.* Philadelphia: W.B. Saunders.

Gioella, E., and Bevil, C. 1985. *Nursing care of the aging client.* Norwalk, Conn.: Appleton-Century-Crofts.

Hannigan, L. 1978, January. Nursing assessment of the integumentary system. *Occupational Health Nursing* 10:19 – 22.

Hardy, M. 1990a. A pilot study of the diagnosis and treatment of Impaired Skin Integrity. *Nursing Diagnosis* 1(2):57 – 63.

Hardy, M. 1990b. Impaired Skin Integrity: Dry Skin. In M. Maas, K. Buckwalter, and M. Hardy, *Nursing diagnoses and interventions for the elderly.* Menlo Park, Calif.: Addison-Wesley.

Hassey, K. 1987. Skin care for patients receiving radiation therapy for rectal cancer. *Journal of Enterostomal Therapy* 14:197 – 200.

Herman, L., and Gilchrest, B. 1989. Pruritus in the elderly. *Geriatric Medicine Today* 8(2):23 – 44.

Hogstel, M.O. 1983. Skin care for the aged. *Journal of Gerontological Nursing* 9(8):431 – 437.

Hylen, A., Karlsson, E., Svanberg, L., and Walder, M. 1983. Hygiene for the newborn — to bath or to wash? *Journal of Hygiene* 91:529 – 534.

Kuller, J., Lund, C., and Tobin C. 1983. Improved skin care for premature infants. *Maternal Child Nursing* 8:200 – 203.

Lindell, M., and Olsson, H. 1990. Personal hygiene in external genitalia of healthy and hospitalized elderly women. *Health Care for Women International* 11:151 – 158.

Lund, C., Kuller, J., Tobin, C., Lefrak, L., and Franck, L. 1986. Evaluation of a pectin-based barrier under tape to protect neonatal skin. *Journal of Obstetric, Gynecologic, and Neonatal Nursing* 15(1):39 – 44.

McConn, R. 1987. Skin changes following bone marrow transplantation. *Cancer Nursing* 10(2):82 – 84.

Malkiewicz, J. 1981, December. The integumentary system. *RN* 44:55 – 60.

Nightingale, F. 1946. *Notes on nursing.* Facsimile of first edition. 1859. Philadelphia: Stern and Company.

North American Nursing Diagnosis Association. 1989. *Taxonomy I. Revised 1989.* St. Louis, Mo.: NANDA.

Parent, L. 1985. Therapy of skin problems in the elderly. *U.S. Pharmacist* 10(4):48 – 54.

Parth, C., and Kapke, K. 1983. Aging and the skin. *Geriatric Nursing* 4(3):158 – 162.

Pearson, L.J., and Kotthof, M.K. 1979. *Geriatric clinical protocols.* Philadelphia: J.B. Lippincott Co.

President's Message. 1990. ET nursing's window of opportunity. *Journal of Enterostomal Therapy* 17(3):95 – 97.

Seitz, J., and Newman, J. 1988. Factors affecting skin condition in two nursing populations: Implications for current handwashing protocols. *American Journal of Infection Control* 16(2):346 – 353.

Shelley, W., and Shelley, E. 1982. The ten major problems of aging skin. *Geriatrics* 37(9):107 – 113.

Spoor, H.J. 1958, October. Measurement and maintenance of natural skin oil. *New York State Journal of Medicine,* 3292 – 3299.

Tindall, J., and Smith, J. 1963. Skin lesions of the aged. *Journal of the American Medical Association* 186:1039 – 1042.

Tobin, C. 1984a. Part II: Dispelling common myths. *Neonatal Network* 3(3):24 – 27.

Tobin, C. 1984b. Part III. Stoma care. *Neonatal Network* 3(3):28 – 35.

Walther, E.M., and Harber, L.C. 1984. Expected skin complaints of the geriatric patient. *Geriatrics* 39(12):67 – 80.

Watt, R. 1986. Nursing management of a patient with a urinary diversion. *Seminars in Oncology Nursing* 2(4):265 – 269.

Weiner, E.M., Beiser, S., Giudice, R., Kanat, E., Kaplan, E., Kauth, B., and Stone, D. 1983. Treating the dry skin syndrome. *Journal of the American Podiatry Association* 63(11):571 – 581.

Urosevich, P.R. (ed.) 1981. *Nursing photobook.* Horsham, Penn.: Nursing 81 Books, Intermed Communications.

3

FEEDING

NANCY J. EVANS

Every careful observer of the sick will agree in this that thousands of patients are annually starved in the midst of plenty, from want of attention to the ways which alone make it possible for them to take food.

Florence Nightingale

The word *nutrition* derives from the Latin "to nurse, feed or care for." Taylor (1988) describes nutrition as an art as well as a science but suggests that modern medicine and modern society attach more value to nutrition as a science. Gavan, Hastings-Tolsma, and Troyan (1988) state that "little is as basic to the human experience as nutrition and many of our earliest memories are embedded within the context of feeding." Eating and maintaining a sense of well-being are basic human instincts. Professional nurses have always been concerned about human responses, focusing on health care maintenance, recovery from illness, and promotion of well-being (Leininger 1988). Nutritional well-being of patients has been a constant concern of nurses.

The complexity of health care today demands that nursing practice be based on sound theory; however, this is tempered by those who suggest that no amount of scientific theory ever got food into a patient, and nurses should be encouraged to value the humanistic skills that result in patients' being fed (Taylor 1988). There is no denying the technological advances of modern medicine where nutrients can be given to patients in a mechanized, highly technical way. Enteral and parenteral nutrition have added a new meaning to the word *feeding* and are lifesaving therapies for patients who are unable or unwilling to take in food orally. Caretakers should not use these therapies for individuals with a functional gastrointestinal tract who might ordinarily eat if given the opportunity and the proper assistance.

DESCRIPTION OF THE INTERVENTION

Feeding, defined by Webster, is to give food or to supply nourishment. Feeding can be described as a set of specific actions taken by oneself or a caretaker to ensure adequate nutrient intake to sustain life. The success of Feeding is influenced by physiological and psychological factors. The ability to take in nutrients is dependent on complex neuromuscular coordination, as well as individual cognitive abilities. The desire for food determines the quantity and quality of food intake and is not entirely dependent on physiological need.

Components of Feeding

Hunger is a familiar set of sensations stimulated by the depletion of nutrient stores; it can be viewed as a protective mechanism. Hunger is associated with the physiological need to eat and is accompanied by various physical responses, including rhythmic contracts of the stomach, tight or gnawing feelings in the stomach, and vague feelings of tension or restlessness (Guyton 1991). The lateral hypothalamus is described as the hunger center (Vick 1984).

The experience of hunger may be disrupted by situations that distract or reduce the individual's mental awareness (Anderson 1982). For example, the stress of illness, injury, surgery, and/or emotional distress may disrupt the hunger response. Many patients may be alert to the feelings of hunger but are unwilling or unable to respond. For example, aphasic or cognitively impaired patients may be unable to communicate verbally and do not eat unless the caretaker is sensitive to their nonverbal cues.

Appetite is the psychological desire to ingest food that usually accompanies hunger (Vick 1984). It is an affective state, associated with pleasure rather than physiologic need. Although the term is often used interchangeably with *hunger,* *appetite* is defined as a desire for a specific type of food. This desire for food is shaped by an individual's past experience, cultural traditions, and economic situation (Donoghue, Nunnally, and Yasko 1982). The appetite center, located in the hypothalamus, receives messages from the cerebral cortex such as vision, smell, taste, and touch, and is therefore subject to some degree of conscious control.

Physical ability determines if a patient can independently complete the task of feeding. It requires smooth, well-coordinated motions of the arms and hands. The activity requires energy; a 70 kg man expends up to 2.5 kcal/min during eating (Caldwell and Kennedy-Caldwell 1981).

Mechanical aspects of food ingestion also determine the success of feeding patients. Once food is made available to an individual, the success of safe nutrient intake is largely dependent on the effectiveness of chewing and swallowing. Mastication, necessary to prepare foods for digestion, is controlled by muscles that are innervated by the motor branch of the fifth cranial nerve (Guyton 1991). The condition of the oral mucosa is critical to the ability to take in food. The oral mucosa must be moist, with adequate saliva production to facilitate and aid in the digestion of food. The oral mucosa may be altered by infection, medications, chemotherapy, radiation, and surgical procedures.

The swallowing mechanism is a complex set of precisely timed movements that result in the safe passage of food into the stomach. Table 3 – 1 describes the three stages in the swallowing mechanism: voluntary stage, pharyngeal stage, and esophageal stage. Both chewing and swallowing are controlled by an intricate neuro-

TABLE 3 – 1. STAGES OF THE SWALLOWING MECHANISM

STAGE	FUNCTION
Voluntary	Food is moved into the pharynx by action of the tongue against the palate
Pharyngeal	Presence of food in the pharynx stimulates swallowing receptors: trachea closes, esophagus opens, peristaltic wave carries food into esophagus
Esophageal	Esophagus accepts food from pharynx Esophagus transports food bolus by peristaltic action into the stomach

Source: A. C. Guyton, *Textbook of medical physiology* (Philadelphia: W. B. Saunders, 1991).

TABLE 3–2.   CRANIAL NERVE FUNCTION IN THE CHEWING AND
SWALLOWING MECHANISM

CRANIAL NERVE	NAME	FUNCTION	OUTCOME LOSS
Fifth	Trigeminal	Controls muscles of mastication; provides sensation to face, teeth, gums, and tongue	Loss of sensation; inability to move mandible
Seventh	Facial	Provides the sense of taste; controls the muscles of the face	Increased salivation; pouching of food in cheeks
Ninth	Glossopharyngeal	Transmits sensation to the tongue, pharynx, and soft palate; influences sense of taste, production of saliva, and swallowing	Decreases sensation of taste and salivation; diminishes or inhibits gag reflex
Tenth	Vagus	Controls sensation in larynx, base of tongue, pharynx, palate, and their muscles	Increased difficulty swallowing; nasal regurgitation; reduced or lost gag reflex
Twelfth	Hypoglossal	Controls the extrinsic and intrinsic muscles of the tongue	Inability to position food for chewing, resulting in pouching.

Source: P. A. Donahue, When it's hard to swallow. Feeding techniques for dysphagia management, *Journal of Gerontological Nursing* 16(4) (1990):9.

muscular network, and damage to the cranial nerves that control this system results in specific loss of function (Table 3–2).

Clinical Implications of Malnutrition

Malnutrition starts when patients do not eat enough to meet their needs (Jee-jeebhoy 1990). If patients are unable or unwilling to eat, nurses must quickly intervene to prevent the rapid depletion of the body's protein and energy reserves. Nurses must appreciate the deleterious outcomes that can result from patients' not being fed.

Malnutrition in the hospital setting is well documented. When questioned, almost any clinician will support the importance of nutrition, yet the prevalence and degree of malnutrition in hospitalized patients have been reported to vary from 30% to 50% (Bistrian et al. 1974, 1976). Malnutrition is associated with increased morbidity and mortality (Studley 1936; Buzby et al. 1980).

The result of inadequate intake from either total or partial starvation is a mobilization of the body's available energy stores. The quick energy sources available in muscle and liver glycogen supply only 24 hours to 48 hours of fuel. Adipose tissue provides a more abundant source of fuel for the body and in normal-weight individuals can supply energy for about 2 months (Cahill 1988). Total unstressed starvation will result in a weight loss of 15% over a 3-week period. In stressed starvation, a patient will sustain weight losses similar to total unstressed starvation when receiving as much as 50% of calories needed (Hill and Beddoe 1988). In early unstressed starvation, a great deal of muscle protein is catabolized daily to provide fuel; however, within a few days, the body is able to reduce the amount of muscle catabolism and ketoadapt in order to maintain muscle mass. In stressed starvation,

TABLE 3–3. CONSEQUENCES OF MALNUTRITION

ORGAN SYSTEM	PATHOPHYSIOLOGY	CLINICAL OUTCOME
Cardiac	Decreased cardiac muscle mass	No evidence of cardiovascular disturbance
Pulmonary	Decreased diaphragm weight Decreased respiratory strength Decreased endurance	Inability to clear secretions; decreased exercise tolerance; inability to wean from ventilator
Immune function	Decreased cell-mediated immunity Delayed cutaneous hypersensitivity	Increased incidence and severity of infection; delayed wound healing
Wound healing	Decreased collagen synthesis	
Skeletal muscle strength	Alterations in muscle contraction relaxation response Decreased muscle endurance	Fatigue; inability to perform activities of daily living

Source: J. M. Kinney et al. (eds.), *Nutrition and metabolism in patient care* (Philadelphia: W. B. Saunders, 1988).

this regulatory function is impaired, and skeletal muscle will continue to be catabolized, resulting in further depletion of protein stores. The cost of unrelenting negative protein-energy balance is evident in organ dysfunction and negative clinical outcome (Table 3–3).

The relationship between nutritional status and patient outcome is evaluated in terms of morbidity and mortality. To define this relationship, one must be sure that objective measures accurately predict nutritional status. Mullen (1981) developed a prognostic nutritional index (PNI) that incorporated four measurements (albumin, transferrin, triceps skinfold, and delayed hypersensitivity) to calculate relative risk of mortality and morbidity. This model accurately classified as high or intermediate 89% of patients who eventually developed complications after major gastrointestinal surgery.

IDENTIFICATION OF INTERVENTIONAL TOOLS

Feeding as an intervention requires a specific plan that targets the deficit or cause of impairment. The ultimate goal is to provide adequate nutrients to prevent malnutrition. A secondary goal is to restore the patient's independence in this basic self-care activity. Assessment of the individual for a feeding plan should include a nursing history and physical exam. A thorough nursing history will determine the presence of risk factors and guide the clinician in a more focused assessment of the specific feeding impairment.

Identification of High-Risk Situations

Metabolic demands of hospitalized patients are increased due to the stress of illness. Nurses must be able to identify patients who cannot meet these demands independently. Deficits occur in the physical ability to coordinate muscles to bring food to the mouth, the mechanics of chewing and swallowing, or the ability to understand the task of feeding. Table 3–4 lists some common high-risk situations that require a more focused assessment.

Anorexia is a well-documented problem in cancer patients (Sigal and Daly 1990). Possible pathophysiologic causes include sustained stimulation of receptors in the gastrointestinal (GI) tract resulting in early satiety, release of tumor by-

TABLE 3–4.   HIGH-RISK SITUATIONS

Neuromuscular impairment

Cerebral vascular accident	Parkinson's disease
Myasthenia gravis	Immobility
Multiple sclerosis	Trauma to upper extremities
Amyotrophic dystrophy	Spinal cord injury

Anorexia
Chronic illness: cancer, COPD
Treatment (chemotherapy, radiation therapy)
Depression

Cognitive deficits
Psychiatric illness
Confusion state
Dementia
Organic brain syndrome

Sensory perceptual deficits
Age
Medications
Cerebral vascular accident

products, difficulty swallowing, and/or fatigue (Knox 1983). Treatment-related causes of anorexia occur because of alterations in taste, oral inflammation, nausea and vomiting, infection, and fatigue. Other causes can be anxiety and depression associated with the diagnosis of cancer.

Decreased appetite is common in patients with chronic lung diseases (Openbrier and Covey 1987). Although the etiology is unclear, anorexia may be caused by dyspnea, fatigue, coughing, increased sputum production, and side effects of medications (Dougherty 1988).

The frail elderly are particularly at risk for impaired feeding. They may not have the manual dexterity, energy, or ability to feed themselves. Conditions that affect their ability to eat include arthritis, recurrent strokes, neurological disorders, sensory perceptual deficits, fractures, and poor oral conditions. Anatomical changes that occur in the very old may also affect feeding—for example, decreased ability to swallow related to decreased saliva and dehydration, dilated esophagus, decreased peristalsis in the esophagus, decreased secretion of acid in the stomach, and hiatal hernia, which is common in obese elderly women (Hogstel and Robinson 1989).

The context in which the Feeding takes place can affect nutrient intake. Like many other nursing activities, Feeding is influenced by the development of a therapeutic relationship. Norberg and colleagues (1988) observed feelings of anxiety in the caregiver when a patient refuses to eat. It is an extremely stressful situation for a caregiver when the patient is refusing to eat since discerning if the patient is refusing or simply unable to eat is difficult. This study observed how caretakers in 24 Swedish nursing homes conceptualized food refusal and how they treated patients who refused food. In the 143 nursing interviews, there were 138 accounts of food refusal, which represented 72% of the time interviewees were able to describe an event of a patient's refusing food. The types of food refusals included were physical reasons, such as the patient was too ill or could not perform the eating activities or had GI complaints; psychological reasons where caretakers felt the patient wished to die or did not understand the situation; and cultural reasons, which included food taboos and lack of acquaintance with certain types of food presented. The investigators identified the lack of a therapeutic nurse-patient relationship and suggested a more consistent patient care assignment so that caregivers were more familiar with individual patients and more confident in interpreting the behavior.

Backstrom, Norberg, and Norberg (1987) studied feeding difficulties in chronically ill patients at 24 Swedish nursing homes. The aim of the nursing care for patients with eating problems was to help maintain or regain independence in feeding. Over a 4-week period there was a median of 16 to 20 feeders for each patient. The average duration of feeding in the totally dependent patients was 20 minutes, and difficulty feeding was reported in 81% of the feeding encounters. Caregivers described the process of feeding as dependent on the psychosocial aspects of the feeding situation. Dealing with impairments of sensory perception and cognition resulting in feeding problems requires a detailed knowledge of the patient and his or her disease, as well as continuity of care.

Clearly patients with eating problems can create such anxiety that caregivers often rotate these assignments to reduce the stress level. Athlin and Norberg (1987) described the development of the interaction between the patient and the caregiver in the patient assignment system by observing six severely demented women and four caregivers. Feeding problems were described as impaired reflexes, as well as lack of purposeful behavior. Caregivers documented impaired communicative behavior and verbalized overwhelming concern in interpreting the patient's behavior. Often the caregiver was not sure if the patient could understand the attempt to communicate.

Assessment of Feeding Impairment

There is often a great deal of anxiety related to assessing why the patient will not eat. It can be difficult to identify if the problem is physical or psychological. Emotional problems may be related to the patient's feelings about not eating. In the hospital setting, where patients lack control over their environment, eating may be one area where they feel they can exercise some decision-making power (Ross 1987). Furthermore, they may be angry at the diagnosis and displace their anger onto eating behavior. Additionally, the depression or despair related to a situational event can take the appetite away.

It is important to explore the patient's feelings about not eating. A subjective assessment should include the patient's own description of hunger and appetite.

Assessing the level of consciousness will alert the nurse to patients at risk for aspiration. Patients who are obtunded are obviously in danger of aspiration. The patient's cognitive abilities must be assessed since this will have an impact on the ability to understand and complete the task of feeding independently. Demented, disoriented, or confused patients, although alert, are at risk for feeding problems because they do not understand the importance of eating and have a propensity for being distracted.

Assessing the patient's physical ability to feed and identifying patients with impairments is imperative for planning successful interventions. Table 3–5 reviews key assessment criteria and suggests possible etiologies for deficits. Assessing the time needed to eat may identify patients who are slow. The pace of eating varies among individuals; however, patients who routinely take longer than 60 minutes to complete a meal may be partially dependent feeders and require assistance. In some patients, the ability to bring food to the mouth may be inconsistent. They often start out feeding themselves without problems but quickly tire. Poor coordination results in food landing on the patient's bed, meal tray, or floor but never reaching the patient's mouth. Patients who are not able to see the tray may leave various foods untouched. Patients who cannot handle utensils will eat those foods

TABLE 3–5. ASSESSING THE PATIENT'S ABILITY TO EAT

ASSESSMENT CRITERIA	POSSIBLE ETIOLOGY OF IMPAIRMENT
Time it takes to eat	Dysphagia, fatigue, fear of choking
Ability to bring food to the mouth	Neuromuscular impairments, decreased endurance, fatigue
Ability to see all food on tray	Visual field cuts: Cerebrovascular accident (CVA), glaucoma cataracts, diabetic retinopathy
Ability to handle eating utensils	CVA, neuromuscular impairment, immobility, missing limbs, external devices, casts
Ability to chew food	Ill-fitting dentures, oral infections, poor oral hygiene, trauma, surgery to oral cavity
Ability to swallow food	Neurological impairment, cranial nerve damage

Source: J. M. Buelow and P. Jamieson: Potential for altered nutritional status in the stroke patient, *Rehabilitation Nursing* 15(5) (1990):260.

on the tray that can be easily picked up with the fingers and leave behind foods that require utensils. If chewing is a problem and proper menu selection has not occurred, patients will favor liquids and soft foods.

Identifying patients at risk for swallowing difficulties and recognizing those with abnormal swallowing is a critical piece of assessing feeding problems. Ensuring the safety of patients by preventing potential aspirations is critical.

Signs of abnormal swallowing include packing food in the cheeks, drooling, throat clearing during a meal, frequent coughing during a meal, and fluid leaking from the nose after swallowing.

IDENTIFICATION OF ASSOCIATED NURSING DIAGNOSES

Six nursing diagnoses are pertinent to the intervention of Feeding:

1. Altered Nutrition: Less Than Body Requirements
2. Feeding Self Care Deficit
3. Impaired Swallowing
4. Altered Thought Processes
5. Impaired Physical Mobility
6. Sensory/Perceptual Alterations

Altered Nutrition: Less Than Body Requirements is defined by Carpenito (1983) as a state in which the individual experiences or is at risk of experiencing reduced weight related to inadequate intake of nutrients. Several etiological factors are dysphagia, cancer, anorexia, and absorptive disorders. Hypermetabolic or hypercatabolic states result in demands that are difficult to meet. Depression and social isolation affect the psychological desire to eat.

Feeding Self Care Deficit characterizes the individual with impaired motor function or cognitive function, which causes a decreased ability to feed oneself (Carpenito 1983). Neuromuscular impairments such as Parkinson's disease, muscular dystrophy, myasthenia, muscular weakness, and central nervous system tumors are contributing factors. Visual disorders occur with glaucoma, cataracts, or cerebrovascular accidents. Situational factors are immobility, trauma, or the placement of external fixating devices that restrict arm movement. The elderly may experience decreased visual and motor abilities, as well as muscle weakness and changes in taste and appetite. The assessment should be focused on self-feeding abilities: the ability to swallow, chew, use utensils, and visualize the food.

Impaired Swallowing is a serious obstacle to safe nutrient intake, and patients will need to relearn how to swallow correctly. Patients with severe impairments in thought processes may be totally dependent on someone feeding them during this crisis period. Strategies will support the patient until he or she is ready for more independent behavior.

Nursing interventions for all diagnoses focus on strategies to ensure that patients take in adequate nutrients to avoid malnutrition.

SUGGESTED PROTOCOLS FOR USING THE INTERVENTION

Feeding, an independent nursing intervention, has been a cornerstone of nursing practice since the days of Florence Nightingale. Nurses are involved in the day-to-day care of patients and are highly aware of feeding difficulties. They are present during mealtimes and are able to assess what patients are able to eat and try to discern any problem with eating. A successful Feeding intervention ensures that the patient safely takes in adequate nutrients to meet metabolic demands.

General strategies to improve nutritional intake relate to choices of menu and the accessibility of dietitians on the wards during mealtime. Patients should have a choice of menu to avoid food monotony. Dietitians should be accessible on the wards during mealtimes to help assess individual preferences. Kitchen facilities should be available at the unit level to increase patient choices. Dedicated refrigeration and microwave supplies for patients encourage patients' families to bring foods that are appealing to patients and allow more flexible mealtimes.

Appetite is often impaired in a hospital setting for a variety of reasons and obstructs the desire for food intake. Several strategies can be used to maximize or enhance an individual's appetite. First, the nurse can create a pleasant environment during mealtime. This can be done by clearing the area of unsightly bedpans, urinals, suctioning equipment, or dressing supplies. Reducing other noxious stimuli includes adequate pain relief prior to meals and avoidance of invasive procedures immediately prior to a meal.

Appetite can be enhanced by taste, smell, and vision. Taste alterations can occur from injury after radiation to the oral cavity, surgical resection to the tongue, medication, and oral infections. Oral hygiene is important to maximize the optimal function of taste buds. Routine mouth care should include the following:

1. Cleansing the mouth after each meal and at bedtime.
2. Use of a soft-bristle toothbrush.
3. Rinses with warm saltwater.
4. Avoidance of alcohol-containing mouthwash.
5. Avoidance of glycerine and lemon juice.

The ability to smell prepared foods will also stimulate the appetite. Although patients cannot participate in food preparation, offering them a chance to smell food prior to meals may stimulate appetite. Nurses can also reduce all noxious odors that might negatively affect appetite, allow patients to see the food to help stimulate their appetite, position the food so that it is visible, and describe the different foods. Description is especially important for patients with visual impairment.

Eating is ordinarily a time for social interaction (Sanders 1990), yet patients are usually given meals in their own rooms. Creating social contact by feeding patients in a central area may be one option, as is encouraging family and friends to visit during mealtimes. Patient care assignments should be designed so that patients requiring Feeding can be assigned to the same caregiver as much as possible. As the patient and caregiver develop a therapeutic relationship, the Feeding will become a more pleasurable and successful experience for both.

Patients with sensory, perceptual deficits require specific nursing actions to ensure adequate food intake. The nurse should be sure any corrective lenses are on and properly fitted and describe the food and its location on the tray. The use of different colored trays and dishes is helpful to patients with these deficits. Arranging the food in a clocklike pattern is an easy way to orient the patient to the position of various foods on the tray. Describing the position of foods is imperative for patients with visual field cuts. Food should not be placed to the blind side.

Cognitive impairments can result in the patient's misunderstanding the task of eating or being unable to complete the task because of a short attention span. These patients require frequent cuing and close supervision. The following nursing actions are useful steps in feeding patients with cognitive impairments:

1. Create a quiet, unhurried environment.
2. Explain the procedure.
3. Orient the patient to the purpose of feeding equipment.
4. Provide frequent cuing to the patient (e.g., "Mrs. S, pick up the toast" or "Mr. S, chew the food in your mouth").
5. Provide several small meals for patients with short attention spans.

Various neuromuscular impairments can make the seemingly simple activity of Feeding difficult or impossible. Occupational therapy can be consulted for assistance in planning the Feeding intervention and correct use of assistive devices. Patients with physical impairment should be allowed adequate time for eating and privacy, be positioned at a 90-degree angle with the meal tray at elbow height, and be provided assistive devices (e.g., plate guards, built-up spoons).

Another physical factor that can affect patients' ability to feed themselves is endurance. They may be able to start the task but are quickly fatigued and cannot complete the task. The individual's ability to maintain a level of performance is related to the functioning of the cardiovascular, respiratory, neurological, and musculoskeletal systems. Creative planning by the nurse can provide rest periods prior to mealtimes. Rest periods should be scheduled prior to meals after activities such as physical therapy and ambulation. Assisting in meal setup by opening packages and cutting food enables patients to conserve energy for eating.

Chewing and swallowing dysfunction are frequent additional reasons for difficulties in eating. Dysphagia accompanies various neurological insults. A team approach has been described in the literature in the successful management of patients with swallowing impairments (Emick-Herring and Wood 1990). Speech pathologists can be helpful in localizing the impairment and suggesting useful strategies. The nurse must also understand the complexity of normal swallowing mechanisms in order to plan appropriate interventions.

The following four steps should be taken prior to Feeding to assess patient readiness:

1. Assess the level of consciousness; the patient must be alert.
2. Assess the patient's gag reflex by tickling the back of the throat.
3. Have the patient produce an audible cough.
4. Have the patient produce a voluntary swallow.

Feeding should take place in a calm, adequately supervised environment. Patients should be positioned in a normal eating position with the feeder clearly visible. Some patients may have difficulty in moving the food bolus from the front to the back of the mouth. Food should be placed in the unaffected side of the mouth. If the tongue is damaged or impaired, assistive devices such as adapted feeding syringes will move food toward the pharynx, where the swallowing reflex (if intact) takes over. Once the food bolus makes it to the pharynx, the patient should tilt the chin down, to decrease the risk of aspiration. Massaging the throat on the affected side helps stimulate the tactile areas that initiate the swallowing reflex. Patients who have difficulty coordinating chewing, breathing, and swallowing should be instructed to hold the head forward and hold the breath before swallowing. After the food is put in the mouth, the nurse should watch the thyroid cartilage to see if the patient has swallowed and inspect the mouth before introducing more food into the oral cavity. Allowing sufficient time between each mouthful will ensure that patients adequately chew and swallow the food. Nurses must be alert for signs the patient is becoming fatigued, restless, or agitated. Suction equipment should always be available in case of an emergency, and nurses should know how to perform the Heimlich maneuver.

EVALUATING THE INTERVENTION

The intervention of Feeding is used to maintain or improve the nutritional status of patients. Nurses design creative strategies to assist or support the individual's ability to take in nutrition. One aspect of evaluation may be the achievement of independence in feeding. Evaluation of the success of the intervention must also include objective measures of nutritional assessment.

A thorough comprehensive nutritional assessment must be completed initially to establish a baseline and evaluated serially to document the success of the nursing intervention. A comprehensive nutrition assessment allows the practitioner to diagnose the presence of malnutrition and identify the severity of malnutrition. Assessment should consist of the following:

1. Medical/surgical history
2. Physical exam: Height, weight, skinfold thickness, somatic muscle mass
3. Visceral protein status: Albumin, prealbumin, transferrin
4. Energy expenditure: Estimated/measured
5. Nitrogen balance

Muscle and fat depletion is often obvious on physical exam of patients who are moderately to severely depleted. They appear cachectic, with wasting of fat stores. Bony prominences are obvious in the ribs and scapulae, and the arms and legs appear spindly. The waist is pinched in, and there is temporal wasting. Height and weight help to determine if someone is at or below the ideal or usual body weight. Skinfold thickness and midarm circumference indicate the degree of fat and somatic muscle depletion. Biochemical levels define the presence and severity of visceral protein depletion. Table 3–6 identifies common nutritional assessment parameters used to determine the presence and severity of malnutrition. Downward trends in these measures should alert the nurse to reevaluate the nursing care plan.

TABLE 3–6.   DEGREE OF MALNUTRITION

INDICATOR	NORMAL	MILD	MODERATE	SEVERE
Albumin (gm/dl)	>3.5	3.0–3.5	2.4–2.9	<2.4
Transferrin (mg/dl)	>200	150–200	100–150	<100
Prealbumin (mg/dl)	>20	10–15	5–10	<5
Weight (% ideal body weight)[a]	90–120	80–90	70–80	<70
Weight (% usual weight)[b]	96–120	85–95	75–84	<75

Source: S. Curtas, Nutritional assessment. In C. Kennedy-Caldwell and P. Guenter (eds.), *Nutrition support nursing core curriculum*, 2d ed. ASPEN, Silver Spring, Maryland, 1988 (pp. 29–41).
[a] Current weight/ideal weight×100.
[b] Current weight/usual weight×100.

Energy expenditure defines the caloric needs of individuals. It can be estimated by using the Harris and Benedict (1919) equation:

$$\text{Basal Energy Expenditure (male)} = 66.47 + (13.75 \times \text{weight}) + (5.0 \times \text{height}) - (6.76 \times \text{age})$$

$$\text{Basal Energy Expenditure (female)} = 655.10 + (9.56 \times \text{weight}) + (1.85 \times \text{height}) - (4.68 \times \text{age})$$

Energy expenditure can also be measured by using indirect calorimetry, a more accurate measure in critically ill patients and a more accurate way to determine the energy requirements of patients (Feurer et al. 1984). Nitrogen balance evaluates the degree of catabolism and the adequacy of protein intake. In normally nourished individuals, the nitrogen balance should be 0; however, in many disease states and/or catabolic conditions, increased losses and decreased intake disrupt this equilibrium, resulting in a negative nitrogen balance. Calorie counts document intake and compare it to the documented protein and energy needs.

The purpose of conducting a nutritional assessment is to make a nutritional diagnosis. Marasmus is defined as the wasting of body fat and skeletal muscle with a sparing of the visceral protein stores. This is often seen in prolonged starvation, chronic illness, anorexia, and the elderly (Grant et al. 1981). Overall dietary intake may be poor, but despite the low overall intake, there is a relatively adequate protein-to-calorie ratio. These patients appear malnourished on physical examination. Kwashiorkor is defined as the wasting of visceral proteins with a preservation of fat and somatic muscle. This is often seen in periods of acute illness where there is a decreased protein intake and a catabolism of skeletal muscle. Affected patients can have normal or above normal anthropometric measures, but their serum proteins are depleted. They usually have increased extracellular water, pitting edema, and, in severe depletion states, ascites and anasarca. Some patients have a mixed marasmus-kwashiorkor, with aspects of both. This combination is associated with the highest risk of morbidity and mortality. Interestingly, malnutrition assessed by appearance is often consistent with diagnoses made by specific objective studies. Various researchers have found approximately 80% agreement between a subjective global nutritional assessment and the more traditional objective measures such as anthropometrics and serum proteins (Hirsch et al. 1991; Baker et al. 1982). They do suggest the accuracy of the assessment may be related to the level of clinical expertise and the degree of malnutrition.

CASE STUDY

RT, a 79-year-old female, was admitted to the hospital because of mild dehydration and malnutrition. She has a history of chronic organic brain syndrome/dementia and arthritis.

RT lives alone in an apartment and has no living relatives nearby. She has been homebound for the last 6 months because of increasing pain in her hands, back, and knees. RT is followed by a local visiting nurse, who has been providing Meals-on-Wheels and homemaker services.

RT appears thin but not wasted. She is 5 feet, 4 inches; her current weight is 108 pounds — 86% of her ideal body weight and less than her usual 125 pounds. RT is alert, oriented to person. Serum protein values are as follows: albumin 2.9 mg/dl, prealbumin 9 mg/dl, and transferrin 120 mg/dl.

RT states she has no appetite because of severe pain in her joints (8 on a scale of 1 to 10). The nurse's aide reports RT takes no initiative in feeding herself. Assessment of RT's mouth revealed poor oral hygiene. Her gag reflex was intact, and she could produce an audible cough and a voluntary swallow. The nursing diagnoses are: Altered Nutrition: Less Than Body Requirements, Feeding Self Care Deficits, and Impaired Physical Mobility, secondary to joint pain.

The first step in the Feeding intervention is treating RT's pain, which is contributing to her anorexia. Pain management should be timed so she is comfortable during mealtimes. The nurse has documented that the patient can safely swallow; however, RT is unable to feed herself because of limited mobility in her upper extremities. She is a partially dependent feeder and will need assistance in meal setup (opening cartons, cutting meats). Each meal should be supervised, and the environment should be calm and unhurried, with no distractions. The nurse should provide frequent cuing and simple commands to direct RT in the task.

Later evaluation reveals that RT describes an increased appetite. Objective measures of nutritional status are improved. With close supervision and frequent commands, she can now feed herself. Because of limited social support at home, RT is being evaluated by social services for placement in a nursing home.

SUMMARY

Providing nutrition, or Feeding, is deeply rooted in our culture as a symbol of caring and compassion (Knox 1989). It is a basic need that evokes a great deal of emotion and sense of moral duty. Yet this usually pleasurable experience can become painful, humiliating, and even dangerous for some patients. Nurses using Feeding as an intervention must have a strong theoretical knowledge base regarding the physiological and psychological components of nutrient intake. This theoretical knowledge must be combined with the art of nursing to design creative patient care plans.

REFERENCES

Anderson, J. 1982. The significance of hunger to nursing. In C. Norris (ed.), *Concept Clarification in Nursing* (pp. 192–222). Rockville, Md.: Aspen Publications.

Athlin, E., and Norberg, A. 1987. Caregivers' attitudes to and interpretations of the behavior of severely demented patients during feeding in a patient assignment care system. *International Journal of Nursing Studies* 24(2):145–153.

Backstrom, A., Norberg, A., and Norberg, B. 1987. Feeding difficulties in long-stay patients at nursing homes. Caregiver turnover and caregivers' assessments of duration and difficulty of assisted feeding and amounts of food received by the patient. *International Journal of Nursing Studies* 24(1):69–76.

Baker, J.P., Detsky, A.S., Wesson, D., Wolman, S., Stewart, S., Whitewell, J., Langer, B., and Jeejeebhoy, K.N. 1982. Nutritional assessment. A comparison of clinical judgment and objective measurement. *New England Journal of Medicine* 306(16):969–972.

Bistrian, B.R., Blackburn, G.L., and Hallowell, E. 1974. Protein status of general surgical patients. *Journal of the American Medical Association* 230:858–860.

Bistrian, B.R., Blackburn, G.L., Vitale, J., Cochran, D., and Naylor, J. 1976. Prevalence of malnutrition in general medical patients. *Journal of the American Medical Association* 235:1567–1570.

Buelow, J.M., and Jamieson, D. 1990. Potential for altered nutritional status in the stroke patient. *Rehabilitation Nursing* 15(5):260–263.

Buzby, G.P., Mullen, J.L., Matthews, D.C., Hobbs, C.L., and Rosato, E.F. 1980. Prognostic nutritional index in gastrointestinal surgery. *American Journal of Surgery* 139:160–167.

Cahill, G.F., Jeejeebhoy, K.N., Hill, G.L., and Owen, O.E. 1988. Starvation: Some biological aspects. In J.M. Kinney, (eds.), *Nutrition and metabolism in patient care* (pp. 193–204). Philadelphia: W.B. Saunders.

Caldwell, M., and Kennedy-Caldwell, C. 1981. Normal nutritional requirements. *Surgical Clinics of North America* 61(3):489–507.

Carpenito, L.J. 1983. *Nursing diagnosis: Application to clinical practice.* Philadelphia: J.B. Lippincott Company.

Curtas, S. 1988. Nutritional assessment. In C. Kennedy-Caldwell and P. Guenter (eds.), *Nutritional support nursing core curriculum,* 2d ed. (pp. 29–41). American Society for Parenteral and Enteral Nutrition. Silver Spring, Md.

Curtas, S., Chapman, G., and Meguid, M. 1989. Evaluation of nutritional status. *Nursing Clinics of North America* 24(2):301–313.

Donahue, P.A. 1990. When it's hard to swallow. Feeding techniques for dysphagia management. *Journal of Gerontological Nursing* 16(4):6–9.

Donoghue, M., Nunnally, C., and Yasko, J. 1982. *Nutritional aspects of cancer care.* Reston, Va.: Reston Publishing Company.

Dougherty, S. 1988. The malnourished respiratory patient. *Critical Care Nurse* 8(4):13–22.

Emick-Herring, B. and Wood, P. 1990. A team approach to neurologically based swallowing disorders. *Rehabilitation Nursing* 15(3):126–132.

Feurer, I.D., Crosby, L.O., and Mullen, J.L. 1984. Measured and predicted resting energy expenditure in clinically stable patients. *Clinical Nutrition,* 3, 27–34.

Gavan, C.A., Hastings-Tolsma, M.T., and Troyan, P.J. 1988. Explication of Newman's model: A holistic systems approach to nutrition for health promotion in the life process. *Holistic Nursing Practice* 3(1):26–38.

Grant, J. 1981. Current techniques of nutritional assessment. *Surgical Clinics of North America* 61(3):437–464.

Guyton, A.C. (ed.). 1991. *Textbook of medical physiology,* 8th ed. Philadelphia: W.B. Saunders.

Harris, J.L., and Benedict, F.G. 1919. *A biometric study of basal metabolism in man.* Publication 279. Washington, D.C.: Carnegie Institute.

Hill, G.L., and Beddoe, A.H. 1988. Dimensions of the human body and its compartments. In J.M. Kinney, K.N. Jeejeebhoy, G.L. Hill, and O.E. Owen, (eds.), *Nutrition and metabolism in patient care* (pp. 89–118). Philadelphia: W.B. Saunders.

Hirsch, S., de Obaldice, N., Peterman, M., Rojo, P., Barrientos, C., Iturriaga, H., and Bunout, D. 1991. Subjective global assessment of nutritional status: Further validation. *Nutrition* 7(1):35–38.

Hogstel, M.D., and Robinson, H.B. 1989. Feeding the frail elderly. *Journal of Gerontological Nursing* 15(3):16–20.

Jeejeebhoy, K.N. 1990. Assessment of nutritional status. In J. Rombeau and M. Caldwell (eds.), *Clinical nutrition enteral and tube feeding,* 2d ed. (pp. 123–127). Philadelphia: W.B. Saunders.

Kinney J.M., Jeejeebhoy, K.N., Hill, G.L., and Owen, O.E. 1988. *Nutrition and metabolism in patient care.* Philadelphia: W.B. Saunders.

Knox, L.S. 1983. Nutrition and cancer. *Nursing Clinics of North America* 18(1):97–110.

Leininger, M.M. 1988. Transcultural eating patterns and nutrition: Transcultural nursing and anthropological perspectives. *Holistic Nursing Practice* 3(1):16–25.

Mullen, J.L. 1981. Consequences of malnutrition in the surgical patient. Surgical Clinics of North America 61(3):465–487.

Nightingale, Florence. 1859. *Notes on nursing: What it is and what it is not.* London: Harrison & Sons.

Norberg, A., Backstrom, A., Athlin, E., and Norberg, B. 1988. Food refusal amongst nursing home patients as conceptualized by nurses' aides and enrolled nurses: An interview study. *Journal of Advanced Nursing* 13:478–483.

Openbrier, D.R., and Covey, M. 1987. Ineffective breathing pattern related to malnutrition. *Nursing Clinics of North America* 22(1):225–247.

Ross, B. 1987. Helping the patient who won't eat. *Nursing* 17(4):29.

Sanders, H.N. 1990. Feeding dependent eaters among geriatric patients. *Journal of Nutrition for the Elderly* 9(3):69–74.

Sigal, L.K., and Daly, J.M. 1990. Enteral nutrition and the cancer patient. In J. Rombeau and M. Caldwell (eds.), *Clinical nutrition: enteral and tube feeding,* 2d ed. (pp. 263–280). Philadelphia: W.B. Saunders.

Studley, H.O. 1936. Percentage of weight loss: A basic indicator of surgical risk in patients with chronic peptic ulcer. *Journal of the American Medical Association* 106:458.

Taylor, M. 1988. Food glorious food. *Nursing Times* 84(13):28–30.

Vick, R.L., 1984. *Contemporary medical physiology.* Reading, Mass.: Addison-Wesley.

Yen, P.K. 1983. Special help for eating problems. *Geriatric Nursing: American Journal of Care for the Aging* 4(4):257–259.

4

INTERMITTENT CATHETERIZATION

JANET P. SPECHT
MERIDEAN L. MAAS
SALLY WILLETT
NANCY K. MYERS

Intermittent Catheterization is the introduction and removal of a catheter at regular intervals to empty the bladder, leaving the client catheter free. It is performed by the client or a caregiver and can be used by clients in their homes or in institutions. The catheterization can be done using clean or sterile procedures. The purposes are to eliminate residual urine in the bladder, reduce urinary infections because of the reduction of residual urine, prevent incontinent episodes, regain bladder tone, and increase client control of urinary elimination and self-care. Intermittent Catheterization is one intervention for specific types of urinary incontinence and for persistent urinary infections that may also cause incontinence. It is an effective nursing intervention for Overflow Incontinence, Reflex Incontinence, and Urge Incontinence secondary to infection and inflammation of the bladder.

Interventions for urinary incontinence are critical for nurses' repertoire of treatments because of the prevalence of urinary incontinence in both the community and institutions. Nurses are frequently the health professionals who discover and assume responsibility for treating and managing the problem. At least 10 million adult Americans suffer from urinary incontinence. Approximately 30% of community-resident elderly and at least half of all nursing home residents have urinary incontinence (Smith and Newman 1990). In acute care settings, the incidence varies from 5.5% to 48% (Palmer 1988), with settings reporting higher incontinence rates having a higher proportion of elderly patients. In a study of 18,084 patients of general physician practitioners in Great Britain and one of the few studies including children, Thomas, Plymat, and Blannin et al. (1980) found a 6% incidence of incontinence among children aged 5 to 14 years old, a 5% incidence in patients aged 15 to 64 years, and a 10% incidence among patients aged 65 years and older.

The nursing intervention Intermittent Catheterization has a research base but is seldom used by nurses to treat incontinence. Despite its potential to promote continence and to provide an alternative to indwelling catheters, it has received little attention in the nursing literature. Indwelling catheters are frequently used in nursing homes as the only intervention for incontinence. Although severe side effects, including urinary tract infections and severe fistulas, can result, indwelling catheters are used in approximately 10% to 30% of incontinent individuals living in long-term-care institutions (Ouslander, Kane, Vollmer, and Menezes 1985). In a survey of three Massachusetts nursing homes, Ribeiro and Smith (1985) found that 40% of the 412 residents had an indwelling urinary catheter.

LITERATURE REVIEW

Intermittent Catheterization was introduced after World War II as a bladder training technique for paraplegic and quadriplegic patients (Champion 1976). At that time, Intermittent Catheterization was conducted only under sterile conditions by a physician. Patients were catheterized at frequent intervals throughout the day. The procedure worked much as a bladder drill. Thus, the rationale for the intervention is to train the bladder, prevent inhibition of the detrusor muscle by an indwelling catheter, and promote bladder muscle tone (Comarr 1972). Early studies showed that patients trained in such a manner for about 7 weeks were able to void normally (Guttman and Frankel 1966). Guttman and Frankel published results of an 11-year study of 476 paraplegic and quadriplegic patients for whom sterile Intermittent Catheterization was used and demonstrated that 62% remained infection free and most patients regained normal voiding. In addition, there was a low incidence of hydronephrosis, vesicoureteral reflux, and calculosis. Studies by Bors (1967), Walsh (1967), and Lindan and Bellomy (1971) also demonstrated a high percentage of sterile urine, a lack of complications, and success with regaining continence without continued catheterization. Only Pelosof et al. (1973) reported any negative findings using intermittent catheterization. He found two cases of hydronephrosis and recommended that renal function tests be performed prior to initiating Intermittent Catheterization.

The introduction of Intermittent Catheterization has been the biggest single advance in the management of neurogenic urinary elimination difficulties because it allows regular emptying of the bladder and the ability to remain catheter free (Oliver 1990). The procedure was modified based on studies by Lapides, Diokno, Silber, and Lowe (1972) and Champion (1976) and is now taught as a clean, not sterile, self-catheterization used for bladder training as well as for other clients for whom nerve supply to the bladder is disrupted.

Clean Intermittent Catheterization is a technique in which patients self-catheterize or are catheterized by caregivers at regular intervals. It has been recommended for use in clients with urinary retention related to a weak or atonic detrusor muscle (as in diabetic neuropathy), overflow incontinence related to blockage of the urethra (as in benign prostatic hypertrophy), and with reflex incontinence related to spinal cord injury (Lapides, Diokno, Gould, and Lowe 1976; Ouslander et al. 1985; Ouslander and Uman 1985; Urinary Incontinence 1986). Since the late 1970s, the technique of intermittent clean self-catheterization has become widely adopted for the long-term management of people with persistent large residual urine volumes (Oliver 1990).

The rationale for clean Intermittent Catheterization is based on the assumption that the blood supply to the bladder must be maintained in order to promote the bladder's ability to fight infection. The emphasis is not on maintaining sterility but on frequent emptying of the bladder to prevent ischemia. Bladder overdistention slows bladder circulation, predisposes the bladder to infection, and prevents normal bladder muscle contraction. Thus, frequent clean catheterization of the bladder prevents overdistension, allows the bladder to fight infection, and promotes reestablishment of bladder muscle tone (Horsley, Crane, and Reynolds 1982). The technique has been shown to reduce the incidence of complications associated with indwelling catheter use (Ouslander et al. 1985).

Lapides and colleagues (1976) reported a review of 218 patients who were taught clean Intermittent Catheterization. The subjects' ages ranged from 4 to 84 years, with 145 subjects between 21 and 84 years of age. A number of different diagnoses related to voiding difficulties and incontinence were represented in the sample. The results of the survey were that for clients experiencing Reflex Incontinence or Overflow Incontinence, clean Intermittent Catheterization combined with anticholinergic and alpha-adrenergic medication alleviated incontinence as well as chronic perineal dermatitis (Lapides et al. 1976). Confirming the findings of Lapides and his colleagues, Champion (1976) followed seven patients for 1 year who used clean Intermittent Catheterization and who had previously been managed with sterile Intermittent Catheterization. Urine specimens and renal function remained unchanged after use of clean compared to sterile Intermittent Catheterization for all of the patients. In summary, the studies of Lapides and colleagues (Lapides, Diokno, Silber, and Lowe 1971; Lapides, Diokno, Lowe, and Kalish 1973; Lapides, Diokno, Gould, and Lowe 1975; Lapides, Diokno, Gould and Lowe, 1976), Hasham, Meyer, Altshuler, Butz, Norderhaug, and Uehling (1975), Champion (1976), and Kass, McHugh, and Diokno (1979) provide support for the use of the clean Intermittent Catheterization intervention for treatment of Reflex, Overflow, and Urge Incontinence due to infection without complications of exacerbated urinary tract infection or compromised renal function, as long as catheterizations are frequent enough to maintain 300 cc or less urine volume in the bladder.

Most work with children has been done with those suffering from spina bifida (Kaye and Van Blerk 1981) and spinal injury patients (Pearman 1976). More recently, the intervention has been used for all categories of children with incomplete bladder emptying. Altshuler, Meyer, and Butz (1977) instituted a clean intermittent self-catheterization program in 1973 with pediatric spinal-cord-injured and melomenigocele patients, aged 2 to 17 years, at the University of Wisconsin Hospitals. Parents of young children were taught the procedure, and older children learned self-catheterization. Criteria for inclusion in the study were a bladder capacity of over 50 cc, some anal sphincter tone, and grossly undamaged kidneys and ureters. Although the children did not always regain continence without use of the intermittent catheter, all were able to remain dry between catheterizations. The clean intermittent self-catheterization intervention did provide a means for the children to manage their own urinary elimination. Most were able to learn quickly, the intervention allowed them to avoid wet clothing, and they were spared the embarrassment of accidents and odors that usually accompany incontinence. Further, the children were able to participate in more activities characteristic of their age groups, the intervention was not expensive, and the equipment needed was minimal and nonrestrictive of activities and socialization. Other studies in children (Hasham et al. 1975; Kass et al. 1979) indicate that age is not a contraindication for the use of the clean Intermittent Catheterization intervention, although equipment and the techniques may be somewhat different.

Specht, Tunink, Maas, and Bulechek (1991) reported good success in regaining continence with the use of clean Intermittent Catheterization at the Iowa Veterans Home with clients who had atonic bladders. However, they point out the need for further testing in the elderly, since much of the research with the intervention has been done with children and young adults. It is unclear whether complications might be more common in a geriatric population (Ouslander et al. 1985). Palmer (1990) advocates the use of Intermittent Catheterization when surgical or pharmacologic intervention is inappropriate or unsuccessful for the voiding dysfunction with large volumes of postmicturition residual urine, which becomes increasingly common with advancing age. If Intermittent Catheterization will keep the older adult continent, whether in an institutional setting or in the community, every effort should be made to ensure that this is done (Palmer 1990). Older persons often require Intermittent Catheterization less often than younger people with voiding problems because residual urine accumulates more slowly in the older bladder (Oliver 1990).

Nurses are often skeptical of the intervention of Intermittent Catheterization, fearing it will lead to infections or cause trauma to the urinary tract. There are mixed recommendations about the use of clean versus sterile technique, particularly in situations where the client is institutionalized or not performing self-catheterization. Nurses struggle particularly with the idea of clean versus sterile technique. Some sources recommend that while patients are in institutions, the sterile procedure be used to prevent cross-contamination (Long 1991). However, no studies have been reported that compared the use of the two forms of the Intermittent Catheterization intervention in institutions, making this comparison an important area for nursing research.

Clearly, there is a strong research base for the use of Intermittent Catheterization by nurses to treat Reflex Incontinence and Overflow Incontinence, to prevent Urge Incontinence resulting from urinary tract infection, and to avoid the use of indwelling catheters. The research base provides strong support for the clean Intermittent Catheterization nursing intervention, which has the added advantages of flexibility, convenience, and low cost for clients across settings. These advantages are also important for the use of the intervention by nurses who are more likely to prescribe and implement the intervention when it is not costly and requires a minimum of equipment and time.

NURSING DIAGNOSES AND CLIENT GROUPS

The nursing intervention Intermittent Catheterization is proposed to treat specific nursing diagnoses of urinary incontinence. Assessment and diagnosis of the specific urinary incontinence diagnosis is essential for the appropriate prescription of Intermittent Catheterization. There are five urinary incontinence diagnoses in the NANDA taxonomy: Reflex Incontinence, Urge Incontinence, Stress Incontinence, Functional Incontinence, and Total Incontinence (Carroll-Johnson 1989). Specht, Tunink, Maas, and Bulechek (1991) define two additional diagnoses: Overflow Incontinence and Iatrogenic Incontinence. Although iatrogenesis of incontinence can result in one of the five NANDA diagnoses or overflow incontinence, it is useful to identify Iatrogenic Incontinence as a distinct diagnosis in order to encourage early detection and correction, which is most often a discontinuation of the offending nursing or medical treatment. Intermittent Catheterization is usually effective in the treatment of Overflow Incontinence, Reflex Incontinence, Urge Incontinence due to urinary tract infection and inflammation, and Iatrogenic Incontinence when retention and bladder overflow are manifested. All of these diagnoses can be observed in clients of all age groups; however, Overflow, Urge, and Iatrogenic Incontinence are most common among elderly clients, and Reflex Incontinence is most common among younger adults and children who are more prone to spinal cord damage due to accidents or congenital anomalies.

Overflow Incontinence occurs when the bladder becomes sufficiently overdistended that voiding attempts result in frequent, small amounts of urine, often in the form of dribbling. The causes are bladder hypotonia due to impaired bladder neuromusculature and bladder outlet obstruction. Large amounts of residual urine, hesitancy, slow stream, passage of infrequent, small volumes of urine (dribbling), a feeling of incomplete bladder emptying, sudden leakage of urine related to bending or turning, dysuria, and a palpable full bladder are common signs and symptoms seen with all etiologies of Overflow Incontinence.

Urge Incontinence is involuntary urination that occurs soon after a strong sense of urgency to void (Carroll-Johnson 1989). Heightened urgency results from bladder irritation, reduced bladder capacity, or overdistention of the bladder. The irritation of the bladder stretch receptors causes spasms and emptying. The common signs and symptoms for Urge Incontinence are the ability to identify the urge to void and precipitancy. Urine loss is larger and more prolonged than with Stress Incontinence.

Reflex Incontinence is the involuntary loss of urine caused by completion of the spinal cord reflex arc (bladder contraction) in the absence of higher neural control (Carroll-Johnson 1989). Bladder filling or perineal or lower abdominal stimuli precipitate reflex bladder contraction. Voiding is observed when a specific and predictable volume is reached with no reported sensation of urgency or voiding (Wheately 1982).

Iatrogenic Incontinence results from physician- and/or nurse-controlled factors, such as restraints, medications, fluid limitations, bed rest, and intravenous fluids. Without the treatment, the client would be continent; thus, assessment data for the diagnosis include onset of incontinence coincident with the initiation of medical or nursing treatments that can influence control of urine.

PROTOCOL FOR INTERVENTION

The first step of the intervention protocol is to perform a comprehensive assessment of the client in order to determine the specific nursing diagnoses of urinary incontinence. Detailed discussion and tools for assessment are reported by Specht et al. (1991). Many clients, especially the elderly, have two or more specific incontinence diagnoses. Thus, Intermittent Catheterization will often be prescribed along with another nursing intervention (e.g., Kegel exercises for Stress Incontinence).

The next step of the intervention protocol is to teach the client, the family, or staff caregivers the basic rationale for Intermittent Catheterization as a nursing intervention to treat the specific nursing diagnosis of incontinence. The basic rationale is that overdistention of the bladder (150 cc for clients aged 1 to 5 years, 240 cc for ages 6 to 9, more than 300 cc for ages 9 years and older) (Lowe 1982) causes bladder wall ischemia and interferes with the bladder's ability to fight infection, as well as interfering with the bladder's muscle contractility. Thus, if the bladder volume is kept equal to or less than 300 cc in older children and adults, continence is promoted by preventing urinary tract infection, kidney damage due to reflux of urine up the ureters, and the ineffectiveness of detrusor muscle contractions to empty the bladder. Clients, family members, and/or staff are also taught not to force fluids because increased fluids contribute to bladder overdistention and, thus, to incomplete bladder emptying.

Assessment for clients who will benefit from Intermittent Catheterization will also include notation of manual and mental ability to perform the catheterization procedure or the availability of a family member or staff caregiver who can perform the procedure, willingness of the client to do self-catheterization at regular intervals or to have someone else do it, 100 cc or greater bladder capacity of the client to prevent too frequent catheterization and an intact and unobstructed urethra (Lapides et al. 1976).

Next, the abilities of the client to perform self-catheterization are assessed, along with the setting within which the client resides and the availability of family or staff to perform the Intermittent Catheterization if the client is unable. A candidate for clean intermittent self-catheterization must have the manual dexterity to manipulate the catheter and must be motivated to perform the technique frequently throughout the day (usually when the bladder has distended with approximately 300 cc of fluid) and in any number of settings. Caregivers must possess these same qualities. A determination must be made whether to use clean or sterile Intermittent Catheterization. Although there is an insufficient research base to evaluate the potential untoward effects of clean Intermittent Catheterization in all settings, we believe that the use of the clean technique enhances the maintenance of the needed frequency of catheterizations, it is more cost-effective, and is more convenient in all settings. The advantages of frequent emptying of the bladder using the clean technique are expected to more than offset any increased risk of infection. Bacteria carried into the bladder will be quickly inactivated by the healthy bladder tissue (Lapides et al. 1975). Therefore, the use of clean Intermittent Catheterization is recommended.

The person (client or other) who will be doing the catheterization must be taught catheterization technique along with care of the equipment. A detailed clean catheterization procedure and instructions for teaching self-catheterization are provided in Tables 4 – 1 and 4 – 2. The person should successfully demonstrate the skill to the prescribing nurse. If the client is to do self-catheterization, having a full bladder while practicing the technique will help him or her learn more quickly. Before attempting the procedure, the client, family member, or staff person needs to be familiar with the equipment and body structures. For women doing self-catheterization, it is often helpful to use a mirror to visualize the vulva, labia and meatus. Catheter size is dependent on the age of the client. A 12 to 14 French catheter is recommended for adults. Red rubber catheters are more flexible and cause less trauma. Lubrication (water-soluble gel) should be used when catheterizing males. For persons who complain of discomfort with catheterization, xylocaine gel can be used as a lubricant.

Patients are frequently maintained on antibacterial medication for a period of 2 or 3 weeks, as well as on anticholinergic or cholinergic medications to assist bladder control (Horsley, Crane, and Reynolds 1982). An attempt should be made to sterilize the urine with antibacterial chemotherapy (e.g., furantoin, ampicillin, or sulfamethoxazole) when the intermittent catheterization begins (Lapides et al. 1975). Anticholinergics (e.g., oxybutynin chloride or propantheline bromide) are prescribed for patients with uncontrolled bladder contractions evidenced by incontinent episodes between the catheterizations. The cholinergics (e.g., bethanechol chloride) are used for persons who have atonic and partial motor paralytic bladders. The nurse should discuss the assessment data of the client's incontinence problem and the plan for treatment with the client's physician to obtain the needed supportive medical therapy.

Prescribing the frequency of catheterization is the crucial step in the Intermittent Catheterization protocol. Catheterization every 3 hours and once during the night is recommended for most adults; however, the frequency is determined by the amount of urine obtained at each catheterization. The frequency must be adjusted so that the volume of urine obtained is 300 cc or less. If more than 300 cc is

TABLE 4–1. PROCEDURE FOR CLEAN SELF-CATHETERIZATION

MALE	FEMALE
Items needed Red rubber catheter Prepared container with Alconox and water (1 tablespoon Alconox to 1 gallon water) Large container for urine collection—calibrated	**Items needed** Red rubber catheter Prepared container with Alconox and water (1 tablespoon Alconox to 1 gallon water) Lubafax (optional) Large container for urine collection—calibrated Mirror
Procedure 1. Place 1 gallon water in a container large enough to hold catheters. Add 1 tablespoon Alconox. 2. Place catheters in Alconox solution and allow catheters to soak at least 1/2 hour. 3. Wash hands well. 4. Remove catheter from Alconox solution and rinse well with tap water. Place in a convenient clean place. 5. Squirt a small amount of Lubafax on tip of catheter. 6. Pick up penis with left hand, and with right hand insert tip of catheter into penis. (Right hand will be used to pick up penis if you are left-handed.) Continue to advance catheter until urine starts to flow. From this point advance catheter approximately 1 inch more. Since a small catheter is used it may be necessary to crede bladder while catheter is in place. 7. Continue until urine stops flowing. 8. When bladder is empty, remove catheter slowly, pausing at any point where urine starts to flow again. After catheter is completely removed, wash and place in Alconox solution. 9. If you wish to take catheters outside the home, rinse catheter well in tap water after it has soaked in Alconox for at least 1/2 hour. Wrap catheter in Saran Wrap.	**Procedure** 1. Place 1 gallon water in a container large enough to hold catheters. Add 1 tablespoon Alconox. 2. Place catheters in Alconox solution, and allow catheters to soak at least 1/2 hour. 3. Wash hands well. 4. Remove catheter from Alconox solution and rinse well with tap water. Place in a convenient clean place. 5. Assume position with legs separated, mirror in place so meatus can be easily seen. 6. Take catheter in right hand (left if left-handed), and separate labia with left hand. Lubafax may be squirted on catheter if desired. Insert tip of catheter into urethra. Continue to advance catheter until urine starts to flow. From this point, advance catheter approximately 1 inch more. Since catheter may be small, crede bladder while catheter is in place. 7. When bladder is empty, remove catheter slowly, pausing at any point where urine starts to flow again. After catheter is completely removed, wash and set aside to be placed in Alconox. 8. If you wish to take catheter outside the home, rinse catheter, which has soaked in Alconox solution, and wrap in Saran Wrap. Be sure catheter is rinsed well in tapwater so that no Alconox solution remains.

obtained, the interval between catheterizations must be shortened; similarly, if the volume of urine is substantially less than 300 cc, the interval can be lengthened.

Urinalysis and renal function tests are performed prior to initiating the Intermittent Catheterization intervention. Urinalysis should be repeated after 3 days of catheterizations, 5 days after the discontinuation of antibacterial medication, and every 2 weeks to 1 month thereafter. Renal function tests should be done every 6 months. Finally, the effectiveness of the Intermittent Catheterization must be continuously evaluated. A detailed record must be kept of the catheterization schedule, fluid input, and amount of urine obtained with each catheterization. Any voidings by the client must also be recorded, including the time and amount of urine voided. The nurse must closely monitor these data along with medications and the client's attitude and motivation regarding the intervention. The desired outcomes of no incontinence episodes, absence of urinary tract infections, social enhancement, and voiding without incontinence are also monitored.

TABLE 4–2.   TEACHING INTERMITTENT SELF-CATHETERIZATION TO FEMALE PATIENTS

Patient should have a full bladder.

Before attempting the procedure, familiarize patient with

1. Catheter
2. Visualization of vulva in the mirror
   —Clitoris
   —Urethra
   —Vaginal outlet

Assuming her to be right-handed, she

1. Holds labia apart with the second and fourth fingers of her left hand.
2. Applies considerable pressure with the third finger, palpating urethral meatus until she is certain that she can feel the urethra without looking.
3. Releases the pressure but does not move finger.
4. With right hand, holds the catheter about 1/2 inch from the tip, directing it slightly forward, and inserts it into the urethra under her finger until the urine flows.

Have the patient remove the catheter as soon as the urine flows.

Thereafter, she is taken to the bathroom where she will practice several times until she feels comfortable about the procedure.

Have her sit with the full part of her hips forward but not so far as to lose balance. Some patients do better sitting backward on the toilet. Some do best standing, with one foot resting on the toilet.

If patient is having difficulty palpating urethra, sometimes success is achieved by occluding the vaginal outlet with two fingers or inserting a tampon.

Emphasize the following:

1. This is just a trick to learn.
2. Hold labia minora apart and direct catheter upward.
3. Urethra will not disappear.
4. Do not get angry with oneself—self-defeating.
5. Never do it if too nervous—stop, do something else, and then come back to it.

Some little girls can see their urethra while sitting on the toilet so there is no need to palpate.

Materials needed = 14F clear plastic catheter

Reprinted from a procedure developed by Bette S. Lowe, R.N., E.T., Nurse Clinician, Section of Urology, Department of Surgery, The University of Michigan Medical Center, Ann Arbor, Michigan, published by Grune & Stratton.

CASE STUDIES

Case Study 1

Mr. DS is a 70-year-old man who has been living in a long-term-care facility for the past 7 years. He is alert and oriented but suffers from a number of chronic conditions: degenerative joint disease with maximal involvement of the left knee, left residual paresis from a cerebovascular accident (CVA) suffered in 1979, chronic obstructive lung disease, hypertension, diabetes, and a history of alcoholism. He is 5 feet, 10 inches tall and weighs 290 pounds. From April 1985 to January 1990 Mr. DS has had urinary symptoms the majority of the time, among them difficulty getting a stream started, dribbling, and voiding in small amounts, with a diagnosis of recurrent bladder infections. In 1986 he complained of increased dribbling to the point of needing to change his clothes regularly. In January 1987, a transurethral resection of the prostate (TURP) was performed for benign prostatic hypertrophy with bladder neck obstruction, found to be the cause of the recurrent urinary tract infections. In April 1987 he was still having some problems with dribbling, but it seemed improved. From January through September 1988, he had no urinary tract infections and little dribbling or incontinence. In October 1988 the dribbling increased, which Mr. DS thought was the result of taking a prescribed diuretic.

Exasperated with the continued dribbling and wetness and the difficulty in maintaining his hygiene, Mr. DS demanded an indwelling catheter so he could remain dry. However, when he had an indwelling catheter in place, he had increased difficulties with urinary tract infections. Because he wanted to remain mobile, he wanted a leg bag on in the daytime, making it impossible to maintain a closed system of drainage and increasing his risk for infection. He had an indwelling catheter intermittently until September 1989, when he had an indwelling catheter continuously until January, 1990. Evaluations at the Genitourinary (GU) Clinic at the Veterans Administration Medical Center (VAMC) recommended removal of the catheter, but Mr. DS refused to be without the catheter because the dribbling continued. At the time of his evaluation in the GU Clinic in November 1989, he was diagnosed with hyperspastic bladder/hypertonic neurogenic bladder. A cystoscopy and cystometrogram were done, which showed mild hypertrophy of the prostate, inflamed bladder, and a small-capacity bladder with uninhibited contractions. His bladder capacity was 120 cc, and his first detrusor contraction was at 70 cc of urine volume in the bladder. He was told at the clinic that nothing could be done about the dribbling and that he should not use an indwelling catheter.

Mr. DS returned to the long-term-care facility where he resided. He was unable to wear the condom catheter recommended at the VAMC because of his small penis and obesity. He again insisted that he have an indwelling catheter. Following a comprehensive assessment of his presenting signs and symptoms, his primary nurse made the following nursing diagnoses: Urge Incontinence due to chronic infection and inflammation and small, hyperactive bladder; overflow incontinence due to mildly enlarged prostate; and Reflex Incontinence due to sacral nerve damage secondary to CVA. His nurse determined to use the intervention of Intermittent Catheterization to treat the three problems by correcting the etiologies of recurrent urinary tract infections and bladder neck obstruction and to control bladder and premature reflex bladder emptying. A urinalysis was obtained showing 1 plus *Escherichia coli* bacteria. His blood urea nitrogen (BUN) and creatinine were within normal limits. Mr. DS was agreeable to try anything that might help. He had a large urine output —usually 1000 cc to 2000 cc every 8 hours. He was asked to restrict his fluid intake to 2500 cc in 24 hours, a substantial reduction for him. In consultation with the physician, a 2-week series of Macrodantin, 50 mg b.i.d. was initiated and Ditropan two times per day was initiated to help to control the uninhibited bladder contractions. Clean, rather than sterile, Intermittent Catheterization was used to enhance compliance with the frequent catheterizations required and to decrease the time required to carry out the procedure. Because Mr. DS's obesity and limited range of motion made it impossible for him to perform the procedure himself, the procedure was done by licensed nurses.

Before initiating the Intermittent Catheterization procedure and to form the basis for the schedule of catheterizations/voiding, a 3-day urinary elimination record was completed to determine the number and frequency of incontinence episodes; the number, frequency, and amounts of voidings; and Mr. DS's intake. Because he was nearly always wet from the constant dribbling, the Intermittent Catheterization schedule was initially set up for every 2 hours with a protocol to have him void immediately prior to each catheterization. Instructions on the nursing prescription sheet were as follows:

1. Wash hands before beginning the catheterization.
2. Remove catheter from the Betadine solution and rinse with tapwater. Place catheter on a clean paper towel.
3. Position the resident comfortably supine.
4. Put on disposable gloves.
5. Lubricate tip of catheter.
6. Insert catheter and allow bladder to drain until urine stops flowing. Remove the catheter slowly when the bladder is empty.
7. After the catheterization is done, cleanse the meatus with soap and water.
8. Record urine output.

Instructions for care of the catheter between uses were:

1. Wash the catheter with baby shampoo and water. Rinse with running water.
2. Place the catheter in a covered pan containing Betadine solution until the next use.
3. Change Betadine solution daily and change the pan weekly.
4. Use 10 cc of Betadine to 100 cc of tapwater.

The amounts of voiding, the amount of urine obtained with catheterization, and the number of times incontinent or wet during the 2-hour intervals were recorded. The procedure was implemented on January 16, 1990, midday. During the first 2 days of the intervention, 300 cc of urine was obtained in one catheterization. Mr. DS had only two incontinent episodes; they occurred when he was absent from the unit and did not return for the catheterization. The positive results were shared with the staff and Mr. DS, and the schedule was changed to 3-hour intervals.

For the next 10 days, the 3-hour interval was used, with more than 300 cc obtained from only one catheterization. Many catheterizations resulted in no urine or volumes of less than 50 cc. There were no incidents of incontinence, and Mr. DS's voidings steadily increased in volume. The schedule was then changed to every 6 hours. Amounts of Mr. DS's voidings continued to increase, and during the next 2 weeks he had only three incontinent episodes, all occurring during the day when he drank large amounts of fluid and delayed toileting because of social activities. On February 19, the Intermittent Catheterization procedure was discontinued. Monitoring of incontinent episodes continued through March 10 with no further incidents of incontinence observed. In March, his BUN and creatinine remained within normal limits, and a urinalysis was negative. Mr. DS regained continence and voided on his own with no symtoms of urinary infection or dribbling. Mr. DS and the nursing staff were pleased with these outcomes.

Case Study 2

Mr. JL is a 71 year-old-widower who has lived in a long-term-care facility for the past three years. He had a fracture of the sixth thoracic vertebrae of the spine with paraplegia following a fall from a roof in 1987. He also has a history of rectal ulceration, chronic obstructive lung disease, and cardiac arrythmias. Since he was taught at a Veterans Administration rehabilitation center following his fall, Mr. JL has been doing clean Intermittent Catheterization to manage his Reflex Incontinence. He performs the catheterization every 6 hours. He has enough upper body control to carry out the procedure independently. However, he has had continuous asymptomatic urinary tract infections (UTI). Upon investigation, it was found that he was doing inadequate cleansing of the catheter between catheterizations, causing recurrent UTIs. Mr. JL's BUN and creatinine are within normal limits. Monitoring was ordered by the primary nurse to evaluate whether the corrected catheter cleansing technique cleared his UTI. Because the UTI persisted, monitoring of the amounts of urine obtained with each catheterization was initiated. A pattern of large amounts of urine in the bladder was observed, causing pressure in the bladder and eliminating the infection-controlling effect of adequate blood flow to the bladder wall. The interval between Intermittent Catheterizations was changed to every 4 hours, and he was placed on bacterial suppressant chemotherapy to control the UTI. Mr. JL has no incontinent episodes between catheterizations and values the control that clean self-intermittent catheterization gives him.

This case study illustrates the use of Intermittent Catheterization to manage Reflex Incontinence when it is anticipated that the client will always need to manage urinary elimination with catheterization. It also illustrates the need for continued follow-up and evaluation to ensure that the procedure is carried out correctly with the desired outcomes achieved.

SUMMARY

Intermittent Catheterization is a nursing intervention for the nursing diagnoses Reflex Incontinence, Overflow Incontinence, and Urge Incontinence secondary to bladder infections and inflammation, and Iatrogenic Incontinence that is manifested by the other diagnoses. It is a versatile intervention that can be used across settings and can be performed by the client, family members, or other caregivers. The intervention holds promise as an alternative to indwelling catheters and can result in the correction of long-term incontinence. We recommend the clean procedure, although the effects of its use, compared to the sterile procedure, need more clinical research. One of the hardest obstacles to overcome with this intervention is the resistance to the required frequency to maintain less than 300 cc of urine in the bladder. Because of convenience, clients and caregivers are anxious to do the procedure less often. The use of the clean procedure helps to ameliorate this problem to some extent because less equipment and time are required to perform the procedure. Some clients are clearly opposed to catheterization even for collection of data needed to diagnose the incontinence problem. Intermittent Catheterization is not a viable option for these persons. Evaluation of the effectiveness of Intermittent Catheterization by monitoring the amounts of urine voided, the amounts obtained with catheterization, the number of incontinent episodes, urinary infections, and renal function is essential to ensure that the desired results are obtained, for providing feedback and encouragement to the client and caregivers, and for monitoring for untoward effects.

A research base is developing for the use of Intermittent Catheterization by nurses to treat specific types of urinary incontinence. Nurses need to use the intervention more and share the results of clinical trials in the literature. The clean Intermittent Catheterization intervention needs to be tested further with clients of all ages and in all settings. Continued nursing research is needed to build the clinical knowledge of nurses for the treatment of the devastating condition of incontinence using the nursing intervention of Intermittent Catheterization.

REFERENCES

Altshuler, A., Meyer, J., and Butz, K.J. 1977. Even children can learn to do clean self-catheterization. *American Journal of Nursing* 77(1):97–101.

Bors, E. 1967. Intermittent catheterization in paraplegic patients. *Urology International* 22:236–249.

Carroll-Johnson, R. 1989. *Classification of nursing diagnoses: Proceedings of the 8th National Conference.* Philadelphia: Lippincott.

Champion, V.L. 1976. Clean technique for intermittent self catheterization. *Nursing Research* 25(1):13–18.

Comarr, A.E. 1972. Intermittent catheterization for the traumatic cord bladder patient. *Journal of Urology* 107(5):762–765.

Guttman, Sir L., and Frankel, H. 1966. The value of intermittent catheterization in the early management of traumatic paraplegia and tetraplegia. *Paraplegia* 4; 63–84.

Hasham, A.I., Meyer, J., Altshuler, A., Butz, M., Norderhaug, K., and Uehling, D.T. 1975. Clean intermittent catheterization for meningiomyelocele. *Wisconsin Medical Journal* 74:117–118.

Horsely, J.A., Crane, J., and Reynolds, M.A. 1982. Intermittent catheterization: *CURN Project: Michigan Nurses' Association.* New York: Grune and Stratton.

Kass, E.J., McHugh, T., and Diokno, A.C. 1979. Intermittent catheterization in children less than six years old. *Journal of Urology* 121:792–793.

Kaye, K., and Van Blerk, P.H. 1981. Urinary continence in children with neurogenic bladders. *British Journal of Urology* 53:241.

Lapides, J., Diokno, A.C., Silber, S.J., and Lowe, B.S. 1971. Clean, intermittent, self catheterization in the treatment of urinary tract disease. *Transactions of the American Association of Genito-Urinary Surgeons* 63:92–95.

Lapides, J., Diokno, A.C., Silber, S.J. and Lowe, B.S. 1972. Clean, intermittent, self catheterization and treatment of urinary tract disease. *Journal of Urology* 107:458.

Lapides, J., Diokno, A.C., Lowe, B.S., and Kalish, M.D. 1973. Followup on unsterile, intermittent, self catheterization. *Transactions of the American Association of Genito-Urinary Surgeons* 65:44–47.

Lapides, J., Diokno, A.C., Gould, F.R. and Lowe, B.S. 1975. Further observation of self catheterization. Transaction of the American Association of Genito-Urinary Surgeons, 67:15–17.

Lapides, J., Diokno, A.C., Gould, F.R., and Lowe, B.S. 1976. Urinary tract infection in women: Part 2. *Journal of Practical Nursing* 26:25–27.

Lindan, R., and Bellomy, V. 1971. The use of intermittent catheterization in a bladder training program. *Journal of Chronic Disease* 24(12):727–735.

Long, M. 1991. Managing urinary incontinence. In W.C. Chenitz, J.T. Stone, and S.A. Salisbury (eds.) *Clinical gerontological nursing: A guide to advanced practice* (pp. 203–215), Philadelphia: W.B. Saunders.

Lowe, B.S. 1982. Intermittent catheterization procedure. Section of Urology, Department of Surgery. University of Michigan Medical Center, Ann Arbor, Michigan.

Oliver, L. 1990. The neurogenic bladder. In K. Jeter, N. Faller, and C. Norton (eds.), *Nursing for continence.* Philadelphia: W.B. Saunders Company.

Ouslander, J., Kane, R., Vollmer, S., and Menezes, M. 1985, July. *Technologies for managing urinary incontinence.* (Health Care Technology Case Study 33. OTA-HCS 33. Washington, D.C.: U.S. Congress, Office of Technology Assessment.

Ouslander, J., and Uman, G. 1985. Urinary incontinence: Opportunities for research, education, and improvements in medical care in the nursing home setting. In E.L. Schneider, *The teaching nursing home.* New York: Raven Press.

Palmer, M.H. 1988. Incontinence: The magnitude of the problem. *Nursing Clinics of North America* 23(139):139–157.

Palmer, M.H. 1990. Incontinence in the elderly. In K. Jeter, N. Faller and C. Norton (eds.), *Nursing for continence.* Philadelphia: W. B. Saunders Company.

Pearman, J.W. 1976. Urological followup of ninety nine spinal-cord injured patients initially managed by intermittent catheterization. *British Journal of Urology* 48:297.

Pelosof, H.V., et al. 1973. Hydronephrosis: Silent hazard of intermittent catheterization. *Journal of Urology* 110(10):375–377.

Ribeiro, B, and Smith, S. 1985. Evaluation of urinary catheterization and urinary incontinence in a general nursing home population. *Journal of American Geriatric Society* 33(7):479–481.

Smith, D.A., and Newman, D.K. (eds.). 1990. Urinary incontinence: A problem not often assessed or treated. *Focus on Geriatric Care and Rehabilitation* 3(10):1–9.

Specht, J., Tunink, P., Maas, M., and Bulechek, G. 1991. Urinary incontinence. In M. Maas, K. Buckwalter, and M. Hardy (eds.), *Nursing diagnoses and interventions for the elderly.* Redwood City, Calif.: Addison-Wesley.

Thomas, T., Plymat, K., and Blannin, J. et al. 1980. Prevalence of urinary incontinence. *British Medical Journal* 281:1243–1245.

Urinary Incontinence. 1986. Proceedings of the 1986 NANDA Conference. Unpublished report.

Walsh, J.J. 1967, September 27. Further experience with intermittent catheterization. *Proceedings Annual Clinical Spinal Cord Injury Conference* 17:134–140,

Wheatley, J. 1982. Bladder incontinence: Four types and their control. *Postgraduate Medicine* 7(1);75–82.

5

BOWEL MANAGEMENT

AUDREY M. McLANE
RUTH E. McSHANE

DEFINITION AND DESCRIPTION

Bowel Management is a progressive program of elimination designed to regulate and control Bowel Incontinence. The complexity of a Bowel Management program depends on the type of bowel dysfunction, the patient's functional status, support systems, life-style, and the environment. For all types of bowel dysfunction, patient goals include: to produce a soft, formed stool; to defecate at a regularly scheduled time, place, and interval; to eliminate or minimize spontaneous stools (incontinence); to prevent constipation, impaction, and diarrhea; and to complete the bowel routine in 30 to 45 minutes.

A well-planned Bowel Management program is based on a detailed history of a patient's previous pattern of elimination and current medical problem; clinical validation of an altered bowel elimination pattern, including contributing factors (nursing diagnosis); digital examination of the rectum to assess anal sphincter tone and to establish presence or absence of stool; review of medical evaluations and current medications; and temporary use of laxatives and enemas to produce a clean bowel (McLane and McShane 1991).

Components of a Bowel Management program include: understanding of continence and incontinence mechanisms; diet modifications to achieve desired stool consistency and to trigger gastrocolic-duodenocolic reflex; regular physical exercise; instruction and practice of pelvic floor exercises (PFE); temporary medications and use of digital stimulation; development and implementation of a daily toileting regime; instruction of patient and family or caretaker; and flow sheets for documentation and evaluation. An effective Bowel Management program usually requires from 6 to 8 weeks to produce a soft, well-formed stool within 1 hour of the designated time (Alterescu 1986; Davis, Nagelhout, Hoban, and Barnard 1986; Hanak 1990).

LITERATURE RELATED TO COMPONENTS OF BOWEL PROGRAM

Understanding of Continence/Incontinence Mechanisms

An understanding of the mechanisms underlying normal elimination and bowel dysfunction is required to instruct and assist a patient to regulate and control bowel elimination. Stool moves into the rectum in response to stimulation of the vagus nerve, which contracts the colon. As the rectum distends, the internal anal

TABLE 5-1.   NEUROGENIC BOWEL TYPE: CONTROL AND REFLEX

	UNINHIBITED BOWEL	REFLEX BOWEL	AUTONOMOUS BOWEL
Cerebral control	Decreased	Absent	Absent
Sphincter control	Decreased	Absent	Absent
Bowel sensation	Intact	Decreased or absent	Absent
Saddle sensation[a]	Intact	Decreased or absent	Decreased or absent
Bulbocavernosus reflex[b]	Intact or increased	Increased	Absent

[a] Perianal sensation elicited by response to pinprick or light touch; suggests intact sensory function at the sacral spinal cord level (Cannon 1981, p. 227).
[b] Palpable contraction of the bulbocavernous and ischiocavernous muscles and a visible contraction of external anal sphincter. A positive reflex indicates reflex bowel function will return after a period of spinal shock (Cannon 1981, p. 227).

sphincter relaxes, the urge to defecate is perceived, and conscious effort must be made to avoid bowel incontinence by contracting the puborectalis muscle and the external anal sphincter. Since the rectum can accommodate to fecal material, defecation may be delayed, but stool will harden in the rectum in the presence of chronic distension (Alterescu 1986; Wald 1989).

Stool consistency and volume are important factors in maintaining continence. Small pellets of stool entering the rectum do not produce distension and hence do not alert the individual to defecate. Large volumes of liquid stool entering the rectum quickly overcome the continence mechanism (Pemberton and Kelly 1986). To remain continent, individuals must be motivated, must have intact anorectal sensation, must be able to store feces through compliance, must be able to contract the puborectalis and external anal sphincter muscles, and must have access to a toileting facility.

Central nervous system (CNS) damage from disease or trauma may compromise bowel function and lead to stool retention and/or incontinence. Since the process of defecation is controlled by the somatic and autonomic nervous systems, voluntary bowel control is altered when motor and/or sensory pathways are compromised. Impaired cerebral control (unawareness of urge to defecate and inability to inhibit defecation) and/or impaired anal sphincter sensation or control result in fecal incontinence (Sharkey and Hanlon 1989).

If damage occurs to the CNS, bowel function is initiated and regulated without mediation by the cerebral cortex. The condition is referred to as a neurogenic bowel. Five types of neurogenic bowel have been identified, but only three are common: uninhibited, reflex, and autonomous neurogenic bowels. Motor paralytic and sensory paralytic bowel types are rarely seen. The types of neurogenic bowel dysfunction are defined by the level of injury or disease and response to sensory and motor tests (Table 5-1). A paralytic ileus usually follows spinal cord trauma and is part of the phenomenon known as spinal shock. A Bowel Management program is not begun until bowel sounds return. A lubricated, gloved finger inserted into the rectum will elicit contraction of the internal anal sphincter if the reflex arc is intact. The presence of soft or impacted stool can be assessed at the same time. Prior insertion of an anesthetic cream must precede stimulation of the anal sphincter if a patient has a spinal cord injury at or above the T-6 level, since autonomic dysreflexia can occur.

Autonomic dysreflexia (AD) is a syndrome that refers to an acute episode of unchecked sympathetic reflex activity occurring in 80% of patients with cervical and high thoracic lesions above the T-6 spinal cord segment. AD patients with lesions as low as T-8 have been reported in a few studies (Rudy 1984). AD is a clinical emergency, with immediate treatment required to prevent convulsions, cerebrovascular accident, respiratory arrest, and myocardial accident. It is characterized by severe hypertension with extremes of systolic blood pressure as high as 300 mm Hg and diastolic pressure increases up to 175 mm Hg. The reflex sympathetic vasoconstriction is produced by sensory impulses from the bladder, rectum, or pelvic viscera, which stimulate the sympathetic nervous system as the sensory impulses move up the cord. The lesion blocks the sensory impulses, prevents interpretation by higher nervous centers, and blocks as well reflex inhibition of the sympathetic activity by higher nervous centers (Eichner and Curtis 1990; Sharkey and Hanlon 1989). Vasoconstriction below the lesion and compensatory vasodilation above produce the complex set of signs and symptoms characteristic of autonomic dysreflexia:

Hypertension	Trouble breathing or stuffy nose
Feeling anxious or nervous	No temperature but chills
Throbbing or pounding headache	Cool clammy skin below level of injury
Blurred vision	Perspiring above level of injury
Slow pulse rate	Red flushed face with profuse sweating
Nausea	Piloerection (goose bumps) upper body

The immediate nursing intervention is to elevate the head of the bed so that orthostatic hypotension will occur (contraindications to elevation are unstable spinal injury or cervical traction). Blood pressure must be monitored every 3 minutes to 5 minutes while attempting to remove the sensory stimulus. If careful bladder and catheter assessment rule out a distended bladder, the anal area should be anesthetized with Nupercaine ointment and the rectum checked carefully for constipation or impaction. An impaction must be removed gently (Markman 1988). (The specific medical treatment for AD can be found in standard neurosurgical or rehabilitation nursing texts; see Martin, Holt, and Hicks 1981; Rudy 1984; Dittmar 1989.)

Bowel function is classified as uninhibited when lesions are cortical or subcortical above the C-1 vertebral level (e.g., cerebrovascular accident, multiple sclerosis, and specific types of brain trauma and tumors). Upper motor neurons (UMNs) located in the cerebral cortex, internal capsule, brainstem, or spinal cord are damaged, while lower motor neurons (LMNs) located in the anterior gray matter throughout the spinal cord are spared. Bowel sensation and saddle sensation are intact, and the bulbocavernosus reflex is intact or increased (Table 5 – 1). Awareness of the urge to defecate and voluntary control of the anal sphincter are decreased because the brain is unable to interpret sensory impulses to defecate. Activation of the sacral reflex produces defecation and is accompanied by a sense of urgency. Digital stimulation is discouraged because it is painful (Cannon 1981; Sharkey and Hanlon 1989).

Reflex neurogenic (automatic) bowel function is associated with spinal cord lesions above the T-12 to L-1 vertebral level (e.g., quadriplegia, high thoracic paraplegia, and multiple sclerosis). The lesions affect UMNs and sensory tracts but spare LMNs. In most instances, bowel sensation and saddle sensation are decreased or absent, and the bulbocavernosus reflex is increased (Table 5 – 1). Complete or incomplete nerve pathway interruption occurs between the brain and spinal cord with loss of voluntary control of defecation and the anal sphincter. Sacral nerve segments S2-S3-S4 are intact, permitting the reflex arc to function in response to rectal distension from accumulated feces. Fecal incontinence occurs suddenly, without warning, as a mass reflex. A stimulus-response type of bowel control can be developed using the mass reflex. Incontinence episodes between mass reflex emptyings are infrequent due to parasympathetic innervation (via sacral segments), which maintains external anal sphincter tone. Persons with injuries below T-5 and intact abdominal muscles may use those muscles to bear down to increase pressure within the abdominal cavity to help open the external anal sphincter in coordination with contraction of the rectal portion of the bowel. Manual pressure and digital stimulation may also be used (Cannon 1981; Sharkey and Hanlon 1989).

Autonomous neurogenic (flaccid) bowel function occurs with spinal cord injuries or lesions at or below the T-12 to L-1 vertebral level (e.g., paraplegia, intervertebral disk syndrome, tumors, and spina bifida). The lesions affect the LMNs. Saddle sensation is decreased or absent, and the bulbocavernosus reflex is absent (Table 5–1). Cerebral control of defecation and voluntary control of the anal sphincter are absent. Since the lesion directly involves the S2-S3-S4 segments and destroys spinal reflex arc activity, no reflex emptying of the bowel occurs. Both the internal and external anal sphincters lack tone; therefore, with little or no resistance to stool in the rectum, incontinence occurs frequently (Cannon 1981; Sharkey and Hanlon 1989).

Idiopathic fecal incontinence is a neurogenic type of fecal incontinence found in 80% of incontinent patients who have no evidence of a generalized neurologic disorder (Penninckx 1987). A denervation injury that produces abnormalities of the pelvic floor and external sphincter is thought to be the underlying mechanism resulting from chronic straining, childbearing, childbirth, or rectal prolapse (Loening-Baucke 1990). A minor degree of bowel incontinence or seepage following a hemorrhoidectomy may result from removal of a portion of vascular tissue in the anal cushions. The highly vascular anal cushions are formed by folds in the thick anal lining and interdigitate to plug the anus at rest (Gibbons, Bannister, Trowbridge, and Read 1986).

Despite a high degree of motivation, for many individuals maintaining continence is a challenge. The absence of intact anorectal sensation, damage to internal or external anal sphincters or the puborectalis muscle, changes in rectal compliance, or poor access to a toileting facility may be difficult to overcome.

Diet Modifications

A diet high in fiber is an essential component in the prevention and treatment of a wide variety of bowel dysfunctions. Whole grain cereals and breads, legumes, nuts, leafy vegetables, and raw fruits with skins are examples of high-fiber foods. Some fruits, such as bananas and prunes, have laxative properties as well as being high in fiber. The fiber serves as a bulking agent and helps to hold water. The net result is a stool that remains soft and bulky during its passage through the bowel, provided 2500 mL of fluid are ingested every day (McLane and McShane 1986).

Regular meals and a well-balanced diet help develop a systematic bowel routine and decrease episodes of spontaneous stools. Three servings of vegetables and fruits (two raw with skins) are recommended daily. Cereals, baked goods, and meatloaf can be enriched with unprocessed bran and wheat germ, both inexpensive sources of fiber. Gradual addition of dietary fiber prevents the side effects of flatulence, distension, and diarrhea (Sharkey and Hanlon 1989).

Certain foods increase or decrease intestinal transit time. Overconsumption of dairy products and refined foods, such as white bread and white rice, increases the risk of constipation. An increased risk of diarrhea is associated with overconsumption of caffeine, spicy foods, and alcohol. Davis et al. (1986) recommend a breakfast free of fatty acids to trigger the gastrocolic-duodeno-colic reflex. Fatty acids slow down the digestive process and delay reflex stimulation.

The adequacy of a diet for nutrients, balance, and facilitation of elimination must be determined. The patient's diet, fluid intake, appetite, and physical condition require careful assessment. Evaluation of preonset habits includes personal food preferences, vegetarianism, and ethnic, cultural, and religious influences on diet (Hui 1983).

Physical Exercise

Physical activity and regular physical exercise increase gastrointestinal motility and help to regulate and control bowel dysfunctions. Persons with disabilities must be taught how to perform activities of daily living (ADLs) with minimal assistance. As functional improvement continues, many can be taught how to shift their weight in bed or in a wheelchair. The arms of a wheelchair can be used to raise the body for a few moments if upper arm strength can be developed. Doing push-ups on the toilet seat while doing a Valsalva maneuver is an effective technique to speed up bowel action for many quadriplegics and paraplegics. Patients can be taught how to do abdominal massage, proceeding from the right groin upward, across the abdomen, and down to the left groin to stimulate and hasten bowel action (Cannon 1981).

Pelvic Floor Exercises

Pelvic floor exercises (PFEs) are repetitive contractions and relaxation of the anal sphincter and the puborectalis muscles (25 to 30 times) three times daily. Each contraction should be maintained for 3 seconds or 4 seconds and then repeated in staccato machine-gun fashion without tensing the muscles of the legs, buttocks, or abdomen (McCormick and Burgio 1984). If contractions are maintained for 1 minute, sphincters tend to fatigue and then go into a refractory stage (Penninckx 1987). PFEs are a component in the management of incontinence associated with neuromuscular disorders, incontinence following rectal surgery (e.g., hemorrhoidectomy), and so-called idiopathic incontinence.

PFEs may be incorporated as a component of biofeedback training, a trial-and-error learning process used to help patients recognize rectal distension and provide a visual display of external anal sphincter contractions. Wald (1989) identified the following prerequisites for successful biofeedback training: a motivated patient with the ability to comprehend and follow directions, some degree of rectal sensation, and the ability to generate a squeeze pressure. He described a success rate of 70% for patients who meet the criteria, with most incontinent adults responding after one training session, including patients with diabetes, nondeforming trauma, sphincter surgery, and idiopathic incontinence. Some researchers are less enthusiastic about the effectiveness of biofeedback (Penninckx 1987; Loening-Baucke 1990). Wald emphasized the need for component analysis and controlled outcome studies to identify the mechanisms by which biofeedback works. This recommendation was supported in another review of biofeedback studies. The authors pointed out that effectiveness did not entirely depend on the variable trained. They concluded that nonspecific treatment effects, such as emotional support by staff or behavioral modifications, may be equally important in the efficacy of biofeedback training for fecal incontinence (Bielefeldt, Enck, and Wienbeck 1990).

Temporary Medications and Use of Digital Stimulation

Laxatives and enemas are temporary measures used to ensure a clean bowel prior to the initiation of a Bowel Management program for most types of bowel dysfunction. Diarrhea associated with irritable bowel syndrome, infection, lactose intolerance, and use of antibiotics is an exception. A stool softener, such as dioctyl sodium sulfosuccinate (Colace), and bulk-forming agents may be used as part of a Bowel Management program. Colace 100 mg two to three times a day may be given initially and the dose adjusted to produce a stool of the desired consistency. A bulking agent, such as Metamucil, may be necessary until dietary adjustments provide a patient with sufficient natural fiber.

Suppositories (dulcolax and glycerin) act by irritating the bowel wall, which results in reflex peristalsis and emptying of the bowel. Suppositories must be inserted at room temperature and placed in contact with the bowel wall to produce the desired effect. Manual removal of some stool may be necessary to ensure proper placement. Both suppositories have disadvantages; dulcolax suppositories may cause injury to mucous membranes, and glycerin suppositories, although milder, may produce abdominal cramping. After establishing the reflex-response defecation pattern, digital stimulation may be substituted for suppositories. A well-lubricated, gloved index finger is used to perform digital stimulation to relax the internal anal sphincter. Rotation against the anal sphincter wall for 30 seconds to 2 minutes will relax the sphincter. The finger is removed, and reflex peristalsis produces evacuation (Sharkey and Hanlon 1989). Digital stimulation to perianal skin may initiate reflex activity and sphincter relaxation.

Development and Implementation of a Toileting Routine

Timing is the critical element when a predictable pattern of elimination is the desired goal. If suppositories are part of the routine, they are inserted within 1 hour of the triggering meal, usually breakfast, to take advantage of gastrocolic and duodenocolic reflexes, which are strongest when the stomach is empty (Lewis 1988; Davis et al. 1986). Fatty acids must be excluded from the triggering meal since they delay reflex stimulation and slow digestion. Some patients may require anorectal stimulation to trigger reflex relaxation of the internal anal sphincter. Rectal stimulation may be done by the patient or caretaker and usually results in sphincter relaxation in about 30 seconds. Fifteen minutes after the triggering meal or after rectal stimulation, the patient should be placed on the toilet or commode or in a side-lying position for evacuation of feces. Rectal stimulation may be repeated a second time if the first attempt does not produce results. Sitting on a toilet or a commode should be limited to 20 minutes. Stool softeners and bulking agents may be used if stool consistency is too firm and feces are difficult to expel. A minimum of 2500 to 3000 mL of fluids are required in order for stool softeners and bulking agents to be effective.

Instruction of Patient and Family/Caregivers

Instruction of patients and family members or caregivers is an ongoing part of a Bowel Management program. Patients with functional disabilities or spinal cord injuries must become proficient in directing others in their Bowel Management and other aspects of daily living. Family members or caregivers are familiar with the environment within which the patient will be living and are able to identify potential barriers that require modification of a program or modification of the home environment. Their understanding of and participation in all aspects of patient care and their emotional support may make the difference in a patient's or family member's decision to return home or to seek placement in a nursing home.

Patients and family members will benefit from understanding all of the components of Bowel Management — diet, fluids, exercise, and toileting routine. In some situations, caregivers must develop skill in the insertion of suppositories, anorectal digital stimulation, and manual removal of feces. If a patient has an injury at or above the T-6 vertebral segment, family members or caregivers must be taught how to recognize and treat AD.

Flow Sheets for Documentation and Evaluation

Flow sheets are needed for documentation and evaluation of a Bowel Management program because of its complexity and the prolonged time period required for implementation of the various components. Sharkey and Hanlon's "record of bowel movements" (1989, p. 219) is an example of a bowel elimination record that could be used. It includes the following items: date and time, description of bowel movement, medications, suppositories, and diet. Each component of the Bowel Management program is followed by a list of abbreviations for the descriptors. Type and frequency of exercise, including pelvic floor exercises, desired frequency (goal), time of triggering meal, type and time of rectal stimulation, place of evacuation, and amount of assistance required, could be added to maintain a more complete record. Flow sheets provide a quick summary of a patient's daily, weekly, and monthly progress with a minimum of writing.

DIAGNOSTIC ASSESSMENT

Evaluation of bowel dysfunction begins with a history of a patient's current pattern of bowel elimination and perceived change in pattern associated with an alteration in health and/or functional status. History of a patient's pattern of elimination includes consistency, frequency, and size of bowel movements; associated symptoms of pain, urgency, and excess flatulence; frequency of diarrhea, incontinence, and constipation; past history of anorectal surgery or trauma, diabetes, inflammatory bowel disease, neurological disease, and laminectomy; and number and complications of vaginal deliveries.

Patients presenting with idiopathic fecal incontinence may require anorectal manometric assessment, including anal resting pressure, maximal squeeze pressure, rectal sensations and elastic properties of the rectal wall, and responses of internal and external sphincters to rectal distension. Rectal infusion of saline is used to assess overall function of continence mechanisms (Loening-Baucke 1990; Bielefeldt, Enck, and Wienbeck 1990). Proctoscopy and rectoscopy are used to rule out anal fistula and inflammatory bowel disease (Penninckx 1987). Rosen et al. (1986) described a bedside method for evaluation of the anal sphincter and the puborectalis muscle. The lubricated index finger of the examiner is placed approximately 7 cm into the rectum and is hooked posteriorly. The patient is instructed to tighten the muscles to avoid defecation. The puborectalis muscle should move anteriorly, narrowing the anal canal and constricting the finger.

Incontinence frequently accompanies other bowel dysfunctions, such as diarrhea, colonic constipation, and fecal impaction. Colonic constipation, fecal impaction, and incontinence can all be viewed as stool retention disorders. Groups at risk for developing bowel dysfunctions and related nursing diagnoses are summarized in Table 5 – 2.

TABLE 5-2.   POPULATIONS AT RISK FOR BOWEL DYSFUNCTIONS

AT-RISK GROUPS	RELATED NURSING DIAGNOSES
Economically deprived, disabled, elderly, persons living alone, homebound, terminally ill	Colonic constipation, perceived constipation, Bowel Incontinence
Spinal cord injury (UMN)	Bowel Incontinence
Spinal cord injury (LMN)	Stool retention/Bowel Incontinence
Irritable bowel syndrome, inflammatory bowel disease	Diarrhea (may alternate with constipation), Bowel Incontinence
Postpartum (multiparas), laminectomy, hemorrhoidectomy, sphincter surgery, diabetes, trauma, chronic straining	Idiopathic Bowel Incontinence
Institutionalized frail elderly, prolonged immobility	Fecal impaction, Bowel Incontinence

SUGGESTED PROTOCOL FOR BOWEL MANAGEMENT

Tentative goals and components of a bowel control program must be shared with the patient and family members or other caretaker prior to its initiation. Delineation of goals and selection of components are based on the patient's functional status, nursing diagnosis, patient environment, and patient, family, and caregiver preferences.

1.   Provide each person with a list of components and associated goals (Table 5-3), and use the list to guide a discussion of how the bowel program would progress.

2.   Try to identify the primary caregiver, and elicit information about potential barriers to home care.

3.   Allay initial anxiety as much as possible by being alert to areas of information that seem unusually stressful for anyone. Try to find out what there is about the subject matter that heightens anxiety.

4.   Learn the patient, family members', and caregiver's level of knowledge about bowel elimination, and correct misunderstandings.

5.   Assist the patient in selecting the time of day for bowel evacuation. Discuss gastrointestinal reflexes and the triggering meal.

6.   Assist the patient in selecting a comfortable place for the bowel program. Point out the advantages of a toilet or bedside commode (e.g., effects of gravity). Position the patient on the left side if the bed must be used.

7.   Demonstrate the insertion of suppositories or digital stimulation if that is part of the bowel program. Gently rotate a gloved and lubricated index finger in the rectum for 30 to 60 seconds. Gently remove some stool in the rectum prior to inserting a suppository. Set up a time for a return demonstration.

8.   Assist the patient to a toilet or commode 15 to 20 minutes after the triggering meal. Limit time on the commode to 20 minutes. Digital stimulation may be repeated (if part of program) if defecation does not occur.

9.   Demonstrate abdominal massage and how to do push-ups while the patient is on the toilet or commode.

10.   Use mild soap and water to clean skin in the perianal area. Use some type of ointment, such as Desinex or A&D, to protect skin if it looks red.

11.   Discourage the use of laxatives and enemas.

12.   Provide written information about a high-fiber diet and use of bulk forming agents, such as Metamucil. Alert the patient to notice gas-forming foods and foods that cause diarrhea or constipation, and delete them from the diet.

TABLE 5–3. COMPONENTS AND GOALS OF A BOWEL
MANAGEMENT PROGRAM

COMPONENTS	GOALS
Understanding of continence/in-continence mechanisms	To complete an accurate diagnostic assessment To identify type of bowel dysfunction To prevent and treat complications
Diet modifications	To achieve desired stool consistency To trigger gastrocolic-duodenocolic reflex
Pelvic floor exercises	To strengthen anal sphincters To prevent episodes of incontinence
Physical exercise	To stimulate peristalis To strengthen upper arms to aid in transfer
Progressive use of suppositories and digital stimulation	To avoid irritation of colon To stimulate reflex peristalis To relax internal anal sphincter To avoid stool retention and drying of stool
Plan and implement toileting routine	To coordinate triggering meal with use of suppositories or rectal stimulation To take advantage of gastrointestinal reflexes To schedule time for assistance with transfer from bed to commode or toilet To agree upon stool frequency (e.g., every other day)
Instruction of patient, family, or caregiver	To identify primary caregiver To facilitate successful home care of patient
Flow sheets for documentation and evaluation	To ensure accurate and complete documentation of care To recognize any change in pattern of elimination To facilitate evaluation of effectiveness of care

13.   Provide written instructions about pelvic floor exercises if they are part of a bowel program: "Contract and relax anal sphincter without tensing muscles of buttocks, legs, or abdomen. Do this 25 to 30 times, three times a day. Maintain contraction for only 3 seconds or 4 seconds."

14.   Assist the patient to select exercises and implement a program of daily physical exercise. Coach the exercise session as needed.

15.   Provide written instructions about when to call the nurse for assistance: "Blood or excessive mucus in stool; unable or unwilling to eat food and drink sufficient liquids; severe constipation or diarrhea that lasts more than 2 days; pain or fullness in abdomen; perianal skin breakdown; any concerns or questions about program."

16.   Provide flow sheets and assist the patient, family member, and caregiver with keeping timely and accurate records of diet, exercise, stools, and so forth.

17.   Change only one component of a bowel program at a time.

18.   Provide written instruction about signs and symptoms of Autonomic Dysreflexia for patients with cervical and high thoracic lesions. Include ways to prevent its occurrence and emergency treatment. Stress the life-threatening nature of AD.

CASE STUDIES

Case Study 1

JA, a 37-year-old woman, was the mother of five children, and the wife of RA, a farmer who raised wheat in a midwestern state. JA was referred by her family physician to the continence clinic at a medical center 30 miles from her home.

The admission interview was conducted by a registered nurse. JA reported use of continence aids to manage frequent seepage of stool, which began after a hemorrhoidectomy. Surgery was performed 4 days after a vaginal delivery of her fifth child, a boy weighing 10 pounds, 2 ounces. The hemorrhoids were very painful throughout the last trimester of pregnancy and during the delivery. JA elected to have the surgery done in the immediate postpartum period because her oldest daughter was home from college for the summer.

JA was 5 feet, 5 inches, weighed 128 pounds, and reported that she ate three meals a day without between-meal snacks. A description of foods eaten in an average day revealed that her diet was low in fiber. She ate fruit with every meal but disliked raw and green vegetables and whole grain cereals and breads.

Frequent episodes of constipation (two to three times a month) were reported. Mornings were very busy in JA's household, and she often delayed responding to an urge to defecate because the children needed her. She used milk of magnesia almost every week to prevent or treat constipation.

JA's primary exercise was caring for husband, the children, and her home. She and her husband went bowling every Wednesday evening and visited her parents every other Sunday after church. The remainder of their social life revolved around their family life and the children's activities.

Anorectal manometric assessment and proctoscopy were done by Dr. I, who reported a less than normal maximal squeeze pressure, intact internal and external anal sphincters, a small rectal fissure, and perianal redness. Dr. I suggested a trial of pelvic floor exercises, addition of fiber to her diet, use of Desitin ointment for perianal redness, and regular physical activity three times a week. He recommended that she return in 2 months, and if she had not improved he would begin a course of biofeedback. JA expressed relief that she did not require additional surgery and agreed to follow Dr. I's recommendations.

Nurse R reviewed Dr. I's findings with JA and responded to her questions about biofeedback. Patient goals were mutually agreed upon and included decrease in seepage of stool, decrease in use of milk of magnesia, reduction in number of episodes of constipation, and healing of perianal area.

Written instructions about how to do pelvic floor exercises were discussed. JA was told to contract and relax the anal sphincter and puborectalis muscles 25 to 30 times three times a day and in conjunction with a bowel movement. She was instructed to hold the contractions for no more than 3 seconds or 4 seconds without tensing the muscles of the legs, buttocks, or abdomen.

Diagrams were used to help JA understand the physiology of normal bowel elimination. She was encouraged to respond to the urge to defecate without delay. A list of high-fiber foods, sample recipes, and easy ways to increase fiber in the diet gradually were discussed. The function of fiber in conjunction with 2500 to 3000 mL of fluids daily in the production of a soft, formed stool was emphasized. The temporary use of a bulk-forming agent, such as Metamucil, was suggested until diet modifications could be made.

Nurse R prepared a flow sheet for JA to document her diet, exercises, and bowel movements. The flow sheet serves as feedback and helps to reinforce changes in behavior. Suggestions were given for improving rectal hygiene, including cleansing the area with mild soap and water and using Desitin ointment to prevent skin breakdown. Ways to increase exercise were reviewed with JA, who expressed interest in swimming at the local high school, which was open to adults twice a week.

JA telephoned 2 months later and cancelled her appointment because the baby was ill. She reported progress in all areas: stool seepage was rare; laxative use was reduced (no milk of magnesia for 3 weeks); stools were softer and easier to pass; episodes of constipation were reduced; Metamucil was used every day; and some progress had been made in increasing fiber (whole wheat bread was used instead of white). She had been too busy to start swimming but hoped to have time in the near future.

Case Study 2

JR, a 19-year-old student, was a victim of a hit-and-run accident that occurred while he was riding a motorcycle to a part-time job at a local newspaper. He was admitted to the neuro intensive care unit of the university hospital with a concussion, multiple cuts and contusions, and a spinal cord injury at the T-10 vertebral level. He remained in spinal shock for 6 days and was transferred to an intermediate-care neurological unit 7 days after admission.

JR's parents, two older brothers, and a younger sister took turns driving 94 miles each way from their rural home in another state to be with him. JR's major concerns were his damaged motorcycle and missing his final exams. He felt confident that he would regain use of his lower extremities and control over bowel and bladder functioning. He was indifferent about learning anything related to a Bowel Management program or Intermittent Catheterization since he considered his situation temporary. He cooperated with his caregivers but remained a passive recipient of care. He instructed family members to come after lunch so they would not be around during his bowel care, which was done after breakfast. JR tolerated a light diet by his ninth day postinjury, and bowel sounds indicated return of peristalsis. JR reported that constipation had been a problem preinjury. Metamucil was given each morning to help produce a soft formed stool.

MA, the primary nurse for JR, enlisted the help of the family to begin learning about his care. The oldest brother obtained JR's permission to learn about the Bowel Management program so that JR could leave the hospital sooner and complete his recovery at home. The components and goals of the program were shared with the brother and JR, who still showed reluctance to become involved in self-care activities. The nurse crossed out the components on the list that were not appropriate for JR.

MA suggested evacuation of JR's bowel every other day. Initially a mild laxative, Senokot, was given every other night, and a glycerin suppository was used the following morning. JR was turned on his left side, and 20 minutes later, perianal digital stimulation was used to help evacuate the stool. MA used a well-lubricated gloved finger to check the rectum for complete evacuation. On two occasions, manual removal of some stool was required. During the procedure, MA described what she was doing and responded to questions posed by JR's brother. Abdominal massage was demonstrated, and a series of daily exercises were agreed upon, including active range of motion of upper extremities and passive range of motion of lower extremities.

During the next 2 weeks, JR's brother took over the bowel care with supervision by the nurse. Glycerin suppositories were replaced by rectal stimulation, Senokot was discontinued, and a bedside commode was used for stool evacuation. A high-fiber diet was substituted for the Metamucil. Flow sheets used for documentation were reviewed, and it was noted that JR had only one spontaneous stool between the alternate-day bowel program.

On the twenty-seventh day postinjury, JR reported the return of some feeling in his legs. Subsequently he became more interested in participating in self-care activities. He required a minimum of instruction since he had been listening to the nurse instruct his brother. Within a week, JR was telling caregivers how to proceed with his bowel care. On day 38 postinjury, JR was transferred to a rehabilitation setting closer to his home. A copy of the bowel program and copies of the preceding week's flow sheet were used for discharge planning and accompanied JR to the new setting.

RECOMMENDATIONS FOR PRACTICE AND RESEARCH

Since fecal incontinence is a major factor in the decision to institutionalize a family member, objective assessment of anorectal parameters should be done prior to nursing home placement. Patients with anatomic deficits might be candidates for surgical intervention. A summary of physical signs, objective measurements, relevant history, and response to intervention strategies should accompany a patient's transfer to a new setting, home, rehabilitation hospital, or nursing home. The comprehensive information can be used to guide the selection of components of an effective Bowel Management program and serve as a baseline for systematic clinical evaluation of one Bowel Management intervention (see Penninckx 1987 or Maas and Specht 1991 for an assessment guide).

The paucity of research (both medical and nursing) in the control of bowel dysfunctions, especially incontinence, is a cause for concern. The actual number of persons suffering from Bowel Incontinence is unknown. Since individuals at risk for developing Bowel Incontinence are well known, epidemiologic studies need to be done to determine the actual incidence of bowel incontinence. Intervention components should be tested in high-risk groups to determine the effectiveness of preventing incontinence (e.g., teaching multiparas with a history of constipation how to do pelvic floor exercises). The emotional support of health professionals and family members/caregivers and behavior modification strategies are variables that require a higher priority in nursing's research agenda. Bowel Management programs for persons with spinal cord injuries need to be tested for their effectiveness. The needs of family members and other caregivers must be considered in developing and implementing plans of care.

The burden of incontinence falls on patients, families, health care professionals and resources, and the environment. The development, distribution, and acceptance of "continence aids" is a poor substitute for programs that regulate and control bowel dysfunctions.

REFERENCES

Alterescu, V. 1986. Theoretical foundations for an approach to fecal incontinence. *Journal of Enterostoma Therapy* 13:44–48.

Bielefeldt, K., Enck, P., and Wienbeck M. 1990. Diagnosis and treatment of fecal incontinence. *Digestive Diseases* 8:179–188.

Cannon, B. 1981. Bowel function. In N. Martin, N.B. Holt, and D. Hicks (eds.), *Comprehensive rehabilitation nursing* (pp. 224–241). New York: McGraw-Hill.

Davis, A., Nagelhout, M.J., Hoban, M., and Barnard, B. 1986. Bowel management: A quality assurance approach to upgrading programs. *Journal of Gerontological Nursing* 12(5):13–17.

Dittmar, S. 1989. *Process of rehabilitation nursing.* St. Louis: C.V. Mosby Co.

Eichner, S., and Curtis, R.L. 1990. Alterations in motor function. In C. Porth (ed.), *Pathophysiology: Concepts of altered health states,* 3d ed. (pp. 893–928). Philadelphia: J.B. Lippincott.

Gibbons, C.P., Bannister, J.J., Trowbridge, E.A., and Read, N.W. 1986. Role of anal cushions in maintaining continence. *Lancet* 1(8486):886–888.

Hanak, M. 1990. *Education guide for spinal cord injury nurses.* New York: American Association of Spinal Cord Injury Nurses.

Hui, Y.H. 1983. *Human nutrition and diet therapy.* Belmont, Calif.: Wadsworth Health Science Division.

Lewis, N.A. 1988. Nursing management of altered patterns of elimination. *Journal of Home Health Care Practice* 1:35–42.

Loening-Baucke, V. 1990. Biofeedback therapy for fecal incontinence. *Digestive Diseases* 7:112–124.

Maas, M., and Specht, J. 1991. Bowel incontinence. In M. Maas, K.C. Buckwalter, and M. Hardy (eds.)., *Nursing diagnosis and interventions for the elderly* (pp. 169–180). Redwood City, Calif.: Addison-Wesley Nursing.

McCormick, K.A., and Burgio, K.L. 1984. Incontinence: An update on nursing care measures. *Journal of Gerontological Nursing* 10(10):16–19, 22, 23.

McLane, A.M., and McShane, R.E. 1986. Elimination. In J.M. Thompson et al., *Clinical nursing* (pp. 2059–2075). St. Louis: C.V. Mosby Co.

McLane A.M., and McShane, R.E. 1991. Constipation. In M. Maas, K.C. Buckwalter, and M. Hardy, *Nursing diagnoses and interventions for the elderly* (pp. 147–158). Redwood City, Calif.: Addison-Wesley Nursing.

Markman, L.J. 1988. Bladder and bowel management of the spinal cord injured patient. *Plastic Surgical Nursing* 8(4):141–145.

Martin, N., Holt, N.B., and Hicks, D. 1981. *Comprehensive rehabilitation nursing.* New York: McGraw-Hill.

Ozer, M.N., and Bayless, J.E. 1987. Managing your bowels. In L. Phillips, M. Ozer, P. Axelson, and H. Chizeck (eds.), *Spinal cord injury: A guide for patient and family* (pp. 111–123). New York: Raven Press.

Pemberton, J.H., and Kelly, K.A. 1986. Achieving enteric continence: Principles and application. *Mayo Clinic Proceedings* 61:586–599.

Penninckx, F.M. 1987. Faecal incontinence. *International Journal of Colorectal Disease* 2:173–186.

Rosen, L., Khubchandani, I.T., Sheets, J.A., Stasik, J.J., and Riether, R.D. 1986. Management of anal incontinence. *American Family Physician* 33(3):129–137.

Rudy, E.B. 1984. *Advanced neurological and neurosurgical nursing.* St. Louis: C.V. Mosby Co.

Sharkey, E.L., and Hanlon, D. 1989. Bowel elimination. In S. Dittmar (ed.), *Process of rehabilitation nursing.* St. Louis: C.V. Mosby Co.

Wald, A. 1989. Disorders of defecation and fecal continence. *Cleveland Clinic Journal of Medicine* 56(5):491–501.

6

POSITIONING

JENNIFER M. LOEPER

The ability to move around is critical to performing self-care independently. Through movement, we communicate our emotions and intentions and perform those tasks needed for survival.

When an insult occurs to the central nervous system, movement is impaired. It may be temporary or permanent, depending on the location and severity of the insult. At this point, it becomes imperative that the caregiver initiate a plan that minimizes the impact of the insult and maximizes the remaining functions related to movement.

Positioning, by definition, implies a proactive response to the hazards of immobility. It is a method of maintaining posture in order to prevent contractures and pressure ulcers. It includes not only the posture assumed when standing but also when sitting and lying down.

For the purpose of this discussion, attention will be focused on those who suffer a neurological insult to the central nervous system and less on patients who are immobilized because of treatment-related or maturational limitations or because of an acute episode of illness.

In order to treat a patient with impaired mobility, what goes on not only in therapy but also during the rest of the day is of primary importance to the caregiver. If the patient moves abnormally during the day when not in therapy, no gain can be achieved or maintained. Positioning is a key factor in extinguishing abnormal movement and promoting successful rehabilitation of the patient.

PHYSIOLOGY OF MOVEMENT

The past education of nurses in the care of the immobilized patient was based on the idea that once a stroke or damage to a neuron occurred, or the central nervous system was injured, the loss was permanent, and nothing could be done to promote recovery. All compensatory techniques and nursing activities were focused on the "good" side, and the impaired side of the body was neglected. It is now known that this approach only reinforced the patient's neglect of that side.

In order to understand the rationale behind the Positioning of a patient with impaired mobility, it is necessary to examine the physiology of movement and the developmental sequence of motor activity.

Karl and Berta Bobath, pioneers in the treatment of adult hemiplegia, along with other researchers, have developed an approach designed to retrain the affected side of the body. The goal of treatment is to suppress abnormal patterns of movement while promoting normal postural control. This goal is achieved in part by correct positioning of the patient at all times (Gee and Passarella 1985).

Reflex mechanisms go through stages of development from spinal to cortical levels of activity (Johnstone 1978). Tonic reflexes are those that respond to stimulation of the sensory nerve endings. This is the most basic response. At the other end of development are the cortical reflex mechanisms, which give the individual voluntary control over a response.

Muscle tone is present to some degree in all voluntary muscles. Tone is higher in the muscles that hold the body in an upright position—the antigravity muscles. These muscles are located in the extensors of the lower limbs, trunk and neck, the forearm flexors, and shoulder depressors. Muscle tone, reflexive in nature, is a response to stimuli and weight transference.

Balance reactions and smooth movement depend on normal postural tone. Various postures depend on the ability to move body parts in a sequential manner; those needed for the task are stimulated, and those not needed are inhibited, and the movement is accomplished. Balance is important because everything we do is against gravity and requires constant body readjustment to maintain balance. K. Bobath (1990) describes this as the "normal postural reflex mechanism"; it functions in an intact adult brain and supports the refined movement.

Children have a central nervous system that is immature and primitive in response to any stimuli. The small child's body responds automatically and mechanically. As the child matures, higher centers are more developed, refined, and exhibit more inhibition over movement. The tasks accomplished are more sophisticated and complex. When an injury occurs to the brain, the reflexes again become more primitive in nature. The lower centers lose the control of the higher centers, and the reflexes become exaggerated. A lesion in the central nervous system, especially of the upper motor neuron, interferes with normal postural control. The result is abnormal patterns of coordination of movement, posture, and muscle tone. Since inhibition of patterns of activity occurs in the higher centers, inhibition is lost, and spasticity results.

A pattern of spasm develops in which retraction of the affected shoulder with depression and internal rotation occurs. The forearm is flexed and pronated. The pelvis retracts, and the leg externally rotates. The hip, knee, and ankle extend on the affected side with inversion and plantar flexion of the ankle. The trunk flexes laterally toward the affected side (Loeper et al. 1986).

Synergies—combined contractions of muscles that work together as a unit without cortical control—develop that are primitive in nature and abnormal in the adult. Usually a synergistic pattern of tonic contraction develops as a result of excessive tone in the antigravity muscles. For example, in the upper limb when an attempt to lift the arm is made, the flexor synergy of an elevated and retracted scapula, abducted and externally rotated shoulder, flexed elbow, supinated forearm, flexed wrist, and flexed and adducted fingers and thumb is seen. Correct positioning is used to inhibit the excessive tone until cortical control can be reestablished (Davies 1985).

These movement patterns should not be confused with spasticity, an involuntary response to a stimulus. Synergies are voluntary patterns of movement used when a person performs a task. The synergies are stereotyped movements, and the effort used by the patient is always the same regardless of the demand (Davies 1985).

The goal of rehabilitation is to reduce to a minimum the spasticity that may develop. At the same time, because there is a lack of cortical control, spasticity will develop (Johnstone 1978). Therein lies the challenge for the nurse. One method of controlling spasticity is Positioning—in this case, Positioning that uses the antispasm pattern of control at all times. The antispasm pattern consists of (1) protraction of the shoulder with external rotation, (2) forearm extension with supination, (3) finger extension with abduction, (4) protraction of the pelvis with internal rotation of the leg, (5) hip, knee, and ankle flexion, and (6) elongation of the trunk on the affected side.

Immobility, once thought of as a treatment modality, has been proved to present additional hazards to an already compromised patient. Immobility, whether it is treatment induced or a result of the maturational process, can induce contractures in the joints as soon as 3 days. It becomes necessary to begin a Positioning program early in the patient's course of recovery.

Most of the nursing research about Positioning deals with the effects of immobility on the body. Positioning is seen as a countermeasure to the adverse effects of immobility. Nursing, in collaboration with physical and occupational therapy, has researched and developed Positioning programs, especially with newborns in the intensive care units and for patients with insults to the neurological or cardiovascular systems (Fay 1988).

NURSING DIAGNOSES AND CLIENT GROUPS

The nursing diagnosis most appropriate for the intervention of positioning is the North American Nursing Diagnosis Association listing of Impaired Physical Mobility related to alteration in upper and lower limbs. By its very definition, Impaired Physical Mobility is the state in which the individual experiences or is at risk of experiencing limitation of physical movement (Carpenito 1987). A secondary diagnosis that can be considered is Potential for Injury: Physiologic related to increased susceptibility to muscle contractures and impairment of skin integrity due to pressure ulcer development.

The group of patients that is at risk for this diagnosis are those with neuromuscular or musculoskeletal impairment. The person nursing who is most aware of needing the Positioning intervention is the individual who is bedridden or hospitalized and/or who has suffered an insult to the central nervous system—for example, a stroke, brain injury, or spinal cord injury. The population that is less often addressed but still is in need of a positioning program are individuals who, through the maturational process, have a treatment-related impairment, such as a cast or splint that restricts movement, and patients who have pathophysiological impairments, such as multiple sclerosis or lupus.

IMPLEMENTING THE INTERVENTION

Initially, a thorough assessment of the patient is done in order to establish the positioning parameters. Issues taken into consideration include the reason for immobility, whether the patient is able to participate in and/or comprehend the Positioning program, and the degree of physical impairment. Data collected may include the patient's level of consciousness, amount of pain, level of sensation, muscle function, condition of skin, presence or absence of muscle spasticity, and/ or contractures. Once a thorough assessment has occurred, a plan is developed based on the assessment and the resulting nursing diagnosis.

The plan may be so formal that a specific Positioning schedule on a timed basis included in the plan of care is developed, or it may be less formal and driven by the patient's response to certain positions. Standard positioning seems to indicate that a change of position needs to occur every 2 hours. The frequency depends on a number of variables, including comfort, pain, amount of spontaneous movement, condition of skin, amount of sensation, and presence of edema. For these reasons, some people may need to change position every 30 minutes, while others can tolerate a single position for 4 hours. If the patient is unable to communicate or is severely impaired physically, more frequent changes may need to occur.

As a plan is developed, good posture is the standard by which positioning is measured. Good lying posture consists of spinal alignment, knees slightly flexed, feet at right angles in the same direction as the patellae, and spinal curves maintained with hips at about 150 degrees. Good sitting posture permits the feet to rest flat on the floor, hips and knees flexed to right angles, body weight borne on the ischial tuberosities, and the spine directly above the ischia. The trunk is in good alignment, with the arms being supported at elbow level, either by armrests on the chair or resting on a table (Loeper et al. 1986).

An individual who has had a central nervous system insult will experience either weakness or paralysis. Whatever the cause, the presenting symptoms are treated in the same manner although not necessarily to the same degree. Additional compensation for the deficits each person displays are a part of the basic care plan. The nurse, with the input from physical and occupational therapists, develops a Positioning schedule based on the person's needs.

A patient who has a weak or paralyzed side often tends to neglect it. Attention must be focused on this side in order to regain maximum use. These recommendations support this idea by giving sensory input to the weaker side. The goal of care is to reeducate the affected limbs.

Persons recovering from a cerebrovascular accident or a closed-head injury develop synergistic patterns of movement that dictate their activity. Position these patients by placing their limbs "out of synergy." The positioning suggestions that follow assume the patient is an ideal candidate with no added challenge and should be adhered to when possible. Occasionally a patient's preexisting condition may alter the outcomes initially established. Prior fractures with misalignment, arthritis, or skin breakdown may need to be considered and taken into account when developing a Positioning plan.

Supine Bed Positioning

Placing a patient supine is one of the most frequently selected options when beginning a plan of care. The affected upper extremity should be in an abducted position, with the shoulder protracted and externally rotated. The elbow and wrist are extended, while the forearm is supinated. The hand can be left alone if it is resting in an open position. If high tone causes the hand to be drawn into a fist, the patient should be fitted with a night resting splint. Rolled washcloths or other soft devices should not be placed in the hand because they increase feedback into the hand and promote a spastic wrist and finger flexion.

The upper extremity can be positioned by placing a small pillow under the scapula that extends to the arm and supports it in an abducted and slightly elevated position. Place this pillow between the arm and the trunk to prevent the arm from pulling into the synergy if the patient moves, coughs, or yawns.

The lower extremity usually moves into an extensor synergy, which consists of pelvic retraction and elevation, hip extension and internal rotation, knee extension, ankle plantar flexion, and foot inversion. To counteract this, the patient's hip will need to be protracted slightly flexed and held in a neutral position. Flex the knee slightly. Place a flat pillow under the hip to protract the hip with one end of the pillow brought down to position the knee. A footboard used with a patient with spasticity will tend to promote a plantar response or increase the extensor spasticity and should be avoided.

Positioning on the Unaffected Side

If a patient is positioned on the unaffected side, the shoulder is protracted while the affected arm is placed forward on pillows. Extend the elbows and wrist, and place the forearm in neutral or slight pronation. If the hand is fisted, it requires use of a night resting splint.

Protract the affected lower extremity and slightly flex the hip. Place the knee in a few degrees of flexion, and support the leg on pillows. Extent the unaffected leg, and position it behind the upper leg.

If the bed sags, as many beds do, shortening of the trunk on the affected side is encouraged. A small pillow is placed under the unaffected side between the crest of the pelvis and the rib cage. This lengthens the affected side of the trunk and discourages truncal imbalance.

When positioning someone on the unaffected side, use a small pillow under the head to promote neck flexion laterally and stretch the muscles on the affected side.

Positioning on the Affected Side

Lying on the affected side is vital to promoting recovery of function. For Positioning, the affected shoulder is protracted, and the arm is maintained in neutral rotation. The elbow and wrist are extended, and the hand, if open, is left alone. If fisted, it is placed in a night resting splint. A firm cone will suffice while waiting for an appropriate resting splint. The large end of the cone should be on the little finger side, the small end between the thumb and index finger.

Position the lower extremities with the hip of the affected side protracted. The hip and knee are slightly flexed. The upper leg is fully extended and in line with the trunk. Place pillows between the legs to maintain good alignment. Some patients are unable to tolerate full side lying due to arthritic joints, skin problems, or intolerance of the position. For these patients, place pillows just behind the back to allow the patient to roll back against them.

When the patient rolls into the side-lying position on the affected side, care must be taken to protract the scapula in order to avoid pain and trauma to the shoulder joint.

While the patient is lying on the affected side, the problem of trunk shortening is not an issue because now the sag of the bed will lengthen the affected side of the trunk.

Prone Positioning

Many older people or people with respiratory problems may not tolerate the prone position. It does, however, provide hip extension and shoulder retraction and for this reason is a desirable alternative.

For some patient populations, such as those with amputations, spinal cord injuries, closed-head injuries, or skin problems, prone positioning may be very helpful to avoid development of contractures or pressure ulcers.

Position the patient prone in the center of the bed with the feet hanging over the end of the mattress. Do not place the feet against the footboard; rather, allow the feet to hang free. Make sure that the shoulders and hips are in direct alignment with each other. The arms are placed in an alternating position, with one arm overhead and the other arm straight along the side. The face is usually turned toward the overhead arm.

Wheelchair Positioning

The first consideration in wheelchair positioning is to provide a firm back and a firm seat. Firm surfaces allow the pelvis to be centered and stable. A lumbar roll or other support device will provide the patient with the support needed to maintain a proper lordosis. Keep the patient against the firm back and base by using a hip belt, crossing the hip joint at a 45-degree angle. All too frequently, belts are incorrectly placed at the waist or the top of the pelvis. This encourages posterior pelvic tilt and discourages dynamic trunk mobility. If these patients continue to have trunk shortening after the adaptations, a lateral trunk support will be necessary. A pad can also be added behind the scapula or pelvis to discourage retraction on the affected side.

Since the goal of care is to provide a patient with the most functional sitting position, the hips should be at a 90-degree to 95-degree angle, and knees and ankles should be at a 90-degree angle. Feet should be well supported on the footrests. When a stroke or head-injured patient wheels the chair, it is essential that the seat be close enough to the ground to allow the foot to touch the floor without requiring the patient to slide forward in the chair. This may mean that a low seat chair should be ordered.

Upper-extremity positioning is based on the stable, well-supported pelvis and trunk. Many upper-extremity problems are solved with a firm chair back and base. Other necessary equipment may include a lapboard to support the arm, a splint to maintain an open hand, or a cone fixed to the lapboard to maintain the arm in neutral rotation. If persons do not require a lapboard, it is essential that the armrest reach the elbow so the patient does not need to lean toward one side for support.

Finally, a critical component of the Positioning program for patients using wheelchairs is an adequate wheelchair cushion. Assessment for an appropriate cushion is done early in the evaluation process in conjunction with physical and occupational therapists. The cushion promotes good alignment and posture while maintaining skin integrity.

Evaluation

Evaluation is the final step in implementing the nursing care plan for Positioning. Evaluation is ongoing and based on the patient's response. One key indicator is the patient's progress toward the functional outcomes. One would expect to see a decrease in the spastic tone and the flexor or extensor synergies. The patient would continue to progress toward the maximal level of independence and become more participative in daily care. If there is a deterioration of the abilities or an increase in spasticity, the program must be adjusted to address these issues.

CASE STUDY

Mrs. C is a 68-year-old woman who suffered a stroke that left her with left-side hemiplegia. She is 5 feet, 2 inches and weighs 90 pounds. Her appetite is poor, and she often leaves most of her food on the tray. She dislikes getting into a chair and prefers staying in bed because she tires so easily. She spends a lot of time watching television, which is located on the right side of her room. Her sacrum now has a reddened area, and there is a spot on her left heel as well. Her left arm is pulled into flexion, and her hand tends to remain fisted.

The issues to consider when developing a nursing diagnosis include the fact that she has impaired mobility of her left side, her nutritional status is marginal, and she is considered a high-risk patient for pressure ulcer development. The most appropriate diagnoses for Mrs. C are Impaired Physical Mobility related to an alteration in upper and lower limbs and Altered Nutrition: Less Than Body Requirements.

A nursing plan of care was developed to address these issues. Specifically, a Positioning schedule was developed and implemented to prevent further impairment and promote optimal functional recovery of her left side. Initially Mrs. C was repositioned every 2 hours while she was in bed. Lying on her back was avoided because of the reddened areas on her sacrum and her left heel. When she was positioned on her left side, her shoulder was protracted and the left arm in a neutral rotation with the elbow and wrist extended. Her hand at this point would remain open of its own accord. Her lower extremities were flexed at the hip and knee. The left hip was protracted, and pillows were placed between her legs to protect her bony joints.

When Mrs. C was placed on her right side, her shoulder on the left side was protracted and her arm supported forward on pillows. Her elbow and wrist were extended, and her forearm was in neutral. Her left leg was protracted and slightly flexed at the hip. Her left knee was flexed and supported on pillows. Her right knee was extended and positioned behind the left.

The sitting position was avoided until the reddened areas cleared. She was transported to therapies by a cart and wore protective boots. She ate her meals while lying on her side, and needed assistance with preparing her foods and liquids.

The television was moved so that she could watch it while lying on either side.

Mrs. C's nutritional status needed to be addressed. She needed both a high-calorie and a high-protein diet. Collaboration among the nurse, dietitian, and family was initiated. Her favorite foods were determined and provided by both the family and dietary department. It was supplemented with snacks that added calories and protein. A swallowing consultation was orded to rule out any swallowing difficulties.

As the redness disappeared on Mrs. C's sacrum, she was allowed to sit for short periods of time. It was at this point that she was wheeled to the dining room for her meals in order to promote socialization and increase her food consumption.

Mrs. C's tolerance for sitting and side lying increased during her hospitalization. Prone lying was unsuccessful due to an increase in her anxiety level. She stated she never slept on her stomach at home and had no desire to begin now. When she was discharged on day 32 of her admission, she was sent to an intermediate-care area with the long-term goal of returning home.

CONCLUSIONS

Positioning is the key intervention in preventing problems associated with Impaired Mobility. In the individual who has had a cerebral insult, Positioning is the difference between success or failure in achieving the goals of rehabilitation. If the individual has contractures or spasticity that is not controlled, participation in the rehabilitation process is limited.

For the patient who has treatment-induced immobility, Positioning prevents the complications. Skin integrity is maintained, adequate ventilation and circulation are promoted, and the recovery process is shortened.

Since the nurse is the one member of the health care team who sees the patient 24 hours a day, it becomes vital that the nurse develop a Positioning plan upon the patient's admission. Collaboration with the physical and ocupational therapists can help the nurse intervene appropriately and speed the patient's recovery.

REFERENCES

Bobath, B. 1990. *Adult hemiplegia: evaluation and treatment.* 3d ed. London: Heinemann Medical Books.

Boroch, R. 1976. *Elements of rehabilitation in nursing: An introduction.* St. Louis: C. V. Mosby Co.

Carnevali, D. and Bruekner, S. 1970, July. Immobilization: reassessment of a concept. *American Journal of Nursing* 70(7):1502–1507.

Carpenito, L.J. 1987. *Nursing diagnosis: Application to clinical practice.* 2d ed. Philadelphia: J.B. Lippincott.

Davies, P. 1985. *Steps to follow: A guide to the treatment of adult hemiplegia.* Berlin: Springer-Verlag.

Dittmar, S. 1989. *Rehabilitation nursing: Process and application.* St. Louis: C.V. Mosby.

Duncan, P., and Badke, M.B. 1987. *Stroke rehabilitation.* Chicago: Year Book Medical Publishers.

Fay, M.J. 1988, April. The positive effects of positioning. *Neonatal Network* 6(5):23–28.

Gee, Z., and Passarella, P. 1985. *Nursing care of the stroke patient.* Pittsburgh: AREN-Publications.

Johnstone, M. 1978. *Restoration of motor function in the stroke patient.* New York: Livingstone.

Johnstone, M. 1980. *Home care for the stroke patient: Living in a pattern.* New York: Livingstone.

Loeper, J., Flinn, N., Irrgang, S., and Weightman, M. 1986. *Therapeutic positioning and skin care.* Minneapolis: Sister Kenny Institute.

Nesbitt, B. 1988, July. Nursing diagnosis in age-related changes. *Journal of Gerontological Nursing* 14(2):7–12.

Olson, E.V., Johnson, B.J., Thompson, L.F., McCarthy, J.A., Edmonds, R.E., Schroeder, L.M., and Wade, M. 1967, April. The hazards of immobility. *American Journal of Nursing* 67(4):780–797.

Palmer, M., and Wyness, M.A. 1988, February. Positioning and handling: Important considerations in the care of the severely head-injured patient. *Journal of Neurological Nursing* 20(1):42–49.

Sanford, M. and Fowler, C. 1989, September–October. Positioning the patient with an abductor pillow. *Orthopedic Nursing* 8(5):21–23.

Wing, A., Lough, S., Turton, A., Fraser, C. and Jenner, J.R. 1990, February. Recovery of elbow function in voluntary positioning of the hand following hemiplegia due to sroke. *Journal of Neurology, Neurosurgery, and Psychology* 53(2):126–134.

7

PRESSURE REDUCTION

BARBARA J. BRADEN
NANCY BERGSTROM

Pressure Reduction refers to an abatement of the pressure exerted over parts of the body that interface with another surface for the purpose of controlling the transfer of pressure to deeper tissues. This so-called external mechanical load may be experienced as either normal (direct) pressure or tangential loading (shear) (Bennett, Kavner, Lee, Trainor, and Lewis 1984).

The primary objectives of Pressure Reduction as a nursing intervention are to maintain capillary blood flow and prevent the development of pressure sores by diminishing the intensity and duration of pressure to which the skin and its supporting structures are exposed. Provision of comfort is sometimes a secondary objective.

Pressure Reduction is an intervention that may be achieved by repositioning to achieve temporary pressure reduction or relief or altering the physical properties of the support surface.

Reduction of pressure at the interface of a support surface is usually achieved by providing a surface for sitting or lying positions that disperses pressure over a larger surface area of the body, thereby reducing pressure over bony prominences. Complete pressure relief at a support surface-bony prominence interface is difficult, if not impossible, to achieve. Pressure relief over a given bony prominence, however, may be achieved for a period of time by frequent repositioning.

LITERATURE RELATED TO THE INTERVENTION

The relationship of pressure to tissue necrosis has been studied extensively, and several features of this phenomenon are well documented. One important feature is that low external loads of prolonged duration are at least as likely to damage tissues as high pressure of shorter duration (Daniel, Priest, and Wheatley 1981; Dinsdale 1974; Husain 1953) and that muscle is much more susceptible to the destructive effects of pressure than normothermic skin (Daniel, Priest, and Wheatley 1981).

A great deal of variability has been found in the intensity and duration of pressure that is required to produce necrosis. It appears that the amount and duration of pressure required to damage the skin can be mediated by intrinsic and extrinsic factors that alter the ability of the tissues to tolerate pressure (Braden and Bergstrom 1987) (Figure 7–1).

Friction is a classic example of a factor that alters tissue tolerance for pressure. Dinsdale (1974) found that when the skin of normal swine was pretreated with

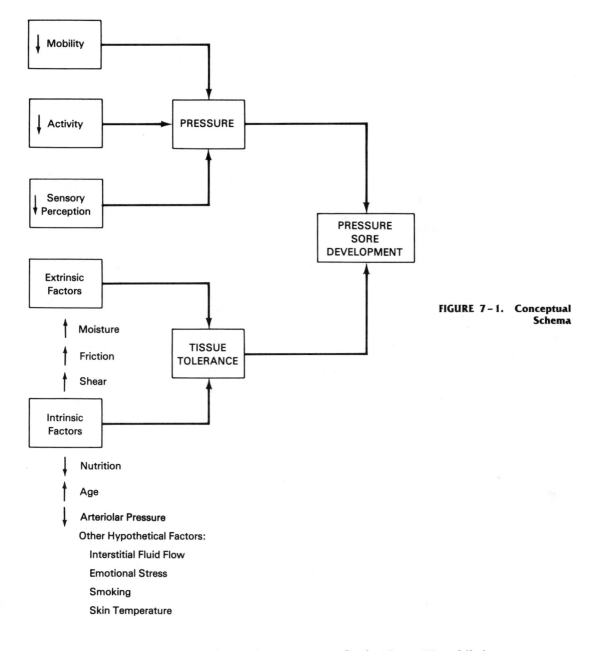

FIGURE 7 - 1. Conceptual Schema

friction, it ulcerated after being subjected to pressures of only 45 mm Hg, while in the absence of friction, a pressure of 290 mm Hg was required to produce ulceration.

Other examples of factors that alter tissue tolerance abound. Maceration of the skin from excess exposure to moisture can decrease tissue tolerance by decreasing the skin's tensile strength (Flam 1987), and certain sources of moisture, such as loose stools, are particularly harmful. Normal changes in the mechanical properties of collagen and elastin that occur with aging can increase the compressibility of the tissues (Kenney 1982; Krouskop 1983) and make the tissues more susceptible to both direct pressure and shearing forces (Bennett et al. 1984). Persons who are undernourished and underweight have tissues that deform more easily and therefore tend to develop higher interface pressures than persons who are overweight

(Ferguson-Pell 1990). Finally, blood pressure has been found to affect capillary dynamics to the extent that subjects who were hypertensive have been able to withstand higher external loads before vascular occlusion occurred than those subjects who were normotensive (Bergstrom and Braden 1991; Larsen, Holstein, and Lassen 1979). These and many other individual differences can contribute to diminished tissue tolerance and therefore to differences in the intensity and duration of pressure required to produce necrosis.

Because there is no single answer to questions regarding the intensity and duration of pressure required to produce tissue necrosis at various sites on the human body, certain generalities apply to preventive protocols. Frequent repositioning as a means of temporary pressure relief or reduction has long been the backbone of preventive protocols. Frequent pressure relief is essential not only to prevent direct tissue injury but also to allow occult tissue injury to heal before repetitive subclinical pressure insults lead to perceptible skin breakdown. Norton, McLaren, and Exton-Smith (1962) found that a program of repositioning high-risk patients every 2 hours or 3 hours was successful in decreasing the number and severity of pressure sores as compared to similar groups receiving local skin care (creams and cleansers only). Still, nine of these patients developed pressure sores that might have been prevented by more frequent turning or a pressure-reducing support surface.

There is some evidence that small shifts in body weight might be important in preventing pressure sores. Exton-Smith and Sherwin (1961) studied the relationship between pressure sore development and the mean number of spontaneous body movements that elderly patients newly admitted to a geriatric unit made from 11:00 P.M. to 6:00 A.M. Of the 50 subjects studied, 10 subjects had, on the average, fewer than 20 spontaneous body movements per night, and 9 of these developed a pressure sore. Only 1 other subject developed a pressure sore, and, while her mean movement score was 23, erythema developed on a night the score fell to 15, and a frank sacral sore was seen 2 nights later when the score for that night had fallen to 7. Twenty-eight of the 50 subjects had a mean nightly movement score of greater than 50, and, of these, 9 had mean scores of greater than 110. Because of instrumentation artifact that occurred with major movements, the movements recorded in the lower ranges have been assumed to represent small shifts in body weight.

Several investigators have attempted to demonstrate that protocols incorporating small shifts in body weight (whether provided by the nurse or by the patient) are effective in preventing pressure sores. Brown and colleagues (Brown, Boosinger, Black, and Gaspar 1985) studied 15 at-risk subjects; 7 received usual care and 8 received usual care and small shifts in body weight. None of the subjects receiving small shifts in weight developed pressure sores, while 1 of the 7 subjects receiving usual care developed two pressure sores. Other investigators, using instrumented wheelchair seating, attempted to demonstrate that pressure sore development in spinal-cord-injured patients would be related to the frequency of small shifts in body weight performed by the patient (Merbitz, King, Bleiberg, and Grip 1985; Patterson and Fischer 1986). They found instead that no pressure sores developed despite widely varying and sometimes multihour periods of exposure to sitting pressures exceeding the usual acceptable intensity level. None of these studies, however, had a large enough sample to warrant acceptance or rejection of small shifts in body weight as a preventive strategy.

Other investigators have examined the effect of various body positions on interface pressure. Garber, Campion, and Krouskop (1982) found that the traditional side-lying position in which the superior leg is flexed (55-degree to 65-degree hip flexion, 80-degree knee flexion), positioned ahead of the midline of the body, and supported by a pillow produced very high trochanteric pressures in normal and spinal-cord-injured subjects. Significant reduction in trochanteric pressure ($p < .001$) was achieved in spinal-cord-injured subjects when the superior leg was extended (30-degree hip flexion, 35-degree knee flexion) and positioned behind the midline of the body. Seiler, Allen, and Stahelin (1986), in a related study, examined differences in transcutaneous Po_2 (tc Po_2) at the site of the trochanter when subjects were positioned in a 90-degree lateral position and a 30-degree lateral position on a normal hospital mattress and on a "super-soft" mattress. They found that, regardless of mattress, trochanteric tc Po_2 decreased significantly from baseline when positioned in the 90-degree lateral position but not when the subject was positioned in the 30-degree lateral position. Consequently, these researchers recommend the 30-degree lateral position with the patient's leg position determined by comfort alone.

While good positioning and frequent repositioning can do much to prevent pressure sores, it may also be necessary to provide a support surface that reduces interface pressure over bony prominences. In the literature, these surfaces are generally categorized as mattress (or wheelchair) overlays, mattress replacements, or specialty beds. Mattress overlays and mattress replacements are considered to be either static (foam, gels) or dynamic (alternating pressure surfaces). Specialty beds are described as either low air loss or air fluidized. Investigators evaluate these surfaces in either clinical trials or in laboratory studies utilizing such measures as interface pressures, skin oxygen tension, or blood flow. Both types of studies are important, but the strongest evidence would come from large randomized clinical trials.

There is a common and persistent perception that a support surface interface pressure that exceeds 32 mm Hg will lead to closure of the capillary bed and result in ischemic injury. This figure represents the mean blood pressure obtained by Landis (1930) through cannulation of the arteriolar limb of capillaries in the finger nailbeds, but interface pressures of 32 mm Hg obtained at other body sites cannot be assumed to protect against closure of the capillary beds at that site. Transmission of load through tissue and muscle mass may decrease or increase depending on the body site and characteristics of the tissue at that site for any specific person (Ferguson-Pell 1990; Le, Madsen, Barth, Ksander, Angell, and Vistnes 1984). For this reason and a myriad of others, an interface pressure of 32 mm Hg should not be viewed as an absolute standard for evaluation of support surfaces.

Interface pressure values may, however, be used as an index to compare pressure reduction capabilities of support surfaces in circumstances where similar subjects and identical instruments and protocols are assured.

Mattress overlays, mattress replacements, and specialty beds are commonly used to achieve pressure reduction. Research into the effectiveness of these devices is difficult to evaluate because differences in surfaces, subjects, instrumentation, and protocol invalidate many comparisons. There are a few areas, however, on which findings converge:

1.   Almost any surface tested reduced pressure below that of a standard hospital mattress (Bliss, McLaren, and Exton-Smith 1967; Goldstone, Norris, O'Reilly, and White 1982; Jacobs 1989).

2.   Foam overlays that were 2 inches to 3 inches thick did not compare favorably to other pressure-reduction surfaces (Stapleton 1986), including thicker foam surfaces (Krouskop 1986).

3.   Gel-filled overlays and mattresses reduce pressure better than most foam overlays (Berjian, Douglass, Holyoke, Goodwin, and Priore 1983; Krouskop 1986).

4.   The air-fluidized bed results in substantial pressure reduction and appears to be beneficial in healing pressure sores, although results are not always dramatic (Allman, Walker, Hart, Laprade, Noel, and Smith 1987; Bennett, Bellantoni, and Ouslander 1989; Jackson, Chagares, Nee, and Freeman 1988).

Other characteristics must be considered in a surface intended to reduce pressure and prevent pressure sores. According to Ferguson-Pell (1990), the following factors need to be appraised:

Moisture accumulation and moisture resistance
  • Heat accumulation or loss
  • Sufficient stability to allow for ease of turning, shifting, and transferring
  • Frictional properties of the surface and cover
  • Cost, durability, and maintenance requirements
  • Flammability
  • Safety

Since different products have differing abilities to reduce pressure, these additional factors may be used to evaluate the advantages and disadvantages of certain surfaces under individualized circumstances. For example, although there is some evidence that gel pads are somewhat more effective than thick foam in reducing pressure, gel pads or mattresses are heavy, difficult to handle, and contribute to heat loss. This last factor would be a distinct disadvantage for a thin, elderly person who might become very cold if placed on gel but a distinct advantage for a person who is overweight and prone to heat accumulation.

In addition to these characteristics, nurses will be interested in whether special linens or bed-making procedures are necessary and if the surface is easy to clean, disinfect, and/or deodorize. Safety issues to consider include whether the surface increases the risk of falls because it raises the level of the support surface above or even with the side rail or is so slick that linens become a sliding board when patients are leaving the bed or chair.

IDENTIFICATION OF INTERVENTION TOOLS

Instruments are available to measure the level of interface pressure and the effects of that pressure. These instruments include electropneumatic pressure sensors, laser Doppler flowmetry, and transcutaneous Po_2, but these are primarily research tools rather than clinical tools. In this instance, screening tools to determine presence and level of risk are the primary clinical tool used to determine when the intervention of Pressure Reduction is appropriate.

Rating scales are the most common screening tools used by nurses to identify patients at risk for pressure sore development. Rating scales have the advantage of being low in cost and noninvasive, but a critical evaluation of their reliability and predictive validity is necessary before implementation in a clinical setting. The commonly accepted measures of predictive validity for screening tests are sensitivity, specificity, predictive value of positive results (PVP), and predictive value of negative results (PNP) (Lilienfeld and Lilienfeld 1980; Larson 1986). Sensitivity is a measure that indicates, among all subjects who developed a pressure sore, the proportion of those who were identified by the screening tool as being at risk. Specificity is a measure that indicates, among all subjects who did not develop a pressure sore, the proportion of those who were identified by the screening tool as being at low or no risk. Sensitivity and the PNP are both influenced by the number of false-negatives, while the number of false-positives influences specificity and the PVP.

The ideal screening test would be 100% sensitive and 100% specific, but this is rarely achieved, even by tests intended for diagnosis rather than screening. This ideal is still less likely to be achieved when the condition is preventable. Nevertheless, these performance estimates are essential to determining appropriate usage in clinical decision making. Several instruments designed to predict the risk of pressure sore development have been reported in the literature, but only the Norton and the Braden Scale have undergone sufficient testing to justify use (Norton, McLaren, and Exton-Smith 1962; Bergstrom, Braden, Laguzza, and Holman 1987).

The Norton Scale has been studied extensively (Goldstone and Goldstone 1982; Goldstone and Roberts 1980). This tool consists of five parameters — physical condition, mental state, activity, mobility, and incontinence — each rated from 1 to 4, with one- or two-word descriptors for each rating. Scores range from 5 to 20, with a score of 14 indicating the onset of risk and a score of 12 or below indicating a high risk for pressure sore formation. Interrater reliability was not reported, but in two studies of predictive validity ($N = 59$, $N = 40$) sensitivity ranged from 89% to 92% and specificity ranged from 36% to 57% (Goldstone and Goldstone 1982; Roberts and Goldstone 1979).

The Braden Scale (Bergstrom et al. 1987; Bergstrom, Demuth, and Braden 1987; Braden and Bergstrom 1989) has also been developed to predict the risk for pressure sore development. The scale is composed of six subscales reflecting sensory perception, skin moisture, activity, mobility, nutritional intake, and friction and shear. All subscales are rated from 1 to 4, with the exception of the friction and shear subscale, which is rated from 1 to 3. Each rating is accompanied by a description of criteria for rating. Potential scores range from 4 to 23. Interrater reliability for 86 pairs of observation by a graduate student and a registered nurse primary caregiver was reported to be $r = 0.99$ ($p < .001$). In two studies of predictive validity in hospitalized patients ($N = 99$, $N = 100$), sensitivity was 100%, and specificity ranged from 90% to 64% at a cut score of 16. Taylor (1988) and Smith et al. (1991) compared the predictive validity of the Braden Scale with other often-used instruments and concluded that it had a higher degree of reliability and validity.

IDENTIFICATION OF ASSOCIATED NURSING DIAGNOSES AND APPROPRIATE CLIENT GROUPS

Strategies to reduce pressure should be instituted for persons who have existing pressure sores or are at risk for developing pressure sores. Some of these strategies are also appropriate for persons experiencing pressure-related discomfort or pain with movement. Nursing diagnoses directly associated with these client groups are Impaired Skin Integrity, Potential Impaired Skin Integrity, Pain, and Chronic Pain. Other nursing diagnoses associated with the need for Pressure Reduction are secondary to the diagnosis Impaired Skin Integrity or Potential Impaired Skin Integrity. The following represent examples (but not an exhaustive list) of diagnoses that indicate increased risk for Impaired Skin Integrity: Activity Intolerance,

Impaired Physical Mobility, Altered Nutrition: Less Than Body Requirements, and Altered (Peripheral) Tissue Perfusion.

SUGGESTED PROTOCOL

Pressure Reduction is not a dichotomous intervention (the nurse chooses to intervene or not intervene). The degree of intervention is highly related to the functional status of the patient, the specific etiology of the reduced functioning, and the activities in which the patient will be engaged. For this reason, strategies will be described using a level of activity and mobility for initial screening and total Braden Scale scores to differentiate further the level of risk.

Patients at risk for pressure sores should be identified on admission to health care facilities and services. All individuals at risk for developing pressure sores by virtue of their bedfast or chairfast status should be assessed using a clinical assessment tool to determine the level of risk and other associated risk factors. This assessment should take place within 24 hours to 48 hours of admission. Following the initial assessment, reassessment should take place at periodic intervals, depending on the rapidity with which the condition changes and whenever a major change occurs in the condition. The following schedules may be useful:

Intensive care: Every shift when the condition is unstable; daily or less when the condition is stable.

Medical-surgical settings: Every other day when condition is stable; and when the condition changes (e.g., surgery, medical complications).

Home care: Every visit until the client is stable and when the condition changes.

Nursing homes: Weekly for 1 month or until the condition is stable; when the condition changes; and monthly after the first month as long as the condition does not change.

Risk assessment should be done using an adequately tested risk assessment tool like the Braden Scale or the Norton Scale. The Braden Scale for Predicting Pressure Sore Risk (Bergstrom et al. 1987) has demonstrated reliability and validity, has been tested in numerous clinical settings with easily achieved interrater reliability, and requires little time to administer (less than 1 minute when administered by the primary caregiver). (Figure 7–2). The Norton Scale does not have operationalized levels for each of the subscales, and reliability has not been demonstrated through clinical studies. For this reason, the Braden Scale is recommended as the basis for risk assessment and clinical decisions related to pressure reduction.

Pressure sore risk increases as scores on the Braden Scale decrease. Scores of 15 to 16 indicate mild risk, 12 to 14 moderate risk, and below 12 serious risk. The most important initial intervention for any level of risk is pressure reduction. The manner in which pressure reduction is achieved depends on the level of risk as indicated by the mobility and activity subscales of the Braden Scale. This can be refined by an understanding of the sensory perception and friction and shear subscales. Individuals who are at mild to moderate risk based on scores of 2 or 3 on the activity or mobility subscales and who have other risk factors (e.g., incontinence or malnutrition) may need more protection from pressure than individuals without the additional risk factors.

It is also essential to remember that in a program of pressure sore prevention or treatment, Pressure Reduction protocols address only one aspect of the problem, albeit the most crucial aspect. Risk factors that affect tissue tolerance must be

Patient's Name _____   Evaluator's Name _____

	1	2	3	4	Case 1	Case 2	Case 3
SENSORY PERCEPTION ability to respond meaningfully to pressure-related discomfort	**1. Completely Limited:** Unresponsive (does not moan, flinch, or grasp) to painful stimuli, due to diminished level of consciousness or sedation. OR limited ability to feel pain over most of body surface.	**2. Very Limited:** Responds only to painful stimuli. Cannot communicate discomfort except by moaning or restlessness. OR has a sensory impairment which limits the ability to feel pain or discomfort over 1/2 of body.	**3. Slightly Limited:** Responds to verbal commands, but cannot always communicate discomfort or need to be turned. OR has some sensory impairment which limits ability to feel pain or discomfort in 1 or 2 extremities.	**4. No Impairment:** Responds to verbal commands. Has no sensory deficit which would limit ability to feel or voice pain or discomfort.	4	3	2
MOISTURE degree to which skin is exposed to moisture	**1. Constantly Moist:** Skin is kept moist almost constantly by perspiration, urine, etc. Dampness is detected every time patient is moved or turned.	**2. Very Moist:** Skin is often, but not always moist. Linen must be changed at least once a shift.	**3. Occasionally Moist:** Skin is occasionally moist, requiring an extra linen change approximately once a day.	**4. Rarely Moist:** Skin is usually dry, linen only requires changing at routine intervals.	2	1	1
ACTIVITY degree of physical activity	**1. Bedfast:** Confined to bed.	**2. Chairfast:** Ability to walk severely limited or non-existent. Cannot bear own weight and/or must be assisted into chair or wheelchair.	**3. Walks Occasionally:** Walks occasionally during day, but for very short distances, with or without assistance. Spends majority of each shift in bed or chair.	**4. Walks Frequently:** walks outside the room at least twice a day and inside room at least once every 2 hours during waking hours.	2	2	1
MOBILITY ability to change and control body position	**1. Completely Immobile:** Does not make even slight changes in body or extremity position without assistance.	**2. Very Limited:** Makes occasional slight changes in body or extremity position but unable to make frequent or significant changes independently.	**3. Slightly Limited:** Makes frequent though slight changes in body or extremity position independently.	**4. No Limitations:** Makes major and frequent changes in position without assistance.	3	3	2
NUTRITION usual food intake pattern	**1. Very Poor:** Never eats a complete meal. Rarely eats more than 1/3 of any food offered. Eats 2 servings or less of protein (meat or dairy products) per day. Takes fluids poorly. Does not take a liquid dietary supplement. OR is NPO and/or maintained on clear liquids or IV's for more than 5 days.	**2. Probably Inadequate:** Rarely eats a complete meal and generally eats only about 1/2 of any food offered. Protein intake includes only 3 servings of meat or dairy products per day. Occasionally will take a dietary supplement. OR receives less than optimum amount of liquid diet or tube feeding.	**3. Adequate:** Eats over half of most meals. Eats a total of 4 servings of protein (meat, dairy products) each day. Occasionally will refuse a meal, but will usually take a supplement if offered. OR is on a tube feeding or TPN regimen which probably meets most of nutritional needs.	**4. Excellent:** Eats most of every meal. Never refuses a meal. Usually eats a total of 4 or more servings of meat and dairy products. Occasionally eats between meals. Does not require supplementation.	3	3	3
FRICTION AND SHEAR	**1. Problem:** Requires moderate to maximum assistance in moving. Complete lifting without sliding against sheets is impossible. Frequently slides down in bed or chair, requiring frequent repositioning with maximum assistance. Spasticity, contractures or agitation leads to almost constant friction.	**2. Potential Problem:** Moves feebly or requires minimum assistance. During a move skin probably slides to some extent against sheets, chair, restraints, or other devices. Maintains relatively good position in chair or bed most of the time but occasionally slides down.	**3. No Apparent Problem:** Moves in bed and in chair independently and has sufficient muscle strength to lift up completely during move. Maintains good position in bed or chair at all times.		2	1	1
				Total Score	16	13	10

FIGURE 7–2. The Braden Scale for Predicting Pressure Sore Risk

controlled or ameliorated when possible, and protocols for local care of pressure must be assiduously followed.

Pressure Reduction Strategies

Pressure reduction may be achieved through a variety of nursing activities and assistive devices: frequent repositioning, the use of pillows or wedges to keep bony prominences from direct contact, heel and other specific contact point protective devices, monitoring the elevation of the head of the bed, using trapezes and other lifting devices, mattresses, overlays and replacements, seat cushions, and specialty beds. Nurses who are involved in making facility or agency-wide decisions concerning specific support surfaces should seek published data. The most useful data are provided by clinical trials showing that subjects using the device of interest develop fewer pressure sores than a group of subjects receiving basic nursing care. When these types of data are not available, comparisons of interface pressures for various surfaces can be used with caution.

Mild Risk

Mild risk is present when Braden Scale scores are 15 or 16 or activity and/or mobility subscale scores are 2 or 3. If other major risk factors not measured by the Braden Scale (low blood pressure, elevated temperature, fecal incontinence, advanced age, severe emaciation) are present, the nurse should advance to strategies appropriate at the next level of risk. Repositioning-related strategies may include using a turning and positioning schedule. If the patient is thin and has poor muscle tone, only 30-degree lateral turns should be employed. More assistance may be needed with positioning during the night or anytime sedatives or narcotics are being used. Mattress overlays would not be expected to be necessary unless it is desirable for patient comfort, in which case, a foam overlay of 2 inches or 3 inches may be sufficient. Individuals having difficulty with bed mobility may benefit from heel or elbow pads or a trapeze to reduce friction when repositioning in bed. Comfort may be increased through the use of pillows or other padding in lean individuals.

Moderate Risk

Moderate risk is present when Braden Scale scores are between 12 and 14 points, or activity and/or mobility subscale scores are no higher than 2. Repositioning should be done with assistance and with attention to good body mechanics, using pillows and pads to protect bony prominences and heel and elbow protectors as needed for comfort. Lateral positioning should not exceed 30 degrees. Legs should be supported on pillows with the heels off the mattress when the patient is lying in the recumbent position. Mattress overlays, such as 4-inch foam, static or alternating air pads may be desirable, but they do not reduce the importance of a documented repositioning schedule or the use of other protective devices. Trapezes and foam heel and elbow pads may be useful in reducing friction.

High Risk

High risk is present when Braden Scale scores are below 12 points or activity and/or mobility subscale scores are below 2. This level of risk is even greater when other risk factors are present (e.g., hypotension, hyperpyrexia). Turning schedules should include either increased frequency of turns or assisted frequent, small shifts in body weight, and lateral turns should not exceed 30 degrees. High-quality foam wedges and pads should be used in positioning. When patients can tolerate the prone position, it should be added to the turning schedule because it allows the most common sites of pressure sore formation (sacrum, trochanters, heels) to be totally relieved of pressure while also preventing flexion contractures of the hips. Impeccable padding and positioning are required if the prone position is to be employed. Gel pads or mattresses may be used depending on the individual patient. Molded padded boots may be used to protect the heels from excessive pressure. Specialty beds are not generally required to prevent pressure sores in high-risk patients when adequate nursing care is available unless these specialty beds are useful for preventing additional problems.

Actual Impairment of Skin Integrity

The aggressiveness of pressure-reduction strategies in persons with existing pressure sores depends on the stage and size of the pressure sore (Figure 7 – 3), the circumstances under which the pressure sore developed, and the individual characteristics of the patient.

Superficial pressure sores (Stage I, Stage II) can usually be managed by devising a turning schedule that avoids all pressure over the site of the sore, especially if the patient was at only mild risk when the sore developed. The plan for Pressure Reduction should be adjusted incrementally upward from the conditions under which the sore developed. For example, if the sore developed when frequent repositioning was being faithfully but solely employed, it may be necessary to add a 4-inch foam mattress to the plan of care. If the Braden Scale score is declining or indicates moderate or high risk, pressure-reducing strategies should follow the same protocol recommended for prevention at that level of risk.

Full-thickness sores (Stage III, Stage IV) may require more aggressive pressure reduction to heal, particularly if they are large. As recommended for the superficial sores, complete pressure relief must be provided at the site of the sore for healing to occur, and if the Braden Scale score is declining or indicates moderate risk, pressure-reducing strategies should follow the same protocol recommended for prevention at that level of risk. When the Braden Scale score indicates high risk and/or the sores are very large and/or other major risk factors not measured by the Braden Scale (low blood pressure, elevated temperature, fecal incontinence, advanced age, severe emaciation) are present, a low-air-loss or air-fluidized bed should be considered.

SPECIAL CONSIDERATION: GOALS OF PATIENT CARE

All individuals found to be at risk for pressure sores should have routine, systematic (head-to-toe) examination of the skin. The frequency of this examination will vary with the level of risk and the independence of the individual. As a rule, daily examination of the skin may be adequate in inpatient settings, especially when this is coupled with evaluation of specific sites that become accessible during repositioning. The condition of the skin should be documented on the record daily in acute-care and weekly in long-term-care settings. Tools to guide evaluation and documentation of skin condition are abundant, and one that is similar to those used in most clinical settings and has been tested and documented to be reliable and valid is shown in Figure 7 – 3 (Bergstrom 1990). It is to document the skin condi-

Pressure Sore Data Collection Questionnaire
Skin Assessment Tool (Nurse II)

Name _____   ID Number _____

DATE OF OBSERVATION: _____   _____

	Month	Day	Year

ASSESSMENT SITE*   SKIN CONDITION

	Size	Depth	Stage
1) Back of head	_____	_____	_____
2) Right ear	_____	_____	_____
3) Left ear	_____	_____	_____
4) Right scapula	_____	_____	_____
5) Left scapula	_____	_____	_____
6) Right elbow	_____	_____	_____
7) Left elbow	_____	_____	_____
8) Vertebrae (upper-mid)	_____	_____	_____
9) Sacrum	_____	_____	_____
10) Coccyx	_____	_____	_____
11) Right iliac crest	_____	_____	_____
12) Left iliac crest	_____	_____	_____
13) Right trochanter (hip)	_____	_____	_____
14) Left trochanter (hip)	_____	_____	_____
15) Right ischial tuberosity	_____	_____	_____
16) Left ischial tuberosity	_____	_____	_____
17) Right thigh	_____	_____	_____
18) Left thigh	_____	_____	_____
19) Right knee	_____	_____	_____
20) Left knee	_____	_____	_____
21) Right lower leg	_____	_____	_____
22) Left lower leg	_____	_____	_____
23) Right ankle (inner/outer)	_____	_____	_____
24) Left ankle (inner/outer)	_____	_____	_____
25) Right heel	_____	_____	_____
26) Left heel	_____	_____	_____
27) Right toe(s)	_____	_____	_____
28) Left toe(s)	_____	_____	_____
29) Other (specify)	_____	_____	_____

*Assess and record each site each observation time. Mark site(s) on figure below.

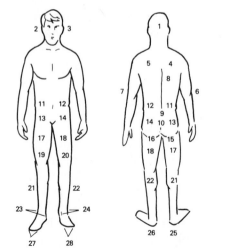

Stage Key

Stage 0   No redness or breakdown
Stage 1   Erythema only: redness does not
           disappear for 24 hours after
           pressure is relieved
Stage 2   Break in skin such as blisters
           or abrasions
Stage 3   Break in skin exposing
           subcutaneous tissue
Stage 4   Break in skin extending through
           tissue and subcutaneous layers,
           exposing muscle or bone
Stage 9   Dark necrotic tissue. (Use this
           rating until tissue sloughs,
           then continue staging.)

Revised 3/2/89 © Nancy Bergstrom

FIGURE 7–3. Pressure Sore Data Collection Questionnaire Skin Assessment Tool (Nurse II)

tion since this documentation is necessary to demonstrate the effectiveness of nursing actions in meeting the goals of pressure reduction.

In addition, the overall goals for the patient must be considered when selecting the methods to be used to prevent or manage the treatment of pressure sores. Patients who are recovering from acute illness, are chronically ill, and/or are in rehabilitative care should have access to the best preventive-treatment strategies necessary. When patients are terminally ill and pressure sores may be a sign of general physical decline, the goal of care should be kept in mind. Terminally ill patients may have comfort as a goal. To meet this goal, less disruption and movement may be desired, and Pressure Reduction may involve more attention to support surfaces and less attention to turning schedules. The key point is that the goal of care should be known and a rational plan developed. Neglect is not to be condoned.

CASE STUDIES

Braden Scale scores for the case studies are shown in Figure 7-2.

Case Study 1

Mrs. L is a 75-year-old woman who suffered a fractured hip in a fall at the grocery store and has been admitted to an extended-care facility 5 days after hip-pinning surgery. She had a Braden Scale score of 16 when risk was assessed the day following admission, with a score of 2 on the activity, mobility and friction, and shear subscales. These scores were awarded since she is chairfast and too weak to make or maintain major changes in position or to lift up when moved. She had no deficits in sensory perception but was incontinent at night. She had been eating over half of all meals served but did not have a big appetite and was underweight for her height. Because she was so light, she had a tendency to slide down in bed. Her temperature had been within normal range since admission, but her blood pressure had been only 106/74 mm Hg.

The plan for Pressure Reduction included a scheduled turning program that specified lateral turns not to exceed 30 degrees and head of bed elevation not to exceed 30 degrees. Ordinarily at this level of risk, a meticulous turning schedule would have been sufficient, but because Mrs. L had several additional significant risks (low body weight, low blood pressure), the nurses decided to use a mattress overlay as well. Elbow and heel protectors were ordered to prevent friction injuries from occurring, but Mrs. L was deemed to have too little upper arm strength to benefit from a trapeze. Nutritional supplementation, scheduled nighttime toileting, and a program of mobilization were also instituted.

Case Study 2

Mr. S was a heavy-set 80-year-old widower who had a cerebrovascular accident at his daughter's home. On initial examination, he had right-sided hemiplegia and some mental clouding. He could move his left side, but since it was his nondominant side, he could not use his left extremities effectively and required several people for lifting when repositioning. He was unable to swallow, and, when this did not improve in 24 hours, a nasogastric tube was inserted and enteral feedings begun. Because he could not call for assistance with toileting, an external catheter was put in place, although it was accidentally displaced on occasion. His blood pressure was stabilized at 140/86 mm Hg. He was given a Braden Scale score of 13 with a score of 1 on activity and friction and shear subscales, a score of 2 on mobility, and a score of 3 on sensory perception, nutrition, and moisture.

The primary nurse decided to replace the standard hospital mattress with a thick foam mattress. A trapeze and lift sheet were placed on the bed to facilitate repositioning. A scheduled turning program that included lateral turns not to exceed 30 degrees was instituted. Since Mr. S experienced some regurgitation when the head of the bed was elevated to 30 degrees, it was elevated to 45 degrees. The turning schedule was adjusted to restrict the time Mr. S spent in the supine position to 1 hour per turn.

Case Study 3

Miss W suffered a severe head injury in a car accident and was admitted to a skilled nursing facility in a chronic vegetative state following several weeks of stabilization in an acute-care hospital. She was incapable of voluntary movement but moaned and winced occasionally and had some spastic movements in her lower extremities. The gastrostomy feedings she was receiving resulted in occasional liquid stools but eliminated earlier problems of regurgitation that had been experienced with the nasogastric tube. Her skin was frequently moist because of bouts of profuse perspiration, and her total Braden Scale score was 10.

The scheduled turning program included the usual lateral turns not to exceed 30 degrees and head of bed elevation not to exceed 30 degrees. Because there was no possibility of eventual mobilization, the schedule also included positioning in the prone position for 1 hour or 2 hours every shift as a means to prevent hip flexion contractures and to provide multihour pressure relief on other bony prominences. Foam wedges were ordered to facilitate positioning, and foam-padded boots were obtained to prevent foot drop and decrease heel pressure. A thick foam mattress replacement was placed on the bed, and a schedule for periodic replacement was written in the Kardex. The osmolality of the gastrostomy feedings were adjusted to prevent the liquid stools. Bowel elimination was facilitated with glycerin suppositories on Monday, Wednesday, and Friday.

SUMMARY

Nurses have struggled for many years with prevention and treatment of pressure sores, and Pressure Reduction has been the cornerstone of these efforts. Frequent repositioning is the nursing strategy traditionally utilized as a means to achieve pressure reduction. An assortment of high-tech approaches have also become available, consisting primarily of specialty beds, but these are quite costly. Developing a rational plan of nursing actions that is effective in reducing pressure and appropriate to the individual's level of risk can be cost-efficient but requires knowledge of the scientific base for this intervention. This knowledge, in conjunction with good nursing judgment concerning its appropriate application, will bring nursing closer to the goal of eliminating pressure sores from all health care settings.

REFERENCES

Allman, R.M., Walker, J.M., Hart, M., Laprade, C.A., Noel, L.B., and Smith, C.R. 1987. Air-fluidized beds or conventional therapy for pressure sores. *Annals of Internal Medicine* 107(5):641–648.
Bennett, L., Kavner, D., Lee, B.Y., Trainor, F.S., and Lewis, J.M. 1984. Skin stress and blood flow in sitting paraplegic patients. *Archives of Physical Medicine and Rehabilitation* 65(4):186–190.

Bennett, R.G., Bellantoni, M.F., and Ouslander, J.G. 1989. Air-fluidized bed treatment of nursing home patients with pressure sores. *Journal of the American Geriatric Society* 37(3):235– 242.

Bergstrom, N. 1990. Nursing assessment of pressure sore risk. Research proposal funded by National Institutes of Health, National Center for Nursing Research.

Bergstrom, N., and Braden, B. 1991. A prospective study of pressure sore risk among institutionalized elderly. Manuscript.

Bergstrom, N., Braden, B., Laguzza, A., and Holman, A. 1987. The Braden Scale for predicting pressure sore risk. *Nursing Research* 36(4):205–210.

Bergstrom, N., Demuth, P.J., and Braden, B.J. 1987. A clinical trial of the Braden Scale for predicting pressure sore risk. *Nursing Clinics of North America* 22(2):417–428.

Berjian, R.A., Douglass, H.O., Jr., Holyoke, E.D., Goodwin, P.M., and Priore, R.L. 1983. Skin pressure measurements on various mattress surfaces in cancer patients. *American Journal of Physical Medicine* 62(5):217–226.

Bliss, M.R., McLaren, R., and Exton-Smith, A.N. 1967. Preventing pressure sores in hospital: Controlled trial of a large-celled ripple mattress. *British Medical Journal* 1(537):394–397.

Braden, B. and Bergstrom, N. 1987. A conceptual schema for the study of the etiology of pressure sores. *Rehabilitation Nursing* 12(1):8–12, 16.

Braden, B.J., and Bergstrom, N. 1989. Clinical utility of the Braden Scale for Predicting Pressure Sore Risk. *Decubitus* 2(3):44–51.

Brown, M.M., Boosinger, J., Black, J., and Gaspar, T. 1985. Nursing innovation for prevention of decubitus ulcers in long term care facilities. *Plastic Surgical Nursing* 5(2):57–64.

Daniel, R.K., Priest, D.L., and Wheatley, D.C. 1981. Etiologic factors in pressure sores: An experimental model. *Archives of Physical Medicine and Rehabilitation* 62(10):492–498.

Dinsdale, S.M. 1974. Decubitus ulcers: Role of pressure and friction in causation. *Archives of Physical Medicine and Rehabilitation* 55(4):147–152.

Exton-Smith, A.N., and Sherwin, R.W. 1961. The prevention of pressure sores: Significance of spontaneous bodily movements. *Lancet* 47(2):1124–1126.

Ferguson-Pell, M.W. 1990. Seat cushion selection: Technical considerations. *Journal of Rehabilitation Research and Development,* clin. suppl. 2:49–73.

Flam, E. 1987. Optimum skin aeration in pressure sore management (abstract). *Proceedings of the Annual Conference of Engineering in Medicine and Biology,* 29,84.

Garber, S.L., Campion, L.J., and Krouskop, T.A. 1982. Trochanteric pressure in spinal cord injury. *Archives of Physical Medicine and Rehabilitation* 63(11):549–552.

Goldstone, L.A., and Goldstone, J. 1982. The Norton score: An early warning of pressure sores? *Journal of Advanced Nursing* 7(5):419–426.

Goldstone, L.A., Norris, M., O'Reilly, M., and White, J. 1982. A clinical trial of a bead bed system for the prevention of pressure sores in elderly orthopaedic patients. *Journal of Advanced Nursing* 7(6):545–548.

Goldstone, L.A., and Roberts, B.V. 1980. A preliminary discriminant function analysis of elderly orthopaedic patients who will or will not contract a pressure sore. *International Journal of Nursing Studies* 17(1):17–23.

Husain, T. 1953. An experimental study of some pressure effects on tissues, with reference to the bed-sore problem. *Journal of Pathology and Bacteriology* 66:347–358.

Jackson, B.S., Chagares, R., Nee, N., and Freeman, K. 1988. The effects of a therapeutic bed on pressure ulcers: An experimental study. *Journal of Enterostomal Therapy* 15(6):220–226.

Jacobs, M.A. 1989. Comparison of capillary blood flow using a regular hospital bed mattress, ROHO mattress and Mediscus bed. *Rehabilitation Nursing* 14(5):270–272.

Kenney, R.A. 1982. *Physiology of aging: a synopsis.* Chicago: Year Book Medical Publishers.

Krouskop, T.A. 1983. A synthesis of the factors that contribute to pressure sore formation. *Medical Hypotheses* 11(2):255–267.

Krouskop, T.A. 1986. The effect of surface geometry on interface pressures generated by polyurethane foam mattress overlays. A compilation of reports by the Rehabilitation Engineering Center at the Institute for Rehabilitation and Research, Houston.

Landis, E. 1930. Studies of capillary blood pressure in human skin. *Heart* 15:209–228.

Larsen, B., Holstein, P., and Lassen, N.A. 1979. On the pathogenesis of bedsores. *Scandinavian Journal of Plastic and Reconstructive Surgery* 13(2):347–350.

Larson, E. 1986. Evaluating validity of screening tests. *Nursing Research* 35(3):186–188.

Le, K.M., Madsen, B.L., Barth, P.W., Ksander, G.A., Angell, J.B., and Vistnes, L.M. 1984. An in-depth look at pressure sores using monolithic silicon pressure sensors. *Plastic and Reconstructive Surgery* 74(6):745–754.

Lilienfeld, A.M., and Lilienfeld, D.E. 1980. *Foundations of epidemiology.* 2d ed. New York: Oxford University Press.

Merbitz, C.T., King, R.B., Bleiberg, J., and Grip, J.C. 1985. Wheelchair push-ups: Measuring pressure relief frequency. *Archives of Physical and Medical Rehabilitation* 66(7):433–438.

Norton, D., McLaren, R., and Exton-Smith, A.N. 1962. *An investigation of geriatric nursing problems in hospitals.* London: National Corporation for the Care of Old People.

Patterson, R.P., and Fisher, S.V. 1986. Sitting pressure-time patterns in patients with quadriplegia. *Archives of Physical and Medical Rehabilitation* 67(11):812–814.

Roberts, B.V. and Goldstone, L.A. 1979. A survey of pressure sores in the over sixties on two orthopaedic wards. *International Journal of Nursing Studies* 16:355–364.

Seiler, W.O., Allen, S., and Stahelin, H.B. 1986. Influence of the 30 degrees laterally inclined position and the "super-soft" 3-piece mattress on skin oxygen tension on areas of maximum pressure—implications for pressure sore prevention. *Gerontology* 32(3):158–166.

Smith, D.M., Winsemius, D.K., Besdine, R.W. 1991. Pressure sores in the elderly: Can this outcome be improved? *Journal of General Internal Medicine* 6(1):81–93.

Stapleton, M. 1986. Preventing pressure sores—an evaluation of three products. *Geriatric Nursing* 6(2):23–25.

Taylor, K.J. 1988. Identification of patients at risk for pressure sores. *Journal of Enterostomal Therapy* 15(5):201–205.

8

SLEEP PROMOTION

FELISSA L. COHEN
SHARON L. MERRITT

Interventions relating to Sleep Promotion are used to address problems caused by sleep pattern disturbances. The exact nature of Sleep Promotion activities depends on the underlying cause of the sleep disruption.

Sleep pattern disturbance has been defined as a disruption in sleep time that results in feelings of discomfort, interferes with the individual's usual life-style, or both (Kim, McFarland, and McLane 1989). Persons with such a disturbance have a change in their sleep cycle that is inconsistent with their biological or emotional needs (Carpenito 1989) and experience this disturbance when their sleep-wake cycle is inconsistent with the norms for a particular developmental age group or conflicts with environmental or sociocultural expectations (Carrieri, Lindsey, and West 1986).

Various defining characteristics (symptoms) of disturbed sleep have been described (Carpenito 1989; Johnson 1989; Lo and Kim 1986; Kim, McFarland, and McLane 1989) (Table 8–1). Subjective complaints relate to reported changes in the sleep pattern and the way the person feels during the day (or normal waking hours) as a result of the sleep disruption. Objective defining characteristics reflect various changes in mood and behavior, as well as some physical signs, that may be associated with disturbed sleep.

THE SLEEP-WAKE CYCLE

Sleep is a complex process consisting of several stages governed by the interaction of neurochemical systems and endogenous circadian and ultradian pacemakers. The most widely accepted sleep stage classification is that of Rechtschaffen and Kales (1968). It consists of different stages of consciousness that includes REM (rapid eye movement or desynchronized) sleep, NREM (non–rapid eye movement or synchronized) sleep, and wakefulness. There are four stages of NREM sleep. Stage 1 NREM sleep is the usual transition between waking and sleeping, accounting for 5% to 10% of total sleep time. Stage 2 NREM sleep accounts for 45% to 55% of the total sleep time in adults. Stages 3 and 4 NREM sleep are characterized by slow electroencephalogram (EEG) waves, are called slow wave or delta sleep, and account for 10% to 20% of total sleep time. REM sleep periods account for 20% to 25% of total sleep time. In REM sleep, there are wide variations in pulse, respiration, blood pressure, brain temperature, cortical blood flow, and oxygen consumption, as well as atonia of major muscles. The rapid eye movements and muscle twitches that occur may be related to dreaming that occurs during REM sleep.

TABLE 8–1. DEFINING CHARACTERISTICS ASSOCIATED WITH A SLEEP PATTERN DISTURBANCE

SUBJECTIVE	OBJECTIVE
Verbalizes difficulty in falling asleep	Mood alterations, such as anxiety, depression, apathy
Awakens earlier or later than desired	Restlessness
Interrupted sleep	Irritability
Complains of not feeling well rested	Listlessness
Verbalizes complaints of pain or anxiety at night	Lethargy
Verbalizes restlessness during sleep	Disorientation
Complains of daytime sleepiness	Agitation
Reports altered sleep pattern	Mild, fleeting nystagmus
Verbalizes fatigue during the day	Hand tremor
Reports dozing during the day	Ptosis of eyelid, thick speech, dark circles under eyes, frequent yawning

In normal adults, sleep usually begins in NREM, progressing from stage 1. REM sleep usually occurs after a change from stage 3 or 4 NREM to stage 2 NREM. Sleep usually consists of recurring alterations between REM and NREM stages occurring in 70-minute to 120-minute cycles with 4 cycles to 6 cycles per night. In the first third of a typical night, stages 3 and 4 NREM sleep predominate; in the last third, stage 2 NREM and REM sleep predominate, and stage 4 NREM sleep may be absent (Baker 1985; Cherniack 1981; Kryger, Roth, and Dement 1989).

Developmental differences exist for the amount of time spent in each stage and for total sleep time. Infants have the longest total sleep time and the highest percentage of REM sleep, while in the elderly there is a reduction of total sleep time, an increase in stage 1 NREM sleep, and decreases in REM, stage 3, and stage 4 NREM sleep (Baker 1985; Cherniack 1981; Kryger, Roth, and Dement 1989).

SLEEP DISORDERS

Alteration of sleep patterns or disturbed sleep are frequent complaints made by patients both inside and outside hospitals. The actual prevalence depends on the population surveyed and other methodological factors. When grouped together, sleep disturbances are complaints voiced by 15% to 33% of the population (Spiegel 1981). They may be symptoms of sleep-related disorders (for example, excessive daytime sleepiness in narcolepsy and sleep apnea) or secondary to insufficient sleep or other medical, toxic, or environmental conditions. Sleep disturbances are generally thought of as disorders of the initiation and maintenance of sleep, disorders of excessive somnolence, disorders of the sleep-wake cycle, and dysfunctions that are associated with sleep disruption such as nightmares or sleepwalking (Association of Sleep Disorder Centers, 1979). About 20% of employed workers in the United States work evenings or nights or rotate shifts (Toufexis 1990). Disturbances of the sleep pattern may also be related to mental illness. Early-morning wakening is viewed as a symptom of importance in evaluating depression and can be of use not only in the diagnosis of depression but also in assessing the response to treatment.

Insomnia is a common complaint; it is a symptom, however, and not a disease by itself. It is a perception by the person that his or her sleep is not normal. Nighttime sleep difficulties are only part of the picture. The daytime effects of disturbed sleep may include fatigue, sleepiness, impaired functioning, depression, anxiety, and other mood changes. It is sometimes difficult to establish whether poor sleep causes disturbed daytime functioning or whether psychological disturbance is part of the daytime symptomatology and the sleep effects are part of that picture (Kryger, Roth, and Dement 1989). Insomnia must be assessed in terms of duration, severity, and nature. Acute or transient insomnia lasts for several days and is seen in previously normal sleepers experiencing a stress, such as schedule change, jet lag, personal problems, or an acute stress such as hospitalization. Short-term insomnia lasts for 1 week to 3 weeks and may be associated with situational problems at work, with the family, or due to illness. It can be precipitated by grief, illness, or anxiety. Careful management using sleep hygiene techniques is critical in order to prevent persistent or chronic insomnia, a condition that has continued for more than 3 weeks, and even months or years, and may be due to psychiatric, medical, or environmental conditions, which include conditioned insomnia and drug or alcohol dependency (Drugs and insomnia 1984). Hospitalized patients may be victims of sleep deprivation due to endogenous causes, resulting from their illness, stress, and drugs, and also to exogenous causes, resulting from environmental disturbances and frequent awakening. Hospitalization is an excellent model for transient or short-term insomnia (Erman 1985). Severity of the insomnia is measured not only by the degree of sleeplessness experienced but more so by the degree of impaired daytime performance and sleepiness that occurs. Because sleep disruption, particularly when it is persistent, is often associated with psychiatric disorders, psychiatric evaluation may be necessary for a complete assessment and treatment of the problem.

A few primary organic disorders of sleep bear mentioning. Narcolepsy is a sleep disorder with a prevalence in the United States of at least 1 in 1,000. The cause is unknown, and symptoms include excessive daytime sleepiness with irresistible sleep attacks and disturbed nighttime sleep that may occur alone or in conjunction with cataplexy (sudden bilateral voluntary muscle weakness lasting from a few seconds to minutes), sleep paralysis (temporary loss of muscle tone between awakening and falling asleep), hypnagogic hallucinations (vivid, terrifying hallucinations often occurring during sleep paralysis), and other visual and sleep-related disturbances (Baker 1985; Cohen 1988). Sleep apneas are central, obstructive, peripheral, or mixed. Symptoms of obstructive sleep apnea (the most common type) include excessive daytime sleepiness, sleep attacks, nocturnal breath cessation and snoring, and snorting and gasping sounds. Nighttime sleep is disrupted and restless. Symptoms are usually noticed before aged 40 years, and many of these patients are obese, hypertensive males. It is a potentially life-threatening disorder (Kales, Vela-Bueno, and Kales 1987).

ASSESSMENT

Prior to initiating nursing interventions aimed at restoring a comfortable pattern of sleep for the individual patient, assessment of the problem is necessary. There is a good deal of variation in the length of sleep a normal person gets during the night; variations may be due to age and sex and are not subject to change by the nurse. In general, sleep is sufficient if there is no subjective complaint and no disruption of daytime (or waking time) performance. The range in hours for "normal" sleep in adults is 5 hours to 10 hours, with 7 hours to 9 hours being most usual. Sleep changes with advancing age. Elderly people tend to sleep less soundly, wake more frequently and for longer times than when they were younger, and awaken earlier in the morning. There may be an increase in daytime napping (Spiegel 1981). Changes are also seen in the sleep stages. The amount and quality of sleep change according to some variables that can be more readily manipulated, such as environmental disturbances that notoriously occur in the hospital: noise due to elevators, suction machines, monitors, and sounds made by other patients and employees; unnecessary awakenings by staff; light; the administration of medications that alter sleep; pain; anxiety; the sharing of their room with a stranger; and so forth.

Assessment of sleep disturbances includes both objective and subjective measures, among them family, medical, and social histories, sleep history, sleep diary, paper-and-pencil measures of sleepiness, and physical examination. Polysomnography and the Multiple Sleep Latency Test (MSLT) may be necessary to make a definitive medical diagnosis (Cohen 1988). Polysomnography involves the simultaneous monitoring of sleep and selected physiological parameters. It usually consists of monitoring the following: EEG (usually with central, occipital and frontal leads), electro-oculogram (EOG) to detect REMs, electromyogram (EMG), usually recorded from muscles under the chin, and other studies, such as electrocardiography (EKG) and respiratory flow measures. Other physiological measurements, such as ear oximetry and esophageal pH, may be added in some instances depending on the reason for the polysomnography. The MSLT is a direct measure of sleepiness. It is generally done immediately following nocturnal polysomnography. The standard study consists of four tests performed at 2-hour intervals beginning 1½ hours to 3 hours after awakening that are geared to measuring the speed of falling asleep (sleep onset latency) in a sleep-producing environment. In the final analysis, only the affected person can indicate his or her satisfaction with sleep (Closs 1988).

If the patient is a regular client of the nurse or has a history on record, some components of the assessment may be obtained from the chart or existing records. Some medications known to contribute to sleep difficulties include adrenergic and dopaminergic agonists, steroids, thyroid hormone, antihypertensives, anticonvulsants, narcotics, cancer chemotherapeutic agents, antidepressants, theophylline derivatives, antipsychotics, central nervous system depressants, and stimulants. Alcohol, tobacco, and caffeine consumption also can cause sleep disturbances (Gregory, Simmons, and Berger 1988). Paradoxically, some medications used to induce sleep can cause rebound insomnia after long-term use (Rall 1990).

A full description of the sleep complaint is important to assess. The patient should be asked to describe the sleep problem: the duration, the circumstances under which it developed, factors that precipitate or accentuate it, previous treatment, and the impact of the problem on their lives and family (Gregory, Simmons, and Berger 1988). If the patient is not sleeping well, a first step is to clarify what is meant by that statement. Is the patient having trouble falling asleep or remaining asleep, or is the quality of the sleep a problem? If the client is awakening during the night, how many times does this occur? Can the client describe what wakes him or her up? A description of the room in which the patient sleeps is important. The nurse needs to find out if the person takes daytime concerns, such as those related to the job, to bed. Is the problem related to some specific recent change, such as a job layoff. Are there other emotional concerns such as those related to interpersonal or family relationships or financial problems that can be contributing to disrupted sleep? Are disturbing dreams or nightmares a cause of awakening, or is the anticipation of them keeping the client from falling asleep? (Cohen 1988; *Patient Care* 1986)

What about physical complaints? Does the person have to get out of bed because he or she needs to use the bathroom? Is the person having trouble falling asleep or staying asleep because of pain, cramping, or other physical reasons? Symptoms such as heartburn or gastric pain may cause difficulty when the person lies down. Shortness of breath, wheezing, or other respiratory symptoms may contribute to problems. The patient may recall awakening because of choking or difficulty in breathing or because of his or her snoring. Does the person complain of discomfort in the feet and legs that is relieved by getting up and walking around (restless legs syndome)?

For longer or chronic sleep disturbances, it is often helpful for the patient to keep a sleep diary. This can be of assistance in establishing the sleep patterns for that individual and/or triggering events that disturb sleep. For the patient with long-standing sleep pattern disturbances, this record should be maintained for several weeks and include actual napping periods, the time the person gets into bed, approximate time of falling asleep, the time of awakening in the morning, medication use and times taken, exercise patterns, mealtimes, cigarettes smoked, alcohol use, quality of sleep, and any feelings of emotional upset such as worry or stresses. Are the sleep problems relatively constant or episodic? How does the person feel the next morning: tired, fatigued, excessively sleepy, or alert? Does the person have periods of falling asleep during the day? What other symptoms are experienced? The nurse should inquire about symptoms that tend to accompany complaints of excessive daytime sleepiness, such as losing muscular control or sleep attacks (Cohen 1988; *Patient Care* 1986).

Sleep difficulties can be caused by disruption of the sleep-wake cycle or circadian rhythm disturbances such as those resulting from jet travel or working rotating shifts. For those experiencing sleep disturbances because of altered sleep-wake cycles, it is important to separate out short- versus long-term alterations (e.g., rapid time zone transitions like jet lag versus chronic shift rotation). If sleep-wake cycle disruptions create major life disturbances, alternative approaches can be tried.

The characteristics of the disturbed nighttime sleep should be described. This information should include the usual amount of sleep per night, the patient's schedule and whether it is regular or irregular, excessive body movements during sleep, snoring, sleep-wake patterns, including daytime naps, disturbing dreams, and whether difficulty is experienced in falling asleep at night or awakening in the morning. It is helpful to question the bed partner or roommate for information on snorting, gasping, or apneic periods, the apparent presence of bad dreams, restlessness, or sleepwalking (Cohen 1988; Kales, Soldatos, and Kales 1980; *Patient Care* 1986).

ASSOCIATED NURSING DIAGNOSES

Sleep Pattern Disturbance is a broad nursing diagnosis that can apply when people experience a primary or secondary sleep disorder (McFarland and McFarlane 1989). Since usual sleep patterns are individual, data collected through a comprehensive, holistic assessment are needed to determine the etiology of the disturbance for each person. Responses to sleep deprivation are also individual and people may exhibit a variety of other nursing problems.

Pain, Fear, and Anxiety may be exhibited by people who have concurrent medical conditions that underlie the sleep disturbance. Fatigue and Altered Role Performance are likely to be present regardless of the reason for the disturbance. Potential for Injury exists if people who are excessively fatigued continue to participate in their usual activities, such as driving a car or working with heavy machinery. When people are deprived of deeper stages of sleep (stages 3 and 4 NREM and REM) over an extended period of time, behavior indicating Sensory/Perceptual Alterations and Altered Thought Processes are often exhibited. Research into the effects of the intensive care unit environment on sleep deprivation has demonstrated that many patients who received less than 50% of their usual sleep time hallucinated and became disoriented, combative, paranoid, and delusional (Thelan, Davie, and Urden 1990). Ineffective Individual Coping and Knowledge Deficit may be present when individuals resort to chronic use of hypnotics and sedatives to control a sleep disturbance. People with a primary disorder that is poorly controlled (e.g., narcolepsy) may experience Ineffective Family Coping and Altered Family Processes, especially if the family members have difficulty believing that excessive daytime sleepiness cannot be voluntarily controlled by the individual experiencing this symptom. People with sleep apnea syndrome experience Impaired Gas Exchange and Ineffective Breathing Patterns that may require extensive medical and nursing therapies, such as ventilation support and airway management to control this disorder.

INTERVENTION

Sleep Promotion is a broad area and is addressed here as three interventions: Sleep Promotion: Hygiene Measures; Sleep Promotion: Environmental Alterations, and Sleep Promotion: Drug Therapy.

Sleep Promotion: Hygiene Measures

Application of sleep hygiene techniques are useful for improvement in sleep and prevention of chronic insomnia. These include such measures as the following:

1.   Establish regular times for bedtime and awakening. Do not stay in bed if a full night's sleep has been obtained. Some believe that arising times should be maintained even if the person had difficulty sleeping the night before; others believe that the person should sleep as long as needed in order to feel refreshed in the morning.

2.   While regular exercise is helpful, strenuous exercise close to bedtime can keep one awake and should be avoided.

3.   Avoid eating heavy meals or spicy foods before bedtime because they can lead to gastrointestinal discomfort. Caffeine and alcohol can disturb sleep and should be avoided. In some cases, caffeine (in coffee and many other products) should be avoided after noon. Hunger can also disturb sleep. Both excessive food and fluid intake should be avoided close to bedtime. A warm drink containing milk, such as cocoa, before bedtime may aid in producing drowsiness.

4.   Encourage restful activities such as reading before bedtime, and avoid stimulating or anxiety-provoking activities.

5.   Establish a bedtime routine with a consistent bedtime and the same activities preceding bedtime, such as a warm bath.

6.   The bedroom environment should be conducive to a good night's sleep. Have the room at a comfortable temperature. The bed itself and pillows should be comfortable, and there should be clean linens. The person should put on comfortable nightwear. The room should be free from excessive clutter, dark, and quiet. If

noise is unavoidable, find alternatives such as white noise or earplugs if necessary, or sometimes the cause can be fixed, such as that due to a sticking door or creaking floorboard. In the hospital, a room away from the nurses' station or housekeeping closet might be quieter.

7. When the person lies down in bed and is ready to try to fall asleep, there should not be the anticipation of an awakening event. The patient should be able to clear the mind and relax. He or she needs to avoid thinking about stressful events and events that await the next day. The nurse can teach progressive muscular relaxation techniques that can be applied at this time, with or without visualization of peaceful and relaxing images such as those with water. Biofeedback, meditation, imaging, and self-hypnosis are other alternatives.

8. Avoid smoking and other tobacco use.

9. If, after a reasonable period of time (usually about 30 minutes) sleep is still elusive, the person should get out of bed and do something else without dwelling on trying to fall asleep. He or she should get back in bed and try relaxing again, repeating this routine as many times as necessary. It is important to avoid the mental association of being in bed with wakefulness.

10. Napping during the day should be avoided because it can disturb the following night's sleep. A patient who needs to rest during the day should do this in a place other than the bed.

11. The bed should not be used as a place for work activities; it is important to maintain its association as a restful, relaxing place (Cohen 1988; Golden and James 1988; *Patient Care* 1986).

Sleep Promotion: Environmental Alterations

For insomnia, environmental alterations can be initiated. In the hospital, nurses can also organize work so as to minimize interruptions, remove restrictive devices, eliminate low-level noises, decrease lights, and eliminate nonessential tasks. Since stimulation is higher in the hospital, where possible, this should be minimized or countered.

For persistent insomnia due to disturbances of the sleep-wake cycle due to shift work, other changes may be needed. For example, the person who works midnight to 8:00 A.M. might plan to sleep on returning home in the morning or later in the afternoon. Different eating and sleeping patterns can be tried for optimal results. Short naps may be useful. Work schedules can be adjusted so that forward rotation (moving from days to evenings to nights) occurs. Timed exposures to special bright artificial light and darkness over 2 to 3 days can be useful in resetting the biological clock (Toufexis 1990). Depending on the degree of perceived difficulties, the person may choose to change the working schedule. Some people may feel that they need "permission" to do this.

For those suffering from rapid time zone transitions or jet lag, behavioral techniques can be utilized in preventive fashion. Before leaving home, the person can gradually shift bedtime in the appropriate direction. In general, adaptation to an eastward flight is longer than to a westward one. Short-term drug therapy may also be useful (Kryger, Roth, and Dement 1989).

Chronotherapy may be used for advanced and delayed sleep phase syndromes. In the first, sleep onset is early, from 8:00 P.M. to 9:00 P.M. with early morning awakening (from 3:00 A.M. to 5:00 A.M.). Systematic advancement of bedtime is used until the desired bedtime is reached. In delayed sleep phase syndrome, in which sleep onset is delayed until 3:00 A.M. to 6:00 A.M. with natural arousal at 11:00 A.M. to 2:00 P.M. bedtime is delayed by 3-hour increments each day, establishing a 27-hour day until the desired bedtime is reached. Then the 24-hour day is reestablished (Kryger, Roth, and Dement 1989).

Sleep Promotion: Drug Therapy

Drug therapy has a place in sleep disturbance treatment when used judiciously. Sedative and hypnotic agents are used for the treatment of insomnia. Sedatives decrease activity, moderate excitement, and have a calming effect. Hypnotics produce drowsiness and facilitate sleep. They are generally central nervous depressants with the exception of the benzodiazepines, which are widely used in the treatment of situational insomnia. Their effects as a group include sedation, hypnosis, decreased anxiety, muscle relaxation, and anticonvulsant activity. Some of the most frequently used are flurazepam (Dalmane), temazepam (Restoril), and triazolam (Halcion). Diazepam (Valium), although not directly used for insomnia, may be used before bedtime in patients taking it for anxiety in order to promote sleep. Unlike the barbiturates, the benzodiazepines, in usual therapeutic doses, have only slight effects on respiration and the cardiovascular system. Short-acting hypnotics (such as triazolam) may be used for those who have difficulty in getting to sleep but stay asleep once it occurs. Thus, depending on whether the problem is getting to sleep or staying asleep is important in determining the appropriate drug (Drugs and insomnia 1984). Relatively common side effects of these drugs as a group include weakness, lightheadedness, impairment of mental and psychomotor skills, memory difficulties, often occurring the next day, headache, blurred vision, dizziness, and gastrointestinal effects. Depending on the time the patient takes the medication and the duration of action, effects such as drowsiness, memory problems, and diminished coordination can occur in the morning. Generally these drugs are most useful for situational insomnia on a short-term basis of a few days. Often they are discontinued after acceptable sleep has occurred for 1 night or 2 nights. Gradual discontinuation may be necessary (Drugs and insomnia 1984; Rall 1990). On a long-term basis, hypnotic agents tend to produce rebound insomnia, with decreasing benefit. Increases in nightmares may be found for a time after withdrawal. Caution is needed for their use with the elderly.

For narcolepsy, effective control of symptoms through drug therapy may be difficult to achieve. Medications include central stimulants such as the amphetamines and their derivatives in order to prevent sleep attacks. Major ones used include methylphenidate (Ritalin), dextroamphetamine (Dexedrine), methamphetamine (Desoxyn), and pemoline (Cylert). Side effects are frequent, and amphetamines disturb nocturnal sleep, especially if taken after supper. For the other prevalent symptoms, tricyclic antidepressants and monoamine oxidase inhibitors are used, but their use can result in nocturnal sleep problems also. Newer agents such as serotonin, norepinephrine, and gamma-aminobutyric acid derivatives are also used but have negative effects on usual nocturnal sleep. Nonpharmacologic approaches such as planned daytime naps and diet adjustments may be successful with individual patients (Cohen 1988; Kales, Vela-Buena, and Kales 1987).

The approach to therapy for persons with life-threatening sleep apnea usually involves adjustment of concurrent or underlying medical and psychological problems, weight reduction if possible in those who are obese, medications in mild cases with protriptyline (a tricyclic antidepressant), nasal continuous positive airway pressure, tongue-retaining devices, and even surgical techniques such as uvulo-palatopharyngoplasty and tracheostomy (Kales, Vela-Bueno, and Kales 1987).

CASE STUDY

Mr. B is a 52-year-old married salesman who works for a large national equipment manufacturer. He was referred to the Sleep Center for evaluation of chronic insomnia of about 20 months' duration. Trials with various hypnotics by his family physician had been unsuccessful in promoting effective sleep.

Mr. B complained of difficulty falling asleep when he got into bed at night, along with feeling excessively sleepy during the day; he had difficulty staying awake during sales meetings and readily fell asleep on the train he took to and from his place of work when he was not traveling out of town. When he did get to sleep at night, he reported awakening frequently — sometimes as often as every hour. During the past 6 months, he reported delaying bedtime because of concern over difficulty falling asleep. Additionally, he reported awakening for the day early in the morning, often as early as 4:00 A.M. On the weekends, he tried to sleep most of the morning and took afternoon naps to "catch up on my sleep."

Mr. B appeared weak and fatigued from lack of sleep, with bloodshot eyes that had dark circles around them. He appeared apathetic although well in control of himself and responded appropriately with a tired, tense smile. He reported that his sleep quality had fluctuated since early adulthood; he attributed this to the travel he did as part of his job, which required him to sleep in different hotel rooms for about half of the working days each month.

A detailed psychosocial history revealed that equipment sales in the company for which he worked had declined during the past 2½ years. Some of the salesmen were laid off or asked to take early retirement. Two of Mr. B's children are grown and on their own, with a 19-year-old daughter who is a sophomore in college and still living at home. About 4 years ago, Mr. B and his wife purchased an older home that they planned on updating; however, plans for renovation had been slower to complete than anticipated due to the extensive amount of work required and the associated costs. For the past year, Mrs. B has been complaining about the time required to complete the rehabilitation and the need to live constantly in disrupted surroundings. Mr. B reported that for the past 2 years, he has been able to maintain his income at approximately the same level by increasing his sales in the areas of parts and service, strategies that he felt protected him from losing his job, and he was reluctant to admit that worries over his job and financial situation could be causing his sleep problems.

Review of the sleep diary kept by Mr. B revealed that he tended to lie in bed upon retiring and think about how he could increase equipment sales in the territory for which he was responsible. He mentally planned sales calls and rehearsed how he would conduct his calls the next day. He also thought about what he could do to keep his boss happy so that he would not lose his job. When he awoke during the night, he often thought about his job and even turned on the light to write his ideas down on the pad of paper he kept at his bedside so he would not forget them. Increasingly, plans for rehabilitating the house were also on his mind at night, and he would think about what could be done to cut corners to reduce costs so that the work could be completed and his wife would be happy. Sometimes he conducted these activities before he went to bed and delayed bedtime so that he would be as sleepy as possible when he got in bed. Even when he seemed very sleepy, he often felt anxious and irritated if he did not fall asleep within 10 minutes of retiring.

Somnographic sleep studies that were conducted for 3 nights revealed less than 4 total hours sleep a night with frequent awakenings. Stage 1 sleep predominated, and REM sleep tended to appear in less than 30 minutes, a pattern of sleep that is typical of depression. Psychological testing revealed a serious, well-defended depression. During extended counseling, Mr. B verbalized for the first time how worried he was about losing his job and how he would meet his financial obligations for his daughter's education and completing the house renovation if he was released from his job. He was also worried that his age would prevent him from finding a comparable position.

A sedating antidepressant and better sleep hygiene techniques improved sleep within 2 to 3 days of being instituted. The nurse helped Mr. B establish regular times for retiring and awakening. He no longer experienced waking excessively early in the morning. At times, he stayed in bed up to an hour longer on the weekends, which helped him to feel somewhat more refreshed in the morning if he had awakened a couple of times during the night. Mr. B increased his exercise by planning and conducting a regular program of vigorous walking. He switched to decaffeinated beverages after his morning coffee. When he did not have to entertain customers for dinner in the evening, he moved his evening mealtime up to 6:00 P.M. to avoid excessive intake close to bedtime. Instead of reviewing his sales plans at bedtime, he began reading popular best-sellers, a habit he had had when he was a college student. Instead of taking any hotel that was available, he began to pay closer attention to environmental comfort by booking the same room in the same hotel as much as possible when traveling. Instead of anticipating the next day's events when he got in bed, Mr. B practiced the progressive relaxation techniques taught to him by the nurse. With the encouragement of the nurse, Mr. B sought career counseling. He reviewed company policies relative to release and retirement should this become necessary. He contacted a number of employment agencies and found, to his surprise, that he would have little difficulty finding a comparable job in his field. He made alternative plans for completing the house renovation with his wife; by cutting back on some earlier plans, both were pleased to discover that the work could be completed at less cost and sooner than anticipated.

At his 9-month follow up, Mr. B was found to be no longer depressed. He was off all drugs and satisfied with the dramatic improvement he had experienced in his sleep pattern. Although he still had some minor difficulty with sleeping while traveling, Mr. B claimed that he was satisfied since he had always had some trouble sleeping when he was on the road.

CONCLUSION

Disorders of sleep are a relatively common patient complaint. These may be primary or secondary to other dysfunction or illness. Both long- and short-term problems may be seen. A necessary first step is accurate assessment of the problem. Sleep hygiene techniques may be coupled with both pharmacologic and environmental alterations to implement the intervention of Sleep Promotion.

REFERENCES

Association of Sleep Disorder Centers. 1979. Diagnostic classification of sleep and arousal disorders. *Sleep* 2:1–137.

Baker, T.L. 1985. Introduction to sleep and sleep disorders. *Medical Clinics of North America* 69:1123–1152.

Carpenito, L.J. 1989. *Nursing diagnosis: Applications to clinical practice.* 3d ed. Philadelphia: J.B. Lippincott.

Carrieri, V.K., Lindsey, A.M., and West, C.M. 1986. *Pathophysiological phenomena in nursing: Human responses to illness.* Philadelphia: W.B. Saunders.

Cherniack, N.S. 1981. Respiratory dysrhythmias during sleep. *New England Journal of Medicine* 305:325–330.

Closs, S.J. 1988. Assessment of sleep in hospital patients: A review of methods. *Journal of Advanced Nursing* 13:501–510.

Cohen, F.L. 1984. *Clinical genetics in nursing practice*. Philadelphia: J.B. Lippincott.

Cohen, F.L. 1988. Narcolepsy: A review of a common, life-long sleep disorder. *Journal of Advanced Nursing* 13:546–556.

Drugs and insomnia. 1984. *Journal of the American Medical Association* 251:2410–2414.

Erman, M.K. Insomnia management. 1985. *Journal of Enterostomal Therapy* 12:210–213.

Golden, R.N., and James, S.P. 1988. Insomnia. *Postgraduate Medicine* 83(4):251–258.

Gregory, J.G., Simmons, E.C., and Berger, B.R. 1988. Approaches to insomnia. *North Carolina Medical Journal* 49:502–504.

Johnson, S.E. 1989. Sleep pattern disturbance: Defining characteristics observable in practice. In R. M. Carroll-Johnson (ed.), *Classification of nursing diagnoses: Proceedings of the Eighth Conference* (pp. 368–370). Philadelphia: J.B. Lippincott.

Kales, A., Soldatos, C.R., and Kales, J.D. 1980. Taking a sleep history. *American Family Physician* 22:101–107.

Kales, A., Vela-Bueno, A., and Kales, J.D. 1987. Sleep disorders: Sleep apnea and narcolepsy. *Annals of Internal Medicine* 106:434–443.

Kim, M.J., McFarland, G.K., and McLane, A.M. 1989. *Pocket guide to nursing diagnoses*. 3d ed. St. Louis: C.V. Mosby.

Kryger, M.H., Roth, T., and Dement, W.C. (eds.). 1989. *Principles and practice of sleep medicine* (pp. 431–432). Philadelphia: W.B. Saunders Co.

Lo, C.K., and Kim, M.J. 1986. Construct validity of sleep pattern disturbance: A methodological approach. In M.A. Hurley (ed.), *Classification of nursing diagnoses: Proceedings of the Sixth Conference* (pp. 197–206). St. Louis: C.V. Mosby.

McFarland, G.K. and McFarlane, E.A. 1989. *Nursing diagnosis and intervention: Planning for patient care*. St. Louis: C.V. Mosby.

Patient Care. 1986. An office work-up for sleep disorders. Patient Care 20(2):20–38.

Rall, T.W. 1990. Hypnotics and sedatives: Ethanol. In A.G. Gilman, T.W. Rall, A.S. Nies, and P. Taylor, *Goodman and Gilman's the pharmacological basis of therapeutics*. 8th ed. (pp. 345–379). New York: Pergamon Press.

Rechtschaffen, A., and Kales, A. 1968. *A manual of standardized terminology, techniques and scoring system for sleep stages of human subjects*. NIHM publication 204. Washington, D.C.: U.S. Government Printing Office.

Spiegel, R. 1981. *Sleep and sleeplessness in advanced age*. New York: S.P. Medical Books.

Thelan, L.A., Davie, J.K., and Urden, L.D. 1990. *Textbook of critical care nursing: Diagnosis and management*. St. Louis: C.V. Mosby.

Toufexis, A. 1990, December 17. Drowsy America. *Time*, 126(26):78–85.

9

CONFUSION MANAGEMENT

JACQUELINE M. STOLLEY
KATHLEEN C. BUCKWALTER

Confusion Management is a complex intervention that depends on the etiology and prognosis of the confusion. Confusion is frequently misdiagnosed and thus mismanaged. It is an important concept to understand because it is socially disabling and makes unusually high demands on medical, nursing, and social resources. Nevertheless, understanding confusion as a concept is difficult in that it is rarely discussed by itself; rather, it is often viewed only as a symptom of another problem, such as dementia. As Nagley and Dever (1989) point out, "While there may be a shared understanding of confusion among practitioners, a clear and concise definition of confusion for scientific study is lacking" (p. 80).

Confusion Management incorporates the provision of symptomatic and supportive measures and treatment to eliminate and/or correct any underlying pathophysiological condition (Foreman 1990). These measures can include such diverse actions as modification of the environment to prevent sensory overload and overstimulation or the correction of fluid and electrolyte imbalances. It is important for nurses to distinguish between reversible (acute) and irreversible (chronic) confusional states and to understand that a person with chronic confusion can also experience an acute episode exhibiting exacerbated symptoms related to physical or environmental etiologies. This chapter focuses on treatment of chronic confusion in institutionalized clients.

REVIEW OF THE LITERATURE

Anything that interrupts or violates the homodynamic equilibrium of person, body, self, and the environment can precipitate confusion. Aged persons are particularly vulnerable to disequilibrium due to losses associated with the aging process and various sociocultural factors that increase the perception of stress (Hall 1986). Wolanin and Phillips (1981) delineated five sources of confusion: compromised brain support, sensoriperceptual problems, disruption in pattern and meaning, alterations in normal physiologic states, and the true dementias. Chronic confusion is usually synonymous with the true dementias.

Chronic Confusion

Although there are 70 different conditions that can cause dementia in the middle and late years (Blass 1982; Katzman 1986), Alzheimer's disease (AD) is the most common, representing 60% of the elderly who are irreversibly demented.

Most of the nursing research devoted to chronic confusional states, and therefore much of this chapter, focuses on AD. This progressive disorder is characterized by losses of memory, intellectual and language ability, and general competency over a period averaging 6 to 15 years and ending in death. Although the most commonly cited figure is that between 4% and 7% of persons aged 65 to 75 years suffer from some form of dementia (Cross and Gurland 1986), recent epidemiological evidence from the East Boston studies of Evans and colleagues (1989) suggests that the percentage may be almost twice as high. The percentage increases dramatically to 25% for those over age 85.

The diagnosis of AD is made by exclusion of other possible causes of dementia (McKhann, Drachman, Folstein, Katzman, Price, and Stadlan 1984). Several other degenerative brain diseases present with behaviors similar to those found in AD, although their etiologies are quite different. Multi-infarct dementia (MID) accounts for about 10% of all dementing illnesses. When infarcts occur, cognitive and functional abilities diminish in abrupt, steplike fashion rather than the gradual, almost imperceptible decline noted in AD. MID and AD coexist in another 17% of the cases of irreversible dementia (Heston and White 1983). Other rare conditions account for 13% of the dementias, including Pick's disease, Cruetzfeldt-Jacob disease, Parkinson's disease, Huntington's disease, normal pressure hydrocephalus, and AIDS.

Symptoms of AD

Symptoms of AD progress in stages or phases. Reisberg (1982) measured the stages of AD with an instrument called the Global Deterioration Scale, which measures deterioration in seven stages with stage 1 being normal, with no cognitive decline, and stage 7 being late dementia, indicating very severe cognitive decline. A simpler method delineates the disease progression into four stages: forgetfulness, confusion, ambulatory dementia, and the terminal or end stage (Hall and Buckwalter, 1987) (Table 9–1).

It is estimated the 600,000 persons with AD reside in nursing facilities (Kosich & Grodon 1982) and that they account for nearly half of the admissions (Burnside 1982). Institutionalization can be considered inevitable as the disease progresses (Berger 1985).

Progressively Lowered Stress Threshold

Because of ego-sensory impairments and diminished perceptual and cognitive processes that interfere with the AD client's ability to interact successfully with the environment, control of the environment is essential for care management. Repetitive behaviors, catastrophic reactions, and inappropriate behaviors are symptoms of this impairment (Roberts and Algase 1988). The Progressively Lowered Stress Threshold Model (PLST) (Hall and Buckwalter 1987) asserts that persons with AD require a modified environment because of declining functional and cognitive abilities. According to the PLST Model, persons with AD have an increasing ability to cope with stress as the disease progresses (Hall and Buckwalter 1987).

Hall (1991) has described three types of behavior that may be present throughout the course of the disease: baseline or normative behavior where the client is still cognitively and socially accessible; anxious behavior, which is a response to stress: and dysfunctional behavior, when excess stress is not reduced and the AD victim cannot process the amount, complexity, or intensity of stimuli. These behaviors

TABLE 9–1. STAGES OF ALZHEIMER'S DISEASE

Forgetfulness	1. Short-term memory losses: Misplace, forget, lose things 2. Compensate with memory aids: Lists, routine, organization 3. Express awareness of problem: Concern about abilities 4. May become depressed: Complicates and worsens symptoms 5. Not diagnosable at this stage
Confusion	1. Progressive memory decline: Interferes with all abilities; short term most impaired, long term follows later 2. Disorientation: Time, place, person, thing 3. Instrumental activities of daily living (IADLs): Money management, legal affairs, transportation difficulties, housekeeping, cooking 4. Denial is common but give clues that fear "losing their mind" 5. Depression more common; aware of deficits and frightened 6. Confabulation and stereotyped word usage: Covering up for memory losses 7. More problems when stressed, fatigued, out of own environment, ill 8. Day care and in-home assistance commonly needed
Ambulatory dementia	1. Functional losses in ADLs (in approximate order of loss): willingness and ability to bathe, grooming, choosing among clothing, dressing, gait and mobility, toileting, communication, reading, and writing skills 2. Loss of ability to reason, plan for safety, and communicate verbally 3. Frustration is common 4. Becomes more withdrawn and self-absorbed 5. Depression resolves as the person's awareness of memory loss and disability decreases 6. Becomes less "accessible" to others—unable to retain information or use past experiences to guide behavior 7. Communication becomes more and more difficult with loss of language 8. Behavioral evidence of reduced stress threshold: Up at night, wandering, pacing, confused, agitated, belligerent, combative, withdrawn 9. Institutional care usually needed
End stage	1. Does not recognize family members or even own image in a mirror 2. No longer walks; little purposeful activity 3. Often mute and may yell or scream spontaneously 4. Forgets how to eat, swallow, and chew; weight loss is common and client may become emaciated 5. Develops problems associated with immobility: Pneumonia, pressure ulcers, urinary tract infections, and contractures 6. Incontinence is common; may have seizures 7. Most certainly institutionalized at this point

correspond to the amount of brain damage and the progression of the disease (Table 9–2).

According to the PLST Model, the losses associated with AD and other irreversible dementias fall into four symptom clusters: cognitive or intellectual losses, affective or personality losses, conative or planning losses, and progressively lowered stress threshold (Hall and Buckwalter 1978) (Table 9–3). Confusion Management is directed largely toward providing supportive care to compensate for these losses and flows logically from the PLST framework.

In planning interventions for persons with AD or other diseases manifested by chronic confusion, the following assumptions are made:

1.   All humans require some control over their person and their environment and need some degree of unconditional positive regard.

2.   All behavior is rooted and has meaning; therefore, all catastrophic and stress-related behaviors have a cause.

TABLE 9-2. BEHAVIORAL STATES ASSOCIATED WITH AD

Baseline	The client remains cognitively accessible. The client possesses a basic awareness of the environment and is able to interact and function, limited only by the amount of neurological deficits. The client also remains socially accessible. The client is able to communicate wants and needs and respond to the communication of others in an appropriate manner.
Anxious	The client becomes anxious when feeling stress. Symptoms of anxious behavior may be complaints of a feeling of uneasiness. Eye contact is poor or absent, and psychomotor activity may increase in response to the avoidance of the noxious stimuli. Communication abilities usually remain intact.
Dysfunctional	The client becomes dysfunctional if stress levels continue or increase. The client becomes catastrophic and cognitively and socially inaccessible. Communication is impaired, and the client is unable to interpret the environment appropriately (Wolanin and Phillips 1981). The client may be fearful and panic stricken and actively avoid the noxious stimuli (Hall 1991). Increased confusion, purposeful wandering, night awakening, "sundowner's syndrome," agitation, fearfulness, panic, combativeness, and sudden withdrawal are exhibited with catastrophic, dysfunctional behavior. The client may experience these symptoms infrequently early in the disease, but with disease progression they increase in frequency and intensity (Hall 1991).

3. The confused or agitated client is not comfortable and should be regarded as frightened. All clients have the right to be comfortable.

4. The client exists in a 24-hour continuum. Care cannot be planned or evaluated on an 8-hour-shift basis. If the client has a problem during the night, some changes need to be implemented during the day (Hall and Buckwalter, 1987, p. 401; Hall 1991).

Interventions for chronic confusion include the provision of symptomatic and supportive measures and are based on the above assumptions. Hall and Buckwalter (1987) set forth the following principles in caring for the chronically confused:

1. Maximize the level of safe function by supporting all areas of loss in a prosthetic manner.

2. Provide the client with unconditional positive regard.

3. Use behaviors indicating anxiety and avoidance to determine limits of levels of activity and stimuli.

4. Teach caregivers to listen to the client, evaluating verbal and nonverbal responses.

5. Modify the environment to support losses and enhance safety.

6. Provide ongoing support, care and problem solving for caregivers (Hall and Buckwalter 1987, p. 404).

Using this framework, nurses can provide effective intervention and care for all clients with chronic confusion, as well as those with acute confusional states.

INTERVENTION TOOLS

An appropriate intervention must take into account the degree of loss of the individual suffering from chronic confusion. Thus, it is important to obtain accurate

TABLE 9-3. SYMPTOM CLUSTERS ASSOCIATED WITH PROGRESSIVE DEMENTING ILLNESS

Cognitive (intellectual)	Memory loss, initially for recent events Loss of time sense Inability to abstract Inability to make choices and decisions Inability to reason and problem solve Poor judgment Altered perceptions and ability to identify visual and auditory stimuli Less expressive and receptive language abilities
Affective (personality)	Loss of affect Diminished inhibitions, emotional lability, spontaneous conversation with loss of tact, loss of control of temper, and inability to delay gratification Decreased attention span Social withdrawal and avoidance of complex or overwhelming stimuli Increasing self-preoccupation Antisocial behavior Confabulation, perseveration Psychotic features, such as paranoia, delusions, and pseudohallucinations
Conative (planning)	Loss of general ability to plan activities Inability to carry out voluntary activities or activities requiring thought to set goals, organize, and complete task Functional loss, starting with high-level maintenance activities such as money and legal management, shopping, and transportation; these progress to losses in activities of daily living, generally in the following order: bathing, grooming, choosing clothing, dressing, mobility, toileting, communicating, and eating Motor apraxia Increased fatigue with exertion or cognition, loss of energy reserve Frustration, refusal to participate, or expressions of helplessness when losses are challenged Increased thought about function tends to worsen performance
PLST (progressively lowered stress threshold)	Catastrophic behaviors Confused or agitated night awakening Purposeful wandering Violent, agitated, or anxious behavior Withdrawal or avoidance behavior, such as belligerency Noisy behavior Purposeless behavior Compulsive behavior Other cognitively and socially inaccessible behaviors (Hall, 1988, p32)

Source: Reprinted with permission. W. B. Saunders Co.
Hall, G. R. 1988. Care of the patient with Alzheimer's disease living at home. *Nursing Clinics of North America,* 23(1): 31–46.

physical, social, and psychological histories of the client to determine premorbid personality and strategies used by the in-home caregiver to provide comfort.

The Mini Mental Status Examination (MMSE) is a useful screening tool for ascertaining the current cognitive level of the client and assessing cognitive loss on an ongoing basis (Folstein, Folstein, and McHugh 1975). This test contains 10 items that measure recent and past memory, temporal orientation, language, quick recall, and ability to abstract and calculate, as well as assess affective and conative losses (Hall 1991). The MMSE is a quick and easy method for nurses to obtain baseline measures of cognitive status and to determine changes over time.

Other parameters that nurses must assess in order to develop interventions are sleep patterns, medication use (especially psychoactive drugs), food intake and weight, socialization before and after institutionalization, episodes of anxious, confused, agitated, purposeful wandering, combative or otherwise dysfunctional behavior, functional level, and family's satisfaction with care.

ASSOCIATED NURSING DIAGNOSES

A number of nursing diagnoses are associated with chronic confusional states. Among the most common are Altered Thought Processes, Impaired Communication, Potential for Injury, Potential for Violence, and Sensory/Perceptual Alteration.

SUGGESTED PROTOCOLS

The intervention of Confusion Management is based on the principles identified earlier (Hall and Buckwalter, 1987) and is specified in more detail in this section. Seven areas are addressed: maximizing safe functioning, unconditional positive regard, determining limits of activity/stimuli, listening, modifying the environment, physical care, and caregiver/family support.

Maximizing Safe Functioning

Nurses must prevent and treat the occurrence of excess disability, defined as a condition that exists when the disturbance of functioning is greater than might be accounted for by basic physical illness or cerebral pathology (Dawson, Kline, Wianko, and Wells 1986). Excess disability is thought to be caused by five factors: fatigue, change in routine (caregiver or environment), multiple competing stimuli, stress or frustration resulting from demands to perform beyond capability, and physiologic causes such as illness, discomfort, pain, or medication reactions. Catastrophic reactions or dysfunctional behavior can result from any of these factors, causing excess disability.

Manifestations of dysfunctional behavior include wandering, night awakening, agitation, fearfulness, panic, combativeness, or sudden withdrawal. Nurses can be alert to anxious behavior that often leads to dysfunctional behavior by observing the client for loss of eye contact and attempts to avoid offending stimuli. Prevention and/or containment of the five factors listed above is a key element of confusion management.

Fatigue

Persons with AD and other chronic confusional states tend to react to stress or frustration by becoming more active, not knowing their levels of fatigue tolerance. In addition, sleep patterns tend to be altered with an upset in diurnal rhythms. Nurses must be alert to this and provide for structured rest periods, which prevents fatigue, allows for a reduction in stress levels, and promotes effective sleep patterns. In addition, rest periods provide the client with time to recover from stressful activities such as morning care and mealtimes.

Quiet times of 40 minutes to 90 minutes should occur midmorning and midafternoon and do not necessarily imply sleep. Since many confused clients resist lying in bed, a reclining chair is ideal for this purpose. Staff members must respect structured rest periods and plan care, activities, and visitation around these periods.

Change in Routine, Caregiver, or Environment

It is important to provide a structured routine for persons with chronic confusion. Because of memory loss and diminished intellectual functioning, the confused client has an increased need for security. Security is enhanced by providing a structured routine, familiar caregivers, and a secure environment. Because the client does not need to rely on planning skills for most activities, the use of a consistent routine is effective (Schwab, Rader, and Doan 1985). For example, bath times, mealtimes, rest periods, and activities should be the same every day. If possible, caregivers should be consistent, providing the client with the security of a familiar face. Room changes are discouraged, as well as the location for activities. The client should not be exposed to changes in the environment (e.g., visits to a shopping mall or a favorite restaurant) unless he or she is cognitively and socially accessible and has experienced no dysfunctional behavior in the past associated with these activities. Decorations during changes in season or holidays provide cues to the client about the time of year. However, these decorations and environmental cues must be more subtle than those for clients who are not cognitively impaired to prevent overstimulation and pseudohallucinations.

Multiple Competing Stimuli

Because chronically confused clients are frequently deficient in cognitive and social accessibility, it is important to modify stimuli and to keep everything simple. Persons with chronic confusion have more difficulty interpreting the environment because of brain damage and sensoriperceptual deficits. For example, many chronically confused persons become distracted and confused when eating in a large group, resulting in their inability to consume appropriate nutrients. Thus, mealtimes should be modified as small group activities, with no more than four persons at a table. Some clients may need to eat alone.

Noise levels on a unit for persons with chronic confusion should be decreased. For example, paging systems and call lights that ring or buzz when turned on should not be used. Staff should be aware that yelling, banging, or even the noise of a disruptive client can be disturbing and become a source of agitation for other clients. Television and radio usage should be carefully monitored.

Pictures and photographs should be simple because persons with chronic confusion frequently misinterpret them as real. Therefore, artwork featuring landscapes and scenery is preferable. Photographs should be of familiar persons and labeled with their name to enable the confused client to identify the person in the photograph.

Visits should be limited to familiar persons and should occur at regular times if possible. Only one or two persons should visit at a time, and large group activities, such as a family reunion, should be avoided unless the client has shown comfort and pleasure with these activities. Visitors should be instructed on appropriate topics to address, especially past events, and be reminded not to "test the resident" or expect him or her to have memories or abilities that no longer are there.

Stress or Frustration

Stress and frustration are frequently the result of the expectations of others that go beyond the client's capabilities. It is important for the nurse to assess the client's cognitive ability before implementing an intervention, so that he or she can function at a maximum level.

Persons with chronic confusion have short-term memory deficits. Research involving reality orientation (RO) has shown that this technique is not beneficial (Hogstel 1979; Nodhturft and Sweeney 1982; Parker and Somers 1983) in that confusion may actually be a denial or defense mechanism necessary to cope with unpleasant realities (Feil 1984; Rader, Doan, and Schwab 1985; Shohan and Neuschants 1985). For these reasons, RO is not recommended. The nurse, however, may use an informal RO approach that will help the client with general orientation. For example, the nurse may say, "It's a very warm day for October." In this way, the client can receive cuing on the general time of year, without the expectation of remembering the exact date or season.

Routines should be simplified and choices limited. A chronically confused person may not be able to understand the concept of getting dressed, but if the nurse simplifies the process with step-by-step directions, the client may function well. For example, the nurse might present a shirt while explaining exactly what behavior is expected: "Put your right arm in this sleeve; put your left arm in the other sleeve. Now button the shirt." In selecting clothing, it is important to give minimal choices, since in AD the decision-making process is impaired. Thus, the nurse may exhibit only two items of clothing for the client to choose from rather than opening the closet and asking the client what he or she wants to wear.

Chronically confused clients frequently become catastrophic and combative because of negative feedback from staff and other clients. The client may wander into another's room and be told, "Get out" or "You're crazy." This negative feedback is confusing to the confused client who has difficulty defining his or her own space and property. Because of disinhibition, the client may not eat properly, failing to use utensils. Rather than correcting the client, the nurse should provide foods that are easily eaten with fingers. If segregation in a low-stimulus unit is not possible, nurses may place red or yellow tape on floors to provide boundaries for the confused client. Yellow cloth drapes fastened with Velcro have been known to keep confused clients in their own rooms or out of others' rooms without using restraints. Identifying a confused client's room with his or her name in large block letters or a photograph easily visible outside the door helps the person to identify his or her own space. Red or yellow are universal colors that say "Stop" or "Caution"; they are also the wavelength of light on the color spectrum most visible to aging eyes. It is important to identify all items of clothing and other property with the client's name.

The use of physical restraints is discouraged for chronically confused persons. Although restraints are frequently used to calm a person or provide safety, they rarely have this effect with confused persons. Rather, they cause dysfunctional, catastrophic behaviors, intensify disorganized behavior, contribute to sensory deprivation, loss of self-image, dependency, and increased confusion, and may precipitate regressive behavior and withdrawal or angry, belligerent behavior (Castleberry and Seither 1982; Gerdes 1968; Mion, Frengley, Jakovcic, and Makino 1989; Misik 1981; Rose 1987). The use of restraints has little or no safety value and may actually be hazardous (Rubenstein, Miller, Postel, and Evans 1983). Restraints may cause problems associated with immobilization, such as bone loss, nosocomial infection, and reduced functional capacity, a particular concern with confused clients who may already be experiencing reduced functional capacity and the potential for immobility. Alternatives to restraints should be employed and include the red and yellow tape and drapes, which can be effective in delineating boundaries and discouraging wandering. Nurses should look for the meaning of behavior if the client wanders or is combative and direct their activities toward that underlying cause. Other alternatives to restraints are to provide comfort measures, manipulating the environment with lighting or functional furniture and appropriate activities. Restraints should be used only if they enable a client to function at the highest level possible, not for the convenience of the staff.

Physiologic Causes

The normal aged individual does not present with physiological disorders in the same manner as younger persons. Because of changes in pain tolerance, temperature regulation, baroreceptors, and so forth, symptoms may not clearly point to a disease process until it has become well progressed. Persons with chronic confusion experience diminished perception, interpretation, and communication, and the cause of excess disability and catastrophic reactions is often the result of deviations in their physiological condition. When a chronically confused person becomes more acutely confused, the nurse should first check for physiological causes, such as pain or the need to urinate or defecate. After ruling out this need, the presence of an infectious process should be investigated. Treatment of pneumonia or a urinary tract infection can result in dramatic improvement, yet the only presenting symptom may be an acute increase in confusion. Similarly, constipation and dehydration can cause an acute episode of confusion, and nurses should prevent these conditions by establishing regular bowel programs and providing adequate fluids. Adequate fluid intake is especially important because the chronically confused person does not always interpret thirst and request fluids.

Other common physiological causes of acute confusion are medications, electrolyte imbalances, and pain. When a confused client experiences an acute episode of confusion, the nurse must first rule out physiological and treatable causes through thorough assessment, consultations with the physician, and observation.

Unconditional Positive Regard

The inability of persons with chronic confusion to interpret the environment and the disinhibition experienced make it important for nurses to employ unconditional positive regard. Staff and others must accept the confused client and avoid giving negative feedback for inappropriate behaviors. Verbal and nonverbal messages can be utilized to communicate acceptance and affection to the confused client. Touch is an especially important form of communication and conveys unconditional acceptance. Studies have shown the positive effects of touch for confused clients, such as an increase in facial expression, eye contact, and body movements relative to being touched (Burnside 1979; Langland and Panicucci 1982).

Bartol (1979) emphasized the use of nonverbal communication in the AD victim and states that nonverbal communication may be sharpened as other abilities decline. The AD victim is responsive to emotional undertones in the environment, touch, facial expression, eye contact, tone of voice, and posture (Bartol 1979). Principles of communication with the client with chronic confusion include the following:

1.   Use short words, simple sentences, and no pronouns (only nouns), and begin each conversation by identifying yourself and calling the person by name.
2.   Speak slowly and clearly, lowering voice tone, not volume, unless the patient is deaf.
3.   If you ask a question, wait for a response, and ask only one question at a time.
4.   If you repeat a question, repeat it exactly.
5.   Utilize self-included humor whenever possible (Bartol 1979).

Using these principles, staff convey unconditional positive regard and act to preserve the confused client's dignity by helping to save face. Unless clients request otherwise, address them by their surname, rather than first name, to convey respect.

Determining Limits of Activity/Stimuli

Staff must assess behaviors indicating anxiety and avoidance to determine appropriate levels of activity and stimuli. In so doing, dysfunctional, catastrophic episodes can be prevented. Anxiety-related behaviors include an increase in psychomotor activity, increased or decreased verbalization, loss of eye contact, complaints of feeling uncomfortable or nervous, and/or an attempt to avoid or retreat from the offensive situation (Nowakowski 1985). Anxiety can often be relieved by providing the appropriate amount and kinds of stimulus according to the client's response and periodic rest periods.

Exposure to television and radio must be minimal and carefully monitored. Persons with chronic confusion have difficulty interpreting the media appropriately and may experience pseudohallucinations, sensing people on television as persons "stuck in a box" or "little people in the room" or a radio voice as an auditory hallucination. If television is used, it is important to evaluate the programs watched. Old movies seem to be comforting to the aged in general and especially to the chronically confused because their long-term memory is frequently intact. Nature shows or movies with beautiful scenery can provide positive diversional activity. Radios should be tuned to stations that play classical music or music of the 1930s and 1940s. It is important to obtain a thorough history when planning activities centered around television and radio. Perhaps the client detests classical music and enjoys country western, in which case the nurse would provide the appropriate programming. Current popular music is unfamiliar and overstimulating (rock and roll, hard rock, and heavy metal) and is definitely not recommended. Activities should be simple and geared toward the client's capabilities. High-stimulation activities should be carefully evaluated, be followed by periods of rest, and include only a small group of clients. One-on-one activities are most effective if geared to the client's cognitive ability and interests.

Because of the progressive deterioration associated with most forms of chronic confusion, it is important for all caregivers (staff as well as family) to remember that it may be impossible for the chronically confused person to learn new material. Short-term memory abilities are greatly diminished or absent, and the ability to comprehend or even relearn can result in frustration. All tasks must be geared toward the client's level of intellectual functioning, consist of short and simple directions, and be rewarding for the client at some level. Chronically confused clients have both good days and bad days, and what was performed proficiently on one day may be an impossible task the next. To plan tasks and activities that maximize strengths while minimizing weaknesses, the nurse and other caregivers need a thorough history of the client's likes and dislikes, premorbid abilities, education, capabilities, and occupation.

Listening

Caregivers must listen to confused clients, evaluating verbal and nonverbal responses in order to prevent anxiety and assess for physiological discomfort. For example, a confused client who continually asks for "Mama" may be expressing a need for nurturing and affection, as well as unconditional positive regard that is generally encompassed by the concept of mother. A confused client who takes food from the plate of another may be communicating that she or he is still hungry. Many families find that if the confused person walks away from them, this may indicate that it is time for the visit to end.

Modifying the Environment

More than a decade ago, Lawton (1977) identified the need for environmental modification that coincides with decreasing competence, in order to maintain and enhance the well-being of confused clients. Similarly, Kruzich (1986) found that environmental factors influence social integration as much as the client's level of physical and psychological functioning. Limited or no use of restraints, stable routine with activities, daily assessment of changes, generous use of touch and affection, skilled nonverbal behavior of staff, and family involvement are essential elements of care for demented clients (Burnside 1982).

The low-stimulus special care unit (SCU) ideally offers opportunities to encourage patient control, to modify but not eliminate stimulation, to individualize the schedule, and to modify the internal environment (Schafer 1985). There are no hard and fast rules for creating and maintaining an SCU for the confused client, but general guidelines may be followed to ensure optimum functioning (Ronch 1987):

1.   Provide a coherent, thematically consistent program of environmental stimulation that promotes and predisposes toward prosocialization and adaptive behavior.

2.   Encourage the client's social interaction with peers, family, and staff with as much autonomy as possible.

3.   Provide a personalized, dignified, safe, and secure environment with maximum predictability.

4.   Employ trained, supervised staff.

5.   Manage wandering, agitation, and so forth as responses to cognitive overload.

6.   Use chemical and/or physical restraints only for the betterment of the client, not the staff.

7.   Provide family support.

8.   Prevent and reduce staff burnout through proper interviewing, orientation, training, ventilation, and relaxation.

9.   Make evaluation of the client a preadmission requirement using current screening techniques.

10.   Provide for continued evaluation of the client.

11.   Be nonjudgmental in analyzing problem behavior and in evaluating the effect of programming on staff and clients.

12.   Encourage the highest degree of client adaptation by meeting a wide range of needs and being responsive to both individuals and groups.

Individualized, consistent, safe, and supportive care is the hallmark of effective SCUs for confused clients, which provides for management of symptoms, environmental adaptation, and caregiver support (Gwyther 1985). Expected outcomes of following these general guidelines are restoration of self-worth, stress reduction, acceptance of cognitive impairment, establishment of a calm, secure community, and focus on client strengths.

In modifying the environment, all of the activities thus far discussed are employed. The SCU is usually a specially designated area of a facility with specially trained staff. By controlling the environment in an SCU, the use of physical and chemical restraints has declined; the incidence of pressure sores decreased; improvement in the performance of activities of daily living occurred; clients' weight increased; interaction and social support among AD patients increased; socialization at mealtime increased; use of tranquilizers decreased; agitation, combative behavior, and wandering decreased; and family satisfaction increased (Cleary, Clamon, Price, and Shullaw 1987; Hall, Kirshling, and Todd 1986; Matthew, Sloan, Kilby, and Flood 1988).

Physical Care

Because of the progressive nature of AD and other dementias, the ability to care for self is diminished to the point that the client is totally dependent by the end stage. Interventions to prevent emaciation, prevent pressure areas, control incontinence, enhance mobility, and meet self-care needs are essential. The focus of this chapter, however, is to address those problems unique to the confused client. Nurses are referred to other chapters (e.g., chaps. 1-7), focusing on these problems.

Caregiver and Family Support

Caregivers of persons with chronic confusion can become exhausted in view of the inexorably progressive nature of the disease. Confused clients rarely give positive feedback for care. Education for staff caregivers should incorporate the principles outlined, as well as stress management techniques to prevent burnout. Family must be supported through support groups and education about the stages of the disease. Involving the family in planning and implementing care provides for good family-staff-client relations and helps to facilitate a feeling of usefulness for family members and comfort for the client. Information, support, and education are the primary strategies to facilitate caregivers in caring for the chronically confused.

CASE STUDY

Mary is a 77-year-old female who was admitted to the SCU of a local nursing facility 2 years ago with a diagnosis of Alzheimer's disease, diagnosed 5 years previously. She is in the third stage of AD, moving quickly to the fourth. She had been living in her home in Michigan with live-in help until her admission, but her mental condition has deteriorated so much that it was unwise to keep her at home. She became increasingly dependent in her activities of daily living (ADLs), began wandering, and experienced night wakening. Her caretaker was unable to cope. It was felt that Mary should be placed near her younger son in Iowa. Mary's only other diagnosis is emphysema with no presenting symptoms and for which she is not treated. Mary takes only a multiple vitamin daily and medication as needed for constipation.

Mary is dependent in all ADLs. Her son visits infrequently because Mary no longer recognizes him, and it is distressing for him to see her with such cognitive decline. Most of the day, Mary wanders around her room, chattering and tearing the bedsheets off the beds. She does respond to her name and seems to recognize her frequent caregivers, whom she wants to touch and hug.

Mary's speech is jargon, with many words meaningless to others. When focused by staff, she will follow simple directions, dance with staff, and even hum along to old songs when staff are singing to her. Mary hates to be left alone and will eat only if she can sit on someone's lap or at least very near the person. She will not nap unless someone lies in bed with her to get her to sleep.

Mary's communication is limited. At times her speech is spontaneous — "Leave me alone," when someone is doing something she does not like, such as combing her hair — and profanity comes easily, illustrating the lowered inhibitions frequently observed in persons with AD. Sometimes she cries for no apparent reason but accepts the comfort offered by the staff. Mary detests bathing or showering, and this is one of the most difficult aspects of her care. Staff members are very affectionate with Mary, and she seems appreciative of this acceptance.

Mary responds well to touch, her main form of communication. Her attention is focused only on certain cues: touch, imitation of her chattering, and singing. She listens briefly when her name is called, and when in distress, Mary is able to make appropriate sounds. Her language and reality base have been altered because of her cognitive deficits, but she is able to interpret affection and caring with an appropriate response. According to her family, Mary has never wanted to be alone, and this social response remains intact. She frequently reaches out for caregivers as they pass her by. Her attention span is poor, but hugging, dancing, or singing will maintain her focus for several minutes. She is unable to participate actively in communication unless directed by staff. Her major strength is her love of human contact and the warm manner in which she responds to touch. When utilizing the intervention of Confusion Management for Mary, her primary mode of communication must be considered. Touch and affection are employed to get her attention and to comfort her when she is distressed. The staff members of the nursing facility were able to utilize several of the activities that flow from the PLST model:

1. Always call Mary by name when communicating with her. Identify yourself. In this way, Mary's attention can be focused, even if only for moments, and her social role can be preserved.

2. Use touch and hugs whenever possible except when Mary is not receptive (when she is angry). Mary is particularly dependent on nonverbal language and is able to participate actively in physical touch and communication.

3. Use exaggerated facial expressions and gestures when communicating. This will enhance verbal communication with nonverbal cues.

4. Mimic Mary's jargon to get her attention; then proceed with the task at hand.

5. Sing with Mary, and perhaps dance with her too, in order to have an effective quiet time together, especially if Mary has been upset.

6. Make sure Mary is an active participant in communication and other interactions.

7. Redirect inappropriate behavior. If she is angry or hostile, leave and return in 5 minutes, or have another caregiver take over. Because of impairments in communication, it is fruitless for staff to explain or reason with her. Utilize whatever communication abilities Mary possesses at the time, and do not expect more than that of which she is capable.

8. Provide for rest periods. It is frequently necessary for a caregiver to lie in bed with Mary in order to get her to rest.

9. Provide for safety. Keep all toxic materials, such as cleaning fluids, perfumes, and even some plants, out of reach. Assess her walking ability and provide for rest if she seems unsteady.

SUMMARY

Clients with chronic confusion experience losses in both the cognitive and physical domains. By maximizing strengths and minimizing losses, the nurse can intervene to promote an optimum level of functioning for these individuals. Clients must be viewed holistically, and activities that focus on diversion, self-care, anxiety, communication, planning losses, memory losses, and the provision of unconditional positive regard must be emphasized.

REFERENCES

Bartol, M.A. 1979. Nonverbal communication in patients with Alzheimer's disease. *Journal of Gerontological Nursing* 5(4):21–31.

Berger, E.Y. 1985, November–December. The institutionalization of patients with Alzheimer's disease. *Nursing Homes*, 22–28.

Blass, J.P. 1982. Dementia. *Medical Clinics of North America* 66:1143–1160.

Burns, E., and Buckwalter, K. 1988. Pathophysiology and etiology of Alzheimer's disease. *Nursing Clinics of North America* 23(1):11–30.

Burnside, I.M. 1979. Alzheimer's disease: An overview. *Journal of Gerontological Nursing* 3:(4):14–20.

Burnside, I.M. 1982, Fall. Care of the Alzheimer's patient in an institution, *Generations* 50:22–23.

Castleberry, K., and Seither, F. 1982. Disorientation. In C.M. Norris (ed.), *Concept clarification in nursing.* Rockville, Md.: Aspen.

Cleary, T.A., Clamon, C., Price, M., and Shullaw, G. 1987. A reduced stimulus unit: Effects on patients with Alzheimer's disease and related disorders. *Gerontologist* 28(4):511–514.

Cross, P.S., and Gurland, B.J. 1986. *The Epidemiology of Dementing Disorders.* Contract report prepared for the Office of Technology Assessment, U.S. Congress.

Dawson, P., Kline, K., Wianko, D., and Wells, D. 1986. Preventing excess disability in patients with Alzheimer's disease. *Geriatric Nursing* 1(6):298–330.

Evans, D.A., Funkenstein, H.H., Albert, M.S., Scherr, P.A., Cook, N.R., Chown, M.J., Hebert, L.E., Hennekens, C.H., and Taylor, J.O. 1989. Prevalence of Alzheimer's disease in a community population of older persons. *Journal of the American Medical Association* 262(18):2551–2557.

Feil, N. 1984. Communicating with the confused elderly patient. *Geriatrics* 39:131–132.

Folstein, M., Folstein, S., and McHugh, P. 1975. Minimental state: A practical method for grading the cognitive state of patients for the clinician. *Journal of Psychiatric Research* 12:189–198.

Gerdes, L. 1968. The confused or delirious patient. *American Journal of Nursing* 68(6):1228–1233.

Gwyther, L.P. 1985. *Care of the Alzheimer patient: A manual for nursing home staff.* Chicago: Alzheimer's Disease and Related Disorders Association, and Washington, D.C.: American Health Care Association.

Foreman, M.D. 1990, May–June. Complexities of acute confusion. *Geriatric Nursing,* 137–139.

Hall, G.R. 1986. Confusion. Unpublished manuscript.

Hall, G.R. 1988. Care of the patient with Alzheimer's disease living at home. *Nursing Clinics of North America* 23:(1):31–46.

Hall, G.R. 1991. Altered thought processed: SDAT. In M. Maas and K. Buckwalter (eds.), *Nursing diagnoses and interventions of the elderly.* Menlo Park, Calif.: Addison-Wesley.

Hall, G.R., and Buckwalter, K.C. 1987. Progressively lowered stress threshold: A conceptual model for care of adults with Alzheimer's disease. *Archives of Psychiatric Nursing* 1(6):309–406.

Hall, G., Kirshling, M., and Todd, S. 1986. Sheltered freedom: The creation of a special Alzheimer's unit in an intermediate level facility. *Geriatric Nursing* 7(3):132–136.

Heston, L., and White, J. 1983. *Dementia: A practical guide to Alzheimer's disease and related illnesses.* New York: Freeman.

Hogstel, M. 1979. Use of reality orientation with aging confused patients. *Nursing Research* 28(3):161–165.

Katzman, R. 1986. Alzheimer's disease. *New England Journal of Medicine* 314:964–973.

Kosich, K., and Grodon, J.H. 1982. Aging, memory loss, and dementia. *Psychosomatics* 23(7):746.

Kruzich, J.M. 1986. The chronically mentally ill in nursing homes: Issues in policy and practice. *Health and Social Work* 11(1):5–14.

Langland, R.M., and Panicucci, C. 1982. Effects of touch on communication with elderly confused clients. *Journal of Gerontological Nursing* 8:152–155.

Lawton, M.P. 1977. The impact of the environment on aging and behavior. In J.E. Birren and K.W. Schale (eds.), *Handbook of psychology and aging.* New York: Van Nostrand Reinhold.

McKhann, G., Drachman, D., Folstein, M., Katzman, R., Price, M., and Stadlan, R. 1984. Clinical diagnosis of Alzheimer's disease: A report of the NINCDS-ADRDA work group. *Neurology* 34:939–943.

Matthew, L., Sloan, P., Kilby, M., and Flood, R. 1988, March–April. What's different about a special care unit for dementia patients: A comparative study and research. *American Journal of Alzheimer's Care and Related Disorders,* 16–23.

Mion, L.C., Frengley, J.D., Jakovcic, C.A., and Makino, J.A. 1989. A further exploration of the use of physical restraints in hospitalized patients. *Journal of the American Geriatrics Society* 37:949–956.

Misik, I. 1981. About using restraints with restraint. *Nursing '81* 11(8):50–55.

Nagley, S.J., and Dever, A. 1989. What we know about treating confusion. *Journal of Applied Nursing Research* 1(2):80–83.

Nodhturft, B.L., and Sweeney, N.M. 1982. Reality orientation therapy for the institutionalized elderly. *Journal of Gerontological Nursing* 8(7):396–401.

Nowakowski, L. 1985. Accent capabilities in disorientation. *Journal of Gerontological Nursing* 11(9):15–20.

Parker, C., and Somers, C. 1983, May–June. Reality orientation on a geropsychiatric unit. *Geriatric Nursing,* 163–165.

Rader, J., Doan, J., and Schwab, M. 1985. How to decrease wandering: A form of agenda behavior. *Geriatric Nursing,* 6(4):196–199.

Reisberg, B., Ferris, S.H., DeLeon, M.J., and Crook, T. 1982. The Global deterioration scale (GDS): An instrument for the assessment of primary degenerative dementia. *American Journal of Psychiatry,* 139(9):1136–1139.

Roberts, B.L. and Algase, D.L. 1988. Victims of Alzheimer's disease and the environment. *Nursing Clinics of North America* 35(2):113–118.

Ronch, J.L. 1987. Special Alzheimer's units in nursing homes: Pros and cons. *American Journal of Alzheimer's Care and Research* 2(4):10–19.

Rose, J. 1987. When the care plan says restrain. *Geriatric Nursing* 8(1):20–21.

Rubenstein, H.S., Miller, F.H., Postel, S., and Evans, H. 1983. Standards of medical care based on consensus rather than evidence: The case of routine bedrail use for the elderly. *Law, Medicine and Health Care* 11(6):271–276.

Schwab, M., Rader, J., and Doan, J. 1985. Relieving the fear and anxiety in dementia. *Journal of Gerontological Nursing* 11(6):8–15.

Shafer, S. 1985. Modifying the environment. *Geriatric Nursing,* 6(3):157–159.

Shohan, H., and Neuschantz, S. 1985. Group therapy with senile patients. *Social Work* 30:69–72.

Wolanin, M., and Phillips, L. 1981. *Confusion: Prevention and care.* St. Louis: C.V. Mosby Co.

SECTION II

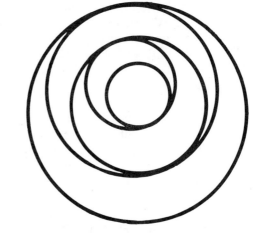

ACUTE-CARE MANAGEMENT

Overview: The Challenge of Nursing in the Acute-Care Setting

GLORIA M. BULECHEK
JOANNE C. McCLOSKEY

Most acute care occurs in hospitals, and hospitals are where most nurses work. In the past decade, hospitals have undergone some dramatic changes: more technology, an increased number of intensive care units, reorganization with more short-term beds, increased use of outpatient clinics and emergency rooms, a shift in payment mechanisms with more health care costs now assumed by the federal government, an influx of new workers, and an increase in specialization. Patients in hospitals are sicker than before, and the care they require is more complex and intensive. To hold down costs, patients are discharged quickly. In such an atmosphere, the challenge to deliver high-quality nursing care is greater than ever. The interventions described in this section are essential for competent care in the acute setting.

In the acute-care setting, patients undergo many stressful tests and procedures. Nurses can help them cope with the stress by using Concrete Objective Information. Concrete Objective Information (previously called Preparatory Sensory Information) "describes both the typical subjective and objective experiences associated with specific health care events." The name of the intervention has recently been changed to reflect research findings that demonstrate the importance of using concrete and objective language. This intervention has a strong research base, although none of the research was conducted earlier than 1970. The majority of the studies for the intervention have been done by nurses, notably by Jean E. Johnson and her colleagues. In Chapter 10, Norma J. Christman, Karin T. Kirchhoff, and Marsha G. Oakley describe the studies and the development of self-regulation theory. They discuss the relative benefits of subjective versus objective information as known from research. Two areas of research have focused on individual differences and combining instructions with the intervention. The authors assert that the most appropriate nursing diagnosis is Potential for Ineffective Individual Coping, and a case study of a woman with this diagnosis scheduled to undergo external radiation therapy demonstrates the implementation of the intervention. The case study implements the use of an audiocassette recording. Concrete Objective Information has low risk for the patient and takes little nursing time. Based on sound research, it should be an intervention that all nurses in acute care settings know how to do and implement frequently.

A related intervention is Truth Telling. Nurses are often in the position in which they have to decide whether a painful truth should be told to a patient. The nurse's dilemma of truth versus deception is thoroughly discussed in Chapter 11 by Debra Livingston and Cassandra B. Williamson. They define Truth Telling as "a process of responsible, caring, and honest communication based on ethical decision making." They propose a truth-telling model that outlines four options for the nurse: whole truth, partial truth, deception, and truth delay. A case study of a woman with symptoms of Alzheimer's disease whose husband and doctor do not want her told illustrates the truth dilemma often faced by nurses. As the authors so well demonstrate, Truth Telling is a complex intervention. It assumes good self-understanding, a sound knowledge base, excellent communication skills, rapport with the patient, and collaboration with other health professionals. Above all, it requires an accurate assessment of the risks, to both the patient who receives the truth and the nurse who tells the truth. More research is needed on the effects of Truth Telling, and the authority of nurses to use Truth Telling as an intervention needs to be acknowledged.

Structured Preoperative Teaching is an intervention frequently preformed by acute-care nurses. According to Betty Patterson Tarsitano in Chapter 12, it consists of standardized information tailored to levels of anxiety. The nurse prepares patients for what to expect postoperatively and to cope with the threat behind the anxiety about surgery. The intervention, which is both structured and flexible, promotes a sense of control over the situation. The research base for the intervention is considerable, with recent research demonstrating that information provision according to anxiety level is more effective than provision of information alone. Tarsitano reviews the research and theoretical literature and supplies an excellent detailed protocol for implementing the intervention according to the patient's anxiety level. A case study completes the chapter.

Crisis Intervention is frequently required in emergency rooms and psychiatric units but should be used in any setting where individuals are in crisis. As Robert J. Kus points out in Chapter 13, crises are normal events for all people. Thus, Crisis Intervention is a psychosocial, not a psychiatric, intervention. Kus overviews three types of crises: developmental, situational, and social. In Crisis Intervention, the nurse assists the client through the steps of problem solving. The goal is to achieve at least the same level of psychological comfort as experienced before the crisis. The process of marshaling their support systems enables many patients to cope more effectively. Thus, the intervention is a form of preventive mental health. As Kus points out, Crisis Intervention is not a 9-to-5 activity, and people in crisis need immediate attention. A nurse who implements this intervention has to be flexible and work in a system that provides for unpredictable and irregular time periods. Kus's case study of a gay alcoholic client in crisis demonstrates that a nurse implementing Crisis Intervention needs good understanding of how to do the intervention and also good knowledge of the crisis situation. Sometimes, as in the case study, the nurse must educate others about the situation. Kus's chapter will help all nurses who work with people in crisis.

Another intervention helpful to those in crises and those experiencing stress is Presence. The presence of the nurse as central to a patient's recovery has long been understood (at least by nurses), but Presence, as a conceptualized, described, and tested intervention, is missing from the literature. While several nursing theorists, most notably J. Patterson and L. T. Zderad, have included the presence of the nurse as a key aspect of successful therapy, little has been done to describe this important intervention. Presence, as delineated by Diane L. Gardner in Chapter 14, has two aspects: the physical ("being there") and the psychological ("being with"). The nurse uses herself as the intervention through such techniques as listening, reassurance, and communication. Gardner describes how Presence is closely aligned with such related concepts as caring, empathy, support, therapeutic use of self, and physical closeness. The fact that Gardner is not clear on whether these concepts are the same or different or merely parts of the intervention, Presence, is due to the scarcity of literature in the area. Through two case studies, both involving patients with Fear and Anxiety, Gardner demonstrates the value of this important nursing intervention.

The sometimes controversial intervention of Therapeutic Touch is discussed in the next chapter by Thérèse Connell Meehan. Developed by Dora Kunz and Delores Krieger in the 1960s, Therapeutic Touch is viewed as an energy field interaction best described using Roger's Science of Unitary Human Beings Model. Meehan reviews the theory and the literature related to the intervention, evaluates research findings, and discusses methodological problems when studing the intervention. Therapeutic Touch does seem to reduce pain and decrease the need for analgesic medication. Whether it increases hemoglobin values and decreases stress is unclear. The author describes the steps of implementation but cautions that nurses need training and experience to carry out this intervention. All nurses should read this chapter, although only those with advanced training and a supportive climate should use it.

A large part of nurses' time in the acute-care setting is spent on medications. Too often, this important activity is viewed as merely assistive to physicians who prescribe the medications. In Chapter 16 on Medication Management, Elizabeth A. Weitzel clearly illustrates that this is an important independent intervention of the nurse that accompanies the more assistive intervention of Medication Administration. Weitzel first reviews literature related to administration of medications by health care providers and then by the topics of error rates, impact of technology, medication review, and supervision of staff. She discusses administration of medication by the patient or family member, including the topic of over-the-counter medications. Four nursing diagnoses are identified as most appropriate for the intervention. Implementation of the intervention involves attention to three interrelated functions: knowledge of the drug and its administration, knowledge of the client and family life-style, and maintenance of good relationships with client, family, physician, and pharmacist. Two case studies illustrate the important role of the nurse to manage the use of medications by their patients.

Chapter 17 on Pain Control by Ada Jacox represents an intervention label at a very abstract level. Jacox overviews the many different types of measures that nurses can use to control pain, including medications, cutaneous stimulation, relaxation techniques, and patient-controlled analgesia. Although much research has been done on pain, the practice of pain management is still poor, due to the lack of well-controlled studies of methods for pain management and the lack of use by practitioners of what is known. What is needed is further identification and testing of specific measures of pain control. The intervention of Pain Control represents the challenge to the nurse of choosing among multiple measures those most likely to benefit a particular patient. To help with this difficult task, Jacox overviews several assessment tools for both adults and children. The use and evaluation of measures to relieve pain is an important aspect of nursing care.

Another important aspect of nursing care is body fluid balance. In the next chapter, Alice S. Poyss defines Fluid Therapy as "the supportive and preventative actions a nurse takes to assist individuals in restoring fluid balance and preventing complications of disease." Fluid Therapy has two objectives: to replace fluid losses and to keep up with ongoing losses. The intervention involves the implementation of the therapeutic intravenous therapy regime and ongoing monitoring of several parameters. Most of the chapter reviews the extensive knowledge base needed to implement the intervention. This is an excellent review of normal fluid balance, thirst and output, and fluid volume imbalances. The author includes an evaluation tool that can be used at the bedside for the ongoing monitoring that is a key feature of the intervention. While the prescription of the specific intravenous fluid is the usual role of the physician, this author has demonstrated that the nursing role in Fluid Therapy is most important for the early detection and prevention of complications and the ultimate success in achieving the desired outcomes.

Infection Control is another intervention that many hospitalized patients who are at risk of infection need. In Chapter 19, Jerri Bryant and Linda J. Lewicki briefly look at the history of Infection Control programs. A table lists references to 10 guidelines that have been developed to prevent and control infections in various areas. The authors focus on the two key aspects of infection control: hand washing and barrier precautions. Three tables help the nurse to decide situations in which hand washing is needed immediately, antiseptic rather than plain soap is required, and masks, gloves, and gowns are required. Two case studies illustrate the use of the intervention.

More attention needs to be given in the acute setting to the impact of the environment on care. An individual's environment includes physical, social, psychological, and cultural factors. Lorraine C. Mion in Chapter 20 describes the intervention of Environmental Structuring as a range of nursing actions that directly or indirectly affect environmental features and conditions. Nurse actions may be focused on physical aspects, nurse-patient interaction, or institutional policies and programs. The intervention can be used for a range of diagnoses, most often involving high-risk groups such as the frail elderly, comatose individuals, infants, or immunocompromised individuals. The interventions should be implemented for specific therapy goals. Three goals are described as examples. The chapter reviews numerous areas of research to support the intervention. The author organizes the reports under institutional design, spaces, sound, and light and color. Four assessment tools to describe environmental features are described.

The last chapter in this section provides a link to succeeding sections; Discharge Planning is about communication between systems of care and among different health care professionals. In the current cost-containment environment, Discharge Planning is receiving a great deal of attention from health care policymakers. The chapter by Kathleen Kelly, Eleanor McClelland and Jeanette Daly addresses current forces driving Discharge Planning, describes the research base for the intervention, and outlines issues for practice and management. While the research demonstrates that Discharge Planning results in reduced length of hospital stay and fewer complications, the focus has been on the use of a discharge planner rather than on identifying the components of the intervention that are responsible for the outcomes obtained. The case study in this chapter helps to identify the components. One issue the authors identify is whether Discharge Planning is best done by a person who specializes in this—a discharge planner—or whether it is an important intervention for all nurses to be familiar with. As we read the chapter, we raised additional questions: Is Discharge Planning as conceptualized here different from managed care? Do all patients need discharge planning? If not, who should get the intervention?

The twelve chapters in this section outline essential acute-care physiological and psychosocial interventions that are often used by hospital nurses. In addition, acute-care nurses often use the interventions in other sections of the book (for example, Surveillance and Patient Teaching). Some of the interventions require system changes so that they are easier to implement, and all of them need more research to determine their effectiveness for particular populations. The challenge in the dynamic acute-care setting is to develop a role that allows nurses to practice and evaluate the effectiveness of these essential nursing treatments.

10

CONCRETE OBJECTIVE INFORMATION

NORMA J. CHRISTMAN
KARIN T. KIRCHHOFF
MARSHA G. OAKLEY

Concrete Objective Preparatory Information is the product of a program of research and theory development spanning approximately 20 years. It is predominantly based on the work of a nurse, Jean E. Johnson, and her colleagues in nursing, although investigators from other disciplines (Wilson 1981; Leventhal and Johnson 1983) have contributed to the empirical and theoretical base of this intervention. Concrete Objective Information, formerly called preparatory sensory information, describes both the typical subjective and objective experiences associated with specific health care events (McHugh, Christman, and Johnson 1982). The name of the intervention was changed to reflect more clearly research findings that documented the importance of describing both the subjective and objective experiences using concrete and objective terminology (Johnson and Lauver 1989; Suls and Fletcher 1985).

Subjective experiences are those known only to the experiencing person. These experiences include the sensory input associated with the event — that is, what will be felt, seen, heard, tasted, and smelled during the experience. The sensory features of the experience are described in unambiguous, or concrete, and objective terms. Evaluative or qualitative adjectives, such as *terrible* or *excruciating,* are not attached to the descriptors of the sensory experiences. The cause of the sensation, when not self-evident, and its temporal features also are described. For example, Concrete Objective Information for a surgical patient includes not only the sensations associated with the surgical incision — tenderness, pressure, smarting, aching — but also the changes in these sensations that occur with movement (may become sharp and seem to travel along the incision) and changes that occur over time (intensity declines with time).

Objective experiences included in Concrete Objective Information are those aspects of the experience that can be observed and verified by someone other than the experiencing person (McHugh, Christman, and Johnson 1982). These aspects of the experience include the timing of specific events associated with the procedure, as well as the nature of the environment in which the procedure takes place. For the example of surgery, description of the objective experiences may include

Revision of this chapter was partially supported by Grant No. 5R29NR01830-03, NCNR, NCI, NIH, to the first author. The authors wish to acknowledge Dr. Jean E. Johnson's helpful comments on an earlier draft of this chapter.

information about the anesthesiologist's visit and when it will occur, the preoperative skin preparation and when it will be done, awakening in the recovery room, and when food and fluids will be permitted. The exact content of the objective aspects of the experience necessarily varies with the specific practices, policies, and environment of the setting in which the procedure takes place. Whatever the exact content, these experiences are described using unambiguous and objective terminology.

THEORETICAL-EMPIRICAL FOUNDATION

Self-regulation theory provides the foundation for understanding the use of Concrete Objective Information as an intervention and for explaining its effects on patients' ability to cope with health care procedures (Johnson and Lauver 1989; Leventhal and Johnson 1983). Self-regulation theory is concerned with the cognitive processing of information and its effects on human behavior. Schema formation is a concept central to self-regulation theory. A schema is a mental, or cognitive, apparatus that structures and stores information from experience (Neisser 1976). It directs the processing of incoming information, the retrieval of information stored from past experiences, the focus of attention, and resulting behavior (Johnson and Lauver 1989).

Further, it is proposed that attentional focus influences the nature of the behavioral response. Because a schema focuses attention, a schema dominated by the objective features rather than the subjective emotional reactions enhances problem-solving approaches in health care experiences (Johnson and Lauver 1989; Leventhal and Johnson 1983; Suls and Fletcher 1985). Since Concrete Objective Information is composed of clear, unambiguous content related to specific aspects of an experience, it eases the processing of incoming information, thereby enhancing interpretation and understanding of the experience (Johnson, Lauver, and Nail 1989). When specific elements (the burning or tingling of an incision) of a more abstract experience (having surgery) are described, patients may more easily draw on past experiences similar to the specific element, increasing their confidence in their ability to cope with the new experience (Johnson and Lauver 1989).

DEVELOPMENT OF SELF-REGULATION THEORY

Preparing patients for stressful health care procedures is a traditional part of nursing practice. Patients usually are given information or instruction thought to ease emotional distress, promote recovery, facilitate adherence to medical regimens, or in some other way enhance health and well-being. Because many of these practices are based on tradition or beliefs inferred from educational theory, they provide little guidance for making clinical decisions about selection of patients who would benefit from the information, the goal to be achieved by providing the information, and the criteria to use in evaluating patient responses to the information. Tests of the effects of Concrete Objective Information and the resulting theory provide guidance in answering these questions when making decisions about patient care.

The definition of Concrete Objective Information has changed as the effects of specific aspects of the informational message have been clarified through the research process. The initial research focused on determining the efficacy of the sensory or subjective component of the message. Because this type of information had not been used with patients, it was initially studied using healthy volunteers in whom a blood pressure cuff was used to induce ischemic pain as the stressful experience (Johnson 1973). As expected, those who were given a description of the typical sensory experiences reported less emotional distress during the experience than those who received only information about the procedure. With some evidence for the benefits of the subjective component of the information, studies in patient populations were initiated.

The early clinical studies focused on the effects of the subjective component of the message, with patients undergoing relatively short-term stressful health care procedures such as gastroendoscopic examination, barium enema, cast removal, and nasogastric tube insertion. The effects of the subjective component were tested against procedural information or a description of the objective experiences (Hartfield, Cason, and Cason 1982; Johnson, Morrissey, and Leventhal 1973) and in some cases also against no information (Hartfield and Cason 1981; Johnson, Kirchhoff, and Endress 1975). These tests permitted comparison of the efficacy of the subjective component to that of the objective component and, in turn, each of these to no information. In other studies, the subjective sensory descriptions were combined with procedural information and tested against no information, instruction in a coping strategy such as relaxation, or health education (Fuller, Endress, and Johnson 1978; Johnson and Leventhal 1974; Padilla, Grant, Rains, Hansen, Bergstrom, Wong, Hanson, and Kubo 1981; Rice, Sieggreen, Mullin, and Williams 1988). In these short-term stressful health care situations, the subjective sensory component alone, as well as when combined with the procedural descriptions, reduced patients' emotional distress during or immediately following the stressful event.

A recent meta-analysis (Suls and Wan 1989) also helps to clarify the effects of the different components of Concrete Objective Information. This statistical comparison of multiple studies done in a variety of clinical and laboratory situations indicated that, in contrast to description of the subjective experience, description of the objective experience produced no benefits over those achieved in control groups. Yet the combination describing both the subjective and objective experiences yielded the strongest effects on reducing emotional distress. From both pragmatic and theoretical perspectives, these findings make sense. Pragmatically, separating subjective experiences from the objective components of an experience may be difficult and artificial, especially for more complex or long-term health care events. From the theoretical perspective, combining both components allows for more complete and accurate schema formation, thus easing interpretation and understanding of the event.

The more complex or long-term situations in which the effects of Concrete Objective Information have been tested include surgery (Hill 1982; Johnson, Christman, and Stitt 1985; Johnson, Fuller, Endress, and Rice 1978a; Johnson, Rice, Fuller, and Endress 1978b; Wilson 1981) and radiation therapy for cancer (Johnson, Nail, Lauver, King, and Keys 1988). From these studies, the importance of including information about the timing of elements in longer-lasting experiences was made explicit (Johnson et al. 1978a). A major contribution of these studies to the development of self-regulation theory was greater understanding of the link between attentional focus and behavioral responses as a function of schema formation in short-term versus long-term health care events.

Compared to tests of the intervention in patients having short-term diagnostic or therapeutic experiences, Concrete Objective Information in these longer and more complex stressful experiences primarily affected outcome indicators reflecting patients' positive problem-solving activities. There were few effects on emotional state. Providing Concrete Objective Information prior to abdominal surgery has been related to shorter hospital stays (Johnson et al. 1978a, 1978b; Wilson 1981), earlier resumption of usual activities (Johnson et al. 1978a, 1978b), and reports of feeling more like one's normal self (Johnson et al. 1985). In patients having radiation therapy for prostatic cancer, Concrete Objective Information was related to lessened disruption in usual recreation and pastime activities (Johnson et al. 1988). Thus, in more complex, long-term health care situations, the positive effects of focusing attention on the concrete objective aspects of the event may become evident only over time (Suls and Fletcher 1985).

Further understanding of how attentional focus on the concrete objective elements of a stressful event improves coping outcomes also was achieved in these long-term studies. Surgical patients given Concrete Objective Information reported perception of increased ability to deal with the experience and a belief that the experience would be less difficult for them (Johnson et al. 1985). Similarity between expectations and experience and understanding of experiences explained the effects of Concrete Objective Information in patients having radiation therapy (Johnson et al. 1988). These findings support the theoretical explanations concerning the means by which Concrete Objective Information produces its effects. With a sense of understanding of the experience and finding experiences similar to what was expected (evidence of schema formation), patients are better able to select coping strategies to deal with the experience.

In short-term situations, there may be few problem-solving behaviors patients can use other than those used to cooperate with the procedure or to control their emotional response. Thus, studies of Concrete Objective Information in these situations reflect the outcomes of patients' behavioral attempts to cooperate and to control their emotional response. In the more long-term stressful events, patients' behavioral options are less restricted. Here the research findings suggest that over time, patients who receive Concrete Objective Information are better able to select coping strategies so as to lessen disruption of or speed resumption of usual daily activities. In summary, the research and theory suggest that a schema, which focuses attention on the concrete objective elements of stressful health care experiences rather than on the emotional, reactive components, helps patients know what to expect and increases their understanding of the experience, thereby enhancing their ability to cope with the experience.

INDIVIDUAL DIFFERENCES

Some investigations of the effects of Concrete Objective Information have attempted to identify if specific groups of patients especially benefit from this intervention. Questions have been asked as to whether patients' coping style or their level of pre-event emotional distress influences their response to Concrete Objective Information (Miller and Magnan 1983; Rainey 1985; Sime and Libera 1985; Watkins, Weaver, and Odegaard 1986; Wilson, Moore, Randolph, and Hanson 1982). Because the findings of these studies vary, it is not clear that a particular style of coping—for example, avoider or sensitizer—or that level of pre-event distress influences patients' responses to Concrete Objective Information. More research and theory development are necessary to clarify the effects of such individual difference variables on self-regulation of coping behaviors. It is important, however, to note that no clear evidence indicates that Concrete Objective Information produces negative effects in certain groups of patients.

COMBINING INSTRUCTIONS AND CONCRETE OBJECTIVE INFORMATION

Another area of study important to nursing practice concerns the effects of combining Concrete Objective Information with instruction in specific coping strategies such as relaxation (Wilson 1981; Wilson et al. 1982; Fuller et al. 1978), ambulation techniques (Johnson et al. 1978a, 1978b, 1985), and distraction (Johnson et al. 1985). Review of studies that investigated the effects of combining the information with instruction in a coping strategy suggests that such a combination was effective where the instruction provided a behavior not already part of the patient's repertoire of coping strategies (Hill 1982; Johnson et al. 1978a, 1978b; Padilla et al. 1981). Further, the newly learned behavior was compatible with that supported by the Concrete Objective Information intervention. For example, teaching ambulation techniques to preoperative patients is intended to increase ambulation and thereby speed recovery, the same behavior and outcome affected by Concrete Objective Information.

Instances in which combining Concrete Objective Information and instruction in a coping strategy did not produce additive effects (Fuller et al. 1978; Johnson et al. 1985; Wilson 1981) may be related to incompatible behavioral responses, the presence of an existing, effective strategy, or the need to use competing cognitive processes. For example, relaxation is intended to decrease activity, whereas other strategies, such as ambulation and leg exercises, increase activity that aids recovery. In other instances — for example, pelvic examination (Fuller et al. 1978) — the patient may have well-established behaviors that are used in preference to, or are incompatible with, the new technique. Finally, some combinations of information and instruction may not be effective because they require patients to use competing cognitive processes. The combination of Concrete Objective Information and distraction may be an example of such a situation (Johnson et al. 1985). Concrete Objective Information draws attention to unpleasant stimuli, and distraction requires avoiding unpleasant stimuli. Selective attention to only certain unpleasant stimuli may not be easily achieved.

INTERVENTION TOOLS—SENSORY DESCRIPTORS

Only typical sensory experiences are included as a part of Concrete Objective Information. Because they are subjective experiences, the descriptors must be obtained from interviews with patients who have undergone the procedure. Only those sensory experiences reported by at least 50% of the patients interviewed are included in the preparatory information for future patients (McHugh et al. 1982).

The sensory descriptions available because of their use in research studies are listed in Table 10–1. Not included in the table are the descriptors for the sensory experiences of patients having radiotherapy for cancer. These may be found in a report by King, Nail, Kreamer, Strohl, and Johnson (1985). In this instance, readers are referred to the original source of the descriptors, for two reasons. First, the sensory experiences in this patient population are numerous because they vary by site of cancer and the specific tissues or organs exposed to radiation. Second, the temporal changes over the course of treatment are well depicted in the original source. Interested readers also may find an example of Concrete Objective Information in Johnson, Kirchhoff, and Endress (1976).

TABLE 10–1.   DOCUMENTED SUBJECTIVE EXPERIENCE DESCRIPTORS
BY STRESSFUL HEALTH CARE EVENT

STRESSFUL EVENT	DESCRIPTORS
Gastroendoscopic examination (Johnson et al. 1973, 1974)	Intravenous medication; needle stick, drowsiness As air pumped into stomach, feeling of fullness like after eating a large meal Physician's finger in mouth to guide tube insertion
Nasogastric tube insertion (Padilla et al. 1981)	Feeling passage of tube Tearing Gagging Discomforts in nose, throat, mouth Limited mobility
Cast removal (Johnson et al. 1976)	Buzz of saw Feel vibrations or tingling See chalky dust Feel warmth on arm or leg as saw cuts cast; will not hurt or burn Skin under padding will be scaly and look dirty Arm or leg may be a little stiff when first trying to move it Arm or leg may seem light because cast was heavy
Barium enema (Hartfield and Cason 1981)	Lying on hard table Fullness Pressure Bloating Uncomfortable Feeling as if might have a bowel movement
Abdominal surgery (Johnson et al. 1978b; McHugh et al. 1982)	Preoperative medications: Sleepy, lightheaded, relaxed, free from worry, not bothered by most things, dryness of mouth Incision: Tenderness, sensitivity, pressure, smarting, burning, aching, sore Sensations might become sharp and seem to travel along incision when moving Arm with intravenous tube will seem awkward and restricted but will feel no discomfort or pain Tiredness after physical effort Bloating of abdomen Cramping due to gas pains Pulling and pinching when stitches are removed
Tracheostomy (Oermann, McHugh, Dietrich, and Boyll 1983)	When moving about, swallowing, or during suctioning: hurting, pressure, choking
Mastectomy — mean of 5.5 years postoperative (Nail, Jones, Giuffre, and Johnson 1984)	Arm or chest wall pain, "pins and needles," numbness, weakness, increased skin sensitivity, heaviness Phantom breast sensations, such as twinges, itching
4-vessel arteriography (Rice et al. 1988)	Before contrast, medium: table is hard, head taping is uncomfortable, cleansing solution is cold After contrast, medium: hot, burning sensation in face, neck, chest, or shoulders

APPROPRIATE CLIENT GROUPS AND ASSOCIATED NURSING DIAGNOSES

Concrete Objective Information may be given to adults who are to undergo diagnostic or therapeutic procedures. Children aged 6 years or older also benefit as long as they are able to understand verbal description of future events. Although younger children need to be prepared for stressful events, verbal description is not the most appropriate method to convey what they can expect to experience because of their level of cognitive development. Patients who have never experienced the anticipated health care event are the most likely to benefit from Concrete Objective Information (McHugh et al. 1982), although patients who have had previous experience also may benefit because the information may be more accurate than their memories (Fuller et al. 1978). With health care events that occur frequently, such as daily or weekly venipuncture, the patients' past experiences dominate the formation of expectations about the experience.

Because Concrete Objective Information is an intervention that facilitates coping or prevents disruption in coping, it is most useful for potential nursing diagnoses. Currently there are no appropriate diagnoses among the 13 potential diagnoses on the NANDA-approved list (Carroll-Johnson 1989) for which this intervention may be used. Yet as Bulechek and McCloskey (1989) note, one of the criteria nurses use in choosing an intervention is its research base.

When the research findings concerning Concrete Objective Information are evaluated using criteria identified by Haller, Reynolds, and Horsley (1979), the intervention is found to be useful for practice. The beneficial effects of Concrete Objective Information have been replicated in a wide variety of clinical settings, patient groups, and stressful health care events. Through conceptual replication, the research has contributed to the development of nursing knowledge; scientific merit is evident. The use of Concrete Objective Information involves little or no risk to patients, and its beneficial effects on coping with stressful health care experiences have been demonstrated. Nurses have clinical control of preparing patients for diagnostic and therapeutic procedures, and providing Concrete Objective Information is feasible. The cost-benefit ratio is more heavily weighted toward benefit than cost, since it provides a guide for selecting information that has a probability of being effective and replacing information that may not be effective. If many patients need similar preparation and time requirements prove costly, the information may be delivered by use of a group, printed materials, or an audiovisual approach.

Given the research base and demonstrated effects on the outcomes of patients' coping with stressful health care events, we suggest that Concrete Objective Information is most appropriately used for Potential for Ineffective Individual Coping, a modification of the NANDA diagnosis. Risk factors (Bulechek and McCloskey 1989) for such a diagnosis that may be modified by the use of Concrete Objective Information are indicative of possible inadequate schema formation and may include lack of prior experience with the stressful health care event, distant prior experience, fear due to the unknown, and a tendency to focus on emotional aspects of experiences.

Concrete Objective Information also may be used for an actual nursing diagnosis. The research base suggests that it may be an effective intervention for fear related to short-term diagnostic or therapeutic procedures.

PROTOCOL FOR USING CONCRETE OBJECTIVE INFORMATION

A major task in using this preparatory intervention is gathering the appropriate information concerning the two components of the message (McHugh et al. 1982). If the subjective sensory information is not already available from the literature, it must be obtained by interviewing at least 15 patients who have undergone the experience for which the message is being prepared. During these interviews, patients may initially tend to describe their experience in general or emotionally charged terms. It may be necessary to guide them to use more specific and objective descriptors. It also is helpful if specific elements of the procedure are used to guide the interview about sensory experiences. Once these data are collected, they are reviewed for similarities, and sensations reported by 50% or more of the patients are incorporated into the message. Sensations should be described in objective terms; evaluative connotations such as *awful* or *intense* should not be used.

The objective component of the message varies from setting to setting because of variations in practices and policies. Nursing staff observing the event can readily note the sequential elements and environmental changes as they occur.

Combining the information gathered about the two components involves linking the sensory experiences to their causes and ensuring that the temporal qualities—frequency, duration, and change over time—are linked to appropriate sensations and elements of the event. Once the message has been developed, it should be reviewed to make sure that it portrays a clear and objective picture of the event and the experiences a patient may anticipate.

Concrete Objective Information may be delivered verbally by the nurse or by group, printed material, or audiovisual techniques if the cost of time is of concern. One should not be concerned with omitting some of the sensory descriptors when providing the information verbally. Partial sensory description has been found to be as effective as a full sensory description (Johnson and Rice 1974). Neither should one be concerned about the power of suggestion when using this intervention. Subjects given false sensory description did not report experiencing those sensations (Johnson and Rice 1974); patients given sensory information as well as those who were not given it reported experiencing similar sensations (McHugh et al. 1982).

When planning to use Concrete Objective Information with instruction in a coping strategy, it may be wise to consider whether the two interventions are compatible in terms of their effects and the mechanism by which the effects are produced. For example, combining the informational intervention of focusing attention on concrete objective elements with teaching the coping strategy of distraction may not lead to the best outcomes for the patient.

Overall, the outcomes to be achieved by using Concrete Objective Information for a nursing diagnosis of Potential Ineffective Individual Coping are to reduce or eliminate the risk factors or to keep the potential diagnosis from progressing to an actual diagnosis (Bulechek and McCloskey 1989). The research base suggests that the following may serve as specific outcome indicators for evaluating the effects of Concrete Objective Information: emotional response and ability to cooperate, especially for relatively brief procedures; for stressful events of a more sustained nature, resumption or maintenance of usual daily activities; and verbal reports of a sense of understanding of the experience or that the experience was similar to what was expected.

CASE STUDY

Mrs. O was a 62-year-old housewife scheduled to undergo external radiation therapy for early-stage endometrial cancer. She had been in good health up until her diagnosis. She was to receive daily treatments (excluding weekends) of 180 rads over a period of 28 days, resulting in a total dose of 5040 rads. Her treatment was carried out on a linear accelerator in an oncology radiation center of a major university hospital.

Due to the recent diagnosis of cancer and undergoing an unfamiliar treatment experience, Mrs. O was facing a potentially stressful situation. Our goal was to prevent a nursing diagnosis of Ineffective Coping due to the stress of an unfamiliar experience and its side effects. The treatment was Concrete Objective Information delivered by audiocassette recording. The following are excerpts from the recording. The first excerpt is from the information provided prior to Mrs. O's first treatment, and the second is from that given on her third day of treatment.

Excerpt 1. This recording describes the typical experiences that you can expect during your radiation treatments. The description is based on what patients similar to you have told us about what they saw, felt, and heard while having radiation treatment similar to yours.

Before your treatment, you will spend a few minutes in the waiting area of the radiation department. The technician will call you when it is time for your treatment. The treatment room is large. It contains a linear accelerator machine, which houses the radiation source. The machine is big, has a table underneath it, and an "arm" that can be moved. The light in the room is dim; however, you may be aware of fluorescent lights along the wall and you will see small beams of red light coming from the walls. These lights are used to help line up the area of your body to be treated. Below the arm of the accelerator is the table that you will lie on during your treatment. Once on the table, you will be asked to slip your clothes down so that the marks placed on your body during simulation will be visible. The technician will then check your position on the table and will adjust the table itself. You may feel the table move up, down, backward, or forward. Once the machine, the table, and you are in the correct positions, the technician will leave the room, and you will receive the first phase of the treatment. It is important that you lay perfectly still for your treatment. The technician will regulate the treatment from outside the room and will watch you on a television screen. You may notice the television camera on the wall. You will be able to talk to the technician through an intercom.

You will receive radiation doses from the linear accelerator when it is in four different positions: above you, below you, and on each side. The technician will come in and change the machine's position. When it is moving, it will make a clicking and a humming sound like a motor. When it stops moving, the technician will leave the room, and you will hear a buzzing sound for a few seconds. This indicates that you are receiving the radiation. You will feel nothing during the treatment. The total time you will spend in the treatment room will be about 10 minutes. When it is finished, the technician will help you with your clothes and assist you down from the table.

Excerpt 2. Women similar to you have told us about symptoms they've experienced while receiving radiation. While not all of the women experience them to the same degree, most tell us they experience diarrhea, fatigue, and nausea [Christman 1990].

Diarrhea can begin in the second week of treatment and continue throughout your treatment. It is due to the effects of radiation on your bowels. It can occur at all times of the day; however, you may notice it more in the morning or during the evening hours. Your doctor will prescribe medications and give you information about foods to eat to help reduce the diarrhea.

Fatigue, or being tired, can begin in the second week of treatment and will increase as your treatments continue. During your treatments you will notice the tiredness periodically during the day but particularly in the afternoon. Some women also experience periodic nausea or being "sick to their stomach" during the first week of treatment or near the end of treatment. Any nausea you may have is not related to the effects of radiation on your body. More likely it is due to changes in your routine, or it may be related to any feelings or concerns you may have about your treatment.

Mrs. O was an energetic and outgoing woman who had to curtail some of her activities due to her treatment schedule and side effects, but they did not change her daily routine entirely. She modified her social activities and planned more of them in her own home for the morning hours when she felt the best. She was not able to keep up with all the housework but felt comfortable allowing her two daughters to take over the laundry and vacuuming. During the fourth week of treatment, Mrs. O stated that she was glad she knew what to expect during her treatments and that it helped her to plan her daily activities.

CONCLUSION

Clearly Concrete Objective Information is an intervention helpful to patients. The strong research and theoretical base is useful to nurses in making decisions about patient care. It provides guidance for selecting patients who are most likely to benefit from the use of Concrete Objective Information and for identifying criteria appropriate to evaluating its effects. Finally, the theoretical base provides the nurse with a clear picture of the goal to be achieved by using Concrete Objective Information as a nursing intervention.

REFERENCES

Bulechek, G.M., and McCloskey, J.C. 1989. Nursing interventions: Treatments for potential nursing diagnoses. In R.M. Carroll-Johnson (ed.), *Classification of nursing diagnoses, Proceedings of the Eighth Conference* (pp. 23–30). Philadelphia: Lippincott.

Carroll-Johnson, R.M. (ed.). 1989. *Classification of nursing diagnoses, Proceedings of the Eighth Conference.* Philadelphia: Lippincott.

Christman, N.J. 1990. Symptom patterns in women having radiotherapy for gynecologic cancer. Unpublished raw data.

Fuller, S.S., Endress, M.P., and Johnson, J.E. 1978. The effects of cognitive and behavioral control on coping with an aversive health examination. *Journal of Human Stress* 4(4):18–24.

Haller, K.B., Reynolds, M.A., and Horsley, J.A. 1979. Developing research-based innovation protocols: Process, criteria, and issues. *Research in Nursing and Health* 2:45–51.

Hartfield, M.J., and Cason, C.L. 1981. Effect of information on emotional responses during barium enema. *Nursing Research* 30:151–155.

Hartfield, M.J., Cason, C.L., and Cason, G.J. 1982. Effects of information about a threatening procedure on patients' expectations and emotional distress. *Nursing Research* 31:202–206.

Hill, B.J. 1982. Sensory information, behavioral instructions and coping with sensory alteration surgery. *Nursing Research* 31:17–21.

Johnson, J.E. 1973. Effects of accurate expectations about sensations on the sensory and distress components of pain. *Journal of Personality and Social Psychology* 27:261–275.

Johnson, J.E., Christman, N.J., and Stitt, C. 1985. Personal control interventions: Short- and long-term effects on surgical patients. *Research in Nursing and Health* 8:131–145.

Johnson, J.E., Fuller, S.S., Endress, M.P., and Rice, V.H. 1978a. Altering patients' responses to surgery: An extension and replication. *Research in Nursing and Health* 1:111–121.

Johnson, J.E., Kirchhoff, K.T., and Endress, M.P. 1975. Altering children's distress behavior during orthopedic cast removal. *Nursing Research* 24:404–410.

Johnson, J.E., Kirchhoff, K.T., and Endress, M.P. 1976. Easing children's fright during health care procedures. *MCN: The American Journal of Maternal Child Nursing* 1:206–210.

Johnson, J.E., and Lauver, D.R. 1989. Alternative explanations of coping with stressful experiences associated with physical illness. *Advances in Nursing Science* 11(2):39–52.

Johnson, J.E., Lauver, D.R., and Nail, L.M. 1989. Process of coping with radiation therapy. *Journal of Consulting and Clinical Psychology* 57:358–364.

Johnson, J.E., and Leventhal, H. 1974. Effects of accurate expectations and behavioral instructions on reactions during a noxious medical examination. *Journal of Personality and Social Psychology* 29:710–718.

Johnson, J.E., Morrissey, J.F., and Leventhal, H. 1973. Psychological preparation for an endoscopic examination. *Gastrointestinal Endoscopy* 19:180–182.

Johnson, J.E., Nail, L.M., Lauver, D., King, K., and Keys, H. 1988. Reducing the negative impact of radiation therapy on functional status. *Cancer* 61:46–51.

Johnson, J.E., and Rice, V.H. 1974. Sensory and distress components of pain: Implications for the study of clinical pain. *Nursing Research* 23:203–209.

Johnson, J.E., Rice, V.H., Fuller, S.S., and Endress, P. 1978b. Sensory information, instruction in a coping strategy, and recovery from surgery. *Research in Nursing and Health* 1:4–17.

King, K.B., Nail, L.M., Kreamer, K., Strohl, R.A., and Johnson, J.E. 1985. Patients' descriptions of the experience of receiving radiation therapy. *Oncology Nursing Forum* 12(4):55–61.

Leventhal, H., and Johnson, J.E. 1983. Laboratory and field experimentation: Development of a theory of self-regulation. In P.J. Wooldridge, M.H. Schmitt, J.K. Skipper, and R.C. Leonard (eds.), *Behavioral science and nursing theory* (pp. 189–262). St. Louis: Mosby.

McHugh, N.C., Christman, N.J., and Johnson, J.E. 1982. Preparatory information: What helps and why. *American Journal of Nursing* 82:780–782.

Miller, S.M., and Mangan, C.E. 1983. Interacting effects of information and coping style in adapting to gynecologic stress: Should the doctor tell all? *Journal of Personality and Social Psychology* 45:223–236.

Nail, L., Jones, L.S., Giuffre, M., and Johnson, J.E. 1984. Sensations after mastectomy. *American Journal of Nursing* 84:1121–1124.

Neisser, U. 1976. *Cognition and reality*. San Francisco: W. H. Freeman.

Oermann, M.H., McHugh, N.G., Dietrich, J., and Boyll, R. 1983. After a tracheostomy: Patients describe their sensations. *Cancer Nursing* 6:361–366.

Padilla, G.V., Grant, N.M., Rains, B.L., Hansen, B.C., Bergstrom, N., Wong, H.L., Hanson, R., and Kubo, W. 1981. Distress reduction and the effects of preparatory teaching films and patient control. *Research in Nursing and Health* 4:375–387.

Rainey, L.C. 1985. Effects of preparatory patient education for radiation oncology patients. *Cancer* 56:1056–1061.

Rice, V.H., Sieggreen, M., Mullin, M., and Williams, J. 1988. Development and testing of an arteriography intervention for stress reduction. *Heart and Lung* 17:23–28.

Sime, A.M., and Libera, M.B. 1985. Sensation information, self-instruction and responses to dental surgery. *Research in Nursing and Health* 8:41–47.

Suls, J., and Fletcher, B. 1985. The relative efficacy of avoidant and nonavoidant coping strategies: A meta-analysis. *Health Psychology* 4:249–288.

Suls, J. and Wan, C.K. 1989. Effects of sensory and procedural information on coping with stressful medical procedures and pain: A meta-analysis. *Journal of Consulting and Clinical Psychology* 57:372–379.

Watkins, L.O., Weaver, L., and Odegaard, V. 1986. Preparation for cardiac catheterization: Tailoring the content of instruction to coping style. *Heart and Lung* 15:382–389.

Wilson, J.F. 1981. Behavioral preparation for surgery: Benefit or harm? *Journal of Behavioral Medicine* 4(1):79–102.

Wilson, J.F., Moore, R.W., Randolph, S., and Hanson, B.J. 1982. Behavioral preparation of patients for gastrointestinal endoscopy: Information, relaxation, and coping style. *Journal of Human Stress* 8(4):13–23.

11

TRUTH TELLING

CASSANDRA B. WILLIAMSON
DEBRA J. LIVINGSTON

Truthfulness is an ethical consideration in virtually all aspects of nursing. Since nursing is primarily an interaction process, there is constant potential for honesty or dishonesty, distortion, or omission (Livingston and Williamson 1985). Opportunities for Truth Telling occur frequently with such issues as values, the patient's right to information, informed consent, confidentiality, placebo therapy, and reporting unethical behavior. Nurses play a key role in clarifying information for patient decision making. As the most consistent care provider, the nurse is in the front-line position to deliver truthfulness. Patients are increasingly aware of their rights and are requesting to be partners in their health care. Increased patient involvement in health care creates the need for nurses to become responsible, accountable, and authentic. Truth Telling is an important aspect of day-to-day clinical practice.

DEFINITION

Truth Telling is a process of responsible, caring, and honest communication based on ethical decision making. The intent of Truth Telling is to: (1) promote greater coping for the individual, (2) provide increased information for decision making, (3) develop trust in the relationship and in care, and (4) give patients what rightfully belongs to them (Livingston and Williamson, 1985).

RATIONALE FOR THE USE OF TRUTHFULNESS

Truth Telling reflects the value of veracity. When the passage of information is as close to the truth as is possible, then truth is upheld. Truth Telling is based on the belief that the receiver has the right to self-determination — the right to be autonomous. In participatory health care, the patient needs information for decision making. Telling the truth and not deceiving the patient is also required for preserving patients' dignity. In an atmosphere of deception or omission, patients lose respect for their care providers and the health care organization. Truth is the atmosphere in which trust thrives. Bok (1978) states, "If there is no confidence in the truthfulness of others, is there any way to assess their fairness, their intentions

151

to help, or to harm?" (p. 31). Once the patient or family feels they have been lied to or deceived, all information given by the health professional will be suspect. The question is no longer whether to tell but who will tell and how.

THE ROLE OF THE NURSE IN TRUTH TELLING

Truth Telling issues between the nurse and the patient often center around nursing care, illness teaching, medication teaching, and home-going instruction. The role of the nurse in providing information about medical diagnosis and treatment alternatives is more ambiguous.

Laws, professional codes of ethical practice, and the American Hospital Association Patient Bill of Rights clearly establish that patients must be informed. Historically the physician has assumed a paternalistic position over the patient who receives care and the nurse who carries out the treatment plan. Today nurses are in positions to support the patient who awaits medical information, to advocate for the patient to receive information, and to participate in delivering the diagnostic and treatment information the patient is requesting.

TRUTH TELLING CONTINUUM

Truthfulness varies on a continuum, with total truth at one end and intentional lying or dishonesty on the other end. While total or absolute truth seems inaccessible, truth advocates talk about being as truthful as possible. Gadow (1981) believes that health professionals put truth behind a smoke screen, saying that truth is not accessible and therefore no form of truth can be offered. Truth Telling involves using sound judgment when sharing clinical information that clinicians possess or to which they have access.

The potential to misuse truth exists. Using truth to coerce a patient to consent to any form of treatment constitutes misuse. Even if refusal of the recommended treatment could hasten a chronic illness or ultimately death, it is still coercion. An example of truth used to coerce is the use of statistical odds that support the health care professional's choice of treatment but do not answer the real question, What is this patient's set of circumstances and prognosis? Goldie (1982) calls this the most pernicious form of deception stating: "At best this ploy [statistical prognosis] encourages a short lived gambler's euphoria" (p. 128). Moving along the truth continuum, from total truth to partial truth, coercion, and deception, it becomes more difficult to determine where one concept ends and another begins. Is giving a patient partial truth, such as most of the side effects of his medication, being truthful, or is it coercive and thus deceptive?

Deception occurs when we communicate messages that are meant to be misleading. Deception is carried out through gestures, action or inaction, disguise, and silence (Bok 1978). Deception is powerful. It can make a situation appear falsely favorable or falsely unfavorable. Used in health care, deception may deny the patient the right to information for decision making and ultimately increased coping. Lying is an extreme form of dishonesty; it is not recognized as a moral action in health care (Bok 1978). Yarling (1978) talks about the "benevolent lie."

Curtin and Flaherty (1982) describe "therapeutic deception." Both forms of dishonesty purport to be in the patient's best interest.

RESEARCH RELATED TO TRUTH

Nursing Practice

Shipps (1988) notes that Truth Telling is a dilemma for nurses. In her preliminary on Truth Telling, Shipps analyzed 715 real life moral dilemmas submitted by Master's level students enrolled in an ethics course at a large northeastern university. The students represented a sample nursing population of the United States, Africa, Asia, and the Middle East. Shipps analyzed the case studies identifying the types of moral dilemmas and the claimants. Forty-nine percent of the cases studied were classified as truthtelling moral dilemmas; these dilemmas included all situations in which a nurse described himself or herself as in the position of giving or withholding information from the patient. Six types of truthtelling situations were identified by content analysis: physician incompetency; informed consent; withholding information: diagnosis, prognosis; withholding information: general, nurse incompetency; unethical behavior in organization; and placebo.

Shipps (1988) studied ethical decision-making behaviors of nurses when they became aware that a physician was deceiving a patient. She interviewed 41 nurses individually who were asked to recall an incident in which the patient was intentionally misinformed or unintentionally uninformed of his or her condition or treatment by a physician. Thirty-four (83%) of the nurses were able to do so. The most frequent type of situation described was that of withholding information from the patient concerning prognosis or diagnosis. In these situations, 18% of the nurses reported telling the patient themselves. Another 44% reported attempting to obtain the truth for the patient, and 35% remained neutral, doing nothing. The situations reported by the nurses varied considerably but were similar regarding the distress the nurses experienced. Shipps also presented the subjects with four hypothetical dilemmas for discussion and asked each to identify a reaction. Analysis of Truth Telling was best predicted by situational factors as opposed to a consistent pattern of behavior exhibited by individual nurses.

Nurses reported feeling caught in a situation beyond their ability and felt unsure of themselves and their appropriate role. An important finding of this study was that contextual or situational factors were influential in the nurse's moral decision-making process. All subjects described themselves as patient advocates. There was unanimous agreement that it would be best for patients to be informed in all situations, but the nurses were unclear how to accomplish this goal and if they were the best person to tell versus the physician, family or other person.

In a study questioning the use of honesty in nursing practice, Schrock (1980) surveyed 83 undergraduate nursing students and 48 B.S.N. completion students. When given a question concerning deceiving a patient about the purpose of a drug, with multiple reasons for using deception, 60% of those using deception offered acting under coercion as a reason. Twenty-seven percent of those being deceptive lacked the confidence to handle the situation. Schrock implies that nurses often use deception in everyday practice, without justifiable reasons for withholding information.

A survey conducted by Sandroff (1981) showed that most of the 12,500 nurse respondents agreed with the patient's right to be informed and believed it was their duty to protect patients by keeping them informed. A poll of over 5,000 nurses by *Nursing Life Journal* (1983) asked several questions related to truth-telling practices. A majority of nurses reported feeling uncomfortable about giving information to patients. Very few (12%) felt it is always wrong to withhold information from patients. Fifty-two percent of the respondents had deceived adult patients about their medications, although 56% believed such deception is unethical.

Patients' Preferences

Research by Elian and Dean (1985) involving 167 patients with multiple sclerosis revealed that 83% favored knowing their diagnosis, 13% were indifferent, and less than 4% preferred not to know.

In a study of 224 adult patients concerning truth telling and Alzheimer's disease, Erde, Nadal, and Scholl (1988) found that more than 90% of the patients wanted to be told their diagnosis so they could make plans for care, obtain a second opinion, and settle family matters. Studies asking whether cancer patients want to be told also reveal that patients prefer receiving the truth about their diagnosis and treatment (Kelly and Friesen 1950; Bowen 1955).

Physicians and Truth Telling

In a landmark study by Oken (1961) with 219 physicians being asked about telling terminally ill cancer patients their diagnosis, 90% indicated a preference for not telling. In 1983, the President's Commission for the Study of Ethical Problems conducted a telephone survey of 800 physicians and 1250 nonphysician adults to determine attitudes about disclosing health and illness information. Eighty-six percent of the physicians believed their patients wanted the truth. When faced with telling about terminal illness, only 13 percent said they would give a statistical prognosis. In a 1989 study concerning physicians' attitudes toward using deception, 44% of the 109 physicians responding made specific statements about the importance of truthfulness. Eighty-seven percent indicated that deception is acceptable on rare occasions (Novack, Detering, Arnold, Lachian, Ladinsky, and Pezzullo 1989).

ETHICAL DECISION MAKING

The nurse is guided in choosing the best option for truth by weighing ethical principles and professional values. Steele and Harmon (1981) maintain that "values determine the selection made between competing alternatives and therefore they hold a key position in any decision making process" (p. 5). By clarifying the values of everyone involved, the nurse determines whether each person holds honesty as a value. "If the value of truthfulness is a priority, it will be reflected consistently in [patient] care" (Livingston and Williamson 1985, p. 367).

Historically, health professionals have tolerated deception for fear truth may cause harm to the patient. The support for this action is based on paternalism. Paternalism seeks to benefit the patient but denies the patient control of information that may be critical for decision making. It is based on the deontologic principles of nonmaleficence, meaning to do no harm, and beneficence, to do good.

Paternalism does not include the deontologic principle of autonomy. The principle of autonomy also strives for nonmaleficence and beneficence, along with maintaining the patient's right to self-determination. Based on autonomy, what is best would be decided by the patient, not the health professional, assuming the patient is competent and well informed.

Utilitarian principles are based on the outcome of actions and the extent to which these actions produce good. Using utilitarian principles for ethical decision making, the nurse would evaluate a dilemma, approving actions that would produce good over bad, expediency, and/or utility for more than one person. Nurses are often in a position where they are aware of what is happening but hesitate to share their concerns. The nurse must decide whether to be a whistle blower — for example, informing the patient or people with authority in the system of a physician's incompetence. While this may be harmful to the physician, it could benefit this and other patients and the reputation of the institution. The nurse reporting the physician's actions could interfere with the physician's practice but would produce the greatest good for the most.

Judging a nurse's decision-making potential in Truth Telling issues based on the nurse's familiarity with ethical principles and his or her level of moral reasoning via Kohlberg's theory is restrictive and limiting. His cognitive/developmental theory describes six stages of moral thinking. The language of helping, caring for others, and being sensitive to the needs of others fall into the conventional stage, viewed as inferior to his higher post-conventional stage. (Women score lower on moral development when measured by Kohlberg's scale.) Shipps (1988) and Nokes (1989) support C. Gilligan's work, which identifies that moral (and ethical) problems arise from conflicting responsibilities, not competing rights. Kohlberg's theory rests on cognitive development, while Gilligan's theory supports social experiences and relationships as equal to or more important than cognitive development (Gilligan 1982). Shipps's (1988) research found nurses to justify their ethical decision making and behavior within the perspective of justice, caring, or a mixture of both.

Women have different ways of reasoning about moral dilemmas. In nursing, a profession that is predominantly women, those making important clinical decisions must pay attention to the setting in which the problem is being analyzed. Nurses must consider situational factors such as the needs of the patient, family, the institution, and health care team members in order to find the "best fit" solution (Nokes 1989). Nursing cannot let go of or ignore its connectedness to others and to health promotion.

In Shipps's (1988) study, contextual factors (nonmoral, clinical factors) contributed to the complexity of moral choice and influenced the decision-making process of nurses using Truth Telling. Examples of contextual factors include severity of illness, age, mental status, family needs, coping ability, institutional support, relationship with the patient, reputation of professional, and the incidence of occurrence.

LEGAL ISSUES

Over the last six decades, the question of how much medical information is good for the patient has been the subject of many lawsuits (LeBlang 1981). LeBlang identifies a common law trend that favors the maximum disclosure of information.

The trend is toward the physician's duty to inform the patient fully about his or her condition or any information about his or her body. The duty to inform goes well beyond giving the patient what is needed for informed consent. In *Betesh v. USA*, 1974, the court specifically held that the physician was obligated to warn the examinee of any finding that would indicate that the examinee was in danger and should seek further medical evaluation and treatment (LeBlang 1981).

Infrequently health professionals have been found negligent because they have given the patient information related to a medical treatment or condition. Full disclosure of pertinent facts describing the patient's condition is advised.

Shipps (1988), in a personal communication with Marie E. Snyder, an attorney, asked about nurses and legal responsibilities. Shipps writes,

> According to Snyder the best defense a nurse can present in a court of law is to be able to say that all actions she took were done on behalf of the client: to prevent harm and to do good. . . . A defense by a nurse that she acted under order of a physician or in order to maintain the integrity of nurse-to-physician relationship or even to protect the physician-client relationship would be much less likely to succeed. (p. 10)

THE NURSE'S AUTHORITY

In providing care, the nurse has the responsibility and authority to explain procedures and nursing interventions. If the physician chooses to withhold medical information that the nurse assesses as important for the patient to know, the nurse has the responsibility to collaborate with the physician and others concerning the withholding. The nurse has the duty to protect the patient's right to be informed. The 1976 American Nurses' Association (ANA) Code for Nurses with Interpretive Statements strengthens the nurse's position to preserve the patient's right to self-determination and information. According to Section 1.1, Self-Determination of Clients, "Each client has the moral right to determine what will be done with his/her person; to be given the information necessary for making informed judgements, to be told the possible effects of care, and to accept, refuse, or terminate treatment" (ANA). The code implies that Truth Telling, at least involving clinical information giving, is a responsibility of the nurse. "While the Code offers direction, it has not been updated and thus does not not reflect the rapidly expanding role of the nurse" (Livingston and Williamson 1985, p. 370).

According to Yarling (1978), whether to disclose information to a terminally ill patient is a moral, not a medical, decision. Therefore, a physician's medical-scientific expertise does not give his or her opinion any extraordinary value. French (1984) concludes that disclosing information does not belong to any one member of the health team. When a patient requests information regarding his or her condition, the nurse has the moral right and obligation to answer the patient. Trandel-Korenchuk and Trandel-Korenchuk (1986) support this position, stating that the nurse has the moral and legal obligation to keep the patient informed. The nurse incurs the moral and legal obligation to disclose the appropriate information when a provider-patient relationship is established with the individual. Curtin and Flaherty (1982) acknowledge there are risks for the nurse who provides medical information to the patient. They believe nurses have the moral duty to be honest in answering patients' questions and state, "There is no law expressly forbidding nurses to disclose information to patients" (p. 333).

Nursing Diagnosis

Truth Telling is an intervention that applies to any patient group. It supports genuine communication, which is a useful strategy for every nursing diagnosis. In particular, Impaired Adjustment, Body Image Disturbance, Anticipatory Grieving, Knowledge Deficit, and Spiritual Distress would be improved by the nurse who uses Truth Telling. Adjusting to one's illness or hospitalization is easier when the patient is informed about what is happening. Patient teaching would be impossible without providing information. The nurse is in a position to foster the patient's identity control and maintain his or her right to self-determination.

Truth Telling is a communication process to aid disclosure about illness, procedures, and treatments. Other examples of nursing diagnoses in which this intervention may be appropriate are Alteration in Comfort and Pain. Being honest with patients about issues concerning care will diminish anxiety, fear, and helplessness and increase a sense of power and effective coping. When patients are hospitalized, many of their daily choices are controlled by the care providers and the hospital routine. They worry about losing control of their physical well-being. Powerlessness is a nursing diagnosis that improves with Truth Telling. The increased information resulting from this intervention enables patients to have better decision-making ability.

Patients cope less effectively when given either too much or too little information or when the delivery of information is poorly timed. Truth Telling must be carefully planned within the nursing diagnosis of Ineffective Denial. For example, a nurse caring for a patient who is newly diagnosed as HIV positive, would watch for the defining characteristics of Ineffective Denial to measure readiness to receive and process information. The issue is balancing the patient's effective use of Denial and the need for information with the amount of information and when to tell.

Anticipatory Grieving is frequently a nursing diagnosis with terminally ill patients. Truth Telling helps the patient with family and friends prepare for death. Kubler-Ross (1969) writes that terminally ill patients can handle "the awesome truth" when it is delivered with sensitivity, warmth, and directness.

TRUTH TELLING AS AN INTERVENTION

Description of the Model (See Model Figure 1)

The theoretical model with options for Truth Telling was deduced from clinical practice. The Truth Telling model provides nurses with a tool to direct values, knowledge, ethical principles, and the nursing process into a compassionate and logically reasoned response. The foundation of the model is the nurse-patient relationship. The model supports the philosophy of nursing as a humanistic, holistic, and patient-centered practice (Livingston and Williamson 1985). It recognizes that nurses are a pivotal part of health care and must work with the physician and other care providers. The model guides the nurse in determining the amount of truth disclosure and how to deliver the truth. When there is not immediate consensus between nurse, physician, patient, and family regarding truth telling, a truth dilemma exists. When the nurse encounters the truth dilemma, he or she uses professional and legal authority supporting the right to tell. The nurse applies an ethical decision-making process and collaborates with the physician and family.

ASSESSMENT

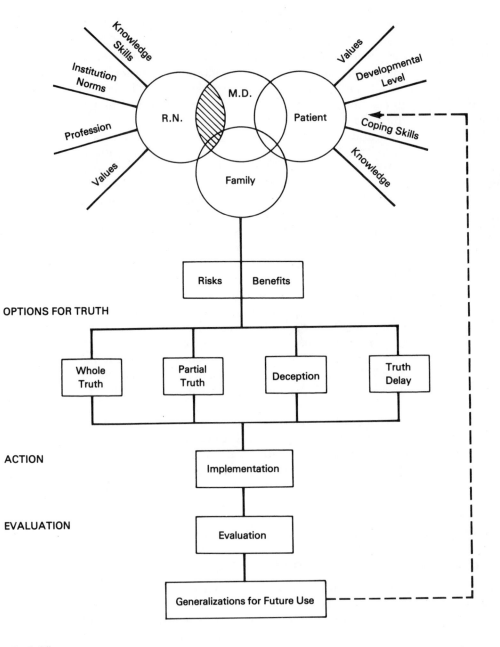

OPTIONS FOR TRUTH

ACTION

EVALUATION

FIGURE 11-1. Truth Telling Model

These activities are vital to the nurse who must decide whether to tell, how much to tell, and who will do the telling.

Assessment is the first stage of the model. The nurse assesses his or her own knowledge and skills, values, and professional duties. In every situation, the nurse must consider the patient, family, and physician's knowledge, values, and desire for truth disclosure. In the second stage, the model identifies four options for truth telling and a risk-benefit analysis of the truth options. Although truth is the most therapeutic response, all four options have clinical application. The third stage of the model is implementation, which requires nursing action. Implementation includes the actual process of telling, the ongoing collaboration with the physician and family, and patient teaching. Evaluation is the fourth stage of the model and directs the nurse to evaluate the effectiveness of the Truth Telling intervention. Evaluation includes generalizations for future use, allows the nurse the opportunity to reflect on the knowledge base, ethical principles, values, and professional actions in this situation. This process of review can influence future care provided to this patient and others.

Assessment

The assessment stage of Truth Telling analyzes the risks and benefits of Truth Telling. It uncovers important information about the patient and allows the nurse to build a trusting relationship essential for helping effectiveness. The information gathered from the patient will assist the nurse and the patient in making the optimal choice for truth. The assessment stage considers all the contextual factors involved in the truth dilemma and will help the nurse select the best option on the truth continuum.

The nurse begins by assessing the patient's values. Does the patient wish to participate in care? How does his or her cultural background influence his or her beliefs about health and illness? How much information does he or she value concerning diagnosis and treatment? Would the patient like to be alone or have someone with him or her when hearing information about the illness? Does the patient prefer the big picture with lots of detail or small amounts of information as it is known?

The nurse will assess the developmental level of the patient, including the age and maturity of the patient and their impact on decision-making ability. Is the patient considered mentally competent? Can the patient make sound decisions? Is he or she able to understand and process information given and to act rationally? The nurse must assess the patient's level of cognitive functioning by noting the patient's ability to read, write, follow simple directions, and recall simple information given. The patient's level of knowledge concerning his or her health status is assessed. What are the patient's concerns? What information does the patient already have? What expectations does the patient have about what will occur? What information does he or she need?

The nurse will assess how well the patient is coping with illness and hospitalization. What is the patient's mental status? Is he or she alert, anxious, confused, sad, passive, aggressive? What is the patient's level of anxiety? What is the level of denial? How has the patient coped with previous difficult situations? Many of these same questions apply when assessing family participation.

To understand the physician's plans regarding Truth Telling, the nurse needs to ask about the value the physician places on the truth and how the physician plans to deliver truth to the patient and the family. The nurse also determines the physician's willingness to collaborate. Does the physician know what is important to the patient and family and what questions they are asking?

The nurse then assesses his or her own competency, which is based on assessment skills, knowledge base, reflection on values and moral issues, communication skills, and rapport with the patient. The nurse must acknowledge his or her authority to tell. Is there support from peers, management, and the institution for telling? The nurse must examine his or her values related to honesty and the patient's rights to self-determination and autonomy. What is the nurse's knowledge base related to this patient's illness? Does the nurse have adequate communication skills to collaborate and deliver the truth? Is the nurse able to provide the necessary time and support needed for all phases of Truth Telling.

After gathering information about the patient, the family, the physician, self, and the institution, the nurse identifies appropriate ethical codes, ethical principles, the patient's rights, and the authority of others. Dealing with these factors, the nurse may confront a truth dilemma: the intersection of all viewpoints regarding ethical principles, legal rights, practice codes, authority, and values. Solving the truth dilemma requires collaboration and group decision making. A risk-benefit analysis of the options for truth will aid in problem solving. At this time, the nurse may compromise his or her position concerning a truth option. This collaboration may take place in a review rounds, a multidisciplinary team meeting, or during an ethical practice committee case review.

Options for Truth

According to the model, the nurse considers the position of others and the patient's position yet makes the final decision about truthfulness as an intervention. The option of whole truth is strongly recommended in most situations. Using whole truth, the intent of the teller is to provide information that is as close to the truth as is humanly possible. Usually whole truth is delivered upon the request of the patient and does not include "compulsive candor" or "truth dumping" (Livingston and Williamson 1985). Choosing this option is clear when the patient, family, nurse, and physician all value truthfulness and the patient has asked for information. It must then be determined who is the best person to do the telling. Considerations include who has the best rapport with the patient and the family and the most knowledge about the illness and treatment plans. In many situations, the immediate effects of whole truth will be discomfort. The intensity and duration of the discomfort must be closely monitored. The patient and family need support and reassurance that they will not be abandoned.

In some situations, delivering whole truth is difficult—for example, when the nurse assesses that the patient wants to know but the family or physician wishes to protect the patient from the bad news. The nurse assesses the patient's capacity for truth and the patient's values and shares this information candidly with the physician and the family. If collaboration does not bring resolution, then the nurse has two choices: select another option for Truth Telling on the continuum or implement whole truth. Either option may incur professional risks. Seeking support from peers, nursing management, and health team members can minimize these risks.

Sometimes the physician wants to give the patient all the information and the nurse has assessed that the whole truth is not in this patient's best interest because of the patient's condition or inability to cope. This situation requires the nurse to present the physician with his or her own assessment of the patient and preferred option for truth. If the physician proceeds with whole truth, the nurse must support the patient and help him or her accept the information.

Partial truth is the second option for truth. The intent of partial truth is veracity. Partial truth allows the nurse to give some information without having to go back to disentangle any false or misleading information. When in doubt about whether the amount of information is adequate using partial truth, ask the patient, "Would it be helpful to know more?" or "What other information would you like?" The nurse must carefully assess the risks and benefits of this option. Gadow recommends less than the whole truth with patients who would be seriously overwhelmed, unable to understand, or are prone to treatment noncompliance. When a patient is noncomplying with treatment, the nurse must question whether the information is partial truth or whether it is meant to coerce (Gadow 1981). Partial truth is an appropriate choice when a patient is using denial to cope with the severity of the medical situation yet is requesting small amounts of information. When there is not an immediate decision that the patient must make regarding treatment, the truth teller may wait until the patient asks for more or shows signs of wanting more information. Eventually the pieces of partial truth will equal whole truth.

Deception is rarely an appropriate option. It is used only when truth endangers the immediate health or well-being of the patient or someone else. For example, a nurse receives a call from a patient threatening suicide with a loaded gun. He states, "I'll use it now unless you promise to keep this a secret." The nurse reassures the patient he or she will not tell and at the same time writes a note to a co-worker, "Please have the police go to patient X!" Another example of when the nurse uses deception is to protect an accident victim who is in intensive care with an acute myocardial infarction. The patient asks, "Is my wife alive?" The nurse knows that the wife did not survive but states, "She is O.K."

When deception is chosen, the risks to the patient and the nurse must be carefully weighed. Deceiving the patient can diminish trust, create anger, and erode the image of the health care system. By not providing accurate information, the patient lacks knowledge he or she may need for problem solving. The use of deception puts into question all information the patient has received. The risks of deception for the nurse include guilt, decreased self-esteem, anxiety about being caught, and additional energy to keep the deception going. If the physician or family has deceived the patient, the nurse is in a truth dilemma. The nurse may feel distressed and will need to consider his or her own decision about truth options. Collaboration is recommended.

There are many forms of deception in the health care arena, ranging from concealment to exaggeration. Placebo therapy is a form of deception. The nurse is forced to decide whether to administer the placebo and what to say if the patient asks, "What is this medication?" or "Why am I taking this?"

Truth delay, the fourth option, is used when the nurse assesses that essential pieces are missing and he or she needs more time. Choosing this option does not remove the nurse from the Truth Telling intervention, but the option does allow more time for assessment, planning, and implementation. If the nurse feels a lack of rapport with the patient or is uninformed about the patient's condition, this option is appropriate. Many nurses lack the confidence to deliver the truth. Truth delay may give the nurse time to prepare a response. It is also used when the nurse is aware the physician has requested that information be withheld until the physician delivers the truth. It is the option of choice when the nurse does not have the time to deliver information or to offer the necessary support to the patient. Using truth delay, the nurse would say to the patient, "I understand the questions you are asking. Someone who is caring for you will get back to you as soon as possible."

Using truth delay, the nurse is responsible for communicating the patient's questions and collaborating with health care team members to plan the Truth Telling intervention. The option of truth delay is like a safety net: allowing the nurse time to identify what is missing and to correct the deficiency. One risk associated with truth delay is increased anxiety for the patient related to the unknown. The patient may also view the delay as deception.

Implementation

Having chosen the best option for truth delivery, the nurse carries out the planned strategy. In the implementation stage, information is provided to the patient and family. The person disclosing the information must have rapport with the patient, be knowledgeable about the patient's condition and the disease process, and possess adequate communication skills. The information must be given at an appropriate time. The timing of information delivery affects the patient's ability to hear the message. The nurse determines a patient's readiness by listening to and watching the patient's responses. Part of timing is allowing for uninterrupted privacy and including significant others as requested by the patient.

Language used should be clear, concise, and at a level the patient is able to understand. Communication skills needed by the nurse include active listening and empathy. Active listening is attending to verbal and nonverbal cues and validating a patient's feelings and underlying concerns. High (1989) states, "Professionals need to be sensitive to the authority and power they possess as listeners" (p. 9). The listener can exploit the patient with a professional dominance with the overuse of eye contact and with touch that is patronizing instead of touch that communicates caring.

Assertive communication by the nurse includes using "I" language in expressing feelings and wants, making soft and caring statements, and using confrontation, defined here as pointing out discrepancies between what the patient or physician believes and their behavior or actions. The patient may say he values truth yet changes the subject every time the nurse talks about his condition or diagnosis.

Teaching the patient to communicate assertively is frequently part of the implementation stage. Assertion skills can increase the patient's sense of control and give him or her the tools necessary to ask more questions or to limit the amount of information being delivered regarding diagnosis and treatment.

Congruence in communication is being truly genuine and without professional armor. The nurse's verbal and nonverbal behavior are congruent when both reflect the same message. Congruence fosters trust in the nurse-patient relationship.

Throughout the implementation stage, the nurse must collaborate with the physician and other members of the health team. A collaborative relationship among the health care team improves patient care. The physician's position and skill in telling information about medical diagnosis directly affects the nurse and the patient. When patients fail to understand, the team needs to give consistent and repeated information. Consistency in truth telling is enhanced by keeping a checklist on the patient's chart. Selekman (1989) recommends a checklist on the patient's chart communicating what the patient has been told about his or her condition, the patient's questions, and the responses of health team members. Additional items on the checklist might be the patient's response to the information and information shared with the family. It is necessary to document all stages of this intervention in order to evaluate the outcome.

Evaluation

Evaluation of the intervention is the last stage of the Truth Telling model. To evaluate this intervention, the nurse reviews the stages of the model to determine if the process of Truth Telling was successful, and whether the outcomes for the intervention were met.

Process evaluation questions include the following:

1.   Were the contextual factors including age, values, and coping incorporated into the decision-making process?
2.   Did the nurse apply ethical principles in the decision-making process?
3.   Did collaboration occur between the nurse and the physician?
4.   Did collaboration occur with the primary caregivers and the family?
5.   Did the nurse/health care team do a risk-benefit analysis of each option for truth?
6.   Was the timing and use of language in delivering information appropriate for the patient?
7.   Was the patient provided adequate support?

Outcome evaluation questions include the following:

1.   Did Truth Telling enhance the well-being of the patient? Was there a decrease in frequency of complaints, decreased restlessness, increased involvement in care, an ability to plan short- and long-term goals, and increased socialization?
2.   What level of learning has occurred? Is the patient able to repeat or demonstrate the information given?
3.   Is the patient participating in the decision-making process? Is he or she asking questions and stating preferences for treatment?
4.   What has the nurse learned during the Truth Telling intervention about self? How will this change his or her nursing practice?

CASE STUDY

At the age of 55, Kay Brown is brought to the emergency room following a car accident. In the emergency room, she is unable to remember her destination, home address, or telephone number. She is admitted to the hospital and immediately taken to the operating room, where her fractured hip is surgically repaired.

Following surgery, she is transferred to an orthopedic unit, where she is frequently visited by her husband. Mrs. Brown is a semiretired high school mathematics teacher, who has been working full time until 2 years ago when her husband retired at age 62. On the second postoperative day, Mr. Brown states that his wife's memory has been declining over the past year.

On the fourth postoperative day, the nurse and physician caring for Mrs. Brown observe more confusion than would be expected and that her confusion is more exaggerated when the television set is on in the evening. The next day, without resolution of confusion, a diagnostic evaluation to rule out dementia, Alzheimer's disease, is requested of the neurology consult team.

The attending physician and Mr. Brown have told the nurse they do not want Mrs. Brown to know her potential diagnosis. They believe that knowing this information would have a negative effect on her sense of well-being and would make her more anxious, unpredictable, and depressed.

When the nurse is with Mrs. Brown, the patient asks, "Why can't I remember your name? Why is my memory getting so poor?" The nurse provides some simple reassurance: "You may be experiencing memory loss due to the surgery and the car accident." The nurse teaches the patient how to transfer and nonweight bear during ambulation. The next morning, the nurse finds the patient showering bearing full weight. During morning report, the night nurse mentions Mrs. Brown has been up wandering about and appears confused about her room location. Based on this information, the postoperative day 4 confusion, and the admission assessment, the nursing diagnoses identified for Mrs. Brown include: Bathing/Hygiene Self Care Deficit, Altered Thought Processes, and Knowledge Deficit (lack of information about condition).

One morning the nurse talks with Mrs. Brown about her health history, her personal and professional life, and her desire to be informed about her condition. The patient describes herself as being very active in her teaching career and her professional organization. She states she maintains the household and feels being in control is important. The nurse asks Mrs. Brown to describe what she knows about her health condition and what changes have taken place in the last year. Mrs. Brown reveals that she has had only one other health problem—skin cancer 5 years ago, involving a mole on her face, which was diagnosed as a malignant melanoma. Since this diagnosis, she states she has worried a lot about melanomas and has a monthly checkup with her doctor. The patient reveals to the nurse she has recently had difficulty with teaching. Her short-term memory is not as good as it used to be. She states she is lost without her list of things to do and asks, "What is wrong with me? Am I going crazy?"

The nurse reflects on her personal and professional values concerning honesty. In 10 years of professional experience, the nurse has valued her role as patient advocate. She has tried to strive for honesty and beneficence. Personally she is dealing with a grandmother who is in a nursing home and has Alzheimer's disease.

The nurse requests a conference with the physician to discuss her assessment data. The nurse presents this information and suggests that they discuss the potential diagnosis of Alzheimer's with the husband and the patient. The physician disagrees with the nurse. The physician has already spoken with the husband, who does not want the patient to know. The physician asks the nurse to withhold information until after the electroencephalogram, magnetic resonance imaging, and neurobehavioral testing are completed. The physician and the nurse agree to use partial truth as a means to deal with the patient's questions: if the patient asks why the tests are being done, they will answer, "These tests will help us understand why you are having problems with your memory." They also record the plan on the front of the chart so other caregivers are consistent with the patient.

Three days later, the test results strongly show the presence of mild-moderate dementia of Alzheimer's type. Another multidisciplinary conference including the husband has been arranged. The nurse presents that Mrs. Brown repeatedly wants information concerning her memory loss and seems embarrassed by her forgetfulness regarding health teaching. In the past she has preferred to be informed about her medical condition. The nurse makes a case for telling the diagnosis so that Mrs. Brown can make appropriate decisions regarding her activities, including teaching. Mr. Brown insists that the tests are wrong and Mrs. Brown does not have Alzheimer's. He states that he does not want her to know that it is even a consideration. The physician responds, "I agree;

this diagnosis is always very difficult to make. Let's not make Mrs. Brown uncomfortable but watch her closely."

The nurse does not agree with the outcome of the conference and feels that the patient has a right to self-determination. She believes that she has developed a sense of trust with the patient and is no longer comfortable avoiding questions the patient asks about her condition. She seeks support from other peers and arranges a nursing care conference with the nurse manager and the geriatric clinical nurse specialist (CNS). The consensus of the care conference participants is to tell Mrs. Brown about her diagnosis. The nurse manager and the CNS openly support the nurse in telling. The nurse analyzes the option for whole truth using a risk-benefit analysis. She determines that the risks of telling include potential deterioration of the nurse-physician relationship and possible anger from Mr. Brown toward her and the institution. Benefits of telling include increased safety for the patient; patient autonomy, including the right to prepare for the future; maintained self-respect for the patient; and understanding family-imposed limits. The nurse benefits by maintaining her values and self-respect.

The nurse goes back to the physician and says, "I have decided after seeking others' opinions to address Mrs. Brown's questions about her condition. My preference is that we would do this together. Otherwise, I will do this myself." The physician refuses to cooperate and states, "I will not participate in this activity. What right do you think you have to interfere with my doctor-patient relationship!" The nurse also discloses to Mr. Brown her intention to tell Mrs. Brown about Alzheimer's disease. She emphasizes that telling will eliminate the burden on Mr. Brown of deception and minimize the related marital friction. The nurse states that he and his wife will have the opportunity to discuss and make decisions together regarding finances, legal matters, disability, and future care. The nurse asks Mr. Brown if he would like to be present when Mrs. Brown is told and asks what he would prefer the illness be called — dementia or Alzheimer's.

After consulting with the geriatric CNS, the nurse has written and verbal information about Alzheimer's to give the patient. The nurse acknowledges her own effective communication skills. Her schedule allows her the time to provide follow-up teaching and support.

Two days later, the patient again asks, "What have you found out about my tests? Why is my memory so poor?" At this time the nurse implements the Truth Telling intervention by giving the patient a simple verbal explanation of the patient's condition and the written materials about Alzheimer's. She stays with the patient and allows time for Mrs. Brown to ask questions. The nurse is empathic when Mrs. Brown responds with shock and sadness: "This is very difficult for you to hear. We will talk about this again. I am here to answer your questions and to help you think about the future. Your husband also knows this information. I encourage you to talk to your doctor and your husband about this." Mrs. Brown thanks the nurse for telling her. She says it clears up the mystery of her day-to-day forgetfulness.

Throughout this intervention, the nurse documents the assessments, actions, and the patient's responses. In the time remaining with the patient, the nurse will measure the success of telling by evaluating the process and outcome of the intervention (G.R. Hall, personal communication about Alzheimer's disease, September 1990).

CONCLUSION

Nurses are constantly faced with complex ethical decisions and truth telling. The model of Truth Telling presented in this chapter can help nurses decide what to do when encountering difficult decisions. The Truth Telling model is a tool to direct values, knowledge, ethical principles, and the nursing process, with four options for delivering the truth: whole truth, partial truth, deception, and truth delay. The nurse's moral reasoning and assessment of contextual factors like age, severity of illness, family needs, and coping ability, are intertwined in his or her ethical decision-making process. How honest a nurse will be in an interaction depends upon the value placed upon truthfulness and the commitment to the issue at hand. The model helps the nurse with decision making regarding the truth dilemma and assists her in choosing an intervention, implementing it, and evaluating the outcome. Using process and evaluation questions, the nurse can determine if her choice of intervention was beneficial, and may guide her future practice. In order to be carried out successfully, the Truth Telling intervention requires a good deal of knowledge, poise, and self-confidence, and a genuine concern for the patient and others. This requires a commitment to assess, monitor, and evaluate each situation thoroughly.

REFERENCES

American Nurses' Association. 1976. *Code for nurses with interpretive statements.* Kansas City, Mo.: American Nurses' Association.

Bok, S. 1978. *Lying: Moral choice in public and private life.* New York: Random House.

Bowen, O.R. 1955. Why cancer victims should be told the truth. *Medical Times* 83(2):793–799.

Curtin, L., and Flaherty, M.J. 1982. *Nursing ethics—Theories and pragmatics.* Bowie. Md; Robert J. Brady.

Elian, M., and Dean, G. 1985. To tell or not to tell the diagnosis of multiple sclerosis. *Lancet* 2:27–28.

Erde, E.L., Nadal, E.C., and Scholl, T.O. 1988. On truth telling and the diagnosis of Alzheimer's disease. *Journal of Family Practice* 26(4):401–406.

Fenner, K.M. 1985. Ethics: Deciding whether to give or withhold information. *Association of Operating Room Nurses Journal* 42(2):278, 280.

French, D.G. 1984. Ethics: Nurse, am I going to live? *Nursing Management* 15(11):43–46.

Gadow, S. 1981. Truth: Treatment of choice, scarce resource, or patient's right? *Journal of Family Practice* 13(6):857–860.

Gilligan, C. 1982. *In a Different Voice.* Cambridge: Harvard University Press.

Gillon, R. 1985. Telling the truth and medical ethics. *British Medical Journal* 291:1556–1557.

Goldie, L. 1982. The ethics of telling the patient. *Journal of Medical Ethics* 8:128–133.

High, D.M. 1989. Truth telling, confidentiality, and the dying patient: New dilemmas for the nurse. *Nursing Forum* 24(1):5–10.

Kelly, W.D., and Friesen, S. 1950. Do cancer patients want to be told? *Surgery* 27:822–826.

Kubler-Ross, E. 1969. *On death and dying.* New York: Macmillan.

LeBlang, T.R. 1981, September. Disclosure of injury and illness: Responsibilities in the physician-patient relationship. *Law, Medicine and Health Care,* 4–7.

Livingston, D., and Williamson, C. 1985. Truth telling. In G.M. Bulechek and J.C. McCloskey (eds.), *Nursing interventions: Treatments for nursing diagnoses* (pp. 365–384). Philadelphia: W.B. Saunders Company.

Nokes, K.M. 1989. Rethinking moral reasoning theory. *Image* 21(3):172–175.

Novack, D.H., Detering, B.J., Arnold, R., Lachian, F., Ladinsky, M., and Pezzullo, J.C. 1989. Physicians' attitude toward using deception to resolve difficult ethical problems. *Journal of the American Medical Association* 26(20):2980–2985.

Nursing Life Ethics Poll Report. 1983. How ethical are you? Part 1. *Nursing Life* 3(1):25–33.

Oken, D. 1961. What to tell cancer patients. *Journal of the American Medical Association* 175:1120–128.

President's Commission for the Study of Ethical Problems in Medicine and Biomedical and Behavioral Research. 1983. *Summing up: Final report on studies of the ethical and legal problems in medicine and biomedical and behavioral research.* Washington, D.C.: U.S. Government Printing Office.

Salzman, L. 1973. Truth, honesty, and the therapeutic process. *American Journal of Psychiatry* 130:1281–1282.

Sandroff, R. 1981. Is it right? Protect the M.D. . . . or the patient? *RN* 44(2):28–33.

Schrock, R.A. 1980. A question of honesty in nursing practice. *Journal of Advanced Nursing* 5:135–148.

Selekman, J. 1989. When the nurse knows and the patient does not: Waiting for a diagnosis. *Holistic Nursing Practice* 4(1):1–7.

Shipps, T.B. 1988. Truthtelling behavior of Nurses: What nurses do when physicians deceive clients. Doctoral dissertation, Boston University.

Steele, S.M., and Harmon, V.M. 1981. *Values in nursing.* New York: Appleton-Century-Crofts.

Trandel-Korenchuk, D.M., and Trandel-Korenchuk, K.M. 1986. Disclosure of information in nursing. *Nursing Administration Quarterly* 10(3):69–73.

Yarling, R. 1978, June. Ethical analysis of a nursing problem: The scope of nursing practice in disclosing the truth to terminal patients. Part II. *Supervisor Nurse*, 28–34.

12

STRUCTURED PREOPERATIVE TEACHING

BETTY PATTERSON TARSITANO

DEFINITION AND DESCRIPTION

Structured Preoperative Teaching consists of planned psychoeducative activities where a registered nurse provides standardized information (sensory, procedural, factual) to presurgical patients and/or family (significant others) according to anxiety and fear levels. The purpose of the information is to help the person perform a certain task or skill to prepare for the postoperative period and to cope with the threat behind the anxiety. The overall goal is to promote positive patient outcomes. The nurse is a supportive, authoritative figure who is familiar with the care of patients and families in surgical settings. The psychoeducative design takes into account the characteristics of the patient and family members (significant others), the abilities and characteristics of the nurse; the focus of the intervention in relation to anxiety and fear levels; distinct properties of the situation; distinct activities of the intervention; the purpose of the intervention; standard information and skills to be provided (procedural, sensory, factual); presentation time; expected measurable outcomes based on valid and reliable clinical indicators; teaching strategies, audiovisual materials, data collection, and recording tools; and documentation of the intervention and the outcomes obtained. Initial preoperative assessment data enable the nurse to identify important concerns of the patient and family, diagnose, and intervene accordingly. The process is then tailored to the particular patient, family, and situation depending on levels of anxiety and fear and coping preferences. The teaching is structured and simultaneous yet flexible and individualized.

LITERATURE REVIEW: GENERAL AND RESEARCH

As early as 1941, nurses were challenged to participate in preoperative instruction of surgical patients, especially the stir-up routine (turning, deep breathing, coughing, and leg exercises (Dripps and Walters 1941). Over the years, preoperative teaching by nurses has become routine, although the challenges posed are no less now than 50 years ago. The complexity of surgery is compounded by such factors as the increasing rises in hospital costs, the concern for cost containment, and the impact of diagnostic related groups (DRGs) on length of hospitalization stays. The delivery time for preoperative teaching has decreased. Some patients are admitted to the hospital the day of surgery; some are admitted on the evening before surgery; some have surgery as an outpatient. Some outpatients and inpatients have general anesthetics, and some do not. Some outpatients are admitted to the hospital after outpatient surgery. Some patients, outpatient and inpatient, who received a general anesthetic may be discharged the day of surgery.

Presurgical patients and family members bring unique characteristics, experiences, and coping preferences to this complex event. Consequently, they appraise the situation differently. Some are threatened; others consider the experience to be a challenge. The same surgical event may be viewed as stressful by one patient but not by another. Some patients are highly anxious, and others are moderately so. Although the patient interprets the event as stressful, family members or significant others may not.

According to Cohen and Lazarus (1983), cognitive appraisals play a major role in determining the effect of stressful events. The ways that patients and families appraise impending surgery affect the stressful impact of the situation, their emotional, physiological, and behavioral reactions, and how they cope. The person's appraisal sets a value on or judges the quality of something. Stress occurs when there is a mismatch between demands and coping resources (Lazarus 1981; Lazarus, Averill, and Opton 1970; Lazarus and Launier 1978).

Coping is the person's behavioral and cognitive efforts to deal with demands and the conflicts between the two (Coyne and Holyroyd 1982). A person determines the effect of a stressful situation by making two cognitive appraisals: primary, where the person judges whether the event is irrelevant, benign or positive, or stressful, and secondary, where the person looks at the situation, determines what he or she can do about it, and matches coping resources and options with the demands of the situation.

Appraisals change continually in response to feedback from the person's thoughts, feelings, and actions and from the situation. Situations judged as irrelevant are considered to have no implications for one's well-being. In situations judged as benign-positive, the event is positive. Situations judged as stressful indicate the demands exceed the person's resources.

There are three types of stress appraisal: harm-loss, threat, and challenge. Harm-loss events are real or anticipated losses of something of important significance. Threatening events refer to situations where there is a possibility of future harm. Events considered to be a challenge occur when the person judges the situation as one that not only demands more than routine resources but also provides an opportunity to overcome a difficulty and to achieve growth and mastery.

Examples of harm-loss and threatening events that people frequently associate with surgical situations include a threat to life itself; concern about loss of important body parts and functions in relation to valued family, sex, and occupational roles; anticipation of pain after surgery; uncertainty in knowing what to expect; loss of control under anesthesia; not being told the truth about the diagnosis; being hospitalized in a large university hospital; and inconsistent and unstructured situations (Auerbach 1973; Baudry and Weiner 1968; Carnevali 1966; Caty, Ellerton, and Ritchie 1984; Cohen and Lazarus 1973; Dumas and Leonard 1963; Graham and Conley 1971; Janis 1958; Johnson and Leventhal 1974; Johnson, Leventhal, and Dabs 1971; Kimball 1969; Lucente and Fleck 1972; Minckley 1974; Speilberger, Wadsworth, Auerbach, Dunn, and Taulbee 1973; Wolfer and Davis 1970; Wu 1973).

Situational and personal factors may change the appraisal of severity of threat-harm appraisals. Factors that contribute to stressful appraisals include emotions associated with the event, such as, anxiety or fear; uncertainty resulting from a lack of accurate information to deal with all aspects of the situation; personal traits that are concerned with the ability to deal with ambiguity; mental abilities; past experiences and education; age; sex; cultural and religious practices; and evaluation of meaning.

Preoperative patients experience varying levels of anxiety and fear. When the perceived threat outbalances the person's perceived resources, increased anxiety results, and the person usually wishes to reduce it. The severity of anxiety and fear sometimes also depends on family members' appraisal of how harmful or threatening the surgery is and what can be done about it. Research findings support the notion that family members and significant others, primarily adults, are very influential in either facilitating or hindering the patient's efforts to take control of uncertain impending events such as surgery (Aradine, Unon, and Shapiro 1978; Dziurbejko and Larkin 1978; Hymovich 1978; Klein, Dean, and Bogdonoff 1968; Litman 1974; McCubbin and Patterson 1982; Melamed and Bush 1985; Minuchin 1974; Mishel 1983; Olson, McCubbin, Barnes, Larsen, Muxen, and Wilson 1983; Silva 1979; Turk and Kerns 1985; Wolfer and Visintainer 1975).

Anxiety is described as a vague, uneasy feeling whose source is often nonspecific or unknown to the person. Fear is a feeling of dread related to an identifiable source that the person validates. Anxiety refers to both a response to a particular situation (state anxiety) and the differences among people when interpreting situations as being threatening (trait anxiety). People who have more than usual trait anxiety also have unusually intense state anxiety in response to stressors, particularly to psychological rather than physical threat (Lamb 1978; Spielberger 1972). The feeling of anxiety is more closely associated with uncertainty than is the feeling of fear. Anxiety is accompanied by well-defined bodily changes, manifested by an increased heart rate and galvanic skin response (clammy hands), muscular tension, especially in the neck muscles, and behavioral manifestations.

The primacy of uncertainty in causes of anxiety was demonstrated by Epstein and Clarke (1970) where people who were told that they had a 5% chance of receiving an electric shock had a higher heart rate and galvanic skin response than people who were told they had a 95% chance.

Janis's (1977) classic study of patients described three levels of anticipatory fear: high, moderate, and low. Surgical patients with high anticipatory fear and with low anticipatory fear have poorer postoperative outcomes than patients with moderate anticipatory fear.

Patients with high anticipatory fear had a history of episodes of anxiety attacks in stressful situations and openly expressed fear preoperatively. They were described as being very verbal in expressing their fear of dying. They admitted their excessive feelings of vulnerability and wanted to delay surgery. They were unable to focus on information. They were described as being constant talkers, directing attention away from surgery-related topics. Some patients had crying or emotional outbursts. They were unable to maintain eye contact or sit still.

Patients with low anticipatory fear appeared most calm and most confident preoperatively, minimizing the possibility of danger and pain. They were described as being outwardly and, surprisingly, cheerful and optimistic about the surgery. They usually indicated they were not worried and appeared to be invulnerable. Most of the patients who showed little or no fear had no previous history of anxiety or panic attacks.

Patients with a moderate amount of anticipatory fear were somewhat fearful before surgery and rehearsed unpleasant occurrences they believed were in store. They sought and evaluated information about activities they would experience from the initial preoperative period through awakening from the anesthetic to the time of discharge. They were responsive to authoritative reassurances from hospital staff but could also reassure themselves when their fears were greatly aroused. They were described as being willing to recognize the reality of the events to be faced and prepared accordingly. They displayed occasional and obvious concern about the surgical procedure, asking questions about specific features of the operation, such as the effects of anesthesia. Their attention span was reasonable but short. They were able to process information.

Janis (1977) calls the psychological process of preparing for an impending event the "work of worrying" (p. 279). He postulates that when a person allows the work of worrying to happen — that is, the person does not avoid anxiety, particularly by denial — the stress associated with the event can be avoided. In order for the work of worrying to be complete, each source of stress must be anticipated and worked through in advance. He proposes that patients with low anticipatory fear have not done the work of worrying. They are not provided with explicit warning information that induces them to face up to what to expect. The patient's failure to worry about the surgery in advance precipitates intense feelings of helplessness postoperatively, as well as resentment toward hospital staff who could no longer be counted on to provide good care.

Providing accurate information in advance of an impending stressful event influences the patient's sense of personal control and coping preferences when dealing with the event. Preparation reduces stress because the patient knows what to expect. Providing specific information, accurately and consistently, which helps to perform common tasks experienced before and after surgery, decreases negative expectations or misconceptions and promotes a sense of control (Abramson, Garber, and Seligman 1980; Auerbach, Martelli, and Mercuri 1983; Bandura 1977; DeCharms 1968; Degner and Russell 1988; Dennis 1990; Fuller, Endress, and Johnson 1978; Glass and Singer 1972; Johnson and Leventhal 1974; Padilla, Grant, Rains, Hansen, Bergstrom, Wong, Hanson, and Kubo 1981).

In the initial steps of the advance preparation, important concerns of the patient and family members should be attended to first since anxiety generated from the concerns may interfere with the patient's ability to process other information needed to feel in control. There are two central points of view as to how control reduces stress: self-regulation, where the patient allows for actual control, reinforces positively, and sometimes decreases the effects of threatening stimuli (Averill 1973; Kanfer and Seider 1973; Seligman 1975); and an increased sense of control in the face of uncertain impending events, leading to increased predictability of what to expect, which reduces stress (Ball and Volger 1971; Klemp and Rodin 1976; Langer 1975).

There are two types of personal control: actual and perceived (Baron and Rodin 1979). Personal control acts as a moderator between the patient's responses and stressful events. The major assumption is that the person is responsible for the outcomes attained through personal efforts. In actual control, the patient is able to influence expected outcomes through selective responding. In perceived control, the patient expects to participate in decision making in order to obtain positive outcomes. With perceived control, the patient has a sense of feeling free to make choices and of being aware of opportunities to select preferred goals and ways to meet the goals and a belief that outcomes or consequences are controlled and influenced by one's own personal actions or capabilities (Bowers 1968; Houston 1972; Pervin 1963; Pranulis, Dabbs, and Johnson 1975; Staub, Tursky, and Schwartz 1971). Individuals who are flexible in their choice of cognitive strategies when dealing with stressful situations can be expected to do better than those who are not (Miller 1990).

Since 1941 an impressive body of accumulated knowledge and research has provided empirical evidence that surgical patients do better when Structured Preoperative Teaching is provided (Archuleta, Plumer, and Hopkins 1977; Carrieri 1975; CURN Project 1981–1982; Egbert, Battit, Welch, and Bartlett 1964; Healy 1968; Hill 1982; Johnson 1975; Johnson, Fuller, Endress, and Rice 1978; Johnson, Rice, Fuller, and Endress 1978; King and Tarsitano 1982; La-Montagne, 1987; Lindeman and Van Aernam 1971; Lindeman and Stetzer 1973; Rice and Johnson 1984; Risser, Strong, and Bither 1980; Schmitt and Wooldridge 1973; Ziemer 1983). However, the evidence provided no precise direction to nurses when planning preoperative teaching programs. In addition, the linkage between the effect of preoperative teaching on positive patient outcomes was tentative.

This uncertainty prompted researchers to examine intervention studies using a series of meta-analytic techniques to determine the effect of nursing activities on patient outcomes. (For further discussion of the analyses, see Devine and Cook, 1983, 1986; Hathaway 1986; Heater, Becker, and Olson 1988; Mumford, Schlesinger, and Glass 1982). Their findings affirmed that preoperative teaching is beneficial. The results indicate that when Structured Preoperative Teaching was provided in consideration of anxiety and fear levels, as compared to routine standard nursing care, positive patient outcomes with associated cost benefits can be expected, including a decrease in length of hospital stay, medical complications, medications used for pain, anxiety, and nausea, and time lost from productive activities after discharge. Better outcomes could be expected when procedural aspects of care were provided for patients with low levels of fear and anxiety and psychological content was the focus of instruction for patients with high levels of anxiety and fear. By balancing the focus of the educational activities with levels of anxiety and fear, the nurse is more likely to influence and inform the patient and family.

INTERVENTION TOOLS

Several teaching tools used in research interventions have been modified for use in hospital situations, including sensory information (Johnson, Rice, Fuller, and Endress 1978) and the stir-up routine of deep breathing, coughing, and leg exercises (Lindeman and Van Aernam 1971). Materials prepared for one setting, however, need to be validated for use in another. Tools with physiological and behavioral indicators for guiding the nurse's assessment of anxiety and fear levels and subsequent intervention activities are not as numerous. Teaching plans used in preoperative teaching programs by nurse educators in hospitals consist of standardized content about the operation and procedures.

The content usually begins with a statement of purpose, which describes to the patient and family what the information is about and its importance in managing both preoperative and recovery situations. A brief summary reinforcing the purpose is given at the end of each presentation. The information is provided in short time frames and presented in a language understandable by the patient and family. To present a more graphic and accurate picture of what can be expected, teaching aids must agree with verbal instructions provided by the nurse and other authoritative figures, such as surgeons and anesthesiologists. The presence of a nurse during audiovisual presentations, including television, is essential for adjusting the focus of the intervention and personalizing standardized instructions. A programmed instruction by Basic Systems (1965) is recommended for use by nurses when planning activities to help the patient cope with preoperative anxiety and fear. The program instructs about (1) recognition of how anxiety develops, the emotional, mental, and physiological effects that occur, the behavior evoked, and anxiety levels and (2) intervention steps where the nurse helps the patient to recognize the anxiety, gain insight into it, and cope with the threat behind it (pp. 130–152).

ASSOCIATED NURSING DIAGNOSES AND CLIENT GROUPS

Presurgical patients admitted for elective surgery and their families or significant others, especially spouses and parents, were the primary focus of preoperative intervention studies. Nursing diagnoses associated with presurgical patients and families for which Structured Preoperative Teaching might be applied include Knowledge Deficit (Specify); Anxiety; Fear; Ineffective Individual Coping; Ineffective Family Coping; and Potential Activity Intolerance.

Protocol for Preoperative Teaching Intervention
of Hospitalized Adults Having Elective Surgery under a General Anesthetic

Step 1. Obtain list of patients to be taught.
Step 2. Obtain the following information before seeing patient.
* Name of Patient_____ DRG #_____
* Name of significant other_____ Phone #_____
* Surgical procedure_____ Operation time_____
* Consent form signed a. Yes _____ b. No _____
* Surgeon_____ Anesthesiologist/Anesthetist_____
* Type of general anesthetic_____
* Preoperative medications a. _____ b. _____
* Immediate preoperative medications a. _____ b. _____
* Risk Classification I _____ II _____ III _____ IV _____
* Previous surgery a. _____ b. _____ c. _____
* Chronic illness a. _____ b. _____
* Occupation _____
* Sex of patient a. Male_____ b. Female_____
* Marital status a. Married _____ b. Widowed _____ c. Divorced _____
        d. Separated _____ e. Never married _____
* Major roles held by patient: a. Breadwinner _____ b. Housekeeper _____
        c. Child care _____ d. Disciplinarian _____
        e. Bill payer _____
* Person taking over roles until patient recovers: a. Spouse _____ b. Relative _____
    c. Friend _____ d. Neighbor _____ e. Other _____
* Adolescents: a. Yes _____ b. No _____
        If yes, living at home? a. Yes _____ b. No _____
* Other children: a. Yes _____ b. No _____
        If yes, living at home? a. Yes _____ b. No _____
* Primary language _____
* Education: a. No formal schooling _____ d. 1 year of college _____
        b. Grade school only _____ e. 2 years of college _____
        c. High school _____ f. 3 years of college _____
        g. 4 years of college _____
Step 3. Proceed to patient's room and establish rapport with the patient and family members (significant others):
* Greet them by name.
* Talk at the patient's level of understanding.
* Speak clearly and distinctly.
* Introduce yourself with your title.
* Explain what you will be doing.
Obtain from patient and family any information not obtained in step 1.
Step 4. Ask patient about:
* What the surgeon has told him or her about the operation.
* What the admission nurse has told him or her about the operation.
* Summarize and clarify information as indicated.

Step 5. Ask patient and family (significant other) about important concerns.
* Validate diagnoses accordingly.
* Intervene where indicated.

Step 6. Provide patient and family (significant other) with teaching booklet about the stir-up routine.

Step 7. Check emotional and behavioral responses of both patient and family (significant other).
* If anxiety level low (normal), proceed to steps 8–12
* If anxiety level moderate, proceed to step 24.
* If anxiety level high, proceed to step 25.

Step 8. Set up slide-tape on deep breathing, coughing, and leg exercises and have the patient and family (significant other) view it. Tell the patient that performing deep breathing, coughing, and leg exercises will benefit him or her in recovery from the operation. The presentation takes about 10 minutes. If the patient will not be doing the complete set of exercises postoperatively, remove those slides from the slide tray.

Step 9. Demonstrate deep breathing.

Step 10. Have patient return demonstration on deep breathing:
* By placing one hand on the abdomen (umbilical area) to exert counterpressure during inhalation and using the other hand to support the area where the incision will be.
* By expanding the abdomen and rib cage on inspiration.
* By inspiring through the nose or mouth.
* By inspiring and expiring slowly, deliberately, and deeply.
* Expiring immediately after inspiration.
* By repeating the exercise three times.

Step 11. Demonstrate coughing.

Step 12. Have patient return demonstration on coughing:
* By coughing immediately after inspiration is completed.
* By coughing three or four times on expiration. The sequence is to inhale, cough, cough, cough.
* By repeating the exercise.

Step 13. Check emotional and behavioral responses. Identify patient's anxiety level:
* If patient's anxiety low (normal), go to step 14.
* If patient's anxiety moderate, go to step 24.
* If anxiety high, go to step 25.

Step 14. Explain leg and foot exercises.

Step 15. Instruct patient to return demonstration in bed:
* With heels on bed, push the toes of both feet toward the foot of the bed until the calf muscles of the leg tighten. Relax both feet. Pull toes toward the chin, until calf muscles tighten. Relax feet.
* With heels on bed, circle both ankles, first to the right and then to the left. Repeat three times. Relax.
* Bend each knee alternately, sliding foot up along the bed. Relax.

Step 16. Record on preoperative checklist the patient's ability to perform deep breathing, coughing, and leg exercises.

Step 17. Summarize, briefly repeating the purpose emphasizing that three exercises—deep breathing, coughing, and leg exercises—will help after surgery. Indicate that nurses will assist postoperatively, but it is important that the patient do them as well as he or she can.

Step 18. Encourage patient to practice deep breathing, coughing, and leg exercises, using the teaching booklet. Indicate that you will return in an hour.

Step 19. In 1 hour, return to patient's room. Check on anxiety level.
* If there is no change, go to step 20.
* If increased to moderate anxiety, go to step 24.
* If increased to high anxiety, go to step 25.

Step 20. Evaluate patient's ability to cough, deep breathe, and do leg exercises. Record on the preoperative checklist.

Step 21. If indicated by anxiety levels and allowed by time frame, continue with providing procedural information. Plan for short sessions. Check anxiety level before, during, and after delivery of content. Continue with instruction as indicated. Explain about:
* Chaplain services
* Preoperative medications
* Tubings and equipment associated with the specific surgical procedure, providing sensory information and using visual aids as needed.
* Early ambulation
* Surgical preparation, enema, douche

Step 22. At end of each brief session, ask the patient to verbalize what was taught.

Step 23. Record what has been taught, the results of the patient's return demonstrations, and the patient's ability to verbalize what was taught.

Step 24. In moderate anxiety the nurse:
* First helps the patient recognize that he or she is anxious by exploring his or her feelings.
* Assists the patient in gaining insight into the anxiety by helping him or her to see the reason for the behavior (anxiety) and for the anxiety (the threat).
* Assists the patient in coping with the threat behind the anxiety by helping the patient to reappraise the threat and to learn new ways of dealing with it.
* Provide essential procedural information.
* Consult with surgeon.
* Record behavior, type of intervention provided and results, and that surgeon was notified.

Step 25. For patients with high anxiety:
* Stay with patient.
* Decrease sensory stimulation.
* Speak slowly and calmly.
* Limit contact with others.
* Consult with surgeon.
* Record behavior manifestations, type of intervention provided, and that surgeon was contacted.

Step 26. Focus on family members (or significant others designated by patient).
* Intervene in anxiety levels, as indicated in steps 25 and 26.
* Repeat all information if necessary.
* Validate diagnoses and intervene accordingly.

CASE STUDY

This case study depicts a patient who has been hospitalized for an elective cholecystectomy. The behavior manifested by the patient is characterized by low (normal) anxiety.

Mr. and Mrs. M's first contact with the preoperative teaching nurse was in Mrs. M's room on the day of admission in the afternoon before the day Mrs. M was scheduled for an elective cholecystectomy. The nurse began the contact by greeting the patient and spouse by their names. She introduced herself and told them that she would be providing them with information about procedures so that they would know what to expect before and after surgery. She also would be showing them how to deep breath, cough, and do leg exercises because these exercises would help Mrs. M recover from the operation.

Before she began the teaching session, the nurse asked if they had any concerns. The nurse already knew that Mrs. M worked part time as an elementary school teacher and that Mr. M was the chief engineer in a consulting firm of engineers. They had three children. Two were living at home: a son, age 14, and a daughter, age 16. One daughter, age 20, was away at college. Although Mrs. M's intolerance of fatty and deep-fried foods increased over the past few months, causing brief episodes of pain and discomfort, except for the birth of her children, this admission to the hospital was her first.

Mrs. M mentioned that she was somewhat afraid and did not know much about hospitals. She was especially concerned about undergoing an anesthetic but jokingly stated that she would rather be asleep than awake during the procedure. She indicated that Mr. M had had a herniorrhaphy two years ago under an anesthetic and recovered well with no complications. None of the children had ever been hospitalized. With a smile, Mrs. M stated that she hoped she would not be in long because the house would be in a mess when she returns home. She was always picking up after her teenagers. No one would eat right either because she was not there to cook. Touching her hand, Mr. M reassured her that although "things would not be the same right now," he would see to it that the house was kept in order. He emphasized that although they would miss her gourmet cooking, she must first take care of herself and "get well fast." The nurse asked Mrs. M about her teaching activities. Mrs. M said that she did not substitute often, so that was no problem, although she would miss the extra money. She admitted concern about whether the incision would inhibit any of her household duties or teaching activities. Also, she was worried about incisional pain and had discussed it with her doctor. The nurse inquired about what the doctor had told her about pain. Mrs. M said, "He told me that I could expect it, but he didn't tell me what I could do about it. I guess I can deal with it okay." The nurse explained to Mrs. M that when she had pain, she should request pain medication. Also, moving about as soon as possible would be helpful in controlling pain. Mrs. M changed the subject and inquired about visiting hours, chaplain visits, a telephone, and the specific time she would be going to surgery.

After about one-half hour of discussion, Mrs. M had displayed normal concerns about the upcoming surgery. Her attention span was reasonable but short. She was able to conduct a conversation with her husband and a nurse she had met for the first time. The nurse then provided Mr. and Mrs. M with a teaching booklet on the stir-up routine, which was standardized for this particular hospital. The nurse carefully provided information to Mrs. M and also to Mr. M, who was also present, about deep breathing, coughing, and leg exercises using slide-tape media. She emphasized that performing deep breathing, coughing, and leg exercises help recovery from the operation. Mrs. M, with some coaching from Mr. M, correctly returned the demonstration immediately after the slide-tape presentation and after the demonstration by the nurse. She was able to do so again 1 hour later under the same nurse's supervision, indicating that Mrs. M was able to process the information. The nurse ended the session by stressing the importance of Mrs. M's participation in ambulation, deep breathing, coughing, and leg exercises for recovery from the operation. The nurse asked Mr. M if he had any questions. She told him that she would return in the morning before surgery to see Mrs. M and would talk to him again.

REFERENCES

Abramson, L.Y., Garber, J., and Seligman, M.E.P. 1980. Learned helplessness in humans: An attributional analysis. In J. Garber and M.E.P. Seligman (eds.), *Human helplessness: Theory and applications* (pp. 3–34). New York: Academic Press.

Aradine, C., Unon, H., and Shapiro, V. 1978. The infant with long term tracheostomy and the parents: A collaborative treatment. *Issues in Comprehensive Pediatric Nursing* 3:29–41.

Archuleta, V., Plumer, O.B., and Hopkins, K.D. 1977. A demonstration model or patient education: A model for the project "training nurses to improve patient education." Boulder, Colo.: Western Interstate Commission for Higher Education.

Auerbach, S.M. 1973. Trait-state anxiety and adjustment to surgery. *Journal of Consulting and Clinical Psychology* 40.

Auerbach, S.M., Martelli, M.F., and Mercuri, L.S. 1983. Anxiety, information, interpersonal impacts, and adjustment to a stressful health care situation. *Journal of Personality and Social Psychology* 44:1284–1296.

Averill, J.R. 1973. Personal control over aversive stimuli and its relationship to stress. *Psychological Bulletin* 80:286–303.

Ball, T.S., and Volger, R.E. 1971. Uncertain pain and the pain of uncertainty. *Perceptual and Motor Skills* 33:1195–1203.

Bandura, A. 1977. *Social learning theory.* Englewood Cliffs, N.J.: Prentice-Hall.

Baron, R., and Rodin, J. 1979. Perceived control and crowding stress. In A. Baum, J. Singer, and S. Valins (eds.), *Advances in environmental psychology.* Hillsdale, N.J.: Erlbaum.

Basic Systems, Inc. 1965. Anxiety: Recognition and intervention: A programmed instruction. *American Journal of Nursing* 65:129–152.

Baudry, F., and Weiner, A. 1968. The family of the surgical patient. *Surgery* 63:416–422.

Bowers, K.G. 1968. Pain, anxiety, and perceived control. *Journal of Consulting and Clinical Psychology* 32:596–602.

Brett, J.L. 1987. Use of nursing practice findings. *Nursing Research* 36(6):344–349.

Carnevali, D.L. 1966. Preoperative anxiety. *American Journal of Nursing* 7:1536–1538.

Carrieri, V. 1975. Effect of an experimental teaching program on postoperative ventilatory capacity. In M. Batey (ed.), *Communicating nursing research: Critical issues in access to data* (pp. 121–141). Boulder, Colo.: Western State Commission for Higher Education.

Caty, S., Ellerton, M.L., and Ritchie, J.A. 1984. Coping in hospitalized children: An analysis of published case studies. *Nursing Research* 33:277–282.

Cohen, F., and Lazarus, R.S. 1973. Active coping processes, coping dispositions, and recovery from surgery. *Psychosomatic Medicine* 35:375–389.

Cohen, F., and Lazarus, R.S. 1983. Coping and adaptation in health and illness. In D. Mechanic (ed.), *Handbook of health care and the health professions* (pp. 608–635). New York: Free Press.

Conduct and Utilization of Research in Nursing (CURN) Project. 1981–1982. *Using research to improve nursing practice.* New York: Grune and Stratton.

Coyne, J.C., and Holroyd, K. 1982. Stress, coping, and illness: A transactional perspective. In T. Mill, C. Green, and R. Meagher (eds.), *Handbook of clinical health psychology.* New York: Plenum Press.

DeCharms, R. 1968. *Personal causation: The internal affective determinants of behavior.* New York: Academic Press.

Degner, L.F., and Russell, C.A. 1988. Preferences for treatment control among adults with cancer. *Research in Nursing and Health* 11:367–374.

Dennis, K.E. 1990. Patients' control and the information imperative: Clarification and confirmation. *Nursing Research* 39:162–166.

Devine, E.C., and Cook, T.D. 1983. A meta-analytic analysis of the effects of psychoeducational interventions on length of postsurgical hospital stay. *Nursing Research* 32:267–274.

Devine, E.C. and Cook, T.D. 1986. Clinical and cost-saving effects of psychoeducational interventions with surgical patients: A meta-analysis. *Research in Nursing and Health* 9:89–105.

Dripps, R.D., and Walters, R.M. 1941. Nursing care of patients: The "stir up routine." *American Journal of Nursing* 41:530–534.

Dumas, R., and Leonard, R.J. 1963. Effect of nursing on the incidence of post-operative vomiting: A clinical experience. *Nursing Research* 12:12–15.

Dziurbejko, M., and Larkin, J. 1978. Including the family in preoperative teaching. *American Journal of Nursing* 78:1892–1894.

Egbert, L.D., Battit, G.E., Welch, C.E., and Bartlett, K.M. 1964. Reduction of postoperative pain by encouragement and instruction of patients. *New England Journal of Medicine* 270:825–827.

Epstein, S., and Clarke, S. 1970. Heart rate and skin conductance during experimentally induced anxiety: Effects of anticipated intensity of noxious stimulation and experience. *Journal of Experimental Psychology* 84:105–112.

Fuller, S.S., Endress, M.P., and Johnson, J.E. 1978. Effects of cognitive and behavioral control on coping with an aversive health examination. *Journal of Human Stress* 4:18–25.

Glass, D.C., and Singer, J.E. 1972. Behavioral after effects of unpredictable and uncontrollable aversive events. *American Scientist* 60:457–465.

Graham, L., and Conley, E. 1971. Evaluation of anxiety and fear in adult surgical patients. *Nursing Research* 20:113–122.

Hathaway, D. 1986. Effect of preoperative instruction on postoperative outcomes. A meta-analysis. *Nursing Research* 35(5):269–275.

Healy, K.M. 1968. Does preoperative instruction make a difference? *American Journal of Nursing* 68:62–67.

Heater, B.S., Becker, A.M., and Olson, R.K. 1988. Nursing interventions and patient outcomes: A meta-analysis of studies. *Nursing Research* 37(5):303–307.

Hill, B. 1982. Sensory information, behavioral instructions and coping with sensory alteration surgery. *Nursing Research* 31:17–21.

Houston, B.K. 1972. Control over stress, locus of control, and response to stress. *Journal of Personality and Social Psychology* 21:249–255.

Hymovich, D. 1978. Incorporating the family into care. *Journal of New York State Nurses Association* 5:9–14.

Janis, I.L. 1958. *Psychological stress: Psychoanalytic and behavioral studies of surgical patients.* New York: Wiley.

Janis, I.L. 1977. Adaptive personality changes. In A. Monat and R. Lazarus (eds.), *Stress and coping: An anthology* (pp. 272–284). New York: Columbia University Press.

Johnson, J.E. 1975. Stress reduction through sensation information. In I.G. Sarason and C.D. Spielberger (eds.), *Stress and anxiety.* New York: Halsted Press.

Johnson, J.E., Fuller, S., Endress, M., and Rice, V. 1978. Altering patients' responses to surgery: An extension and replication. *Research in Nursing and Health* 1:11–21.

Johnson, J.E., and Leventhal, H. 1974. Effects of accurate expectations and behavioral instructions on reactions during a noxious medical examination. *Journal of Personality and Social Psychology* 29:710–718.

Johnson, J.E., Leventhal, H., and Dabbs, J. 1971. Contribution of emotional and instrumental response processes in adaptation to surgery. *Journal of Personality and Social Psychology* 20:55–64.

Johnson, J.E., Rice, V., Fuller, S., and Endress, M. 1978. Sensory information, instructions in a coping strategy, and recovery from surgery. *Research in Nursing and Health* 1:4–17.

Kanfer, F., and Seider, M.L. 1973. Self-control: Factors enhancing tolerance of noxious stimulation. *Journal of Personality and Social Psychology* 25:381–389.

Kimball, C.P. 1969. Psychological responses to the experience of open-heart surgery. *American Journal of Psychiatry* 126:348–359.

King, I.M., and Tarsitano, B.J. 1982. The effect of structured and unstructured preoperative teaching: A replication. *Nursing Research* 31(6):324–329.

Klein, R., Dean, A., and Bogdonoff, M. 1968. The impact upon the spouse. *Journal of Chronic Disability* 20:241–250.

Klemp, G.O., and Rodin, J. 1976. Effects of uncertainty, delay, and focus of attention on reactions to an aversive situation. *Journal of Experimental Social Psychology* 12:416–421.

Lamb, D. 1978. Anxiety. In H. London and J. Exner (eds.), *Dimensions of personality*. New York: Academic Press.

LaMontagne, L. 1987. Children's preoperative coping: Replication and extension. *Nursing Research* 36(3):163–167.

Langer, E.J. 1975. The illusion of control. *Journal of Personality and Social Psychology* 32:311–328.

Lazarus, R.S. 1981. The stress and coping paradigm. In C. Eisdorfer, D. Cohen, and A. Kleinman (eds.), *Theoretical bases for psychopathology* (pp. 28–74). New York: Spectrum.

Lazarus, R.S., Averill, J.R., and Opton, E.M. Jr. 1970. Toward a cognitive theory of emotions. In M. Arnold (ed.), *Feelings and emotions* (pp. 207–232). New York: Academic Press.

Lazarus, R.S., and Launier, R. 1978. Stress-related transactions between person and environment. In L.A. Pervin and M. Lewis (eds.), *Perspectives in interactional psychology* (pp. 287–327). New York: Plenum Press.

Lindeman, C.A., and Stetzer, S.L. 1973. Effect of preoperative visits by operating room nurses. *Nursing Research* 22:4–16.

Lindeman, C.A., and Van Aerman, B. 1971. Nursing intervention with the presurgical patient: The effects of structured and preoperative teaching, *Nursing Research* 20:319–332.

Litman, T. 1974. The family as a basic unit in health and medical care: A social behavioral overview. *Social Science and Medicine* 8:495–519.

Lucente, F.E., and Fleck, S. 1972. A study of hospitalization in 408 medical and surgical patients. *Psychosomatic Medicine* 34:302–312.

McCubbin, H., and Patterson, J. 1982. Family adaptation of crises. In H.M. McCubbin, A. Cauble, and J. Patterson (eds.), *Family stress, coping and social support*. Springfield, Ill.: Charles C. Thomas.

Melamed, B.G., and Bush, J.B. 1985. Family factors in children with acute illness. In D.C. Turk and R.D. Kerns (eds.), *Health, illness, and families*. New York: Wiley.

Miller, S.M. 1990. To see or not to see: Cognitive informational styles in the coping process. In M. Rosenbaum (ed.), *Learned resourcefulness: On coping skills, self-control, and adaptive behavior* (pp. 95–126). New York: Springer.

Minckley, B. 1974. Physiologic and psychologic responses of elective surgical patients. *Nursing Research* 23:392–401.

Minuchin, S. 1974. *Families and family therapy*. Cambridge: Harvard University Press.

Mishel, M. 1983. Parents' perception of uncertainty concerning their hospitalized child. *Nursing Research* 32:324–329.

Mumford, F., Schlesinger, H., and Glass, G. 1982. The effects of psychological intervention on recovery from surgery and heart attacks: An analysis of the literature. *American Journal of Public Health* 72:141–151.

Olson, D., McCubbin, H., Barnes, H., Larsen, A., Muxen, M., and Wilson, M. 1983. *Families—What makes them work*. Beverly Hills, Calif.: Sage.

Padilla, G., Grant, M., Rains, B., Hansen, B., Bergstrom, N., Wong, H., Hanson, R., and Kubo, W. 1981. Distress reduction and the effects of preparatory teaching films and patient control. *Research in Nursing and Health* 4:375–387.

Pervin, L.A. 1963. The need to control under conditions of threat. *Journal of Personality* 34:570–587.

Pranulis, M., Dabbs, J., and Johnson, J. 1975. General anesthesia and the patient's attempts at control. *Social behavior and personality* 3:49–54.

Rice, V.H., and Johnson, J.E. 1984. Preadmission self-instruction booklets, postadmission exercise performance, and teaching time. *Nursing Research* 33:147–151.

Risser, N.L., Strong, A., and Bither, S. 1980. The effect of an experimental teaching program on postoperative ventilatory function: A self-critique. *Western Journal of Nursing Research* 2:484–500.

Schmitt, F.E., and Wooldridge, P.J. 1970. Reduction of anxiety in presurgical patients. *Nursing Research* 22:108–116.

Seligman, M.E. 1975. *Helplessness*. San Francisco: W.H. Freeman.

Silva, M. 1979. Effects of orientation information on spouses' anxieties and attitudes toward hospitalization and surgery. *Research in Nursing and Health* 2:127–136.

Spielberger, C.D. 1972. Anxiety as an emotional state. In C.D. Spielberger (ed.), *Anxiety: Current trends in theory and research* (vol. 1). New York: Academic Press.

Spielberger, C.D., Wadsworth, A.P., Auerbach, S.M., Dunn, T.M., and Taulbee, E.S. 1973. Emotional reactions to surgery. *Journal of Consulting and Clinical Psychology* 40:33–38.

Staub, E., Tursky, B., and Schwartz, G.E. 1971. Self-control and predictability: Their effects on reactions to aversive stimulations. *Journal of Personality and Social Psychology* 18:1157–1162.

Turk, D.C., and Kerns, R.D. (eds.) 1985. *Health, illness, and families*. New York: Wiley.

Wolfer, J.A., and Davis, C.E. 1970. Assessment of surgery patients preoperative emotional conditions and postoperative welfare. *Nursing Research* 19:402–414.

Wolfer, J.A., and Visintainer, M.A. 1975. Pediatric surgical patients' and parents' stress responses and adjustment. *Nursing Research* 24(4):244–255.

Wu, R. 1973. *Behavior and illness*. Englewood Cliffs, N.J.: Prentice-Hall.

Ziemer, M.M. 1983. Effects of information on postsurgical coping. *Nursing Research* 32:282–287.

13

CRISIS INTERVENTION

ROBERT J. KUS

> Tony A, a 26-year-old medical student with one year to go before graduation, has just learned that he is HIV positive. His future has always seemed bright to him; now it appears to be nonexistent, and he is devastated. "I'm not sure that suicide wouldn't be better," he declares.
>
> Wilma S, a 40-year-old unskilled laborer and struggling single mother of three, has just learned that the company where she has been employed for the past six years is closing its plant. "I don't know what to do! Who'd buy my house? This is a one-company town! I just don't know where to turn!"
>
> Lance R, a 28-year-old gay high school teacher, is brought to the hospital emergency room. His blood alcohol level is dangerously high, and he has overdosed on "downers." "It's too much! I just can't seem to cope any more. I wish I were dead."

These three people are all faced with life situations for which they are unprepared. While all have led productive lives and until now have solved the usual problems that have come their way, all are experiencing psychological crises. How each story will end may depend on what help is available. In this chapter, Crisis Intervention, applicable in each of the examples cited, is explored. The discussion here focuses on Crisis Intervention with the individual client rather than with families or other groups.

DEFINITION AND DESCRIPTION

The Concept of Crisis

"A crisis is a state of psychological emergency rendering one's usually effective problem-solving skills useless or greatly diminished" (Kus 1985). Walkup (1974) offers a more elaborate definition. She uses the process or "serial operational" definition advocated by nursing theorist Hildegard Peplau. In so doing, she assumes the client to be a system. In this way, nursing can use Crisis Intervention to treat any type of client: an individual, family, social organization, or community. Crisis, in Walkup's view, is defined in this way:

1.　A change occurs to a system in a dynamic equilibrium.
2.　The system perceives the changes as a disruption of intersystem balance between internal needs and external demands.
3.　The system mobilizes its habitual problem-solving energies (internal resources) and desires situational support (external resources) to attempt to resolve the imbalance.

179

4.   The internal and external resources fail to resolve the problem.

5.   Feelings of helplessness and ineffectiveness result in behavior disorganization (Walkup 1974, pp. 152–153).

Types of Crises

Crises are classified on the basis of their origins. Some writers, such as Hoff (1978) and Riley (1980), classify crises as either maturational or situational. Others add a third type, called social crises by Haber (1982) and adventitious crises by Benter (1979).

Maturational or developmental crises are those that occur "in responses to stresses inherent in predictable life transitions and events" (Haber 1982, p. 309). Specific life span periods, such as childhood, adolescence, and old age, and major social role changes, such as marriage, menopause, and retirement, are examples. Usually maturational crises can be anticipated. Some crises that may be termed developmental can be unanticipated—for example, the process called coming out, which is unique to gay and lesbian individuals. Kus (1990) states that because gay and lesbian children do not usually recognize their sexual orientation until the teenaged years or later and because the early stages of the coming-out process are often fraught with a bewildering array of problems, unanticipated crises can occur.

Situational crises occur when "unanticipated events threaten a person's biological, social, or psychological integrity" (Haber 1982, p. 309)—for example, losing one's job, getting divorced, or losing a loved one. The social or adventitious crisis is a special type of situational crisis resulting from uncommon events that cause multiple losses or severe environmental changes (Haber 1982, p. 309)—for example, being in a fire, riot, or earthquake.

According to Frederick and Garrison (1981), there are usually five phases of human disaster response seen in the adventitious crisis:

1.   The *impact phase,* including the event itself, which is characterized by panic, shock, or extreme fear. The person's judgment and assessment of reality may become minimal, and self-destructive behavior may be seen.

2.   The *heroic phase,* in which friends, neighbors, and emergency teams rally to assist those devastated by the disaster. In this phase, constructive activity may help individuals block out the pain of their losses to some extent, but overactivity may result in burnout.

3.   The *honeymoon phase,* which begins 1 week to several months after the disaster. Life in the community begins anew as money and other forms of help are given to the disaster victims. Psychological and behavioral problems may be overlooked in this phase as those who suffered from the disaster continue to help their neighbors.

4.   The *disillusionment phase,* which lasts from about 2 months to about 1 year —often a time of disappointment, frustration, anger, and resentment as victims begin to compare their neighbors' plights with their own. Victims often manifest their negative feeling states by showing envy, resentment, and hostility toward their neighbors.

5.   The *reconstruction and reorganization phase,* when individuals devastated by the disaster learn to take control of their problems and begin to rebuild their homes, businesses, and lives in a constructive fashion. This phase may last several years.

Clinical Picture

According to Powell and Lively (1981), the individual in crisis often exhibits certain signs and symptoms. Both objective and subjective data are used to help the nurse in assessing the client in crisis.

Objective data include inefficient cognition and motor-behavioral responses. Cognitive responses often seen include decreased perceptual ability, narrowing of focus, thought disorganization, changed ability to solve problems, and decreased ability to perform adequately on the job and in decision making. Objective motor-behavioral responses can be seen in skeletal muscle tension, which includes jerky or rigid movement, restlessness, or constant movement of a body part, or in smooth muscle tension, such as urinary frequency, diarrhea, and vomiting.

Subjective data include alterations in affective and motor-behavioral responses. Among the affective responses are feelings of being overwhelmed by one's problem, helplessness, loss of control, anxiety, guilt, anger, and low self-esteem. Subjective motor-behavioral responses include nausea, insomnia or extreme fatigue and sleep, anorexia or overeating, gastrointestinal pains, headache, backache, neck pain, and chest pain.

Crisis Intervention

"Crisis intervention is the systematic application of problem-solving techniques, based on crisis theory, designed to help the client in crisis move through the crisis process as swiftly and painlessly as possible and thereby achieve at least the same level of psychological comfort as experienced before the crisis" (Kus 1985).

The minimal goal of Crisis Intervention is that the client will function as well after the crisis as before. His or her emotional equilibrium and coping capacity will be restored. Successful Crisis Intervention can also help the client grow beyond the precrisis coping level. During the Crisis Intervention process, the client may learn to focus more effectively on factors that lead to crisis, eliminate expendable life stresses, adopt healthier ways of living, recognize personal strengths and weaknesses, and gain ways of solving problems. Further, when the client's significant others become involved in assisting the client through the crisis, closer bonds may develop, thus lessening the likelihood of recurrent crises. Therefore, Crisis Intervention can also be seen as a form of primary or preventative mental health care, a future-oriented phenomenon.

According to Jacobson, Strickler, and Morley (1968), there are two main types of Crisis Intervention: generic and individual. The generic approach emphasizes the common pattern found in specific crisis events and focuses the interventions on these commonalities. The nurse does not focus on the individual psychodynamics. For example, Lindemann (1944) found that the grief process is composed of fairly predictable stages. Therefore, to help the person do grief work, the nurse need only know the dynamics of this specific type of crisis to be effective. Thus, doing Crisis Intervention with a widow is essentially the same as doing Crisis Intervention with a widower. This approach has the advantage of being practiced on a large scale by both professional and nonprofessional helpers. The disadvantage is that a nurse may be extremely knowledgeable and effective in one type of crisis pattern but ignorant and ineffective in other types of crises.

The individual approach focuses on the individual in crisis and the interpersonal and intrapsychic process of this person (Aquilera 1990, p. 22). This approach is useful when the generic approach fails to help the individual in crisis. Because it is more complex than the generic approach, it is limited to professionals knowledgeable in psychotherapy, such as psychiatrists, psychosocial clinical nurse specialists, psychiatric social workers, and psychologists.

From the nursing perspective, both approaches are valuable. In actual clinical nursing practice, perhaps the most common approach is a combination of the generic and individual approaches. Certainly nurses recognize many crisis patterns and act accordingly. On the other hand, nurses also focus on the uniqueness of the individual and his or her perception of reality, as well as on the host of intervening variables impinging on the client's life. In this chapter, a problem-solving approach to Crisis Intervention will be presented to help nurses assist the maximum number of clients in crisis. This approach is a blend of the generic and individual approaches but focuses more heavily on the generic approach.

A BACKGROUND OF CRISIS INTERVENTION

A Brief History

The two pioneers in the field of Crisis Intervention are Eric Lindemann and Gerald Caplan.

Lindemann formulated his ideas of Crisis Intervention by interviewing persons in bereavement. In his now-classic study (1944), he observed surviving friends and relatives of the hundreds of people killed in the 1943 Coconut Grove nightclub fire in Boston. He noted common patterns or stages in grieving but that some individuals went through the grieving process with relative ease while others had many more difficulties.

From his studies, Lindemann concluded that besides the loss of loved ones, other life crises, such as marriage, might also have predictable patterns. If a helper could intervene early in the crisis, the individual would stand a better chance of getting through the crisis in good mental health. In addition, he believed that mental health workers could intervene in life crises on a community level to help as many people as possible as opposed to the traditional method of intensive one-to-one psychotherapy. In 1946, he and Caplan established just such a Crisis Intervention program, called the Wellesley Project, in the Massachusetts area.

Caplan, in his *Principles of Preventative Psychiatry* (1964), advocated Crisis Intervention as a primary tool to prevent mental illness on a community-wide level. His work has been vitally important in its emphasis on preventative care mental health and on a cost-effective strategy to help the population with everyday life crises. In this work, Caplan noted that most often crises are self-limiting; usually they last from 4 weeks to 6 weeks. During the time of crisis, the individual is vulnerable. On the other hand, it is a time for the possibility of new growth. Much depends on whether the intervention occurs in time. Crisis Intervention is most effective when it occurs in the beginning of the process.

In 1961, a report issued by the Joint Commission on Mental Illness and Health advocated Crisis Intervention. The report showed that too often people in crisis were placed on long waiting lists rather than receiving the immediate help they needed. Following the commission's recommendations, the United States funded the establishment of community-based Crisis Intervention projects. Today, crisis clinics and crisis hot lines are found in even the smallest towns in America.

Benefits of Crisis Intervention

As a mental health strategy, Crisis Intervention is relatively noncontroversial. In fact, its popularity arises out of its many benefits.

First, Crisis Intervention is easy to teach and to learn. Besides health care professionals, Crisis Intervention can be and has been taught and effectively used by a wide range of people, such as bartenders, barbers and beauticians, taxi cab drivers, the police, chemical dependency counselors, clergy, and crisis hot-line workers.

Second, it is cost-effective. Not only does it eliminate costly and time-consuming psychotherapy but also, when used effectively, helps prevent crisis coping from becoming an entrenched life pattern, leading the individual to require hospitalization.

Third, Crisis Intervention can be applied in any setting. It is not limited to a therapist's office or a hospital ward.

Fourth, Crisis Intervention can help the individual in crisis learn new ways of coping with or preventing crisis events in the future.

Fifth, this intervention can save lives. A suicidal client who is assisted through the problem-solving process often finds alternatives to self-destruction and gains rekindled hope.

Sixth, because Crisis Intervention often involves the marshaling of a person's support system, frequently the bonds between the client in crisis and significant others are strengthened. The increased sharing, communication, and understanding can leave the client with a stronger support system after the crisis than existed before.

Finally, because Crisis Intervention is an intervention geared for all persons, it does not carry the same stigma as other forms of mental health therapy.

Guiding Principles

A nurse who is implementing Crisis Intervention should follow certain guiding principles, borrowed from and built on recommendations by Morley, Messick, and Aquilera (1967):

1.   Crisis Intervention is the treatment of choice for persons in crisis. Any idea that it is merely a "Band-Aid" type of strategy done to tide the client over until the "real" therapy can be had should be promptly discarded.

2.   Novices in Crisis Intervention should have adequate supervision by skilled crisis intervention therapists. Crisis Intervention is a clinical skill that requires training and practice, just as such traditional nursing skills, as catheterization or suctioning, do.

3.   The client in crisis should be viewed as a healthy person who is temporarily unable to cope effectively because of overwhelming life stresses. Crisis are normal events. Thus, Crisis Intervention is a form of psychosocial, not "psychiatric," nursing.

4.   Client assessment is more focused than in traditional nursing practice. Rather than delving into all the usual nursing history categories, the nurse focuses on the client's crisis problem and related information, such as support systems.

5.   Both nurse and client must realize that the treatment is sharply time limited and keep their energies focused on solving the crisis.

6,   The nurse deals only with the crisis issue. Extraneous material is not suitable in Crisis Intervention.

7.   The nurse is assertive in intervening. Because crises are self-limiting, time is very valuable.

8.   The nurse must be flexible, playing any role that will help the client—for example, becoming a resource person, consultant, teacher, or message bearer to loved ones.

9.   The goal of Crisis Intervention is always to help the client return to a level of coping that is at least as good as his or her precrisis level of coping.

10.   The nurse should never hesitate to ask for outside consultation if confronted with a crisis situation for which he or she is unprepared. For example, the nurse unfamiliar with the emotional stress associated with the coming-out process of gay people might consult a gay therapist or a therapist or agency knowledgeable about this process.

PROBLEM SOLVING

One of the greatest strengths of Crisis Intervention is that it can be effectively used by nurses and other therapists regardless of their therapeutic orientation or clinical field. Unlike many other nursing interventions, Crisis Intervention has no concrete tools or instruments. However, the crisis interventionist should understand well the stages of the problem-solving process.

Expanding on Dewey's classic *How We Think* (1910), the problem-solving process may be viewed as a series of six steps. The job of the nurse is to assist the client through this process to completion to resolve the crisis.

First, the nurse must help the client identify and describe the problem. Because the client in crisis typically is overwhelmed, he or she often cannot focus clearly enough to identify the specific problem or problems. In short, he or she cannot see the forest for the trees.

Second, once the problem is identified by nurse and client, the nurse can assist the client in generating possible solutions. The nurse may make suggestions if he or she is familiar with alternatives that have helped others in similar crises in the past.

Third, the nurse assists the client in evaluating the possible outcomes or consequences of the alternative solutions. For example, a client in marital crisis might be considering staying with her mate or divorcing him. The nurse might suggest that the client list the positive and negative aspects of each decision.

Fourth, the client decides which alternative will be chosen. It is crucial to remember that it is the client, not the nurse, who must live with this decision. Therefore, it must be the client who makes the decision to act. This is critical to remember because the client is often so vulnerable that any suggestion, no matter how inappropriate for his or her life, is likely to be grasped. The nurse, however, may offer support for whatever decision is made but must reassure the client that support will be forthcoming if the client changes his or her mind. This is easier said than done. For example, in working with abused spouses, it is difficult to support the client's decision to return home to the same setting where repeated batterings have occurred in the past and most likely will in the future. Nevertheless, each person must travel his or her own path through life.

Fifth, the client implements the decision.

Finally, the nurse helps the client evaluate the implementation. Did this solution resolve the crisis? Is the client better off now? If not, the client may have to try another solution.

By going through the problem-solving process with guidance, the client is often better able to do problem solving independently in the future, thus lessening the likelihood of similar crises occurring later.

THE CRISIS INTERVENTION CANDIDATE

Any person experiencing life crises is a candidate for Crisis Intervention. And although some persons have more effective coping and problem-solving skills than others—and are less likely to suffer crisis—life stresses can overwhelm even the strongest among us. Therefore, it is safe to say that everyone is a potential candidate for Crisis Intervention.

Some of the more relevant nursing diagnoses are the following:

Impaired Adjustment
Anxiety
Ineffective Individual Coping
Ineffective Family Coping: Disabling
Fear
Dysfunctional Grieving
Knowledge Deficit (specify)
Powerlessness
Rape-Trauma Syndrome
Social Isolation
Spiritual Distress
Potential for Violence

Any conditions in which a person's problem-solving strategies are found to be ineffective may require Crisis Intervention. For a more comprehensive listing of the types of people with whom Crisis Intervention has been successfully used, readers are directed to the works of Parad, Resnik, and Parad (1976), Ewing (1978), Aguilera (1990), and others.

DOING CRISIS INTERVENTION

To do Crisis Intervention successfully the nurse must recall the principles of crisis theory. An excellent sourcebook in this area is by Infante (1982).

A Synopsis of Crisis Theory

Caplan (1964) identified four phases of a typical crisis:

1. The individual experiences a problem that threatens basic needs. The individual tries to relieve the tension by resorting to traditional problem-solving strategies to end the crisis and thus restore emotional equilibrium.

2. If the individual's usual methods fail, increased tension occurs. He or she becomes disorganized and resorts to a trial-and-error type of solving the problem.

3. If these problem-solving measures fail, the individual experiences an increase in tension, which leads him or her to redefine the problem to fit a past experience or to give up certain of the goals as unattainable. The individual now uses novel or emergency ways of trying to solve the problem.

4.   If these measures fail, tension rises to the breaking point, resulting in major personality disorganization.

There are other points in crisis theory to keep in mind. First, crisis is not pathological. Rather, it is a struggle of the individual to achieve precrisis equilibrium. Whether the crisis will be a growth process or an avenue into genuine pathology often depends on the intervention. Also, the individual in crisis is more amenable to outside intervention than when not experiencing crisis. Furthermore, persons experiencing crisis usually send out signals to others calling for help. Therefore, the crisis interventionist has an excellent opportunity to help the individual learn and grow from this crisis.

Assessment

The assessment in Crisis Intervention is a shorter, more focused form of the traditional nursing assessment. Crisis Intervention is often conducted in 48 hours to 72 hours, with the client's being referred to a more specialized therapist or agency, or it is done in a series of six to eight intense sessions. In addition, because it focuses on the immediate crisis problem and its resolution, many aspects of the usual nursing history are irrelevant.

If the nurse is seeing the client on the first day of the crisis, the client should be assessed for basic physical safety. For example, is the client verbalizing suicidal thoughts? If the client is seen in the community and has to travel after the interview, is he or she in enough control to drive safely? Besides this basic safety assessment, the nurse assesses three other areas: the precipitating event leading to the crisis and the client's perception of the problem, the client's strengths and previous coping skills, and the extent and quality of the client's support system (Haber 1982, p. 313).

To discern the precipitating event and the client's perception of the problem, the nurse asks a number of questions: Why is the client seeking help at this time? What led to the current crisis? How is the client feeling right now? How is the problem affecting his or her life and those of people around him or her? Is the client able to function effectively in his or her basic social roles, such as parent, worker, or student?

In assessing the client's strengths and coping skills, the nurse explores the client's previous ways of dealing with crises and the methods used in attempting to reduce the tension. In addition, the nurse also looks for particular strengths the client may possess. This is crucial in the intervention, as the client often feels ashamed or has low self-esteem for being out of control of life. By cataloging the client's strengths — such as a sense of humor, past resiliency, articulateness, seeking help — the nurse will later be able to use these to reinforce the client's sense of self-worth.

Finally, the nurse assesses the client's support system and the client's use of this system in the present crisis. It is helpful to know, for example, who, if anyone, the client is close to, if there are friends who could help out, and the names of clergy or other helping professionals the client would like to call on.

Planning

Through assessment, the client has already achieved the first step of the problem-solving process: identifying and describing the problem. From the assessment data, the nurse is able to plan specific strategies related to the client's coping abilities, the client's support system and willingness to marshal these forces to help resolve the crisis, the severity or complexity of the crisis, and the nurse's knowledge of this particular type of crisis event.

Intervention

By assessing adequately, it is expected that the nurse has established a trusting and therapeutic relationship with the client. The nurse assures the client that he or she will not abandon the client and will be available until the crisis is resolved: Crisis Intervention is not a 9-to-5 activity. Therefore, the client should have some way of reaching the therapist when not in a formal session.

If the client is in physical danger, the nurse must initiate steps to ensure physical safety. For example, a distraught client may need a ride home or a safe refuge from an abusive spouse. The client with suicidal ideation may need to stay with a friend rather than be alone at home. Often getting the client to promise not to harm self provides enough motivation to help the client from carrying out harmful actions.

The nurse then assists the client through steps 2, 3, and 4 of the problem-solving process: generating possible solutions to the problem, listing the possible consequences of the various solutions, and offering support for the client's decision.

In the fifth step of the problem-solving process, the client implements his or her chosen solution. At this point it is wise for the nurse to be on call in case the client's actions end in failure.

Evaluation

Having carried out the client-chosen plan, the client is assisted by the nurse in evaluating the effectiveness of the solution. The basic question to answer is this: "Are you now at the same level of psychological comfort and coping as you were before the crisis?" Often the nurse will find the client better off now than before; he or she may have deepened friendships and family bonds, found support in self-help community groups not previously known about, or made significant life alterations leading to better mental health. Furthermore, the nurse is able to evaluate the effectiveness of the intervention on the basis of objective data. For example, is the client exhibiting a brighter affect than at the first session, less motor restlessness, and better grooming?

Whether the client will be able to solve problems more effectively in the future is usually known only to the client. Because Crisis Intervention is so time limited, the nurse does not usually learn this information.

CASE STUDY

LR, a 28-year-old high school teacher, was brought to the emergency room of a large southern general hospital by ambulance. On arrival, he was barely conscious. His blood alcohol level was dangerously high, and he stated he had overdosed on "downers" but did not know what kind. He stated, "It's too much! I just can't seem to cope any more. I wish I were dead."

After his medical condition was stabilized, LR was transferred to the acute psychiatric unit. His medical diagnosis was "depression and suicide attempt," and his nursing diagnoses were Ineffective Individual Coping and Impaired Adjustment.

LR was both angry at himself for ending up in the hospital and ashamed of his suicide attempt. While still semiconscious, he told the admitting nurse on the unit that she could not possibly understand him or help him because she was not a gay man. This unit had a gay clinical nurse specialist, a specialist in both gay men's studies and alcohol studies, who was called to see LR.

The assessment revealed that LR was a high school teacher in a small- to medium-sized southern town. Although he accepted being gay as a positive force in his life, he had not disclosed this to his family or colleagues. He was afraid of family rejection, of losing his teaching job if those in authority knew he was gay, and of possible antigay bigotry of the townspeople if his sexual orientation were known. His only gay support system consisted of persons outside his town, many of them living in coastal states many hundreds of miles from where he lived.

LR defined his problem globally: "I'm just too stressed at work. I've gotten so many assignments at school that I'm doing the work of four people." With some probing, it was learned that LR had a severe drinking problem, resulting in past driving-under-the-influence citations, alcoholic blackouts, and over-dosing on pills.

He denied now having suicidal ideation and signed a pledge promising not to harm himself while in the hospital. This document, also containing the promise to tell the nursing staff if he felt suicidal at a later time, was put in his chart. Such action is standard psychosocial nursing practice in acute inpatient settings.

After two 1½-hour sessions, LR defined his crisis as a three-pronged problem: alcoholism; lack of freedom to share self, related to being "in the closet"; and lack of assertiveness in the workplace.

From the data gathered, the priority problem seemed to be alcoholism and alcohol abuse. Fortunately, LR was in a suggestible state, and the usual denial stage found in alcoholics was quickly overcome. I decided to introduce LR to gay-related alcoholism literature and to some Alcoholics Anonymous (AA) readings, especially *Alcoholics Anonymous* (1976), called the "Big Book" by AA members, and to explore options with him, such as joining AA. Furthermore, I planned to teach him about alcoholism as needed and to supply him with positive gay literature while he was in the hospital.

His lack of freedom to share his gay identity and his lack of assertion in telling the school when he had too much work to do were crucial, although secondary, aspects of the problem. Alcoholism is itself a primary disease, not merely a symptom of some other problem. Furthermore, it is always terminal if not arrested.

Finally, my plan called for conducting a miniseminar for the nursing staff related to the gay coming-out process and some of the health problems often experienced in the various stages of coming out.

LR was faced with three main choices to solve the primary problem: continue drinking, cut down on drinking, or abstain from all alcohol. The first choice was readily discarded; drinking led him to the crisis. The second option was also discarded; controlled drinking has been shown to be ineffective in helping alcoholics. This led LR to choose abstinence as the solution.

With his permission, I contacted the local gay AA group. Several men from this group took turns visiting LR in the hospital. Also, his psychiatrist gave her permission for LR to attend the gay AA meetings outside the hospital and to go out for coffee with the members after meetings.

During this time, LR called on his gay friends for support, and the result was overwhelming. Friends began arriving from both coasts and points in between. And because both LR and his friends were extremely popular with both patients and staff, visiting hours on the unit became a time of great joy, laughing, and sharing even for patients who had no visitors of their own. No one was untouched by LR and his friends.

A miniseminar was conducted for the nursing staff. All indicated a great willingness to learn and be as helpful as possible. Following this program, the staff felt freer and more knowledgeable to help LR and LR began being more open with the staff.

When LR first arrived on the unit, he had been intoxicated and reported problems with eating, sleeping, concentrating, and relaxing. After the 4 weeks of Crisis Intervention, his sleeping, eating, and concentration were back to normal. He did have some trouble relaxing, however; he was a high-energy type of individual. His affect was bright, and his outlook on life became extremely positive. He became committed to AA and was an active member of the gay AA group. He was also proud of the fact that his psychiatrist gave him a big hug and told him that she wished all her patients could be like him.

But LR went much further than successfully dealing with his alcoholism. With his new-found lease on life, he decided to tackle the other two aspects of his self-defined problem. First, he told his family and peer teachers that he was gay after deciding that, whatever their reactions to his being gay would be, dealing with these reactions could not be worse than living an "uptight life." His family, his teacher colleagues, and the school principal accepted his disclosure with solid support. In addition, his work load, which the principal agreed had gotten out of hand, was reduced.

LR has celebrated nine AA birthdays since his hospital stay and describes himself as being "really grateful for a second chance at life!"

SUMMARY

Crisis Intervention is a widely applicable intervention. Any condition that renders a person's problem-solving abilities ineffective may require Crisis Intervention. The implementation requires the nurse to assist the patient through the steps of problem solving. To be effective, the nurse needs knowledge of the intervention and the crisis that caused the problem.

REFERENCES

Alcoholics Anonymous. 1976. *Alcoholics Anonymous* (3d ed.). New York: A.A. World Services.
Aquilera, D.C. 1990. *Crisis intervention: Theory and methodology* (6th ed.). St. Louis: C.V. Mosby.
Benter, S.E. 1979. Crisis therapy. In S.J. Sundeen and G.W. Stuart (eds.), *Principles and practice of psychiatric nursing* (pp. 368–386) St. Louis: C.V. Mosby.
Caplan, G. 1964. *Principles of preventative psychiatry.* New York: Basic Books.
Dewey, J. 1910. *How we think.* Boston: Heath.
Ewing, C.P. 1978. *Crisis intervention as psychotherapy.* New York: Oxford University Press.
Frederick, C., and Garrison, J. 1981. Disaster and mental health: An overview. *Behavior Today* 12:32.
Haber, J. 1982. Crisis theory and application. in J. Haber, A.M. Leach, S.M. Schudy, and B.F. Sideleau (eds.), *Comprehensive psychiatric nursing* (2d ed.) (pp. 305–319). New York: McGraw-Hill.
Hoff, L.A. 1978. *People in crisis: Understanding and helping.* Menlo Park, Calif.: Addison-Wesley.
Infante, M.S. (ed.). 1982. *Crisis theory: A framework for nursing practice.* Reston, Va: Reston Publishing Company.
Jacobson, G., Strickler, M., and Morley, W.E. 1968. Generic and individual approaches to crisis intervention. *American Journal of Public Health* 58:339–342.
Kus, R.J. 1985. Crisis intervention. In G.M. Bulechek and J.C. McCloskey (eds.), *Nursing interventions: Treatments for nursing diagnoses.* (pp. 277–287). Philadelphia: W.B. Saunders Company.
Kus, R.J. 1990. Coming out: Its nature, stages, and health concerns. In R.J. Kus (ed.), *Keys to caring: Assisting your gay and lesbian clients* (pp. 30–44). Boston: Alyson.
Lieb, J., Lipstitch, I.I., and Slaby, A.E. 1973. *The crisis team: A handbook for the mental health professional.* Hagerstown, Md: Harper & Row.
Lindemann, E. 1944. Symptomatology and management of acute grief. *American Journal of Psychiatry* 101:101–148.
Morley, W.E., Messick, J.M., and Aquilera, D.C. 1967. Crisis: Paradigms of intervention. *Journal of Psychiatric Nursing* 5:531–544.

Parad, H.J., Resnick, H.L.P., and Parad, L.G. (eds.). 1976. *Emergency and disaster management: A mental health sourcebook.* Bowie, Md; Charles Press.

Powell, S., and Lively, S. 1981. Psychological crisis. In L.K. Hart, J.L. Reese, and M.O. Fearing (eds.), *Concepts common to acute illness: Identification and management* (pp. 340–353). St. Louis: C.V. Mosby.

Riley, B. 1980. Crisis intervention. In J. Lancaster (ed.), *Adult psychiatric nursing* (pp. 528–548). Garden City, N.Y.: Medical Examination Publishing Company.

Walkup, L.L. 1974. A concept of crisis. In J.E. Hall and B.R. Weaver (eds.), *Nursing of families in crisis* (pp. 151–157). Philadelphia: J.B. Lippincott.

14

PRESENCE

DIANE L. GARDNER

DEFINITION AND DESCRIPTION

Just being there is important and helpful. Another's presence conveys to those who are dependent, not well, disabled, or frail the reassurance and comfort that they are not abandoned. Patients frequently experience a diminished energy for self-care, and Presence provides an assurance that a competent caregiver is checking on one and will attend to one's needs. This sense of security is presumed to decrease fear or anxiety and augment coping ability. For example, Schulmeister's (1990) patient reported that he knew how the soldiers felt when they saw Florence Nightingale's lamp because he felt the same way when he saw Schulmeister with her flashlight coming up the driveway.

From the image of the Lady with the Lamp to the modern-day nurse, the presence of the nurse has symbolized professional nursing and has formed the core of the nurse-patient relationship. The effect, both physical and psychological, of the presence of the nurse is hard to capture. It is an elusive concept, challenging to measure in quantitative terms yet recognized by both nurses and their patients. Zderad (1978) stated that Presence is an experience verified by the awareness of both the nurse and the patient. She cited an example from her group therapy work in which spontaneous feedback from a patient demonstrated that the nurse's presence was valued. In this instance, Presence is described in terms of a something-is-going-on-here perception and is validated by having made a difference that was observable by a change in the patient's affective behavior.

A holistic nursing definition of Presence is the physical "being there" and psychological "being with" a patient for the purpose of meeting the patient's health care needs. In this sense, the nurse is an intervention tool in the process of nursing care. It is a dynamic and interactive process, whether conscious or not, based on knowledge and skill in the art and science of skilled caring. Presence is conceived of as a core element of nursing activity. It is the availability of the nurse as helper for the patient. As an intervention, Presence is the nurse's use of self through availability and attention to needs.

The two aspects of Presence, the physical and the psychological presence of the nurse, are intricately interwoven in the reality of nursing care. The nurse's presence for the patient is manifested in three dimensions: the cognitive domain by verbal communication of empathy or understanding of the patient's experiencing; the affective domain by a generation of positive regard, trust, and genuineness, which are evidenced by interpersonal rapport; and the behavioral domain by being physically available as a helper. Presence as a nursing intervention is operationally defined as encompassing all three dimensions.

Concern for the health and welfare of others is central to the profession of nursing. Patients hold an expectation that nurses will enter into a relationship with them characterized by warmth, caring, liking, interest, and respect; Rogers (1962) termed this a "helping relationship." Training and knowledge are required for the nurse to be therapeutically valuable to the patient (Altschul 1979). Paterson and Zderad (1976) stated that nursing, as a clinical art, is transactional; it involves being with and doing with the patient. The patient sees in the nurse the possibility of help, comfort, and support. The nature of the work of nursing continually exposes nurses to the miseries of others. Nurses see the suffering and share the concerns of their patients. Yet as Colavecchio (1982) pointed out, one of the major rewards of direct patient care derives from human contact and from the significance of being present with another during critical times.

RELATED LITERATURE

Despite the use of the term *presence* in the nursing literature and despite an awareness of its centrality to the nurse-patient relationship, little has been done to conceptualize and define this idea formally. Central to the development of the concept of Presence is the work of nursing theorists with a background in psychiatric and mental health nursing. Leininger's research on professional care included an identification of Presence as one of the 99 care constructs whose value may differ across cultures. For example, black patients viewed care as including the use of presence and touch in specific ways (Leininger 1981, 1990). Aamodt (1986) also conceptualized care as being present. Paterson and Zderad (1976; Zderad 1978) can be identified as major theorists for delineation of the concept of Presence. Paterson and Zderad (1976) defined Presence as being available or open in a situation with a wholeness of one's unique individual being. Presence, then, is a gift of the self. Their schema is derived from an existential, phenomenological, humanistic philosophical base. Their thoughts on Presence reflected an emphasis on the psychological aspects of nursing presence: dialogue, empathy, and interactive transactions. In this sense, the nurse uses herself as an intervention tool to create a therapeutic psychological milieu that meets the patient's needs for help, comfort, or support.

The presence of the nurse is the key that opens the door to the nurse-patient relationship, a concept that nurses have recognized and remarked on. In discussing the role of student nurses, Vaillot (1962) noted that they can be a presence to patients. They become so when they are available to patients as opposed to being aloof or being mere spectators in nursing situations. Zderad (1978) sees Presence as basic to the whole process of nursing. Paterson and Zderad (1976) described it as the gift of one's self in interhuman relating. This flows from the nurse's reason for being there: to nurture. There is an implicit expectation that a nurse will extend herself in a helpful way if a patient needs assistance. The presence of the nurse involves openness and availability to what is and to what is not the patient's state of being, weighed against a standard of what ought to be, with the intention of doing something about the difference.

Brodish (1982) has conceptualized the nursing helping relationship in an interaction model. She defined nursing as the therapeutic use of self for the benefit of others after first acquiring the knowledge and the skill necessary to identify needs. What is also needed is an ability to choose strategically among interventions and structure them to respond to the identified needs. Established nursing theorists also have emphasized the conceptualization of nursing as a therapeutic interaction.

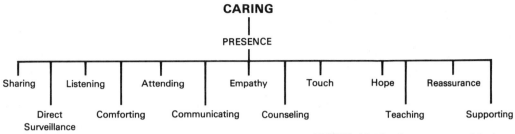

FIGURE 14–1. Components of Caring.

Orlando (1961) theorized that what is unique to nursing is the process involved in interacting with a patient to meet an immediate need. Orem (1971) viewed nursing as an interpersonal process requiring the social encounter of the nurse with a patient and involving a transaction between them. King (1971) defined nursing as a basic interpersonal relationship process of action, reaction, and transaction. In his work with group psychotherapy for survivors of a holocaust, Lifton (1976) identified Presence, defined as a kind of being there or full engagement and openness to mutual impact, as one of three therapeutic principles useful for recovery of mental health.

As a concept, Presence encompasses other interventions, which also are subconcepts of the global caring contruct. Figure 14–1 displays this hierarchy, from caring as a broad, general construct to the general intervention of Presence and then to more specific activities such as listening, touch, and hope. The outcomes of Presence include support, comfort, sustained assistance, encouragement, decreased fear and anxiety, and motivation. Caring is broad enough to include both interactive and noninteractive (in the immediate sense) aspects. Presence implies activities of a direct interactive nature, such as being there, touch, or direct surveillance. It is possible to include under Presence the psychological indirect residual of prior Presence or the anticipation of the help and availability of the nurse in the future, but Presence is primarily viewed as a literal present-tense being there.

Caring and Nurturance

The concept of Presence is a subconstruct of the broad concept of caring or nurturance. Caring is based on an interest in or concern for another human being. It is defined as providing assistance to others in need (Leininger 1980) and as a feeling of compassion, interest, and concern for others (Leininger 1970). The presence of the nurse as a helper is the embodiment of caring in nursing. Greenberg-Edelstein (1986) defined nurturance as the caring and helping that are fundamental to human relationships and groups. Geissler (1990) noted that most nurses would define nurturance as a form of caring that flows from nurse to patient. Both authors argued that *nurturance* is a more inclusive term than *caring* and that nurturance flows two ways. Greenberg-Edelstein (1986) identified five levels of nurturance: unidirectional, elementary, social, therapeutic, and transcending the self. There appears to be little conceptual distinction between the terms *caring* and *nurturance*. However, caring is more of a philosophy than an activity, whereas nurturance has more of an active connotation.

Empathy

Empathy enhances the quality of the nurse's Presence. Egan (1982) described being with, attending to, and listening to another person as potent reinforcers in certain situations. He discussed how, at more dramatic moments of life, simply being with another person is extremely important: another's presence can make a difference in terms of being comforted, even if few words are spoken. Egan believes that helping and other deep interpersonal transactions demand a certain intensity of presence: being fully there is more than physical presence; it is psychological or social-emotional presence as well. He related this to the concept of attending, which he considered to be a basic and important helping skill. Attending and listening skills contribute to effective empathy.

Empathy, or understanding, has been defined as the ability to perceive the meanings and feelings of others and to communicate that understanding to the other person (Gagan 1983). It also includes being able to predict accurately and anticipate the behavioral responses of the other (Kramer and Schmalenberg 1977). Empathy has been perceived as a concept integral to therapeutic nursing and is related to the role of the nurse as the one who creates a caring and helping atmosphere in which healing can be facilitated (Gagan 1983: Stetler 1977). Empathy has been a difficult concept to operationalize. Furthermore, there appears to be a wide range of differences between and among people in terms of their empathic ability (Kramer and Schmalenberg 1977). Research on the empathic ability of nurses has produced mixed results (Gagan 1983). Kramer and Schmalenberg (1977) noted that a relationship exists between helping behavior and empathy; one study found that helping behavior was function of empathic tendency (Mehrabian and Epstein 1972).

Support

The concept of support is also related to Presence. Support is similar to the provision of psychological comfort and has been defined as acceptance. Nursing support is an activity within the context of the nurse-patient relationship; it is one of the basic principles of practice and is thought to be an activity that should be performed by all nurses (Gardner and Wheeler 1981). Gardner and Wheeler studied nurses' perceptions of the meaning of support in their work. Factor analysis showed that the availability of the nurse was an important aspect of support. Critical incident reports elicited behaviors such as sitting and spending time with a patient, which imply the availability of the nurse to the patient. As perceived by the nurses in this study, supportive nursing interventions utilized communication to mediate and alleviate emotional stress.

Corless and Riordan (1990) identified a hierarchy of nursing care activities from the most basic to the complex: assessment and monitoring, therapeutics, physical support and activities of daily living, education, and personal support. As a humanistic aspect of care, Presence would be categorized within the most complex level, personal support. Two research studies included more direct elements of the Presence of the nurse. Gardner and Wheeler's study (1981) on nurses' perceptions of the meaning of support utilized a critical incident technique. Behaviors of availability or nursing Presence, such as sitting and spending time with the patient, were shown to be important in the concept of support. Odell (1981) described a study of loneliness in which she asked adult patients how nurses could help. Her findings indicated that nursing activities that prevent loneliness include the offering of psychological support by initiating short, frequent visits with the patient as an interested and concerned individual. Brief encounters were indeed therapeutic, and included patient requests to "just stop by," "drop in," and "check on me." One respondent indicated, "Just be there when needed."

Therapeutic Use of Self

Presence is closely related to the concept of the therapeutic use of self, which can be traced from the work of Peplau (1952) and has been defined by Uys (1980) as the ability of nurses to employ their entire person or unique individuality and identity scientifically and purposefully as a tool to promote health and to limit disease. Uys (1980) saw the concept of the therapeutic use of self as central to nursing. Krikorian and Paulanka (1982) noted that therapeutic use of self is frequently identified as the nurse's major tool in the nurse-patient relationship. Uys (1980) preferred a broad view of the nurse as a total person in the service of patients. Her operational definition of the therapeutic use of self concept included the four facets of mental, physical, psychosocial, and spiritual aspects. She listed use of physical presence to reassure, encourage, set limits, and motivate as an example of behaviors or skills associated with the use of physical aspects of self.

Physical Closeness and Touch

Physical closeness, nearness, and touching are aspects of Presence in nursing. Caregiving activities are predicated on proximity and bring the nurse into the patient's physical space. Physical closeness was a factor of support in Gardner and Wheeler's (1981) study. In Ricci's (1981) study of personal space invasion in the nurse-patient relationship, anxiety scores of the experimental group showed a definite downward trend, indicating that the intrusion of a nurse into a patient's space had a calming rather than a stimulating effect. Thus, the Presence of the nurse is not generally perceived by patients to be anxiety provoking.

Lynch, Thomas, Paskewitz, Katcher, and Weir (1977) and Thomas, Lynch, and Mills (1975) have studied the effects of different kinds of psychosocial interactions on the cardiac activity of cardiac care unit patients. Cardiac responses to social interaction were monitored in patients who had received the drug curare. They observed abrupt heart rate changes in these patients of up to 30 beats per minute when a nurse simply held the patient's hand and comforted him or her. In this case, Presence was practiced in the form of touch and verbal communication.

In the pediatric literature, a study by Triplett and Arneson (1979) demonstrated that tactile comfort was an effective means of alleviating distress and maintaining trust in young hospitalized children. Sixty-three children between the ages of 3 days and 44 months old who were distressed (crying) at the time of the nurse's comforting were studied to compare techniques. In the verbal-only group, 7 of the 40 techniques were successful in quieting the children, compared with 53 successes of the 60 techniques in the tactile-verbal group. Thus, their data showed a highly significant difference when tactile comfort measures were used.

Summary

No specific nursing research literature describing Presence as an intervention is available. In general, the dimension of the feelings experienced by the patient during the interaction with the nurse has rarely been investigated (Ricci 1981). At this time, evidence for the effectiveness of the Presence of the nurse for the patient must be deduced from related literature and from anecdotal personal experiences about the psychological impact that the reassurance and psychological interaction derived from the Presence of the nurse has on recovery.

INTERVENTION TOOLS

Because of the poor conceptualization of and the paucity of research on Presence, identifiable intervention tools are unavailable. An operational definition of Presence in nursing is the direct availability or interaction of the nurse in the cognitive domain by verbal communication of empathy or understanding of the patient's experience; in the affective domain by a generation of positive regard, trust, and genuineness, which is evidenced by interpersonal rapport; and in the physical domain by being physically involved as a helper. As the nurse assesses the nursing situation, some aspects of Presence may be incorporated into other interventions (Counseling, Teaching, and so forth) or, in certain situations such as social isolation or loneliness, the nurse may choose to use Presence as the intervention of choice.

ASSOCIATED NURSING DIAGNOSES AND PATIENT GROUPS

Presence is a concept that is basic and broad enough to be widely applicable to divergent patient groups and to be useful as an intervention for various nursing diagnoses. For example, the nurse can therapeutically intervene with Presence for adults experiencing loneliness (Odell 1981) and through touch for young children experiencing distress during hospitalization (Triplett and Arneson 1979). Supportive Presence of a nurse has been indicated as making a difference for adult patients newly diagnosed as having inoperable cancer (Gardner and Wheeler 1981), for outpatient male cardiac patients (Ricci 1981), and for psychiatric patients through use of empathic communication (Mansfield 1973). It is theorized that the nurse's presence demonstrates caring, assists copying by implying psychological support, and diminishes the intensity of feelings such as fear, powerlessness, anxiety, isolation, and distress by providing a physical and psychological anchoring of the patient to the nurse as a helpful other.

The availability of the nurse augments the anxious patient's sense of control. The nurse uses the self as an intervention by assisting patients to cope more effectively. The nurse conveys a sense of support by nearness for patients experiencing fear, grief, powerlessness, isolation, or distress. In Presence, the nurse transmits psychological support and comfort to the patient by utilizing techniques such as physical nearness (for example, sitting with the patient) or cognitive-affective awareness of and attending to the patient's needs.

There is some anecdotal evidence that Presence may be a valuable intervention for stigmatized client groups such as persons with acquired immune deficiency syndrome (AIDS). For example, AIDS sufferers report that no one touched them until they were placed on a dedicated AIDS ward under the care of specialized nurses. Further, Presence may be an important nursing intervention in long-term care facilities. In the novel *A Bed by the Window,* Peck (1990) described how patients in a nursing home waited to die until a favorite nurse was on duty so that she could be with them.

Specific nursing diagnoses for which Presence would be most appropriate include the following:

Anticipatory Grieving
Anxiety
Fear

Impaired Verbal Communication
Ineffective Individual Coping
Potential for Injury
Powerlessness
Social Isolation
Spiritual Distress

PROTOCOLS FOR USING PRESENCE

Increasingly the public has begun to define quality in terms of health professionals' time and concern (Curtin 1990). In adult acute nursing care situations, patients' perceptions of competency are a critical dimension. Patients view good care
as including elements of listening, helping, and being there (Murdaugh, Larson,
Gortner, Heinrich, Larson, Orberst, Stone, Therrien, and Watson 1990).

A protocol for effecting the most positive results from Presence begins with an
adherence to caring as a philosophy. The nurse should possess self-awareness, a
commitment to helping others, and a basic knowledge and skill in providing professional care. Beyond this, empathy enriches the experience by enabling the nurse
to identify mentally with patients in order to understand their feelings and the
meaning of their health status. This understanding assists the nurse in structuring
an appropriate and therapeutic mix of activities for meeting identified needs.
Presumably this skill is refined and improved as the nurse gains experience.

Presence is a highly metaphysical concept, and therefore it is hard to reduce to a
concrete protocol. Any protocol for using Presence should allow for patient variables, such as satisfaction, perception of competence, and personal preferences, in
response to the use of the components of the Presence intervention. Further, the
nurse may choose a level of involvement that ranges from a passive, brief encounter to a significant metaphysical interaction.

CASE STUDIES

Case Study 1

DW was a 37-year-old male hospitalized psychiatric patient with a medical
diagnosis of schizophrenia. He had been hospitalized on psychiatric units on
numerous occasions. When not hospitalized, DW had a history of getting into
trouble for unusual behavior, especially for urinating on the floor of his room at
the hotel where he lived. DW was very quiet on the hospital unit. He spent
much of his time lying on his bed in a large ward. He occasionally paced the
halls anxiously, muttering in an angry or fearful tone or stood in the hall
watching what others were doing. He admitted to having auditory hallucinations in the form of voices. DW sometimes told the nurses that others were
going to harm him. His affect was usually flat, and he interacted with others
only minimally. He perceived environmental stimuli, especially people, as
threatening.

The nurse assessed DW's nonverbal communication and diagnosed Fear (retreat to bed) and Anxiety (pacing and muttering). The initial intervention was
an acceptance of these behaviors. The nurse then used Presence with DW.
When the nurse came on the unit, he greeted DW by name. When DW sat in
the dayroom, the nurse would sit nearby and watch television or make brief
comments about activities on the unit. The actual message was nonverbal: that
the nurse was not a threat and that it was safe to be near him. The nonverbal
interaction with DW consisted of being nearby in a nonthreatening position. In
this way, trust could be developed. The nurse utilized his Presence by sitting

with DW in as nonthreatening a manner as possible. The goal of intervention was for DW to be able to choose a greater degree of contact with others and to increase his ability to relate comfortably to others. The nurse was present to DW without demanding interactional responses from the patient, which he was unable to make at the time. At one point, the nurse was called by another patient who needed pain medication. When the nurse arose to go, DW said, "Where are you going? I need you to keep me together!" This verbalization of the meaning of the nurse's Presence indicated DW's active willingness to accept the nurse's Presence in his time of anxiety (Wilberding 1981).

Case Study 2

Michael was a 6-year-old white male who had ingested a caustic lye solution when he was 16 months old. He suffered severe damage to his esophagus and was not expected to survive. He did survive but had to endure multiple hospitalizations and surgeries. The aftermath was a chronic handicapping condition. Michael underwent a colonic interposition at age 4, which was an attempt at surgical correction. Esophageal dilations every 2 weeks were begun to maintain patency of the reconstructed esophagus. Michael is still unable to swallow. He has a tracheostomy and a feeding gastrostomy tube. The esophageal dilations continue. They are now done under general anesthesia because of Michael's level of apprehension and distress.

The nurse assessed Michael's apprehension and distress regarding dilation and diagnosed Fear and Threat related to security and independence needs. The initial intervention included acceptance of his protest behaviors. The nurse then explored alternative coping behaviors with the child and the family. The nurse arranged to stay with the child prior to the procedure, during induction of anesthesia, and after. Michael expressed eagerness for the nurse to remain with him. The nurse accompanied Michael up the elevator to the operating room and remained with him in the operating room during the induction of anesthesia. The nurse remained physically close to Michael, holding his hand and repeatedly giving him verbal reassurances ("I'll be right here"). The actual message was: There is someone present who is focused solely on your welfare.

The goal of the intervention was for Michael to accept induction of anesthesia without intense fear and physical resistance. The nurse was present for Michael to reduce his fear of abandonment in a perceived hostile situation, which thereby helped to decrease traumatic after-effects. As soon as Michael was under the anesthesia, the anesthesiologist who had witnessed the nursing intervention remarked to the nurse about how unusual it was for someone to accompany a child for anesthesia induction. The nurse replied that special permission had been obtained. The anesthesiologist commented about the success of the intervention. He noted that children of Michael's age usually fight anesthesia, yet Michael had remained calm and had fallen asleep quietly. The anesthesiologist was aware of this induction as being less traumatic for the child. The threat and fear of the procedure for the child was apparently alleviated by the Presence of the nurse.

CONCLUSION

Presence as a concept is still abstract and evolving. It will be important to move toward measuring this basic nursing intervention. Basic descriptive studies of a qualitative nature, perhaps using vignettes, should be undertaken to begin the systematic study of Presence. Research could provide a basic understanding of how Presence produces a change in patients and what effects nursing Presence has on patient outcomes. Future research should also explore the link between Presence and nursing competency.

REFERENCES

Aamodt, A. 1986. Discovering the child's view of alopecia: Doing ethnography. In P. Munhall and C. Oiler (eds.); *Nursing research: A qualitative perspective* (pp. 163–172). Norwalk, Conn.: Appleton-Century-Crofts.

Altschul, A.T. 1979. Commitment to nursing. *Journal of Advanced Nursing* 4:123–135.

Brodish, M.S. 1982. Nursing practice conceptualized: An interaction model. *Image* 14:5–7.

Colavecchio, R. 1982. Direct patient care: A viable career choice? *Journal of Nursing Administration* 12:17–22.

Corless, I., and Riordan, J. 1990. Nursing care: A user-friendly approach—Identifying the cutting edge questions. In J. Stevenson and T. Tripp-Reimer (eds.), *Knowledge about care and caring: State of the art and future developments* (pp. 53–64). Kansas City, Mo.: American Academy of Nursing.

Curtin, L. 1990. Touch-tempered technology. *Nursing Management* 21(7):7–8.

Egan, G. 1982. *The skilled helper: Model, skills, and methods for effective helping* (2d ed.). Monterey, Calif.: Brooks/Cole Publishing Company.

Gagan, J.M. 1983. Methodological notes on empathy. *Advances in Nursing Science* 5:65–72.

Gardner, K., and Wheeler, E.C. 1981. Nurses' perceptions of the meaning of support in nursing. *Issues in Mental Health Nursing* 3:13–28.

Geissler, E. 1990. Nurturance flows two ways. *American Journal of Nursing* 90(4):72–74.

Greenberg-Edelstein, R. 1986. *The nurturance phenomenon: Roots of group psychotherapy*. Norwalk, Conn.: Appleton-Century-Crofts.

King, I.M. 1971. *Toward a theory of nursing: General concepts of human behavior*. New York: John Wiley and Sons.

Kramer, M., and Schmalenberg, C. 1977. The first job . . . a proving ground basis for empathy development. *Journal of Nursing Administration* 7:3–20.

Krikorian, D.A., and Paulanka, B.J. 1982. Self-awareness—the key to successful nurse-patient relationship? *Journal of Psychosocial Nursing and Mental Health Services* 20:19–21.

Leininger, M. 1970. *Nursing and anthropology: Two worlds to blend*. New York: John Wiley and Sons.

Leininger, M. 1980. Caring: A central focus of nursing and health care services. *Nursing and Health Care* 1:135–143.

Leininger, M. 1981. *Caring: An essential human need*. Thorofare, N.J.: Charles B. Slack.

Leininger, M. 1990. Historic and epistemologic dimensions of care and caring with future directions. In J. Stevenson and T. Tripp-Reimer (eds.), *Knowledge about care and caring: State of the art and future developments* (pp. 19–31). Kansas City, Mo.: American Academy of Nursing.

Lifton, R. 1976. *The life of the self: Toward a new psychology*. New York: Simon and Schuster.

Lynch, J.J., Thomas, S.A., Paskewitz, D.A., Katcher, A.M., and Weir, L.O. 1977. Human contact and cardiac arrhythmia in a coronary care unit. *Psychosomatic Medicine* 39:188–193.

Mansfield, E. 1973. Empathy: Concept and identified psychiatric nursing behavior. *Nursing Research* 22:525–530.

Mehrabian, A., and Epstein, N. 1972. A measure of emotional empathy. *Journal of Personality* 40:525–543.

Murdaugh, C., Larson, E., Gortner, S., Heinrich, J., Larson, P., Oberst, M., Stone, K., Therrien, B., and Watson, J. 1990. Group II: Adult-acute situations. In J. Stevenson and T. Tripp-Reimer (eds.), *Knowledge about care and caring: State of the art and future developments*. (pp. 127–130). Kansas City, Mo.: American Academy of Nursing.

Odell, S.H. 1981. Someone is lonely. *Issues in Mental Health Nursing* 3:7–12.

Orem, D.E. 1971. *Nursing: Concepts of practice*. New York: McGraw-Hill.

Orlando, I.J. 1961. *The dynamic nurse-patient relationship*. New York: G.P. Putman's Sons.

Paterson, J.G. 1978. The tortuous way toward nursing theory. In *Theory development: What, why, how?* (pp. 49–65). New York: National League for Nursing. (Publ. No. 15-1708).

Paterson, J.G., and Zderad, L.T. 1976. *Humanistic nursing*. New York: John Wiley and Sons.

Peck, M.S. 1990. *A bed by the window*. New York: Bantam Books.

Peplau, H.E. 1952. *Interpersonal Relations in Nursing*. New York: G.P. Putnam's Sons.

Ricci, M.S. 1981. An experiment with personal space invasion in the nurse-patient relationship and its effect on anxiety. *Issues in Mental Health Nursing* 3:203–218.

Rogers, C. 1962. The characteristics of a helping relationship. *Canadian Mental Health*, suppl. 27.

Schulmeister, L. 1990. The lady with the flashlight. *American Journal of Nursing* 90(9):128.

Stetler, C.B. 1977. Relationship of perceived empathy to nurses' communication. *Nursing Research* 26:432–438.

Thomas, S.A., Lynch, J.J., and Mills, M.E. 1975. Psychosocial influences on heart rhythm in the coronary-care unit. *Heart and Lung* 4:746–750.

Triplett, J.L. and Arneson, S.W. 1979. The use of verbal and tactile comfort to alleviate distress in young hospitalized children. *Research in Nursing and Health* 2:17–23.

Uys, L.R. 1980. Towards the development of an operational definition of the concept "therapeutic use of self." *International Journal of Nursing Studies* 17:175–180.

Vaillot, S.M.C. 1962. *Commitment to nursing: A philosophic investigation.* Philadelphia: J.B. Lippincott.

Wilberding, J.Z. 1981. A comparison of two theories of nursing. (96:201 *Conceptual and Theoretical Foundations of Nursing*) (unpublished manuscript). Iowa City: University of Iowa.

Zderad, L.T. 1978. From here-and-now to theory: Reflections on "how." In *Theory development: What, why, how?* (pp. 35–48). New York: National League for Nursing. (Publ. No. 15-1708)

15

THERAPEUTIC TOUCH

THÉRÈSE CONNELL MEEHAN

Some of the earliest symbolism in nursing history reflects the importance of nurses' use of their hands as a mediating focus for their therapeutic intent (Connell 1983). More recently, Mead (1956) has observed that nurses' compassionate use of their hands is one of the unique functions of nursing in modern society. The development and use of Therapeutic Touch as a nursing intervention is one way in which nurses have sought to become more consciously aware of how they use their hands and their potential to facilitate the comfort and healing of their patients.

Therapeutic Touch was developed by Kunz and Krieger (1965–1972) following their systematic observation of the practice of laying on of hands. They were impressed with the practitioner's gentleness and focused intent to help, with the specially developed sensitivity of his hands, and with the fact that ill patients were frequently helped to feel more relaxed, comfortable, and energetic. A nurse, Krieger was especially impressed by the similarity of laying on of hands to the intuitive ways in which nurses have always used their hands in comforting and caring for patients. Building on their observations and their background in Eastern philosophy, Kunz and Krieger developed the theory and technique of Therapeutic Touch, and in 1975 Krieger introduced Therapeutic Touch into nursing practice and literature. Although Therapeutic Touch was derived from the laying on of hands, it is considered to be different in that it is not done within a religious context, the patient's belief in the intervention is not necessary for it to be effective, and it involves a specific, standardized procedure.

DESCRIPTION AND DEFINITION

Therapeutic Touch is viewed as an energy field interaction; as a nursing intervention it is best described using the Science of Unitary Human Beings nursing conceptual model (Rogers 1970, 1990). This model posits that energy fields are the fundamental units of the human being and the human being's environment. From this perspective, nurse and patient extend beyond their physical bodies, each being an energy field pattern within the other's environment. Therapeutic Touch may include physical touch but usually does not. The nurse's hands are held a few inches from the surface of the patient's body because this makes it easier to feel the qualities of the patient as an energy field.

Therapeutic Touch is a knowledgeable and purposive patterning of the patient-environmental energy field process. The nurse begins by assuming a meditative form of awareness called centering, which is fundamental to Therapeutic Touch

201

and is maintained throughout the intervention. It allows the nurse to focus her intent on helping the patient as a unitary whole and to perceive, through her hands, the subtle sensory cues in the energy field patterning of the patient as it extends beyond the patient's body. The nurse assesses the patient by moving her hands about 2 inches to 4 inches from the patient's body, from head to feet, gently attuning to the patient's condition by becoming aware of differences in sensory cues perceived through her hands. The nurse then treats the patient by moving her hands over the patient's body in gentle, downward, sweeping movements, dissipating any areas of tension or congestion and balancing the patient's energy flow. The intervention is done over the patient's clothes, and the patient may sit or lie in any position that is comfortable.

RELATED LITERATURE

Theoretical Rationale

The theoretical rationale used to describe and explain Therapeutic Touch is rooted in philosophical traditions common to many cultures. These traditions posit that aside from the physical matter, separateness, and multiplicity of causal and local events so predominantly evident in ordinary experience, there exists a fundamental, unitary, universal flow of energy within which all matter, consciousness, and events are grounded and interconnected (Weber 1986). Over the past 50 years, the concept of a fundamental, universal energy has become linked to and developed within field theory. Support for the view that energy fields are the basic organizing forces of the universe and that quanta, the solidlike particles of matter, are momentary manifestations of interacting fields is provided by the relativistic quantum field theories of modern physics (Bohm 1973; Capek 1961; Guillemin 1968). Studies of plants, animals, and humans have indicated that energy fields are of fundamental significance in establishing and maintaining pattern and organization in living systems (Burr 1972).

From within this universal energy flows a life-giving, healing energy that is present in all living systems and is composed of intelligence, order, and compassion (Weber 1979, 1986). In a state of health, the healing energy flows with freedom and abundance, whereas in a state of illness, the flow has become blocked and depleted. Conscious awareness of this healing energy and the ability to facilitate its flow within oneself arises through the spiritual dimension of human experience and is considered a natural human potential. Human beings also have the potential to facilitate this flow of healing energy in others, given a relative state of health, the ability to center themselves, and a nonattached intent to help or to facilitate healing in others (Kunz 1985).

The Science of Unitary Human Beings nursing model (Rogers 1970, 1990) was developed from field theory. As energy fields, human being and environment are viewed as unitary phenomena integral with one another in a continuous process of energy field patterning and innovative change. The nurse providing an intervention for a patient is viewed as an energy field pattern integral with the patient's environmental field patterning, and the patient is viewed as an energy field pattern integral with the nurse's environmental field patterning. In Rogers's view, Therapeutic Touch is one example by which "professional practice in nursing seeks to strengthen the coherence and integrity of human and environmental fields and to knowingly participate in the patterning of human and environmental fields for the realization of optimum well-being" (personal communication, June 1988).

Practice Literature

Since the late 1970s, nurses' interest in and use of Therapeutic Touch has been documented in a growing body of literature. Books by Krieger et al. (1979) and Macrae (1988) describe the intervention in detail. The integration of Therapeutic Touch into nursing practice has been described by Boguslawski (1979), Bulbrook (1984), Egan (1985), Fanslow (1983), Hospital Satellite Network (1986), Jurgens, Meehan, and Wilson (1987), Keegan (1988), Keller (1984), Lionberger (1986), Meehan (1990), Miller (1979), and Wyatt (1989). The most frequently reported effect of Therapeutic Touch is a generalized relaxation response, which has led to the belief that it can be effective in helping to relieve a wide variety of symptoms (Borelli and Heidt 1981; Krieger 1979). Its use to reduce pain has been recommended by Boguslawski (1980), Peric-Knowlton (1984), and Wright (1987) and described in detail by Meehan (1990). In addition, it has been reported to be effective in promoting sleep (Braun, Layton, and Braun 1986) and relieving depression (Rowlands 1984) in nursing home residents; calming hospitalized infants (Leduc 1987), patients undergoing anesthesia (Jonasen 1981), and women in childbirth (Wolfson 1984); providing support and comfort for hospitalized children (Finnerin 1981; Macrae 1979), patients with acquired immune deficiency syndrome (Newshan 1989) and patients who are dying (Fanslow 1983; Jackson 1981); and facilitating physical rehabilitation (Payne 1989).

Nurses also report integrating the concepts of centering and focused intent, which underlie their practice of Therapeutic Touch, into a wide range of other nursing activities. Integrating these concepts into activities such as giving a back rub or doing a patient assessment helps the nurse to attune to the patient in a calm and receptive manner and to observe a patient's condition intuitively as well as objectively. In addition, the introduction of these concepts into nurses' practice at a major medical center, through an inservice education program, has been shown to contribute to a significant decrease in work-related stress and emotional exhaustion and increase in personality hardiness and self-actualization (Meehan, Mahoney, Ake, Iervolino, Glassman, Tedesco, and Mariano 1990).

Many nurses who have integrated Therapeutic Touch into their practice report that it has changed their professional lives (Kunz and Krieger 1975–1990, Quinn 1979; Simeone 1985, Woods-Smith 1988). Generally they report feeling more enthusiastic, confident, and satisfied in their work, that their work has become more meaningful to them, and that aside from the frequent stresses of day-to-day practice, they have a greater sense of well-being. Simeone (1985) writes that "the little tasks of nursing seem less tedious and I feel strongly that my relationships with patients have grown more beneficial to both them and me . . . . I still get flustered and frustrated by things that happen on our floor, but I now have a tool to help me revitalize and see things more clearly" (p. 618). These changes are probably brought about through learning the centering meditation, which is basic to the practice of Therapeutic Touch. Learning this relatively simple form of meditation will promote a process of self-healing in the nurse. During the practice of Therapeutic Touch, this meditative perspective brings about an attitude of nonattached compassion and enables the nurse to perceive the inherent beauty of the patient as a unitary whole, aside from whatever the ordinary circumstances of the interaction might be. Such experiences and the development of an underlying meditative perspective inevitably alter the nurse's view of nursing practice and the role it plays in her life.

Research Findings

Research on Therapeutic Touch was initiated by Krieger and has continued to develop, despite a wide range of methodological problems confronted by investigators. The most serious problem in experimental research is to differentiate between the effects of Therapeutic Touch and the placebo effect. Most studies reported after 1983 included a control group that received a mimic Therapeutic Touch intervention, developed and validated by Quinn (1982), as a single-blind placebo control. Full control for the placebo effect through a double-blind design is not possible because placebo effect that arises from implicit and explicit expectation and suggestion by the nurse administering the intervention cannot be eliminated. Some studies have included a control group that received another touch intervention, and some also included a nonintervention group.

Originally Krieger (1975) derived a theory from Eastern philosophy that led her to investigate the effect of Therapeutic Touch on hemoglobin values in ill patients. Although the studies' findings suggested that Therapeutic Touch could have the potential to increase hemoglobin values, methodological problems precluded scientific support for this outcome. Subsequent studies have found no significant relationship between Therapeutic Touch and increased hemoglobin values (Meehan, Mersmann, Wiseman, Wolff, and Malgady 1991) or transcutaneous oxygen blood gas pressure (Fedoruk 1984).

Observations reported by Krieger, Peper, and Ancoli (1979) suggested that Therapeutic Touch could have the potential to promote a relaxation response. Heidt (1981) and Quinn (1984) found that hospitalized patients who received Therapeutic Touch had a significant decrease in anxiety immediately following the intervention. However, in other studies using hospitalized patients as subjects (Parks 1985; Hale 1986; Quinn 1989), no decrease in anxiety was found. In a study of preoperative patients, Meehan et al. (1991) found approximately the same mean decrease in anxiety in the Therapeutic Touch group as was found in the Heidt and Quinn (1984) studies, but this decrease was not significantly greater than in the mimic control group. Fedoruk (1984) found that treatment by Therapeutic Touch was significantly associated with reduction in a behavioral indicator of stress in hospitalized premature infants. However, Randolph (1984) found that healthy females who received Therapeutic Touch while being subject to artificially induced stress had no significant decrease in physiological indicators of stress. Meehan et al. (1991) found that postoperative patients who received Therapeutic Touch morning and evening over a 3-day postoperative period had no significant decrease in anxiety or fatigue and no significant increase in vigor over the intervention period. These findings are confounded by some methodological limitations. For example, Parks's elderly subjects had difficulty completing the anxiety questionnaire, Hale's sample size was very small, Quinn's (1989) findings were confounded by effects of tranquilizing medications, Fedoruk reported variability in lengths of intervention times, Randolph used a modified Therapeutic Touch procedure, and in the Heidt, Hale, and Quinn (1989) studies, the investigators administered the study interventions. In the Meehan et al. study, postoperative measurements were taken several hours following the interventions in an attempt to detect generalized effects. Constructive replication and extension of these studies are needed. To date, scientific support for the view that Therapeutic Touch decreases anxiety beyond a placebo effect and decreases stress is somewhat equivocal.

The assumption that Therapeutic Touch can decrease pain has also been tested. Keller and Bzdek (1986) found that Therapeutic Touch significantly reduced tension headache pain in otherwise healthy subjects immediately following the intervention and 4 hours later. Meehan (1985, 1986) found that Therapeutic Touch could be marginally effective in helping to reduce postoperative pain and that patients waited significantly longer before requesting more analgesic medication. Meehan et al. (1990) found that postoperative patients who received Therapeutic Touch in conjunction with a narcotic analgesic as needed (prn) had no significant decrease in pain over the first 3 hours following the intervention but that patients waited significantly longer before requesting further analgesic medication. Mueller Hinze (1988) found that Therapeutic Touch had no significant effect on experimentally induced pain. Again, methodological limitations confound interpretation of some findings. Measurement of effects were complicated by the facts that in the Meehan study, some patients required analgesic medication before the 1-hour postintervention time was completed; in the Mueller Hinze study, the sample size was very small; and in the Keller and Bzdek study, the principal investigator administered the study interventions. Constructive replication of these studies, and extension to include patients with different types of mild to moderate pain and repeated treatments and measures, is needed. So far, study findings suggest that Therapeutic Touch may have the potential, beyond a placebo effect, to reduce headache pain and decrease the need for prn analgesic medication.

Three qualitative studies concerning Therapeutic Touch have been completed. Lionberger (1985) interviewed 51 nurses who had practiced Therapeutic Touch for at least 6 months and 20 patients. She found that many nurses modified the standardized assessment and treatment phases of the procedure due to difficulty explaining the intervention in environments dominated by the medical model. Lionberger (1986) suggested that Therapeutic Touch be developed as a caring strategy rather than a healing modality. Wyatt (1988) examined conceptual change in 11 nurses who had completed a 2-day advanced continuing education seminar on Therapeutic Touch. Data from surveys and interviews over a 2-month period indicated that while knowledge and application were high 1 week following the seminar, they were not maintained over time due to perceived barriers to implementation in the workplace. Heidt (1990) interviewed and observed 7 nurses who had practiced Therapeutic Touch for at least 3 years and 7 patients. She found that all nurses conformed to the standardized practice procedure, that the primary experience of Therapeutic Touch was that of opening to the flow of the universal life energy, and that during the intervention the patient's experience of Therapeutic Touch frequently paralleled that of the nurse's. More qualitative studies are needed in order to explore and describe the nature of the intervention as it is perceived by nurses and patients.

INTERVENTION TOOLS

The Subjective Experience of Therapeutic Touch Survey (SETTS), a 68-item, self-report tool, was developed by Krieger and Wilcox (Winstead-Fry 1983) to measure how well individuals perform Therapeutic Touch. Their analysis indicated that the tool could reliably distinguish between experienced and nonexperienced practitioners. Extension of this work by Ferguson (1986) indicated that the SETTS could reliably differentiate among experienced practitioners, inexperienced practitioners, and nurses who did not practice Therapeutic Touch and that experienced practitioners were significantly more effective in reducing anxiety in their patients compared with the inexperienced practitioners. Despite some limitations, the SETTS may serve as a guide in selecting nurses who are experienced and effective in the practice of Therapeutic Touch.

The Energy Field Assessment was developed to record specific qualities of the Therapeutic Touch energy field assessment (Wright 1988). This tool is a one-page, three-part form designed to translate the subjective experience of energy field assessment into measurable terms. Wright demonstrated good face, content, and construct validity for the tool. She found significant relationships between location of field disturbance and physical location of pain and between decreased background strength of the field and fatigue but no significant relationship between field disturbance and pain intensity. Although the tool requires further testing, it could serve as a useful guide for nurses learning Therapeutic Touch.

A Therapeutic Touch inservice education course, currently the focus of a demonstration project, has been developed and may serve as a guide to teaching-learning Therapeutic Touch in an acute-care setting (Mahoney, Meehan, Malinski, and Iervolino 1990). The course is designed for beginning practitioners and includes basic theory and practice instruction plus continuing guidance with integrating the intervention into the care of patients.

NURSING DIAGNOSES AND APPROPRIATE PATIENT GROUPS

Because Therapeutic Touch generally promotes relaxation and comfort and thereby facilitates the natural healing process in the patient, it can be used with a wide variety of patient groups. The research literature suggests that Therapeutic Touch may be useful for the diagnoses Pain and Anxiety. The practice literature suggests that Therapeutic Touch may be useful for the diagnoses Ineffective Individual Coping, Fear, Anticipatory Grieving, Impaired Physical Mobility, Powerlessness, and Sleep Pattern Disturbance.

There is essentially no risk in using Therapeutic Touch, but there are some patient groups with which caution is suggested. For many patients, Therapeutic Touch appears to be a new and very different kind of intervention. Therefore, it is generally not wise to use it to treat patients with critical, labile conditions, such as a bleeding intracranial aneurysm awaiting surgery, where absolute quiet is required and it is better not to introduce different and nonessential circumstances. For patients with psychiatric illnesses where the nursing diagnosis Alteration in Thought Processes applies, Therapeutic Touch should be used only by nurses who have had several years' experience with Therapeutic Touch and with caring for such patients and who have excellent clinical judgment. Such patients are often extremely sensitive to close human interaction and to its meaning for them.

RECOMMENDATIONS FOR PRACTICE

These recommendations apply particularly to practice in an acute-care setting and can be adapted for use in other settings. They may seem unnecessarily stringent to some nurses who use Therapeutic Touch and believe that its use is of concern only to the nurse and patient involved. But in most situations, many individuals are involved in patients' care, standards of practice are important, and a clear explanation of Therapeutic Touch as a nursing intervention is necessary to prevent any misunderstandings about its nature and its place in nursing practice. These recommendations are based on 10 years' experience with practice and research of Therapeutic Touch in a major medical center.

Nurses who use Therapeutic Touch should have had at least 6 months' experience in professional practice in an acute-care setting. Their learning of Therapeutic Touch should have been guided by a nurse who has had at least 2 years' experience in using Therapeutic Touch, preferably has a master's degree in nursing, and conforms to the practice guidelines developed by Kunz and Krieger (1975–1990). They should have had 30 hours of instruction in the theory and practice of Therapeutic Touch in a nursing basic or continuing-education program and 30 hours of supervised practice with relatively healthy individuals and have successfully completed written and practice evaluations. They should have a basic understanding of the Science of Unitary Human Beings model and should be able to discuss the references cited for this chapter and all of the peer-reviewed literature related to Therapeutic Touch. They should know the arguments for and against the theoretical rationale underlying Therapeutic Touch and be able to discuss the intervention in terms that can be understood by health professionals and patients who are not familiar with it.

Some colleagues and other health professionals will not be familiar with the theoretical rationale underlying Therapeutic Touch and will consider the intervention quite unconventional. Nurses must ensure that the nursing administrators with whom they work know about Therapeutic Touch as a nursing intervention and have had plenty of opportunity to discuss its use in relation to the range of nursing diagnoses of the particular patient group.

Care must be taken to ensure that the patient's physician or medical team, and other health professionals, also know what Therapeutic Touch is, why the patient will receive it as part of the nursing care plan, and what the expected outcomes are. This is particularly important because Therapeutic Touch is not congruent with the mechanistic, physical-sensory model that underlies medical practice. It is also important because of the implications that the effects of Therapeutic Touch may have for medical interventions such as pain medication. Such exchange of information and discussion can take place through inservice education, staff meetings, and informal meetings.

Procedure

Preparation

When introducing Therapeutic Touch to a patient, it is best to begin with a relatively simple explanation, which can be elaborated upon if necessary. The patient's door or bedside curtains should be closed so that disturbance during the intervention is minimized. The nurse may explain to the patient that during the treatment she will be focusing her attention on her hands and probably will not be talking, but if there is anything that he wants to mention or at any time wants her to stop, he should say so. The patient should be in as comfortable a position as possible, either resting in bed or sitting out of bed. If resting in bed, the patient can lie on his back or side, and the treatment is done over the unimpeded area of the patient and over the bedclothes. If sitting out of bed, it is best if the patient can sit on a stool or sideways on a chair so that the area around the front and upper back of the patient is unimpeded. But this position may be too tiring for some patients, and the intervention can be quite adequately carried out with the patient resting in a high-backed chair. If the patient is sitting on a stool or sideways on a chair, the treatment will be done over the front and upper back of the patient.

The nurse prepares herself to carry out the intervention by centering herself and remains centered throughout the intervention. In centering, she shifts her awareness from a direct focus on her physical environment to an inner focus on what she perceives as the center of life within herself—a center of calm and balance through which she perceives herself and the patient as unitary wholes. Her attitude becomes one of clear, gentle, and compassionate attention to the patient and of focused intent to help the patient but is completely detached from any personal feelings or emotions. She remains quite aware of her physical environment, but this is not the primary focus of her attention. For the experienced practitioner, centering takes less than 5 seconds.

Assessment

The assessment is done in relation to two principles: openness and symmetry. In a state of health, the energy is perceived as a gentle, symmetrical, open flow from head to feet. In a state of illness, the flow is perceived as congested, unsymmetrical, and impeded. The nurse moves her hands, with the palms facing toward the patient and at a distance of 2 inches to 4 inches, over the body of the patient from head to feet in a smooth, light movement. She attunes to the patient's condition by perceiving the pattern of the energy flow through differences in sensory cues in her hands. These cues are extremely subtle and are described by such adjectives as *warmth, coolness, tightness, heaviness, tingling,* and *emptiness.* The nurse notes the overall pattern of the energy flow and any areas of imbalance or impeded flow. Areas of congestion or imbalance are often but not always directly related to areas of illness in the patient's body. The initial assessment is done fairly quickly, in about 30 seconds, but some assessment continues throughout the intervention. After completing the initial assessment, the nurse may, depending on the patient, stop for a moment and tell the patient in general terms her perception of the energy flow and how she will do the treatment.

Treatment

During the treatment phase, the nurse focuses her intent on the specific repatterning of areas of imbalance and impeded flow, using her hands as focal points, for a period of 2 minutes to 10 minutes. Her intent is to dissipate areas of imbalance and facilitate a gentle, symmetrical, open flow. She begins by moving her hands in gentle, sweeping movements from head to feet one time. As she moves her hands over the lower legs and feet, she notes whether there is an open flow of energy in this area. If there is not, she will continue moving her hands over this area or hold the patient's feet physically to facilitate at least some energy flow. Experience has shown that if there is no flow in this lower area at the beginning of the intervention, patterning of congestion in areas over the upper body will be difficult and may feel uncomfortable to the patient.

The nurse then focuses her attention in areas where she has perceived particular imbalances or congestion. For example, if she feels an area of "heat" over the left side of the patient's abdomen, she will project an image of "coolness" as she moves one hand repeatedly through that area, moving the other hand at the same time over the right side of the abdomen and bringing the left and right side into balance.

If she perceives an area of "heaviness" or "tingling" over the patient's chest, she will project an image of a flowing or smoothing movement as she moves her hands repeatedly through the area until she begins to feel the quality of the energy flow change. As she moves her hands through the energy flow, she will at times feel that some of the congestion is clinging to her hands. A brief shake of her hands will dissipate this feeling. To complete the treatment, she places her hands over the area of the solar plexus (just above the waist) and focuses specifically on facilitating the flow of healing energy to the patient.

Length of Intervention

The intervention time depends on the age and needs of the patient. It will range from about 2 minutes for a premature or small infant to 5 minutes to 10 minutes for an adult. Most research studies have used a 5-minute treatment, and generally no more than a 10-minute treatment is needed. Hospitalized patients usually receive the intervention once or twice a day, or they may receive it with each dose of prn analgesic medication. The indications for the intervention and its effects will be recorded in the patient's nursing record.

This outline of the procedure is an elaboration of the operational definition of the intervention used in research studies. It can be supplemented by a much more comprehensive description (Macrae 1988) and by video illustration (Hospital Satellite Network, 1986) and subjective description (Meehan 1990) of practice in an acute-care setting.

CASE STUDY

Mrs. M was hospitalized for a total abdominal hysterectomy because of fibroids. She was 55 years old, otherwise healthy, and of medium build and weight and groomed appearance. She was a widow of 2 years, financially secure, had two grown sons who lived some distance away, and gave the impression of being self-sufficient. She lived an intensely active professional life as a stock analyst for a prominent financial organization and took little time to pursue her more lighthearted interests.

Her surgery was straightforward and her postoperative condition stable. By her third postoperative day, her urinary catheter had been removed, and she was voiding without problem. She had progressed to a soft diet and was able to get out of bed and walk by herself. She reported a moderate amount of incisional pain, for which she received 2 tablets of Percocet every 4 hours to 6 hours. She experienced difficulty sleeping and was prescribed Nembutal 100 mg to settle at night and a repeat dose in 4 hours as needed, which she took. But this had not helped her and a switch to Chloral Hydrate had been made.

Although she was making good physical progress and said that she was "just fine," she was becoming increasingly tense and irritable. Mrs. M's primary nurse took extra time to attend to Mrs. M, using Presence and Active Listening. During this interaction, some of Mrs. M's self-sufficient manner began to melt away. It emerged that she was not sleeping despite the hypnotic medication and was beginning to feel "spaced out." She felt anxious about not being able to cope by herself and profoundly sad about the loss of "part of myself." In addition, although she thought that she had adjusted well to her husband's death, she really missed him now. In her words, "Everything seems just pent up inside of me, and I do wish he was here."

Her primary nursing diagnoses were Anxiety, Pain, and Sleep Pattern Disturbance. The nurse's use of Presence and Active Listening comforted Mrs. M and helped her relax. The nurse explained Therapeutic Touch to her, and Mrs. M said that she would like to try it with her pain medication and instead of her sleeping medication. The first night Mrs. M received Therapeutic Touch when she settled to sleep and again when she awoke at 3:00 A.M. She felt more rested in the morning. On subsequent nights she received Therapeutic Touch when she settled to sleep and slept through the night. She felt that receiving Therapeutic Touch with her analgesic (which had been decreased to Tylenol) facilitated her naturally decreasing need for analgesia. Overall, she began to feel more energetic and also relieved that she could take care of herself again.

For about 2 months after discharge, she continued to receive a Therapeutic Touch treatment once a week at a Saturday morning nursing clinic. She felt that it helped her "get settled into my life again."

CONCLUSION

For many nurses, the use of Therapeutic Touch seems close to the heart of nursing practice. They feel that, to borrow a phrase from Nightingale (1859), it is one way by which they can truly "put the patient in the best condition for nature to act upon him" (p. 110). Others have questioned its appropriateness (Curtin 1980) and effectiveness (Clark and Clark 1984) as a nursing intervention. Further investigation of its nature and effects is clearly necessary and should include a wide range of carefully designed quantitative and qualitative studies. In the meantime, Therapeutic Touch will continue to play a significant role in helping patients, in strengthening nurses' commitment to nursing, and in contributing moments of nurturance and peacefulness in the often stressful and troubled world.

REFERENCES

Boguslawski, M. 1979. The use of therapeutic touch in nursing. *Journal of Continuing Education in Nursing* 10 (4):9–15.

Boguslawski, M. 1980. Therapeutic touch: A facilitator of pain relief. *Topics in Clinical Nursing* 2 (1):27–37.

Bohm, D. 1973. Quantum theory as an indication of a new order in physical law. *Foundations of Physics* 3 (2):144–156.

Borelli, M.D., and Heidt, P. (eds.). 1981. *Therapeutic touch.* New York: Springer.

Braun, C., Layton, J., and Braun, J. 1986. Therapeutic touch improves residents' sleep. *American Health Care Association Journal* 12 (1):48–49.

Bulbrook, M.J. 1984. Bulbrook's model of therapeutic touch: One form of health and healing in the future. *Canadian Nurse* 80 (11):30–34.

Burr, H.S. 1972. *Blueprint for immortality: The electric patterns of life.* London: Neville Spearman.

Capek, M. 1961. *The philosophical impact of contemporary physics.* New York: Van Nostrand.

Clark, P.E., and Clark, M.J. 1984. Therapeutic touch: Is there a scientific basis for practice? *Nursing Research* 33 (1):37–41.

Connell, M.T. 1983. Feminine consciousness and the nature of nursing practice: A historical perspective. *Topics in Clinical Nursing* 5 (3):1–10.

Curtin, L. 1980. Nurse quackery (editorial). *Supervisor Nurse* 11 (3):9.

Egan, E. 1985. Therapeutic touch. In M. Snyder, *Independent nursing interventions* (pp. 199–210). New York: John Wiley.

Fanslow, C.A. 1983. Therapeutic touch: A healing modality throughout life. *Topics in Clinical Nursing* 5 (2):72–79.

Fedoruk, R.B. 1984. Transfer of the relaxation response: Therapeutic touch B as a method for reduction of stress in premature neonates. Doctoral dissertation, University of Maryland. (University Microfilms No. 8509162)

Ferguson, C 1986. Subjective experience of therapeutic touch survey (SETTS): Psychometric examination of an instrument. Doctoral dissertation, University of Texas at Austin. (University Microfilms No. 8618464)

Finnerin, D. 1981. Therapeutic touch for children and their families. In M.D. Borelli and P. Heidt (eds.), *Therapeutic touch* (pp. 64–71). New York: Springer.

Guillemin, V. 1986. *The story of quantum mechanics.* New York: Charles Scribner's.

Hale, E.H. 1986. A study of the relationship between therapeutic touch and the anxiety levels of hospitalized adults. Doctoral dissertation, Texas Women's University. (University Microfilm No. 8618897)

Heidt, P. 1981. Effect of therapeutic touch on the anxiety level of hospitalized patients. *Nursing Research* 30 (1):33–37.

Heidt, P.R. 1990. Openness: A qualitative analysis of nurses' and patients' experiences of therapeutic touch. *Image: The Journal of Nursing Scholarship* 22 (3):180–186.

Hospital Satellite Network (Producer). American Journal of Nursing Company (Distributor). 1986. *Therapeutic touch: A new skill from an ancient practice.* (Videocassette No. 7538) New York: American Journal of Nursing Company.

Jackson, M.E. 1981. The use of therapeutic touch in the nursing care of the terminally ill person. In M.D. Borelli and P. Heidt (eds.), *Therapeutic touch* (pp. 72–79). New York: Springer.

Jonasen, A.M. 1981. Therapeutic touch in the operating room: Best of both worlds. In M.D. Borelli and P. Heidt (eds.), *Therapeutic touch* (pp. 80–84). New York: Springer.

Jurgens, A., Meehan, T.C., and Wilson, H.L. 1987. Therapeutic touch as a nursing intervention. *Holistic Nursing Practice* 2 (1):1–13.

Keegan, L. 1988. Touch: Connecting with the healing power. In B.M. Dossey, L. Keegan, C.E. Guzzetta, and L.G. Kolkmeier. (eds.), *Holistic nursing* (pp. 331–355). Rockville, Md.: Aspen.

Keller, E.K. 1984. Therapeutic touch: A review of the literature and implications of a holistic nursing modality. *Journal of Holistic Nursing* 2 (1):24–29.

Keller, E., and Bzdek, V.M. 1986. Effects of therapeutic touch on tension headache pain. *Nursing Research* 35 (2):101–106.

Krieger, D. 1975. Therapeutic touch: The imprimatur of nursing. *American Journal of Nursing* 75 (5):784–787.

Krieger, D. 1979. *The therapeutic touch: How to use your hands to help or to heal.* Englewood Cliffs, N.J.: Prentice-Hall.

Krieger, D., Peper, E. and Ancoli, S. 1979. Therapeutic touch: Searching for evidence of physiological change. *American Journal of Nursing* 79 (4):660–662.

Kunz, D. 1985. Compassion, rootedness and detachment: Their role in healing. In D. Kunz (ed.), *Spiritual aspects of the healing arts* (pp. 289–305). Wheaton, Ill.: Theosophical Publishing House.

Kunz, D., and Krieger, D. 1965–1972. Healing Workshops. Pumpkin Hollow Foundation, Craryville, N.Y.

Kunz, D., and Krieger, D. 1975–1990. Annual Invitational Workshops on Therapeutic Touch. Pumpkin Hollow Foundation, Craryville, N.Y.

Leduc, E. 1987. Therapeutic touch (letter). *Neonatal Network* 5 (6):46–47.

Lionberger, H. 1985. An interpretative study of nurses' practice of therapeutic touch. Doctoral dissertation, University of California at San Francisco. (University Microfilms No. 8524008)

Lionberger, H.J. 1986. Therapeutic touch: A healing modality or a caring strategy. In P.L. Chin (ed.), *Methodological issues in nursing.* Gaithersberg, Md.: Aspen:

Macrae, J. 1979. Therapeutic touch in practice. *American Journal of Nursing* 79 (4):664–665.

Macrae, J. 1988. *Therapeutic touch: A practical guide.* New York: Knopf.

Mahoney, K., Meehan, T.C. Malinski, V., Iervolino, L. 1990. *Stein Inservice Education Demonstration Project on Therapeutic Touch.* Unpublished project outline. Department of Nursing, New York University Medical Center, New York.

Mead, M. 1956. Nursing—primitive and civilized. *American Journal of Nursing* 56 (8):101–104.

Meehan, T.C. 1985. The effect of therapeutic touch on the experience of acute pain in postoperative patients. Doctoral dissertation, New York University. (University Microfilms No. 8510765)

Meehan, T.C. 1986. *The effect of therapeutic touch on acute pain in postoperative patients: Secondary analysis.* Unpublished report. Department of Nursing, New York University Medical Center, New York.

Meehan, T.C. 1990. The science of unitary human beings and theory-based practice: Therapeutic Touch. In E.A. Barrett (ed.), *Visions of Rogers' science-based nursing.* New York: National League for Nursing.

Meehan, T.C., Mahoney, K., Ake, J., Iervolino L., Glassman, K., Tedesco, P., Mariano, C. 1990. *A professional-self development program for nurses: Final project report to the United Hospital Fund.* Department of Nursing, New York University Medical Center, New York.

Meehan, T.C., Mersmann, C.A. Wiseman, M., Wolff, B.B., and Malgady, R. 1990. The effect of therapeutic touch on postoperative pain (abstract). *Pain* (Suppl. 5), 149.

Meehan, T.C. Mersmann, C.A., Wiseman, M., Wolff, B.B., Malgady, R. 1991. *Therapeutic touch and surgical patients' stress reactions: Final project report to National Center for Nursing Research, NIH.* Department of Nursing, New York University Medical Center, New York.

Miller, L. 1979. An explanation of therapeutic touch using the science of unitary man. *Nursing Forum* 18 (3):278–287.

Mueller Hinze, M.L. 1988. The effects of therapeutic touch and acupressure on experimentally-induced pain. Doctoral dissertation, University of Texas at Austin. (University Microfilms No. 8901377)

Newshan, G. 1989. Therapeutic touch for symptom control in persons with AIDS. *Holistic Nursing Practice* 3 (4):45–51.

Nightingale, F. 1980. *Notes on nursing: What it is and what it is not.* (Replication of original publication by Harrison & Sons, London, 1859). Edinburgh: Churchill Livingstone.

Parks, B.S. 1985. Therapeutic touch as an intervention to reduce anxiety in elderly hospitalized patients. Doctoral dissertation, University of Texas at Austin. (University Microfilms No. 8609563)

Payne, M.B. 1989. The use of therapeutic touch with rehabilitation clients. *Rehabilitation Nursing* 15 (2):69–72.

Peric-Knowlton, W. 1984. The understanding and management of acute pain in adults: The nursing contribution. *International Journal of Nursing Studies* 21:141–143.

Quinn, J. 1979. One nurse's evolution as a healer. *American Journal of Nursing* 79 (4):662–664.

Quinn, J. 1982. An investigation of the effects of therapeutic touch done without physical contact on state anxiety of hospitalized cardiovascular patients. Doctoral dissertation, New York University. (University Microfilm No. 8226788)

Quinn, J. 1984. Therapeutic touch as energy exchange: Testing the theory. *Advances in Nursing Science* 6 (2):42–49.

Quinn, J. 1989. Therapeutic touch as energy exchange: Replication and extension. *Nursing Science Quarterly* 2 (2):79–87.

Randolph, G.L. 1984. Therapeutic and physical touch: Physiological response to stressful stimuli. *Nursing Research* 33 (1):33–36.

Rogers, M.E. 1970. *An introduction to the theoretical basis of nursing.* Philadelphia: F.A. Davis.

Rogers, M.E. 1990. Nursing: Science of unitary, irreducible, human beings: Update 1990. In E.A. Barrett (ed.), *Visions of Rogers' science-based nursing* (pp. 5–11). New York: National League for Nursing.

Rowlands, D. 1984. Therapeutic touch: Its effects on the depressed elderly. *Australian Nurses Journal* 13 (11):45–46.

Simeone C. 1985. Changing practice through therapeutic touch. *California Nurse* 80 (10):618.

Weber, R. 1979. Philosophical foundations and frameworks for healing. *Re-Vision* 2 (2):66–76.

Weber, R. (ed.). 1986. *Dialogues with scientists and sages: The search for unity in science and mysticism.* London: Routledge & Kegan Paul.

Winstead-Fry, P. 1983. *A report to the profession: Nursing research emphasis grant: Families and parenting.* Division of Nursing, New York University, School of Education, Health, Nursing and Arts Professions.

Wolfson, I.S. 1984. Therapeutic touch and midwifery. In C. C. Brown (ed.), *The many facets of touch.* Skillman, N.J.: Johnson & Johnson.

Woods-Smith, D. 1988. Therapeutic touch: A healing experience. *Maine Nurse* 74 (2):3, 7.

Wright, S.M. 1987. The use of therapeutic touch in the management of pain. *Nursing Clinics of North America* 22 (3):704–715.

Wright, S.M. 1988. Development and construct validity of the energy field asessment form. Doctoral dissertation, Rush University. (University Microfilm No. 8821431)

Wyatt, G. 1988. Therapeutic touch: Promoting and assessing conceptual change among health care professionals. Doctoral dissertation, Michigan State University.

Wyatt, G. 1989. Keeping the caring touch in the high-tech maze. *Michigan Hospitals* 26 (5):6–9.

16

MEDICATION MANAGEMENT

ELIZABETH A. WEITZEL

Nurses, in their daily practice, by example and by using every opportunity to help patients make a constructive use and informed choice of all kinds of drugs, can affect the so-called drug problem.

V. Henderson and G. Nite

DESCRIPTION OF THE INTERVENTION

Medication Management is a comprehensive term encompassing the spectrum of knowledge, skills, and interpersonal relationships necessary for the nurse to employ to maximize the effectiveness and minimize the risk of legal drug usage. (Although the illegal use of drugs is of concern to health professionals, it will not be addressed in this chapter.) The role of the nurse in the use of medications is diverse. In addition to the dependent function of administering medications following the orders of a legally qualified health practitioner, there are a number of collaborative and independent aspects.

Sometimes the nurse is responsible for the actual administration of the medication, sometimes the nurse is supervising another staff member, and sometimes the client or family administers the medication.

In addition to knowing why the drug is prescribed, the expected action, and probable side effects, the nurse must be aware of the drug's interactions with other drugs and food, special precautions with the route being used, knowledge of the client, and the knowledge and skill of other staff involved with the administration and monitoring of the medication.

REVIEW OF LITERATURE

Dependent versus Independent Function

The dependent function of the nurse in implementing legally written medication orders is widely accepted. The nurse practice act of many states also recognizes the responsibility of the nurse to monitor health care status and provide health teaching and counseling. These are usually described as collaborative or independent functions, not requiring the written permission of another health professional. Effective practice requires that the nurse integrates the dependent or assistive function of medication administration with the collaborative or independent intervention of Medication Management, appropriately seeking advice or written orders when necessary but also acting on the nurse's own knowledge base.

Knowledge and Skill of the Nurse

The basic nursing education has laid the foundation for the knowledge and skills necessary for Medication Management, including actions of broad classifications of medications, the rudiments of how drugs are absorbed in the body, delivered, metabolized, and excreted, and safe administration of medications by a variety of routes. The constant changes in medications available and their use require nurses to update their knowledge about specific drugs continuously.

As the nurse develops a practice in a specific area, it is important that the knowledge base be expanded in the drugs common to that area, including more detail of the actions of those drugs in the body, common interactions, and side effects—both common and those less likely. The nurse also monitors the effectiveness of the administration modality, being aware of swallowing difficulties with oral administration, adequate retention of the medication with oral, rectal, or vaginal administration, and potential tissue breakdown or damage with topical or parenteral medications.

Error Rates

Fuqua and Stevens (1988), in a literature review on this subject, contend that medication errors are the skeleton in the closet of health care providers. The actual rate of error is not known due to suspected underdetection and underreporting. Several hospital studies cited by Jesse (1981) indicated reported errors in 13% to 18% of all doses administered.

Responsibility for accurate administration of medications is shared by staff nurses, nurse administrators and educators, pharmacists, physicians, and drug manufacturers. This chapter covers the responsibilities shared by nurses. Fuqua and Stevens (1988) found that medication errors were related to the staff nurse variables of inadequate knowledge or medication administration skills, failure to comply with required policy or procedure, and failure in communication. They also found that errors decreased with nursing experience, unless there were increased distractions, interactions, consecutive hours worked, or rotating shifts. However, Bayne and Bindler (1988) found that years of experience was negatively correlated to accurate medication calculation, with nurses having 3 years or less experience the most accurate on a medication calculation test.

Faddis wrote in 1939 that teachers and administrators of nursing are responsible for errors to the extent that they allow conditions to exist that are conducive to making mistakes. Current nursing literature supports this contention. A number of mechanisms for reducing error rates have been reported. One is a severity index for medication errors based on the impact on the client and leading to the appropriate nursing action (Brandt, Deml, Gerke, and Lee 1988).

Other suggestions are aimed at either the agency or the individual employee. The agency is responsible for providing and reviewing policies and procedures that clearly describe correct behavior and define what constitutes a medication error. The agency can also publicize summaries of error rates and common errors and develop a medication deviations committee that includes staff nurses as members. The agency is responsible for pursuing ways of reducing stress and maintaining adequate staffing. There is some evidence that individual behavior can be improved by medication administration training, credentialing, and attendance at a behavior-oriented safety program (Fuqua and Stevens 1988).

Nurses can help physicians, pharmacists, and drug manufacturers assume their share of responsibility by communicating their concerns in a timely fashion.

Impact of Technology

As new technology becomes available, nurses are confronted with changes in all aspects of drug administration, including new routes of administration, different methods of packaging, and new equipment for delivering and monitoring the effects of the drug.

Patient-controlled analgesia is one example of such technology, using an electronically controlled infusion pump connected to a timing device. This pump allows patients to administer small amounts of an analgesic directly into their indwelling intravenous line by pressing a button. The pump can be programmed for the amount of the dose delivered and the frequency of repeat doses. The effectiveness of this device in controlling pain and recording usage has been established in pain research and demonstrated in clinical practice (Giuffre, Keane, Hatfield, and Korevaar 1988).

Another example of technology applied to medication administration includes subcutaneous infusion pumps for analgesia or other medication. These pumps, which can be implanted in the body or worn externally, are effective in hospice home care.

Changing technology is also evident in the increased usage of transdermal patches for a wider variety of medications, now including narcotics, as well as nitroglycerin and scopolamine. Progesterone can be implanted subcutaneously and remain effective for up to 5 years. Nasal spray is being used to deliver a wider range of medications. Aerosol inhalers also deliver a wider range of medications, including nitroglycerin.

Nurses in long-term and home health care are encountering more patients who require knowledge of and skill in dealing with the changes in technology. Three pharmacists describe the multidisciplinary effort to implement a parenteral antibiotic program in the home setting (Kasmer, Hoisington, and Yuniewicz 1987). They have found that, with careful selection of patients, this program is cost-effective and provides several advantages to the patient over prolonged hospitalization.

Even the use of pill boxes with programmable timers requires the nurse to learn new skills and broaden her knowledge base.

Review of Medications

In the acute-care setting, nurses share with doctors and pharmacists the responsibility for review of all the medications prescribed for a particular patient. The purpose of this review is to maximize the effectiveness and minimize the adverse effects of prescribed medications. In home health care and long-term care, this function also emphasizes the review of a continued need for the medication over the long term.

The nurse is likely to be the first to identify that problems have developed with a particular drug, due to proximity to the patient and frequency of contact, which allows the nurse to identify subtle changes in the patient's usual condition. Souter (1990) relates a case in which she advocated for a patient based on subtle changes that she and the patient's wife observed following cardiac artery bypass surgery, ultimately uncovering digitalis toxicity.

As more care delivery systems use the concept of managed care, the role of the nurse in regular review of medications becomes even more crucial. In some respects, review is more effective when one person is familiar with and coordinating all aspects of care.

Supervision of Other Staff

The registered nurse may delegate the administration of certain medications to other staff, but this does not relieve the nurse of responsibility for knowing what drugs the patients in her care are receiving, for what reason, or the patient's response to that medication. It does add the responsibility of overseeing the actions of the staff member to whom this has been delegated, just as it does in any other aspect of care that is delegated. Primary nursing or total patient care has been viewed as one way to avoid this added responsibility. Careful analysis of the needs of the client population and abilities of staff are necessary to determine which staff are best assigned the responsibility of safely administering medications.

Administration of Medications by the Client or Family Member

Most persons spend a very small portion of their lives in a health care institution where staff are administering the medications. Learning to take one's own medication or to administer medication to a family member is crucial to managing chronic disease.

There are several reasons that persons who can correctly demonstrate ability and knowledge in the hospital fail to do so at home. When there seems to be no change in one's overall condition, it might be erroneously concluded that the medication is no longer needed. Cost is also a significant factor in correct usage and continuing to refill prescriptions. A reluctance to take any medication is a factor that may lead to prematurely stopping a medication. When taking the medication interrupts one's life-style, such as urinary frequency with a diuretic, the medication may not be taken as directed. Careful assessment and teaching are needed to combat these problems.

Forgetfulness about the need to take a medication or if the dose has already been taken can also lead to inaccurate use of medications. There are a variety of ways to jog memory or allow for checking whether a dose has been taken, some devised from materials around the home and some commercially prepared. Charts for recording doses taken and containers for daily allotments can help remind and allow for checking on doses consumed.

Patsdaughter and Pesznecker (1988) describe four broad areas of nursing activities related to monitoring medication in the home care setting: communication/coordination with other providers, counseling/discussion, client/family teaching, and direct nursing activities, such as physical or psychosocial monitoring, developing reminders, and conducting pill counts. Their study demonstrated that nurses did not always use the full range of possible nursing activities, perhaps leaving their clients at greater risk than necessary.

Periodic review of all medications, both prescription and over-the-counter and any home remedies being taken, will enhance the effectiveness and decrease the likelihood of significant adverse effects.

Over-the-Counter Medications

Medications legally available without prescription are estimated to be used in over half of all health problems in the United States (Facts and Comparisons Drug Newsletter 1986). One of the problems in the use of these medications is that the only information the user may have received about these drugs is through advertisements, which are often vague and sometimes misleading. The information printed on the package is often in small print, and the important information is difficult to decipher. The user has no knowledge of how this drug may interact with other over-the-counter drugs or with prescription drugs or the effectiveness of the drug for the condition being treated (Forman 1986).

As a number of drugs that previously were available by prescription only now become available in low dosages without prescription, this problem becomes even greater. Nurses have a role in identifying which of these products clients are using and assisting them to receive accurate information about how these products will most likely influence the existing condition.

Home health remedies vary among cultural groups but are generally used by all. Nurses who are aware of the common home remedies being used in their geographic location can inquire about these practices as part of the initial and ongoing assessment. There are also an increasing number of nontraditional (other than allopathic) health practitioners advocating therapies other than prescription medications. The nurse may be able to help the client incorporate these therapies with allopathic therapies or identify components that are dangerous and suggest more appropriate methods (Roberson 1987).

ASSOCIATED NURSING DIAGNOSES

Since the use of medication is so pervasive in modern health care, almost any nursing diagnosis could be related to the intervention of Medication Management. However, a few diagnoses most logically lead to Medication Management as an intervention: Potential for Poisoning, Altered Health Maintenance, Noncompliance, and Knowledge Deficit.

The need for Medication Management with Potential for Poisoning is obvious. In making this diagnosis, the nurse has identified that a person is taking a drug that, given the characteristics of the drug and the condition of the client, has a high potential to lead to drug toxicity. The nurse will need to use knowledge and skill to teach all involved with this situation how the medication is to be administered safely, the factors to monitor that might indicate toxicity, and any action that needs to be taken when these indicators are present.

Altered Health Maintenance by definition refers to "a state in which a person or group experiences or is at risk of experiencing a disruption in health because of an unhealthy life-style or lack of knowledge to manage a condition" (McLane 1987). Knowledge Deficit may be an etiology of this diagnosis, which leads to health teaching and other aspects of Medication Management.

Noncompliance is defined as "the state in which an individual or group desires to comply, but factors are present that deter adherence to health-related advice given by health professionals" (McLane 1987). Again, Knowledge Deficit may be an etiology, and Medication Management, including teaching, may be an appropriate intervention. The person or group must wish to comply for this diagnosis to be applied.

SUGGESTED PROTOCOL FOR MEDICATION MANAGEMENT

Application of Medication Management requires three broad areas of nursing activities; they will be described as separate functions but are actually interrelated: knowledge of the drug and all aspects of its administration; knowledge of the client and family life-style and how taking this medication will affect them; and maintaining open relationships with the client and family, the physician, and the pharmacist.

Knowledge of the Drug and Its Administration

The knowledge about a particular drug or group of drugs increases as a nurse works with clients who are likely to be taking these medications. The nurse reads available literature and consults with the pharmacist and physician to increase knowledge of the intended and adverse effects and details of administration. As clients use medications, the nurse observes the changes in the client and adds this information to the previous knowledge base.

As new technology becomes available, the nurse may deal with a representative of the manufacturer in learning how to use the new equipment, in addition to reading literature available about the product.

Knowledge of the Client and Family Life-style

This area begins with the initial assessment of the client and includes information gathered by other health professionals in their interactions with the client and family. It also requires integrating knowledge of the actions of the medication with information about the client, the family, and their living environment and discussing ways to deal with areas of potential conflict between the prescribed therapy and how the client and family wish to live.

Maintaining Open Relationships

Accurate and pertinent information may be overlooked or unavailable if open communication does not exist among all parties involved. The nurse is often responsible for maintaining this communication and clarifying information. One particular area of concern is interactions that may occur between prescription medications and other prescription medications, over-the-counter medications, home remedies, or food. The pharmacist or other available references should be used until the nurse becomes familiar with common interactions related to medications for which the nurse is responsible.

CASE STUDY

Case Study 1

A 59-year-old man has been admitted to the medical unit following a stay in the intensive care unit. He had a myocardial infarction and has been digitalized for subsequent congestive heart failure. During the second shift you care for him you notice he seems to be slightly confused about recent events, quite different from his behavior yesterday. His chart indicates that over the past 2 days, he has complained of a dull headache that was not relieved by acetaminophen, anorexia, and tingling around the mouth and in the fingers. You assess him and find his pulse has risen from a usual of 80 to 102. He has no pain or fever at this time. He mentions seeing frost on surfaces in the room.

Putting together these symptoms and his recent digitalization and continued administration of digoxin 0.25 mg daily, you suspect he may be starting to become toxic with digitalis. You note that Potential for Poisoning is one of his nursing diagnoses. You confer with the physician when he makes rounds. He orders the digoxin to be held until the results of a serum digitalis level are reported to him. When the level is completed, it is above therapeutic range, and the doctor orders, "No digoxin tomorrow. Begin digoxin 0.125 the following day." The patient responds well and is behaving appropriately in 2 days and is discharged to return home. The doctor leaves a written order with the patient to go to the laboratory and have a repeat serum digitalis level drawn in 1 week.

In addition to teaching this patient about changes in life-style following the myocardial infarction, you will instruct him about the amount and times he will be taking digoxin, how it strengthens his heart, the side effects to look for, and which ones require immediate reporting to the physician. You may discuss ways to remember to take the dose at a regular time each day and to allow for verifying that the dose has been taken. Using printed information sheets, which you review with the patient, will improve his ability to retain the information you have shared, especially if you personalize the information for him. You will also discuss when and how to come to the laboratory for the follow-up serum level.

Case Study 2

A 42-year-old woman seen in the outpatient clinic has been diagnosed having fibromyalgia. The doctor has given her prescriptions for ibuprofen, 400 mg three times a day, and amitriptyline, 10 mg, 1 to 3 tablets, 3 hours before bed. The doctor has asked you to instruct the patient on appropriate use of these medications. You use printed information sheets, personalizing them for this woman. You discuss the advisability of taking ibuprofen with food to reduce stomach irritation, explain why this medication is prescribed, and review the side effects, noting which ones require immediate notification of the physician.

You also use printed information about amitriptyline, reinforcing the doctor's explanation of the desired action being promotion of deeper sleep. You review other aspects of sleep hygiene and the effect of caffeine and alcohol on sleep. You discuss how caffeine might interfere with the effectiveness of amitriptyline and that alcohol will exaggerate morning drowsiness. You discuss this woman's usual pattern of bedtime and awakening to help determine the best time to take the medication to avoid undue nighttime drowsiness and morning carry-over. The patient should not drive after taking the medication, especially until it is known how she will respond to this medication.

She notes that constipation is one of the side effects and comments that she already has problems. You note Constipation as a nursing diagnosis in her record. You discuss the basics of good bowel hygiene, encourage increasing her fluid intake to 2000 cc daily, adding raw fruits and vegetables, and emphasize the gentle exercise routine that has already been discussed with the doctor. You tell her to call if this does not take care of the problem.

SUMMARY

It is appropriate for the nurse to use Medication Management with clients who are taking any form of medication or home remedy to increase the effectiveness and minimize adverse effects. This intervention requires the nurse to have knowledge of and skill in medication administration, action of medications, client and family relationships and life-style, and interpersonal skills with other health professionals. Most of all, the nurse must be willing to act as the client's advocate.

REFERENCES

Bayne, T., and Bindler, R. 1988. Medication calculation skills of registered nurses. *Journal of Continuing Education in Nursing* 19(6):258–262.

Brandt, M., Deml, M., Gerke, M., and Lee, E. 1988. A severity index for medication errors. *Nursing Management* 19(8):80I–80N.

Facts and Comparison Drug Newsletter. 1986. St. Louis: Lippincott.

Faddis, M.O. 1939. Eliminating errors in medication. *American Journal of Nursing* 39(11):1217–1223.

Forman, H. 1986. Patient education and non-prescription drugs. *Patient Education and Counseling* 8:415–418.

Fuqua, R., and Stevens, K. 1988. What we know about medication errors: A literature review. *Journal of Nursing Quality Assurance* 3(1):1–17.

Giuffre, M., Keane, A., Hatfield, S., and Korevaar, W. 1988. Patient-controlled analgesia in clinical pain research measurement. *Nursing Research* 37(4):254–255.

Henderson, V., and Nite, G. 1978. *Principles and practice of nursing* (6th ed.). New York: Macmillan.

Jesse, W. 1981. Medication errors noted as major source of incident reports. *Hospital Peer Review* 39(1):141–143.

Kasmer, R., Hoisington, L., and Yukniewicz, S. 1987a. Home parenteral antibiotic therapy, part I: An overview of program design. *Home Healthcare Nurse* 5(1):12–18.

Kasmer, R., Hoisington, L., and Yukniewicz, S. 1987b. Home parenteral antibiotic therapy, part II: Drug preparation and administration considerations. *Home Healthcare Nurse* 5(1):19–29.

McLane, A. (ed.). 1987. *Classification of Proceedings of the Seventh National Conference.* St. Louis, Mo.: C.V. Mosby.

Patsdaughter, C., and Pesznecker, B. 1988. Medication regimens and the elderly home care client. *Journal of Gerontological Nursing* 14(10):30–33.

Roberson, M. Home remedies: A cultural study. 1987. *Home Healthcare Nurse* 5(1):35–40.

Souter, S. 1990. After the bypass. *Geriatric Nursing* 11(6):271.

17

PAIN CONTROL

ADA JACOX

Pain is one of the most commonly experienced patient problems. It is a pervasive part of many illnesses and a problem with which nurses are expected to deal. Methods for pain assessment and control have been the focus of a considerable amount of nursing research since the mid-1970s. This was evident in a conference for nurse clinicians and researchers held in March 1988 on "Key Aspects of Comfort" where 10 papers on childrens' pain and 10 on adults' pain were presented (Funk, Tornquist, Champagne, Copp & Wiese 1989). It was evident in this and other conferences and publications that nurses are building on each others' work and developing a cumulative body of knowledge about pain. The attention researchers have given to pain has been paralleled in the practice setting, as many nurses have increased the attention given to careful assessment of pain and to its management in children and adults. Similarly, nursing curricula increasingly include consideration of pain in undergraduate and graduate programs.

In spite of the substantial progress made in recent years, the problem of unrelieved pain in children and adults continues to be significant. A National Institutes of Health (NIH 1987) consensus conference on pain concluded that acute pain and cancer pain are significantly undertreated in hospitals and that chronic nonmalignant pain often is overtreated by medication. Although some patients' pain is more difficult to manage than others', in general, unrelieved pain is the result of ineffective management. Marks and Sacher (1973), documenting the incidence of unrelieved acute postoperative pain, reported that 41% of the patients in their study experienced moderate unrelieved pain and 32% had severe unrelieved pain. A later study (Donovan, Dillon, and McGuire 1987) of unrelieved pain in patients on medical surgical units reported that 57.5% experienced "horrible or excruciating pain at some time during their hospitalization." These studies and others have shown that physicians commonly underprescribe analgesics for adequate pain relief and nurses give only 25% to 30% of the medication that is ordered. A similar situation exists with regard to cancer pain in which patients needlessly suffer severe pain that could be better managed. As Oden (1989) noted, the conventional analgesic therapy of intramuscular opiates prescribed on an as-needed basis is poorly effective at controlling a large number of patients' pain.

The problem of poor pain management has its roots in two areas: lack of well-controlled clinical studies of methods for pain management and the lack of use by practitioners of what is known about pain management. Citing lack of clinical research as a problem after noting the increase in research done by nurses may seem paradoxical. Although nurses and other scientists and health professionals have markedly increased the attention given to pain, much remains unknown about how adequate pain management can be achieved. Most research is done to

221

test various drugs for pain relief, with a smaller proportion directed toward the use of nonpharmacological approaches. Furthermore, many of the experimental studies of nonpharmacological approaches have used healthy subjects in whom pain has been experimentally induced. The extent to which findings from experimentally induced pain can be generalized to patients experiencing clinical pain is unknown. Nurses have been among those researchers who have tested various psychosocially based interventions in clinical populations. The second major cause of unrelieved pain has been inadequate use of what is known about pain, as reflected in the studies of unrelieved pain. Whatever the causes of unrelieved pain, it is clear that adequate pain control deserves more attention from nurses and other health care professionals.

An important follow-up of the 1986 National Institutes of Health Consensus Conference is the effort of the American Pain Society (APS), an interdisciplinary organization to which many nurses belong, to incorporate pain assessment and management into hospital quality assurance programs (Max, Donovan, Portenoy, Cleveland, Simmonds, and Evans 1990). The APS advocates incorporating regular monitoring of pain, much in the way that vital signs are monitored, including noting the patient's response to intervention.

Another attempt to improve pain assessment and management is the work being done by an interdisciplinary panel under the auspices of the recently established federal Agency for Health Care Policy and Research. The panel has developed clinical practice guidelines for the management of acute pain and is developing guidelines for the management of pain associated with cancer (AHCPR 1991; Jacox and Carr 1991). These efforts should improve the ability of nurses and others to manage patients' pain more effectively.

DESCRIPTION OF THE INTERVENTION

Effective Pain Control requires a combination of approaches based on patient preference, source and nature of the pain, other individual characteristics of the patient, and modalities available for use in the setting. As Twycross (1978) noted, "In practice a combination of drug, non-drug and common-sense measures are necessary to achieve maximum benefit." The necessity to use a variety of Pain Control measures also was emphasized by McCaffery and Beebe (1989), who have written a practical and useful manual detailing various approaches to pain assessment and management. Achieving adequate pain relief often is a matter of reviewing with the patient what modalities are available and then trying them out until the right combination is found. It requires an individualized approach to determine what works best. Additionally, what works for a patient at one time may not be effective later.

The Pain Control measures briefly described in this chapter include drugs, cutaneous stimulation, relaxation, and psychosocially based approaches such as patient teaching and patient-controlled analgesia. The measures discussed are those most commonly used by nurses and include both those for which nurses have independent authority and those for which responsibility is shared with other professionals. In some states and in some settings, nurses have the authority to order pain-relieving drugs within certain protocols. In other situations, the physician must write the order for the specific drugs to be used and the nurse exercises judgment concerning when and how often to give the drugs. In all situations, the nurse's responsibility is to monitor the patient's reaction(s) to the drugs and to report when the drug, the dose, or the route of administration is ineffective in producing the desired level of pain relief or when the drug produces undesirable side effects. For other measures, such as relaxation, patient teaching, distraction, imagery, and the application of heat and cold, nurses generally initiate the interventions.

ASSOCIATED NURSING DIAGNOSES

The North American Nursing Diagnosis Association's (NANDA) diagnostic categories relevant to Pain Control are Pain and Chronic Pain (NANDA 1990). NANDA's definition for Pain is "a state in which an individual experiences and reports the presence of severe discomfort or an uncomfortable sensation" (NANDA 1990). This definition will not be used as a basis for this chapter since it confuses the concepts of pain and discomfort by making them appear to be synonymous. Although there is overlap between the concepts of comfort and pain (Jacox 1989), in general, the concept of comfort is much broader and is distinctive from the concept of pain.

The distinction between pain and discomfort is evident in a study in which I participated some years ago (Jacox 1979). We asked patients to describe the kinds of experiences they generally considered to be painful events and those they considered to produce discomfort. Thirty events or conditions were selected from patients' responses, and 200 patients were asked to classify each condition. In general, experiences defined as painful included primarily sharp, throbbing, or acute physical sensations. Discomfort had to do with psychosocial situations such as lack of kindness or waiting for a new procedure to be done. Sensations defined as producing discomfort were those that produced pressure or were associated with dullness or aching.

Gordon's (1987) analysis of nursing diagnoses made by nurses showed that discomfort was the third most frequently made diagnosis and Pain was the fourth. She noted the need for clinical studies to determine the relationship between the categories (concepts) of pain and discomfort.

In an attempt to be more precise about the definition of pain, therefore, the definition used in this chapter is "an unpleasant sensory and emotional experience associated with actual or potential tissue damage or described in terms of such damage" (International Association for the Study of Pain, 1986). The categorization of pain described in the report of the NIH Consensus Conference on Pain (NIH 1987) is used here: "Pain following acute injury, disease, or some types of surgery (acute pain); pain associated with cancer or other progressive disorders (chronic malignant pain), or pain in persons whose tissue injury is non-progressive or healed (chronic non-malignant pain). An individual may have more than one type of pain" (p. 35). Acute pain generally lasts from a few seconds to several months, and chronic pain generally lasts longer than several months (American Pain Society 1989). This chapter focuses on measures for acute postoperative pain and chronic malignant pain.

Other nursing diagnoses are associated with the intervention described here because the problem or diagnosis of pain often is interrelated with many other diagnoses. Not only do the problems overlap, but they are interactive or influence each other. A patient who is very anxious, for example, may interpret a noxious stimulus as being painful and then become more anxious. That pain frequently is compounded with anxiety and depression is shown in one study (Craig and Abeloff 1974), which found that more than half of the patients admitted to a cancer research unit showed moderate to high levels of depression and 30% had increased levels of anxiety. The depression that commonly accompanies cancer may produce fatigue, which makes pain more difficult to tolerate. Treatment of the depression may help to relieve both the depression and the fatigue associated with it and thus make it easier for a patient to handle the pain. Pain is not an isolated phenomenon but often must be dealt with as part of several interrelated problems (Jacox and Rogers 1981).

McCaffery and Beebe (1989, p. 36), noting that pain may affect all aspects of a person's life, listed the following eighteen NANDA nursing diagnoses potentially associated with pain:

Anxiety	Feeding Self Care Deficit
Constipation	Bathing/Hygiene Self Care Deficit
Ineffective Individual Coping	Dressing/Grooming Self Care Deficit
Diversional Activity Deficit	Toileting Self Care Deficit
Fatigue	Sexual Dysfunction
Fear	Sleep Pattern Disturbance
Knowledge Deficit	Social Isolation
Impaired Physical Mobility	Spiritual Distress
Powerlessness	Altered Thought Processes

PAIN ASSESSMENT

Basic to selection of measures for Pain Control is a clear description of the patient's pain. Nurses have pioneered in the development of clinical assessment procedures, particularly for the assessment of children's pain. Pain assessment is not something that is done only initially or occasionally but must be done on a regular basis and must be related to the patient's condition and to the interventions being used. Table 17–1 contains an assessment guide for factors to be considered in the evaluation of pain. It contains a summary of factors to consider in a comprehensive pain assessment. Johnson (1977) elaborates on each of these factors.

In addition to verbal questioning of the patient or family, nurses have available numerous simple measures of pain. Three are described here: a simple descriptive scale, a 0–100 numeric scale, and a visual analog scale (VAS). Examples of the three types of scales appear in Figure 17–1.

The terms on a simple descriptive scale may have different meanings for different people, which is a reflection of the subjective nature of pain. A scale in wide use is the 0–100 numeric scale in which there are more choices than in the usual descriptive scale. Different anchors may be used from those shown in the example. A VAS is a line representing a continuum of pain in which only the end point descriptors are used, such as "no pain" and "pain as bad as it possibly could be." Any of these simple measures may be used by clinicians, and nurses in many settings use various modifications of the scales for pain assessment. Also useful for helping patients to indicate the location of pain is a body chart in which the patient is shown the outline of a human body and asked to indicate on it the precise location of the pain.

Pain assessment in children requires different assessment tools because of childrens' more limited ability to conceptualize and communicate. Nurses have contributed in major ways to the procedures and methods available for assessing children's pain. Early work in this area was done by Eland (1985), who used the concept of a figure drawing with front and back views to have children color the location of their pain. Another tool useful with children is the Hester Poker-Chip

TABLE 17 – 1.   Assessment Guide for Evaluation of Pain

A. Characteristics of pain
   1. Location
      a. Areas of pain
      b. Areas without pain
   2. Intensity
      a. Mild
      b. Moderate
      c. Severe
      d. Overwhelming
   3. Quality of pain — words patient uses to describe pain
   4. Chronology
      a. Mode of onset
      b. Precipitating factors
      c. Variations in intensity and quality

B. Pain responses
   1. Physiological responses
      a. Note changes in pulse, blood pressure, respirations
      b. Note presence of dilated pupils, perspiration, nausea, vomiting, pallor
   2. Behavioral responses
      a. Body activity increased or decreased
      b. Protection of painful areas
      c. Body position
      d. Facial expression
   3. Affective responses

C. Pain communication
   1. How does the patient describe the pain and the degree of suffering?
   2. Is the patient groping for a meaning for the pain or does he ascribe some meaning to the pain?
   3. Does the pain interfere with physical activity? Personal relationships?
   4. How does the patient relate pain to the pathology?

D. Coping techniques
   1. Does the patient use any method to control the pain?
   2. If not, what does he do when the pain occurs or increases in severity?

E. Factors that can affect pain
   1. Is fatigue consistently present?
   2. Does the patient appear to be anxious, depressed, frightened?
   3. Is the patient worried about the illness? Does he have questions about it that have not been answered?
   4. What are the patient's expectations in relation to the pain? Does he want complete relief or just enough control to be able to pursue certain activities? What activities have a high priority for him?

F. Sources that should be used in assessing pain include
   1. The patient
   2. Close family members
   3. The medical record
   4. Information about expected pain patterns that occur with the diagnosed pathology

Source: Johnson, M. "Assessment of Clinical Pain," in *Pain: A Sourcebook for Nurses and Other Health Professionals.* A. Jacox (ed.), Boston: Little, Brown and Company, 1977, pp. 159–160.

Scale (Hester 1979). Children as young as 4 years of age are given four or five poker chips and told that they represent pieces of hurt. In one variation of this method, children choose from no poker chips, which means no hurt, to one chip which means a little hurt, up to four chips, which means the worst hurt.

Some of the descriptive scales can be used with children aged 9 years or above, and in some cases even with younger children. Beyer (1989) developed two scales for measuring pain in children. One is a 0–100 numeric scale for older children who understand the numbers, and the second is a six-picture photographic scale for younger children. The photographs show a child experiencing increasing levels of discomfort or distress. The child is told that the picture at the bottom of the scale means "no hurt," and the top picture is the "biggest hurt you could ever have."

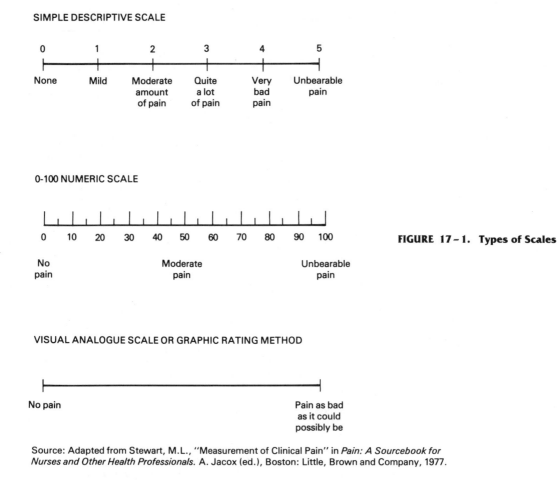

FIGURE 17-1. Types of Scales

Source: Adapted from Stewart, M.L., "Measurement of Clinical Pain" in *Pain: A Sourcebook for Nurses and Other Health Professionals*. A. Jacox (ed.), Boston: Little, Brown and Company, 1977.

PAIN CONTROL

The effectiveness of various measures can be partially explained by the gate-control theory of pain, introduced by Melzack and colleagues (Melzack and Wall 1965). Melzack and others have shown that pain is not only a neurophysiological phenomenon to be explained in terms of a cetain intensity of stimulus always producing the same amount of pain sensation in people. The gate control theory proposes that cognitive and emotional factors influence how pain is perceived and responded to and provides a basis for understanding pain as a mind-body problem. A second major contribution to the theoretical understanding of pain was the discovery that the body secretes opioid-like substances known as endorphins (Snyder 1977). An impulse from the brain triggers the release of endorphins, which bind to opioid receptors in the brain and spinal cord and block transmission of pain signals. Both contributions have advanced substantially the understanding of methods for Pain Control.

Many factors should influence the selection and timing of measures. First is the need to consider the patient's preference, which can be determined by talking with the patient both preoperatively and postoperatively in the case of anticipated surgery or at any time during the course of illness in the case of a patient with pain associated with cancer. Patients should be told that there are multiple ways to manage pain and that generally they do not have to tolerate moderate to severe pain. If measures such as those described in this chapter are ineffective, other methods of control, such as nerve blocks or ablative neurosurgical procedures, can be used.

A second set of factors to be taken into account are other characteristics of the patient, such as the source and nature of the pain, age, previous experience with pain, and methods of pain control that the patient previously has found to be effective. Patients' responses to drugs and to nondrug measures vary widely, and care must be taken to individualize the measures and modify them as necessary.

Whenever possible, it is preferable to prevent pain rather than to wait until it has become moderate or severe before intervening. When pain becomes severe, it causes the patient needless suffering and is more difficult to control. When pain is present most of the time, for example, drugs should be given at regular intervals and in sufficient strength to control the pain rather than given only when the patient requests it, a practice that repeatedly has been shown to be ineffective in many cases. Similarly, when the nurse explains to a preoperative patient how to use simple relaxation methods and emphasizes the importance of communicating the need for pain relief, the patient will be able to participate more actively in pain management following surgery.

Pain Control measures do not have to be used independently of each other. Although there has been little systematic research that has tested combinations of measures (other than combinations of drugs), nurses should not hesitate to use relaxation, distraction, patient teaching, and other methods of Pain Control with or without drugs.

Finally, it is important to understand that effective pain management is dependent on accurate and timely assessment.

APPROACHES TO PAIN CONTROL

Pharmacological Approaches

The use of drugs, singly or in combination, is the dominant approach to Pain Control in acute and chronic cancer pain. Responsibility for use of drugs is shared by physicians, nurses, clinical pharmacists, and patients. In some states and some settings, nurses have the authority to order analgesic drugs within certain parameters or protocols. Whether they have legal authority to order drugs, nurses are responsible for assessing patients' need for drugs, for administering them, for assessing their effectiveness, and for observing for undesirable side effects or complications. Thus, it is important that any nurse working with patients who are experiencing pain be knowledgeable about analgesics.

Three classes of analgesic drugs are used for management of acute pain and chronic cancer pain: nonopioid analgesics, opioid analgesics, and analgesic adjuvants (World Health Organization 1986; APS 1989; McCaffery and Beebe 1989; U.S. Pharmacopeial Drug Information 1991). The following discussion is taken largely from a brief monograph published by the American Pain Society (APS 1989) (available from the American Pain Society, P.O. Box 186, Skokie, IL 60076-0186; [708] 966-0050), which gives details regarding the mechanisms of action, specific drugs in the categories, contradictions for use, and principles of analgesic use.

Nonopioid analgesics include acetaminophen salicylates such as aspirin and nonsteroidal anti-inflammatory drugs (NSAIDS), such as ibuprofen. These drugs are antipyretic and do not produce tolerance, physical, or psychological dependence.

Some NSAIDS are equivalent to aspirin in their pain-relieving effects, and others produce much greater analgesia than aspirin. They can be used alone for relief of pain of mild or moderate intensity or combined with opioids in pain of moderate or severe intensity to reduce the amount of opioid required for adequate pain relief.

Opioids are analgesics that work by binding to opioid receptors in the central nervous system. They include morphine and morphinelike agonists such as codeine and meperidine (Demerol). Meperidine is widely used for pain relief. This is unfortunate because it is short acting, toxic in elderly patients or in patients with impaired renal function, and commonly underprescribed (McCaffery and Beebe 1989; APS 1989). There are many more effective and less toxic drugs, many described in the APS guide on analgesics (1989), which does not recommend Demerol for use in patients who have severe pain.

Analgesic adjuvants are drugs that enhance the effects of opioid or aspirinlike drugs, produce analgesia independently, or counteract side effects of analgesics (APS 1989). They include tricyclic antidepressants, antihistamines, benzodiazepines, caffeine, dextroamphetamine, steroids, phenothiazines, and anticonvulsants.

Patient-Controlled Analgesia

These are methods by which patients control their own administration of analgesia within parameters determined by the health professional. Patient-controlled analgesia (PCA) thus combines psychological (patient control) and pharmacological aspects to produce analgesia.

PCA includes use of many drugs and many routes of administration, from oral to epidural. Recently there has been an increase in the use of mechanical pumps that allow patients to administer opioids or other drugs intravenously or epidurally.

Nonpharmacological Approaches

Nonpharmacological approaches to pain control that are used by nurses include physically based methods such as transcutaneous electric nerve stimulation (TENS), psychosocially based methods such as distraction, and a combination of physically and psychosocially based methods such as relaxation. They can be used alone if they produce an adequate level of pain relief or in combination with drugs to improve pain control or to reduce the amount of drugs needed.

Cutaneous Stimulation

Providing pain relief by sensory stimulation or counterirritation such as rubbing on or near the painful part is a common method of pain relief. McCaffery and Beebe (1989) describe many forms of cutaneous stimulation that nurses can use, including massage, vibration, application of heat or cold, menthol application to the skin, and TENS. TENS provides stimulation through a battery-powered, miniaturized current generator that delivers stimulation pulses transcutaneously to nerve fibers (Sjölund, Eriksson, and Loeser 1990). The pain relief is temporary, and stimulation must be repeated as needed to provide adequate relief. The use of TENS generally requires a physician's order. It has been used effectively to relieve postoperative pain following thoracic, abdominal, and orthopedic surgery. Eland (1989) described its effectiveness in eight children experiencing severe pain associated with cancer.

Relaxation

Relaxation techniques used for pain control range in complexity from simple ones in which the patient is taught to use focused breathing exercises, to those that combine breathing and progressive muscle relaxation, sometimes using meditation or biofeedback techniques. Use of relaxation techniques can help to distract patients from the pain and to gain some sense of control over it. Relaxation exercises also can reduce anxiety and can decrease pain from secondary reflex muscle contractions. Relaxation thus incorporates both physical and psychological dimensions of behavior in achieving pain reduction.

Simple breathing exercises, such as deep breathing, fist clenching, and yawning, can be easily taught to patients pre- or postoperatively or prior to the beginning of a pain-producing procedure. Other relaxation techniques that combine breathing exercises, progressive muscle relaxation, and meditation or imagery can be learned by patients experiencing pain associated with cancer to help with pain management. Details regarding various relaxation techniques are described by McCaffery and Beebe (1989) and by Syrjola (1990).

Patient Education

Patient education includes a number of methods to help patients understand more about their pain and take an active part in its control. In addition to the relaxation techniques, patients can be given information regarding causes of the pain and other methods that they can use to control it.

Providing information regarding the sources of pain and related experiences can help to decrease the anxiety associated with uncertainty and lack of knowledge. Studies by Johnson, Fuller, Endress, and Rice (1978), for example, have illustrated the effectiveness of providing preoperative patients with information regarding the procedures they were going to experience and some of the sensations that commonly accompany the procedure. In this, as in other areas of patient teaching, the information given to patients and when it is given must be individualized to take into account the patient's readiness to learn it.

Other measures useful in pain control are distraction by having patients count backward from 100 or by listening to music; use of imagery to distract and relax; use of acupressure to interrupt pain signals; use of hypnosis; training in coping skills; and cognitive restructuring to monitor negative thoughts and generate more adoptive cognitions.

SUMMARY

Numerous measures can be used by nurses to control pain. They require varying amounts of preparation, time, and equipment, and many have not been tested through rigorous research. Nevertheless, it is important that nurses' approach to pain management be broadly inclusive of many modalities to reflect the complex and individualized experience of pain.

Although increased attention is being given to pain assessment and control by nurses and others, there is still much to learn about one of the most common problems patients experience. The vast array of measures available to nurses and potentially useful in Pain Control must be systematically tested with clinical groups to learn the most effective measures and best combinations for serious patients. The lack of such rigorously conducted research should not, however, deter nurses from using the knowledge that is available and their own experience to improve pain control.

REFERENCES

1991 *Clinical Guidelines for Acute Pain Management: Operative or Medical Procedures and Trauma* (DHHS Pub. No. (AHCPR) 91-0046). Rockville, Md: Agency for Health Care Policy and Research.

American Pain Society, 1989. *Principles of analgesic use in the treatment of acute pain and chronic cancer pain* (2d ed.). Skokie, Ill.: American Pain Society.

Bengt, H.S., Eriksson, M., and Loeser, J.D. 1990. Transcutaneous and implanted electric stimulation of peripheral nerves. In J.E. Bonica (ed.), *The management of pain* (pp. 1832–1861). Philadelphia: Lea & Febiger.

Beyer, J.E. 1989. The Oucher, a pain intensity scale for children. In S.G. Funk, E. M. Tornquist, M.T. Champagne, L.A. Copp, and R. A. Wiese (eds.), *Key aspects of comfort* (pp. 65–71). New York: Springer.

Craig, T.J., and Abeloff, M.D. 1974. Psychiatric symptomatology among hospitalized cancer patients. *American Journal of Psychology* 131:1323.

Donovan, M.L., Dillon, P., and McGuire, L. 1987. Incidence and characteristics of pain in a sample of medical-surgical inpatients. *Pain* 30:69–78.

Eland, J. 1985. The child who is hurting. *Seminars in Oncology Nursing* 1:116–122.

Eland, J.M. 1989. The effectiveness of transcutaneous electrical nerve stimulation (TENS) with children experiencing cancer pain. In S.G. Funk, E.M. Tornquist, M.T. Champagne, L.A. Copp, and R.A. Wiese (eds.), *Key aspects of comfort* (pp. 87–100). New York: Springer.

Funk, S.G., Tornquist, E.M., Champagne, M.T., Copp, L.A., and Wiese, R.A. 1989. *Key aspects of comfort: Management of pain, fatigue, and nausea.* New York: Springer.

Gordon, M. 1987. *Nursing diagnosis: Process and application* (2d ed.) New York: McGraw-Hill.

Hester, N.O. 1987. The pre-operational child's reaction to immunizations. *Nursing Research* 28:250–254.

International Association for the Study of Pain. 1986. Classification of chronic pain: Descriptions of chronic pain syndromes and definitions of pain terms. *Pain* 3 (Suppl.), S1-S225.

Jacox, A.K. 1979. Pain assessment. *American Journal of Nursing* 79:895–900.

Jacox, A.K., and Rogers, A.G. 1981. The nursing management of pain. In L.B. Marino (ed.), *Cancer nursing*. St. Louis: C.V. Mosby.

Jacox, A.K. 1989. Key aspects of comfort. In S.G. Funk, E.M. Tornquist, M.T. Champagne, L.A. Copp, and R.A. Wiese (eds.), *Key aspects of comfort: Management of pain, fatigue, and nausea.* New York: Springer.

Jacox, A., and Carr, D. 1991. Clinical practice guidelines. *Nursing Economics* 9(2).

Johnson, J., Fuller, S., Endress, P., and Rice, U.; 1978. Altering patients' responses to surgery: An extension and replication. *Research in Nursing and Health* 1(3):111–121.

Johnson, M. 1977. Assessment of clinical pain. In A.K. Jacox (ed.), *Pain: A source book for nurses and other health professionals* (pp. 159–160). Boston: Little, Brown.

Max, M.B., Donovan, M., Portenoy, R.K., Cleveland, C.S., Simmonds, M.A., and Evans, W.O. 1991. Standards for monitoring quality of analgesic treatment of acute pain and cancer pain. In M.R. Bond, J.E. Charlton, and C.J. Woolf (eds.), *Proceedings of the VI World Congress on Pain.* Amsterdam: Elsevier, pp. 185–189.

Marks, R.M., and Sacher, E.S. 1973. Undertreatment of medical inpatients with narcotic analgesics, *Annals of Internal Medicine* 78(2):173–181.

McCaffery, M., and Beebe, A. 1989. *Pain: A clinical manual for nursing practice.* Baltimore: C.V. Mosby.

Melzack, R., and Wall, P.D. 1965. Pain mechanisms: A new theory. *Science,* 150–971.

National Institutes of Health. Consensus Development Statement. 1987, Winter. The integrated approach to the management of pain. *Journal of Pain and Symptom Management* 2(1):35–44.

North American Nursing Diagnosis Association. 1990. *Taxonomy I—revised 1990.* St. Louis: NANDA.

Oden, R.U. 1989. Acute post-operative pain: Incidence, severity and the etiology of inadequate treatment. *Anesthesiology Clinics of North America* 7(1):1–15.

Sjölund, B.H., Eriksson, M., and Loeser, J.D. 1990. Transcutaneous and implanted electrical stimulation of peripheral nerves. In J.J. Bonica (ed.), *The Management of Pain* (pp. 1852–1861). Philadelphia: Lea and Febiger.

Snyder, S.H. 1977. Opiate receptors and internal opiates. *Scientific American* 236:44–56.

Stewart, M.L. 1977. Measurement of clinical pain. In A.K. Jacox (ed.), *Pain: A surce book for nurses and other health professionals* (pp. 107–137). Boston: Little, Brown.

Syrjola, K.L. 1990. Relaxation Techniques. In J. Bonica (ed.), *The management of pain* (pp. 1742–1750). Philadelphia: Lea and Febiger.

Tywcross, R.G. 1978. Bone pain in advanced cancer. In D.W. Vere (ed.), *Topics in therapeutics* (4th ed.). Turnbridgewell: Pittman Medical.

United States pharmacopeial drug information volumes I and II. 1986. *Drug information for the health care professional* (11th ed.). Rockville, Md.: U.S. Pharmacopeial Convention.

World Health Organization. 1986. *Cancer Pain Relief.* Geneva: WHO.

18

FLUID THERAPY

ALICE S. POYSS

DESCRIPTION AND DEFINITION

Fluid Therapy is defined as the supportive and preventative actions a nurse takes to assist individuals in restoring fluid balance and preventing complications of disease. Increased use of intravenous therapy has resulted in its becoming commonplace but not without potential for serious hazards. The act of monitoring and assessment is the professional responsibility of the registered nurse (Metheny 1990). The nursing intervention is supportive of medical therapy: managing the patient's illness and promoting and restoring maximum function. Frequent assessment and evaluation of appropriate Fluid Therapy is imperative for the early detection and prevention of patient complications (Plumer 1987).

Abnormalities of body fluid and electrolyte metabolism present certain therapeutic problems. When the mechanisms normally regulating fluid volume, electrolyte composition, and osmolality are impaired, therapy becomes complicated. An understanding of these metabolic abnormalities enables the nurse to make clinical judgments concerning the outcomes of Fluid Therapy. The nurse has the responsibility of recognizing the importance of adverse effects of fluid and electrolyte metabolism. The nurse gathers information through continual physical assessment and monitoring of patient's vital signs. In fluid and electrolyte imbalances, nursing assessment cannot be focused on the problem from the start because fluid and electrolyte disturbances are characterized by myriad symptoms, which cut across all systems. The knowledge the nurse uses in recognizing adverse effects contributes to safe, successful Fluid Therapy in critically ill patients.

RELATED LITERATURE

There are two main objectives of Fluid Therapy: to replace losses that have already occurred and to keep up with ongoing fluid losses. Giving the right amount depends on calculating measurable fluid losses, estimating insensible and third-space losses, factoring in the functional ability of key homeostatic organs, and revising fluid prescriptions according to current indicators of the patient's physical status (Metheny 1990). Intravenous fluids are tailored to meet the deficits in patients' fluid and electrolyte status.

Normal Fluid Balance

Every body system and body organ is used to maintain the internal environment. The lungs, kidneys, heart, adrenal glands, pituitary gland, and parathyroid glands are involved in regulatory mechanisms.

Water is the sole solvent and the most abundant compound in the human body, constituting 40% to 80% of body weight. The body is essentially an aqueous solution in which a vast complex of solutes are distributed in compartments that vary in size and are bounded by lipid membranes. Water is the environment in which the reactions of life occur. The total body water of an individual varies with age, weight, and sex. The amount of water is dependent on the amount of body fat. Body fat is essentially water free; the greater the fat content is, the less is the water content (Maxwell, Kleeman, and Navins 1987).

Fluid housed in the body can be divided into two main compartments: intracellular and extracellular. Intracellular fluid accounts for approximately three-fourths of the body's total body fluid. Intracellular fluid compartments provide the cells with the internal aqueous medium necessary for chemical functions. Extracellular fluid comprises the rest of the body fluid. The extracellular fluid compartments help maintain the internal environment with the nutrients and other substances to the cells, as well as remove the waste materials. This is a constant movement throughout the body, assisting the internal cells in maintenance.

Extracellular fluid includes all body water that is external to all cells, including erythrocytes. Thus, extracellular water includes water inside and outside blood vessels, as well as water that is in the interstitium between cells and water that has crossed epithelial cells (for example, gastrointestinal fluids). Other extracellular water compartments include plasma, interstitial fluid, lymph, inaccessible bone water, and transcellular water (Maxwell 1987). The transcellular compartment is the product of cellular metabolism and consists of secretions such as gastrointestinal secretions and urine. Analysis of the secretions may assist the physician in tracing lost electrolytes and prescribing proper fluid and electrolyte replacement. Excessive fluid and electrolyte loss in this compartment will affect the balance of the two main fluid compartments (Plumer 1987). Interstitial fluid accounts for 15% of total body water. It is the fluid held in the spaces between the cells. Plasma is the fluid component of blood and constitutes the remaining 20% of the extracellular fluid (Maxwell, Kleeman, and Narins 1987).

Water distribution into the various body compartments is dependent on the permeability of the barrier between compartments to water and on the quantity of solute in each compartment. Almost all compartmental barriers in humans are highly permeable to water. Normal intracellular water varies inversely with extracellular sodium; therefore, a decrease in serum sodium creates an increase in intracellular fluid and a decrease in extracellular volume (Goldberger 1980).

The amount of body water loss is easily computed by weighing a patient and noting weight loss: 1 L of body water is equivalent to 1 kg (2.2 lb) of body weight. Weight changes are valuable tools to indicate fluid imbalances (Plumer 1987).

Electrolyte concentration plays a significant role in cellular function and in the distribution of water in the various fluid spaces. If the concentration of ions in either the intracellular or the extracellular fluid space changes, water shifts from the area of lower concentration to the area of higher concentration until the concentrations are again equal. Although the amount and composition of fluid in each compartment remains electrically stable, each compartment is constantly replacing and exchanging ions. This constant interchange of ions and water between the fluid compartments is dependent on the unique structure of the cell membrane, a structure designed to regulate this exchange between the cell and its surrounding environment. Terms related to movement include osmosis, osmolality, active transport, and oncotic pressure (Lancaster 1987).

Osmosis is a special type of diffusion in which water is the chief substance to pass through a selectively permeable membrane (Maxwell 1987). Water moves freely from a weak solution into a more concentrated one. Osmosis stops when both fluids have the same osmolality.

Osmolality is the amount of solute added to water. Osmolality, which measures the number of particles in a solution, can be described as the specific gravity of body fluids. The specifics of osmolality can be summarized as follows (Maxwell 1987):

- The normal osmolality of body fluids is 280 mOsm/kg to 300 mOsm/kg.
- The intracellular and extracellular osmolalities are always equal, and their measurement describes the patient's fluid status.
- Water diffuses from low osmolality to high osmolality.
- Intracellular fluid rapidly reflects extracellular imbalances because of osmotic equilibrium.
- Sodium is the electrolyte that regulates vascular osmotic pressure (Lancaster 1987).

In clinical practice, *osmolality* and *osmolarity* are used interchangeably to refer to the concentration of a patient's body fluid. There is a difference between the two, however. Osmolarity is the concentration of solutes per liter of cellular fluid; osmolality refers to the amount of solutes in total body water (solutes per kilogram of body weight). *Osmolarity* is the appropriate term for use in intravenous Fluid Therapy (Metheny 1990).

Active transport is the force used to move fluids and electrolytes uphill against a concentrated solution. This mechanism uses energy and a carrier substance to move the molecules (Goldberger 1980). An example of active transport is the sodium pump that maintains conduction and contraction in nerve and muscle cells.

Oncotic pressure is a form of osmosis where heavy protein molecules in the plasma are unable to pass through the capillary membranes that keep water in the capillaries. They can also pull it in from the interstitial fluid. This shift of water into (and out of) capillaries is controlled by the balance between oncotic pressure and hydrostatic pressure, the force of the heart's pumping action. The heart's stronger pressure at the end of the capillary pushes some of the fluid electrolytes and nutrients out to bathe the cells, whereas its lesser pressure at the venous end lets the oncotic pressure pull fluid and cellular waste back into circulation (Maxwell 1987). Fluid not returned to the veins in this way slowly passes back into the central circulation through the lymph system. Plasma colloid osmotic pressure is the selective retention of plasma proteins such as albumin and globulin. This lowers the concentration of water and electrolytes, resulting in concentrating plasma albumin. This concentration of plasma proteins determines how the extracellular fluid moves—either intravascular or interstitial (Maxwell 1987).

Thirst and Output: Gains and Losses of Water and Electrolytes

Whether primary or secondary to other conditions, all body fluid disturbances are caused by abnormal differences between gains and losses of water and electrolytes. One mechanism for gaining fluid in a healthy adult is stimulating the thirst center (Maxwell 1987). The body gains water and electrolytes in various ways; water alone is gained by drinking water and by oxidation of foodstuffs and body tissues. Renal regulation of water assists the body in maintaining fluid loss.

The thirst center functions in a manner similar to that of osmoreceptor. When the thirst center is stimulated, particularly by a high extracellular osmolality, water leaves the cells by osmosis, causing them to shrink. The shrinking stimulates signals to the cortex indicating the desire to drink (Goldberger 1980). Although the primary stimulus is that of high osmolality, other patient conditions that suggest other thirst etiologies include the following:

1. Excessive loss of potassium ion (causes cells to shrink).
2. Decreased blood volume.
3. Mucous membrane dehydration.
4. Psychologic states. Research suggests that patients with a diagnosis of schizophrenia have an inherent need to drink water, causing water intoxication (Rinard 1989).
5. Angiotensin II, which is formed in the blood when the kidneys release renin in response to a low blood volume. Angiotensin II stimulates the thirst center as well as the secretion of antidiuretic hormone (ADH) and an increase in gastrointestinal water absorption (Lancaster 1987).

The perception of thirst requires an alert level of consciousness. In the alert person, the thirst mechanisms can compensate when antidiuretic hormone mechanisms fail by causing an awareness of the increased need for fluid to replace that being lost in the urine. Infants, persons with impairment of consciousness, or those with psychologic disturbances may not respond to the stimuli sent out by the thirst center (Rinard 1989). Their bodies may be able to compensate to some extent through ADH secretion mechanisms if these are functioning normally. If both mechanisms fail, body water balance cannot be maintained.

Thirst is not always a reliable indicator of need for fluids. Elderly patients often do not recognize thirst and even if they do may be unable to reach for water (Gaspar 1988). Patients with fluid volume excesses caused by cardiac and renal damage are sometimes quite thirsty. Patients with burns experience great thirst. These needs are met with an oral electrolyte solution, with the quantity carefully measured with the volume of intravenous solutions (Sommers 1990).

The kidneys are the main monitors of fluid balance. They have primary responsibility for regulating the body's water and solute balance. Of the 180 L per day filtered at the glomerulus, about 95% to 99% is reabsorbed throughout the course of the renal tubule. The kidney can produce a concentrated urine or a dilute urine, depending on the needs of the body. Several hormones, notably aldosterone, ADH, parathyroid hormone (PTH), and calcitonin, as well as vitamin D, are important in the regulation of water and solutes (Lancaster 1987). The kidneys control the volume of extracellular fluids by regulating the concentration of specific electrolytes and the osmolality of body fluids (Lancaster 1987).

The hypothalamus balances fluid and electrolytes by secreting ADH to make the body retain water. Too much ADH means too much water retention and a drop in the serum sodium levels (Maxwell 1987).

An overproduction of aldosterone from the adrenal glands causes sodium and water to be retained and potassium to be excreted. Conversely, too little aldosterone causes sodium and water loss and potassium retention (Metheny 1990).

ADH secretion may be stimulated or its activity potentiated by factors such as trauma, pain, stress, anxiety, and medications, such as morphine, meperidine (Demerol), thiazide diuretics, barbiturates, acetaminophen, oxytocin, chlorepropamide, and nicotine. ADH's activity is suppressed peripherally or in the kidney by alcohol, Phenytoin, lithium carbonate and demeclocycline (Karb 1989). Secretion of ADH is also suppressed when the volume receptors in the heart's atria sense increased intravascular volume or when the baroreceptors sense increased blood pressure.

Fluid Volume Imbalances

Fluid Volume Excess

Edema is a detectable accumulation of excess interstitial fluid. It may be confined to a sharply circumscribed area as occurring in local inflammation or angio edema or may be generalized so that interstitial fluid accumulates in virtually every tissue in the body (Metheny 1983).

The existence of edema indicates a disturbance in the normal regulation of extracellular volume. Each of the major disorders associated with generalized edema is characterized by a defect in at least one of the Starling capillary forces and by renal retention of sodium and water (Maxwell 1987). Starling forces include mechanisms that govern the distribution of fluid across capillaries: hydrostatic pressure, decreased colloid osmotic pressure, and increased capillary permeability.

In idiopathic edema, there is an isotonic expansion of the extracellular volume. The extracellular compartment expands in proportion to the fluid infused. The increase in volume of fluid dilutes the concentration of hemoglobin and lowers the hematocrit and total protein levels, but the serum sodium level remains the same (Plumer 1987). Populations at risk for idiopathic edema are the elderly and the early postsurgical or posttrauma patients. Elderly patients have a low tolerance for fluids and electrolytes. Those receiving isotonic saline solutions must be carefully monitored for this complication of Fluid Therapy (Adams 1988).

In patients with cirrhosis, edema is caused by pressure on the vena cava, which impairs the venous drainage from the lower extremities. Low plasma oncotic pressure secondary to hypoalbuminemia may occur when no ascites is present (Adinaro 1987).

In patients with ascites, 10 L or more of fluid can collect in the bowel, resulting in severe extracellular volume loss. Plasma volume is substantially reduced, and hypovolemic shock often ensues. Plasma concentrations of electrolytes are initially preserved; however, the patient becomes thirsty and drinks water, leading to hyponatremia (Adinaro 1987).

The volume of fluid trapped in the intestines can only be estimated. Weight measurements are valueless in detecting the amount of fluid trapped in the bowel. Careful observation of vital signs, the patient's appearance, urinary volume, and specific gravity are significant. Mild tachycardia may suggest an acute fluid loss of 5% of body weight and acute fluid loss greater than 10% of body weight can cause hypovolemic shock (Adinaro 1987).

In severe liver disease, ascites is caused by a decreased plasma albumin, combined with an increased capillary pressure produced by portal hypertension. The combination of both defects allows the albumin-filled fluid to shift out into the peritoneal cavity (Adinaro 1987).

Fluid Volume Deficit

Fluid volume deficit is a result of water and electrolyte loss in an isotonic fashion. Serum electrolytes remain unchanged unless other imbalances are also present.

Fluid volume deficit is most often the result of body fluid loss or fluid collection in the third space. It is also called hypovolemia. The condition is exacerbated by decreased fluid intake. As a result, the extracellular compartment shrinks. This type of deficit is most commonly caused by fluids lost through the gastrointestinal tract and by conditions that cause polyuria and increase in sensible perspiration, respiratory rate and depth, and body temperature. Hypovolemic shock may result from severe loss of extracellular volume. Prolonged severe fluid volume deficit may result in renal failure (Metheny 1983).

The correlation between the volume deficit and physical findings varies depending on the tonicity of body fluids. Patients with isotonic or hypotonic dehydration develop physical findings of volume contraction with smaller deficits of total body water than patients with hypertonic dehydration. However, at least 30 mL/kg, or 5% of body weight, must be lost before volume deficit is evident on examination regardless of the tonicity of body fluids (Goldberger 1980).

In fluid volume deficit, there can be two forms of extracellular defects: isotonic dehydration and hypotonic dehydration. In isotonic dehydration, there is loss of salt and water in proportionate amounts—as occurs, for example, with acute hemorrhage. The intracellular compartment remains unchanged. In hypotonic dehydration, there is hypotonicity of extracellular fluid caused by an osmotic shift of water into cells. The intracellular volume is actually expanded in patients with hypotonic dehydration, and the deficit in extracellular volume is proportionately greater than the overall deficit of total body water (Goldberger 1980).

Other conditions contributing to fluid volume deficit states include gastrointestinal losses, vapor loss from skin and lungs, and iatrogenic treatments. Abnormal gastrointestinal fluid loss can be caused by increased losses in conditions such as vomiting, diarrhea, presence of fistulas, drainage tubes, and gastrointestinal suction. Conditions that interfere with fluid absorption from the gastrointestinal tract, such as obstructions, can also contribute to a loss of extracellular volume. Fluid loss from the skin occurs through perspiration. Extreme water loss occurs when body temperature exceeds 101°F (Maxwell 1987). High temperature and burns increase water loss by evaporation. Water vapor loss via the lungs is increased when conditions exist that are conducive to increasing respiratory rate or depth. An example of increased water vapor loss is that caused by body temperature elevations that produce hyperpnea.

Any disorder or treatment that causes increased urine excretion can lead to extracellular fluid loss. Examples include diuretic use without careful assessment of renal status, conditions such as salt-losing nephritis and hyperglycemia, and hyperosmolar tube feedings. All of these conditions cause polyuria because of the high load of solutes (dissolved substances) causing extracellular fluid to be removed from the plasma, tissues spaces, and from cells in order for the excess solutes to be excreted in the urine. Elevated body temperature increases the amount of metabolic wastes in the body, which requires extra fluid for its excretion by the kidney (Karb 1989).

Patients with fluid volume deficit demonstrate dry mucous membranes and a low urinary output. Neurological manifestations such as confusion and lethargy are symptomatic of prolonged fluid volume loss (Adams 1988).

Sodium Imbalances

Sodium is the major cation in the extracellular fluid compartment. Sodium concentration within the extracellular compartment ranges from 135 mEq/L to 145 mEq/L. Because of its high concentration and inability to cross the cell membrane easily, sodium is the primary determinant of extracellular fluid concentration and the primary regulator of extracellular volume (Maxwell 1987). Sodium is reflective of the body's water balance. Sodium imbalance can occur because of a change of sodium content in the extracellular fluid as a result of conditions such as excessive vomiting or because of a failure of the body to excrete sodium.

An excess of sodium in extracellular fluid is called hypernatremia, also referred to as an intracellular deficit (Metheny 1983). Initial signs and symptoms of uncompensated hypernatremia are the same as those of dehydration and hyperosmolality and hypernatremia. On physical examination, the patient reports thirst, and objectively a red, dry, swollen tongue, elevated temperature, and neurological manifestations are found. Neurological abnormalities such as disorientation, lethargy, irritability, focal or grand mal seizures, and hallucinations are caused by cellular dehydration (Gasparis 1989). In severe cases, permanent brain damage can occur because of subarachnoid hemorrhages as a result of brain tissue contraction.

Causes of hypernatremia include lack of fluid intake largely because of inability to respond to thirst (Gaspar 1988). Other disease states causing hypernatremia include diarrhea, ingestion of salt in abnormal amounts, profuse perspiration, diabetes insipidus, hyperalimentation without fluid correction, increase in loss of water vapor by the respiratory tract, excessive intravenous therapy using sodium-containing fluids, heart disease progressing to congestive heart failure, and chronic renal failure.

Hypernatremia can be prevented by offering fluids at regular intervals or alternate routes such as tube feedings or parenteral therapy; checking for excessive thirst and for an increase in body temperature; checking the mouth, tongue, and mucous membranes and providing mouth care; and monitoring for changes in sensorium, such as restlessness, increased irritability, disorientation, hallucinations, lethargy, stupor, or coma.

Hyponatremia is a condition in which the serum sodium level is below normal. It may be caused by an excessive loss of sodium or by excessive fluid volume. It is generally synonymous with a hypo-osmolar state with a relatively greater concentration of water than sodium. It can be thought of as a condition of water excess resulting in a diluted serum. Hyponatremia may also be associated with a normal extracellular volume because of excessive antidiuretic hormone activity. Hyponatremia may occur in heart failure, nephrotic syndrome, and cirrhosis of the liver. Drugs that impair renal water excretion include nicotine, chlorpropamide, morphine, barbiturates, and Isoproterenol HCL. (Karb 1989).

Sodium losses in disease states are related to gastrointestinal, renal, and third-space fluid losses. Skin losses occur via profuse perspiration and drainage from lesions. Other causes include profuse perspiration with increased fluid intake (athletes), low salt intake, use of diuretics, and aldosterone deficiency caused by adrenal insufficiency (Goldberger 1980). Hyponatremia can also occur when there is a gain in body water as a result of excessive parenteral administration of dextrose and water. In excessive administration of dextrose 5% in water, the body breaks down the dextrose, leaving a hypotonic water solution. This solution pulls potassium and fluid out of the intracellular space into the extracellular compartment, diluting serum sodium and increasing total body volume (Gasparis 1989).

When both sodium and body water are lost, the signs and symptoms are the same as those of extracellular fluid deficit. Pitting edema occurs with patients with hyponatremia associated with intracellular fluid excess.

Early symptoms of chronic hyponatremia caused by a combination of sodium loss and body water gain are those involving the gastrointestinal system, such as anorexia, nausea and vomiting, muscle cramps, fatigue, and dyspnea on exertion. Other symptoms include postural blood pressure changes, poor skin turgor, decreased fullness of neck veins, and flushed skin. Most of the symptoms are related to cellular swelling and cerebral edema, resulting in changes in sensorium with signs of increasing intracranial pressure, lethargy, weakness, confusion, focal weakness, hemiparesis, ataxia, Babinski reflex, convulsions, papilledema, and coma (Metheny 1983).

Intravenous Therapy Replacement

Fluid replacement by the parenteral route is used to correct any preexisting deficit of fluids and electrolytes, maintain fluid and electrolyte balance, or replace losses of electrolytes and fluids, in such conditions as burns, draining fistulas, vomiting, and diarrhea. Patients whose fluid volume is normal at the time therapy is initiated will require a solution to maintain fluid equilibrium. For replacement of an abnormal loss of fluid or electrolytes, replacement fluids are selected with a composition resembling the body fluid lost.

The goal of intervention in fluid replacement is to restore volume to normal without altering the electrolyte balance. Until the 1960s, intravenous therapy was the sole responsibility of the physician. Today hospital policies identify essential guidelines for hospital personnel to follow in inserting and maintaining intravenous lines, as well as preparation and administrating admixtures to patients. Parenteral fluids are classified according to the tonicity of the fluid in relation to the normal blood plasma. The osmolarity of blood plasma is between 280 mOsm/L and 300 mOsm/L. Fluid that approximates 290 mOsm/L is considered isotonic. Intravenous fluids with an osmolarity significantly higher than 290 mOsm/L (+ 50 mOsm/L) are considered hypertonic; those with an osmolarity significantly lower than 290 mOsm/L are hypotonic (Plumer 1987). In a healthy body, the number of cations equals the number of anions. When added together, cations and anions equal 290 mEq/L in extracellular fluid. Intravenous solutions may be equal to (isotonic), less than (hypotonic), or more than (hypertonic) 310 mE/L (Gasparis 1989; Metheny 1990).

The tonicity of the fluid when infused into the circulation has a direct effect on the patient. It affects fluid and electrolyte metabolism and may result in disastrous clinical disturbances. Hypertonic fluids increase the osmotic pressure of the blood plasma, drawing fluid from the cells; excessive infusions of such fluids can cause cellular dehydration. Hypotonic fluids lower the osmotic pressure, causing fluid to invade the cells; when fluid is infused beyond the patient's tolerance for water, water intoxication results. Isotonic fluids cause increased extracellular fluid volume, which can result in circulatory overload (Plumer 1987). Because of the direct and effective role osmolarity plays in intravenous therapy, it is helpful for the nurse involved in the administration of intravenous fluids to be able to identify the patient's osmolarity. The serum osmolarity is calculated by identifying the patient's sodium level, blood urea nitrogen level (BUN), and glucose level and using the following formula:

$$2(NA) + \frac{BUN}{5} + \frac{Glucose}{20} = 280 - 300 \text{ mOsm/L}$$

Each patient's osmolarity should range between 280 mOsm/L and 300 mOsm/L. Identifying the patient's need for hypertonic or hypotonic solutions will aid in assessing the patient's clinical manifestations of imbalances (Gasparis 1990).

Crystaloids are electrolyte solutions named for their potential to form crystals. After being infused into the bloodstream, they act much like extracellular fluid, diffusing through the capillary endothelium to the interstitium as necessary to maintain fluid balance (Plumer 1987).

Colloidal solutions are used as plasma expanders and are obtained from sources other than blood. These solutions exert a colloidal pressure similar to that of plasma proteins. By increasing the colloidal pressure in the vascular bed, fluid is pulled from the extracellular compartments, and the total blood volume is increased. Types of colloidal fluids include normal saline and lactated Ringer's solution; each of these solutions has a sodium concentration similar to that of extracellular fluid. Isotonic fluids have the same osmolarity as intracellular fluid. The fluids fill the extracellular fluid compartment without changing the osmolarity. An example of plasma expander is .9% saline. After colloidal solutions are infused, they are distributed between the extracellular compartment's two divisions. Very little fluid shifts into cells (Plumer 1987).

Hypertonic fluids pull fluid from the intracellular compartment into the extracellular volume. Hypertonic solutions have a lower concentration of free water but a higher osmotic weight (greater than 375 mOsm/L). Types of fluids include 10% to 50% dextrose in water, 5% dextrose in Ringer's solution.

Hypertonic fluids are rarely used without central line monitoring due to the ability of these solutions to cause circulatory overload (Metheny 1990). Hypertonic fluids increase intravascular osmolarity, which results in intracellular and interstitial dehydration.

Hypotonic solutions are used strictly for rehydration states. These solutions give water to dehydrated cells. Hypotonic solutions are given slowly due to shifting of fluid into the cells. Types of fluids include one-half Ringer's solution, D2.5 in water, and .45% PSS. Hypotonic solutions decrease intravascular osmolarity (Plumer 1987).

Colloids are used when the goal is to replace intravascular volume only. Crystalloids are used to replace concurrent losses of water, carbohydrate and electrolytes.

ASSOCIATED NURSING DIAGNOSES

Using Fluid Therapy as a category label for nursing intervention describes objective laboratory tests, physical assessment findings, and subjective information gained from patients. Nurses caring for critically ill adults use this information to develop diagnostic labels for goal-directed care to support the medical treatments of fluid imbalances. A sequence of events can be established instead of using isolated findings to develop nursing diagnoses. There are many groups of critically ill patients who require intravenous fluids. For every group of patients, there are a combination of nursing diagnostic labels one can use to deliver goal-directed nursing care. Head-injured patients are given slightly less fluid to reduce the risk of head injury, whereas patients with fever are given up to 15% more fluids to counterbalance the loss of fluid (Metheny 1990). Both of these groups of patients may be given the diagnostic label of Potential for Injury; although the stimulus for injury is different, the goals to direct nursing intervention to support and monitor fluid balance are similar.

The following are actual and potential problems most applicable to Fluid Therapy:

Fluid Volume Deficit
Fluid Volume Excess
Altered Nutrition
Decreased Cardiac Output
Impaired Gas Exchange
Ineffective Breathing Pattern
Altered Urinary Elimination
Potential for Injury: Cerebral Edema

| Date | Na | BUN | GI | Total | | Gains/ Losses | Average Temperature | Weight |
				Intake	Output			

FIGURE 18-1. Daily Evaluation of Fluid Therapy

EVALUATION TOOLS

The cornerstone evaluation tool useful in Fluid Therapy is the daily intake and output record. However, even carefully maintained records of fluid intake and output are less reliable than an organized and systematized nursing assessment. The most valuable evaluation tool is the nurse, objectively organizing assessment findings from a critically ill patient. Nurses are at an advantage in sequencing assessment findings over time in order to piece together a picture of fluid and electrolyte imbalances and their clinical manifestations. Figure 18-1 details an evaluation tool nurses can use at the bedside in evaluating the patient's fluid status. There are five aspects to this evaluation: the patient's weight, 24-hour total of intake and output, the amount of fluid gained or lost, the average body temperature, and serum laboratory levels pertinent to assessing the patient's osmolarity.

Nurses can assess and monitor the patient's fluid status. The general rule for maintaining fluid balance in a healthy adult is that intake should exceed urine

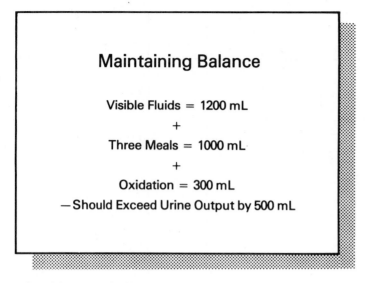

FIGURE 18-2. **Maintaining Balance**

output by 500 mL (Metheny 1983). Nurses can calculate the patient's gain or loss from the 24-hour intake/output record. A sudden rise or fall in a daily weight is a significant sign of a fluid imbalance. Laboratory values of sodium, BUN, and glucose aid in calculating the patient's serum osmolarity. The average daily temperature can assist the nurse in identifying a source of imbalance as in fluid volume deficit (the temperature rises) or identifying the fluid loss. Placing all assessment factors together on one sheet systematically organizes the patient's clinical picture. An organized and systematized assessment of the patient will lead nurses to an accurate nursing diagnosis.

Intake		Output	
• *Normal Daily Intake*		• *Adult Basal State*	
Liquids	1000 mL	1500 ± 500 mL	
Food (Solid)	800 mL		
Oxidation	200 mL	Per Hour: 60 ± 20 mL	
	2000 mL		

FIGURE 18-3.

INTERVENTION

The nursing intervention of Fluid Therapy includes the integration of knowledge of common causes and manifestations of fluid imbalances, as well as recognition of daily fluid requirements in critically ill patients. Organizing nursing assessment and using a Fluid Therapy evaluation tool will facilitate the collection of data. Actions appropriate to evaluating fluid therapy and identifying sources of imbalances will lead to accurate nursing diagnostic labels and goal directed nursing care. Each area that requires monitoring is outlined below.

Intake and Output

All intake and output should be carefully measured and recorded. Hourly urine measurements may be in order if the medical treatment order is to maintain urine output between 30 mL/hr and 50 mL/hr. All body fluids must be measured and recorded for the record. No body fluid should be estimated instead of measured, and ice must be measured as a fluid. Intravenous fluids discarded from shift to shift must be monitored. The fluid lost due to incontinence and perspiration can be weighed, and wound drainage, diarrhea, and any other fluid loss should be measured.

Decreased urinary output can be caused by a deficit of extracellular volume perfusing the kidney. In severe cases of fluid volume deficit, oliguria occurs and may lead to damage to the renal tubules (Lancaster 1987).

Pulse

The quality and the rate of the pulse provides clinical information valuable to assessing fluid and electrolyte changes in the patient. A high pulse pressure, bounding and not easily obliterated by pressure, indicates a high cardiac output. A regular pulse, easily obliterated by pressure, indicates a low blood volume. A bounding, easily obliterated pressure signifies a drop in blood pressure with a wide pulse pressure, indicative of impending circulatory collapse. As the patient's condition deteriorates, the pulse will become rapid, weak, thready, and easily obliterated, signifying circulatory collapse (Plumer 1987).

Respiration

Respirations must be evaluated in terms of rate, depth, and regularity, keeping in mind the respiratory changes that accompany metabolic acidosis and metabolic alkalosis.

Rales present in a patient without known pulmonary disease indicates an accumulation of alveolar fluid and an increased plasma volume, cardiac failure, or both (Metheny 1983).

Blood Pressure

The pulse pressure varies directly with cardiac output. When blood pressure changes are due to blood loss, the systolic pressure falls more rapidly than the diastolic, resulting in a diminished pulse pressure (Metheny 1983). Orthostatic hypotension and an increase in pulse rate when the patient moves from a lying to a sitting or standing position, is indicative of fluid volume deficit. If the condition becomes more severe, the blood pressure decreases even when the patient is supine. This is a result of loss of compensatory mechanisms. Increased pulse rate occurs as a result of the action of the heart to compensate for the decrease in intravascular fluid volume.

Body Temperature

The body temperature is subnormal in fluid volume deficit unless sodium excess is present. In intracellular fluid deficit, the body temperature can rise considerably related to a lack of available fluid for perspiration (Metheny 1983).

Fever causes an increase in metabolism and metabolic wastes. The increase in metabolic wastes requires a solution for renal excretion, therefore increasing fluid loss. Fever also causes hyperpnea, thereby increasing vapor loss through the lungs (Metheny 1983).

Neck Veins

Neck veins are flat with the patient lying supine. Direct measurement of the central venous pressure reveals a decrease in venous pressure. Patients with impaired cardiopulmonary function may have increased venous pressure.

Peripheral Veins

Examination of the peripheral veins provides a means of evaluating the plasma volume. The peripheral veins will usually empty in 3 seconds to 5 seconds when the hand is elevated and will fill in the same length of time when the hand is lowered to a dependent position. Peripheral vein filling takes longer in patients with sodium depletion and extracellular dehydration. Slow emptying of the peripheral veins indicates overhydration and an excessive blood volume, while slow filling indicates a low blood volume and often precedes hypotension.

Skin and Mucous Membranes

Skin turgor and texture is helpful in assessing the state of water balance. When skin over a bony prominence such as the sternum or forehead in an adult is pinched, skin that remains in a raised position for several seconds indicates a deficit in fluid volume (Metheny 1983).

A dry, leathery tongue may indicate a fluid volume deficit or mouth breathing. In order to differentiate between the two, moisture can be checked by placing a gloved finger between where the cheek and gum meet. Dryness in this area indicates a fluid volume deficit (Metheny 1983).

Weight

A sudden gain or loss in weight is a significant sign of a change in the fluid volume. A change in the volume of body fluid can be calculated by weighing the patient daily at the same time of day, on the same scales, with the same amount of clothing. A sudden weight loss or gain of 2 pounds or more in a short time is significant for a change in the patient's fluid status.

Patients with prolonged fluid deficit exhibit altered sensorium caused by a decrease in intravascular fluid volume, which causes a decrease in the perfusion of cerebral cells. The extremities are cold to the touch because of peripheral vaso-constriction.

Other changes include decreased pulmonary artery pressure, decreased cardiac output, decreased mean arterial pressure, and increased systemic vascular resist-ance (Plumer, 1987).

Tube Feedings

Patients receiving full-strength tube feedings, without additional water, are at great risk for developing hypernatremia. Extra water is particularly important when the patient has a fever, a decreased renal-concentrating ability, or extensive tissue breakdown. Sufficient water should be provided if tube feedings are used, to keep serum sodium within normal range. The elderly, because of their decreased renal function, require more water to excrete the prescribed solute load. The general rule is .5 mL of water for every 1 mL of tube feeding (Metheny 1983).

CASE STUDY

LC is a 56-year-old male who returns to your unit following major abdominal surgery. He has a nasogastric tube to low intermittent suction, which drained 800 cc in the recovery room. His blood pH is 7.58. The physician writes for Ringer's solution at 150 cc per hour because he is losing a large amount of electrolytes through his nasogastric tube. In your nursing assessment, you discover LC to have rales and sacral edema. LC's pulse rate is elevated, along with his blood pressure and respirations. Urine output is between 70 mL/hr and 100 mL/hr since returning from the recovery room. His serum osmolarity is 275 mOsm/L.

Along with nursing assessment and monitoring of fluid loss, nursing activities must include the recognition of the inappropriate intravenous solution. The appropriate solution to be hung at this time is dextrose 5% in normal saline; lactated Ringer's solution metabolizes into bicarbonate, therefore elevating an already high blood pH. A complication of infusing lactated Ringer's solution too rapidly is development of a hypo-osmolar state (Metheny 1990). Nurses using the evaluation tool, along with the documented losses of fluids, can collaborate with the physician in prescribing appropriate therapy for this postoperative patient.

CONCLUSION

Nursing actions for Fluid Therapy are in three areas: anticipation for imbal-ances, knowledge of underlying principles, and knowledge of assessment factors in fluid balance. Nurses implementing Fluid Therapy need to monitor patients for fluid imbalances and evaluate the outcomes of the Fluid Therapy. Intelligent, organized nursing assessment and evaluation is necessary to assist patients receiv-ing Fluid Therapy to avoid complications and restore patients to optimum health.

REFERENCES

Adams, F. 1988, July–August. Fluid intake: How much do elders drink? *Geriatric Nursing,* 218–221.
Adinaro, D. 1987. Liver failure and pancreatitis: Fluid and electrolyte concerns. *Nursing Clinics of North America* 22(4):843–852.

Beckwith, N. 1987. Fundamentals of fluid resuscitation. *Nursing Life* 7(3):49–56.

Bowmann, M., Eisenberg, P., Katz, B., and Metheny, N. 1989. Effect of tube-feeding osmolality on serum sodium levels. *Critical Care Nurse* 9(1):22–28.

Chenevey, B. 1987, December. Overview of fluids and electrolytes. *Nursing Clinics of North America*. Philadelphia: W.B. Saunders Co.

Gaspar, P. 1988, July–August. Fluid intake: What determines how much patients drink? *Geriatric Nursing*, 221–224.

Gasparis, L., Murray, E. and Ursomanno, P. 1989, April. I.V. Solutions: Which one is right for your patient? *Nursing* 19, 62–64.

Gasparis. L. 1990, September 24. I.V. dilemmas: Solutions at the bedside. American Journal of Nursing Conference, New Orleans.

Goldberger, E. 1980. *A primer of water, electrolytes and acid-base syndromes.* Philadelphia: Lea and Febiger.

Karb, V. 1989, April. Electrolyte abnormalities and drugs which commonly cause them. *Journal of Neuroscience Nursing* 21(2):125–129.

Lancaster, L. 1987. Renal and endocrine regulation of water and electrolyte balance. *Nursing Clinics of North America* 22(4):761–772.

McConnell, E. 1987. Fluid and electrolyte concerns in intestinal surgical procedures. *Nursing Clinics of North America* 22(4):853–859.

Maxwell, M., Kleeman, C., and Narins, R. 1987. *Clinical disorders of fluid and electrolyte metabolism* (4th ed.). New York: McGraw-Hill.

Metheny, N. 1983. *Nurses' handbook of fluid balance* (3d ed.). Philadelphia: J.B. Lippincott.

Metheny, N. 1990, June. Why worry about IV fluids? *American Journal of Nursing*, 50–55.

Plumer, A. 1987. *Principles and practice of intravenous therapy.* Boston: Little, Brown.

Poyss, A. 1987. Assessment and nursing diagnosis in fluid and electrolyte disorders. *Nursing Clinics of North America* 22(4):773–783.

Reedy, D. 1988, July–August. Fluid intake: How can you prevent dehydration? *Geriatric Nursing*, 224–226.

Rinard, G. 1989, December. Water intoxication. *American Journal of Nursing*, 1635–1638.

Rutherford, C. 1989. Fluid and electrolyte therapy: Considerations for patient care. *Journal of Intravenous Nursing* 12(3):173–182.

Sommers, M. 1990, January. Rapid fluid resuscitation. *Nursing 90*, 53–59.

INFECTION CONTROL

JERRI BRYANT
LINDA J. LEWICKI

DESCRIPTION OF INTERVENTION

Infection prevention and control date back to the mid-1800s when an Australian physician introduced the concept of hand washing in an effort to prevent puerperal fever. At approximately the same time, Florence Nightingale originated hygienic innovations and developed the practice of "fever nursing." Strict attention to personal hygiene and a sanitary environment were the foundations for infection prevention and control.

The modern era of infection prevention and control began in the 1950s when large epidemics of staphylococcal disease occurred in newborn nurseries. Although the epidemics subsided on their own in the 1960s, a more organized approach to infection prevention and control was adopted. During the 1970s virtually every hospital in the United States established a formal infection control program. In 1976 the Joint Commission on Accreditation of Healthcare Organizations (JCAHO) published standards that delineated the requirements for an infection control program. These standards required hospitals to have an ongoing monitoring system (surveillance) for hospital-acquired infections and to develop written policies and procedures for the prevention and control of infection in all areas of the hospital. However, surveillance techniques and the methodology used for rate calculation have never been standardized. Thus, the type, quantity, and quality of nosocomial infection data differ significantly among hospitals.

Formal infection control programs were also aided by the work of the Centers for Disease Control (CDC), which provided training for infection control nurses and produced written guidelines for the hospital environment and for the prevention of urinary tract infection, intravascular device–related infection, pneumonia, and surgical wound infections. In addition, the CDC conducted the Study on the Efficacy of Nosocomial Infection Control (SENIC), which demonstrated that adoption of certain infection control practices could lower infection rates.

The acquired immune deficiency syndrome (AIDS) epidemic forced the CDC to redirect priorities in the 1980s, and it curtailed training and guideline development. Fortunately, the Association for Practitioners in Infection Control (APIC) was able to take on these tasks and continue training and the development of guidelines (Table 19–1).

The Health Care Finance Administration (HCFA) has a generic screen for nosocomial infection as an indicator of quality. Hospitals can be denied Medicare reimbursement because of nosocomial infections.

A detailed description of a comprehensive infection prevention and control

TABLE 19–1.   GUIDELINES FOR INFECTION CONTROL PRACTICE

Centers for Disease Control (CDC)

Wong, E.S., and Hooton T.M. 1983. Guideline for prevention of catheter-associated urinary tract infections. *American Journal of Infection Control* 11:28–33.

Simmons, B.P., Hooton, T.M., Wong, E.S., and Allen, J.R. 1983. Guideline for prevention of intravascular infections. *American Journal of Infection Control* 11:183–193.

Simmons, B.P., and Wong, E.S. 1983. Guideline for prevention of nosocomial pneumonia. *American Journal of Infection Control* 11:230–239.

Williams, W.W. 1984. Guideline for infection control in hospital personnel. *American Journal of Infection Control* 12:34–57.

Garner, J.S., and Simmons, B.P. 1984. Guideline for isolation precautions in hospitals. *American Journal of Infection Control* 12:103–163.

Garner, J.S. 1986. Guideline for prevention of surgical wound infections, 1985. *American Journal of Infection Control* 14:71–80.

Garner, J.S., and Favero, M.S. Guideline for handwashing and hospital environmental control, 1985. *American Journal of Infection Control* 13:110–126.

Garner, J.S., Jarvis, W.R., Emori, T.G., et al. 1988. CDC definitions for nosocomial infections, 1988. *American Journal of Infection Control* 16:128–140.

Association for Practitioners in Infection Control (APIC)

Larson, E., 1988. Guideline for use of topical antimicrobial agents. *American Journal of Infection Control* 16:253–266.

Rutala W.A. 1990. Guideline for selection and use of disinfectants. *American Journal of Infection Control* 18:99–117.

program is beyond the scope of this chapter. Rather, the focus will be on the fundamentals of any program, hand washing, and the use of barrier precautions.

LITERATURE REVIEW

A nosocomial infection is an infection that has its onset during hospitalization and was not present or incubating at the time of admission. Approximately 5% of all patients admitted to acute-care hospitals acquire a nosocomial infection (Haley, Culver, White, et al. 1985a). The annual cost of nosocomial infections in the United States is between $5 billion and $10 billion (Wenzel 1985). It is estimated that one-third of nosocomial infections may be preventable (Haley et al. 1985b).

Direct contact is considered to be the primary mode of transmission of nosocomial infections and the hands of health care workers the most important vehicle for transmission (Weinstein, Nathan, Gruensfelder, and Kabins 1980; Schaberg, Haley, Highsmith et al. 1980; Schaberg, Weinstein, and Stamm 1976). Price (1938) described the existence of two kinds of organisms on the hands: resident and transient flora. Resident flora are organisms that survive and multiply on the skin but are usually of low virulence. They rarely cause infections except when introduced into the body through invasive procedures such as intravascular catheters. Transient flora include many different pathogens. These organisms are not firmly attached to the skin and can be readily removed by hand washing. Thus, the goal of hand washing is to remove transient flora acquired by contact with colonized or infected patients.

Several studies link hand washing to infection. Larson (1988) published a comprehensive review of the hand-washing literature from 1879 to 1986 and found 14 studies linking hand washing to infection. Nine of the studies were retrospective in which interruption in the spread of outbreak strains of microorganisms was attributed to improved hand washing. In five prospective studies, hand washing was the independent variable (cause) and infection the dependent variable (effect). She concluded that the collected evidence from nonexperimental and experimental studies is consistent with the hypothesis that hand washing is causally associated with a reduction in risk of infection.

Barrier precautions have always been an important part of infection prevention and control programs. Prior to the 1980s, precautions were used only for patients diagnosed or suspected of having an infectious disease and were known as isolation precautions. Most hospitals based their isolation policies on guidelines published by the CDC (CDC 1970, 1975; Garner and Simmons 1984). Indeed, the development, interpretation, and enforcement of isolation policies was considered an important task by the majority of infection control nurses surveyed as part of a national task analysis performed by the Certification Board of Infection Control (Shannon, McArthur, Weinstein et al. 1984).

Isolation precautions were initiated in response to a known or suspected diagnosis; thus, isolation precautions were diagnosis driven. In 1984, Jackson and Lynch published an article discussing the exaggerated emphasis on patients labeled "infectious" and the minimal attention paid to general handling of body substances from all patients. Again in 1987, these authors posed the question, "Why not treat all body substances as infectious?" They argued that many infectious diseases are characterized by clinically inapparent cases (such as hepatitis B). Moreover, even infectious diseases with definable clinical symptoms are frequently transmissible during the prodromal phase, before the onset of symptoms.

In 1987, in response to the AIDS epidemic, the CDC developed its system of universal precautions. It recommended that universal precautions be used for the blood and body fluid of all patients. This recommendation was consistent with the arguments put forth several years before by Jackson and Lynch and welcomed by the infection control community. But in a 1988 update on universal precautions, CDC changed its recommendations from all body fluids and delineated those body fluids to which universal precautions applied. They recommended the use of traditional isolation for suspected or known nonbloodborne diseases. This change in recommendations caused much confusion. Hospitals were successfully moving away from traditional diagnosis-driven isolation practices to infection prevention practices used for all patients. The universal precautions system developed by CDC has as its primary goal to reduce the risk of transmission of human immunodeficiency virus and hepatitis B virus to health care workers, whereas the goals of the barrier precaution system advocated by Jackson and Lynch are twofold: to reduce the risk of transmission of nosocomial pathogens (both bloodborne and other) to patients and health care workers.

Barrier precautions should be procedure rather than diagnosis driven. That is, precautions are directed at preventing the transmission of organisms during specific procedures or circumstances (Lynch, Jackson, Cummings, and Bond 1987). This approach takes into account that the source of most nosocomial pathogens is the colonized mucous membranes and secretions of patients, many of whom do not have clinically diagnosed infection. Unlike traditional isolation for which no specific documentation of efficacy exists, the use of barrier precautions for all body fluids from all patients has been demonstrated to reduce nosocomial colonization significantly (Lynch et al. 1990).

NURSING DIAGNOSIS AND APPROPRIATE CLIENT GROUPS

The nursing diagnosis most pertinent to this intervention is Potential for Infection. There are both intrinsic and extrinsic risk factors that influence the risk of nosocomial infection. Intrinsic factors include age, an increasing important variable in the light of an aging population, underlying disease, immobility, nutritional status, and immunosuppressive therapy. There has been a large increase in the number of patients undergoing transplants, such as heart, bone marrow, liver, and even lung. The dramatic increase in patients with acquired immunodeficiency syndrome and the use of drugs and treatments that prolong their life have resulted in a population at risk for infection that did not exist a decade ago.

The most important extrinsic variable has been the explosive increase in diagnostic and therapeutic invasive technology. In addition, the tremendous increase in the number and use of antibiotics has resulted in the development of highly resistant microorganisms.

Any patient, by virtue of hospitalization and exposure to health care workers, is at risk for nosocomial infection; however, the patient's underlying disease and the diagnostic and therapeutic modalities used to provide care greatly affect that risk. The health care worker is also at risk for nosocomial infection, especially blood-borne pathogens. This risk is influenced by the amount of blood exposure and the prevention of injury.

INFECTION CONTROL

Implementation of Infection Control consists of two basic measures: hand washing and the use of barrier precautions.

Hand Washing

Hand washing is the most important measure in the prevention of nosocomial infections. The purpose of hand washing in patient care is to remove microorganisms from the hands that were acquired by recent contact with infected or colonized patients or from environmental sources. The extent of hand contamination varies by type of contact (Table 19–2).

TABLE 19–2. ACTIVITIES RANKED ACCORDING TO THE EXTENT OF HAND CONTAMINATION

CONTACTS UNLIKELY TO CAUSE SIGNIFICANT CONTAMINATION OF THE HANDS[a]	CONTACT LIKELY TO CAUSE SIGNIFICANT CONTAMINATION OF THE HANDS[b]
1. Contact with sterile or autoclaved materials	7. Objects in contact with patient secretions
2. Contact with thoroughly cleaned or washed materials	8. Patient contact in which secretions, such as those from mouth, nose, and rectum, are touched
3. Contact with materials not necessarily cleaned but free from patient contact (e.g., papers, nursing station)	9. Materials contaminated with patient urine
4. Contact with objects handled by patients either infrequently or not expected to be contaminated (e.g., patient furniture)	10. Direct contact with patient urine 11. Materials contaminated with feces 12. Direct contact with feces 13. Materials contaminated with secretions or excretions from infected sites
5. Contact with objects intimately associated with patients but not known to be contaminated (e.g., patient gowns, linens, dishes, bedside rails)	14. Direct contact with secretions or excretions from infected sites
6. Minimal limited contact with patient (e.g., shaking hands, taking pulse)	15. Direct contact with infected patient sites (e.g., wounds, tracheostomy)

Source: Larson, E. 1988. Guideline for use of topical antimicrobial agents, *American Journal of Infection Control* 16:253–266.

Note: 1, Least; 15, greatest.

[a] May not always necessitate handwashing after contact.

[b] Necessitates handwashing immediately after contact; gloving during contact also may be needed.

TABLE 19-3.   INDICATIONS FOR USE OF PLAIN OR ANTISEPTIC SOAP

EXAMPLES	DESIRED EFFECT		
	Mechanical Cleaning[a]	Rapid Reduction of Contaminating and Colonizing Flora[b]	Residual Activity[b]
Routine patient bathing	X		
Routine hand washing in low-risk patient areas	X		
Routine hand washing in high-risk patient areas (e.g., newborn nursery, intensive-care unit, severely immunocompromised, transplant unit)	X	X	X
Preparation of hands before invasive procedures (e.g., venipuncture)	X	X	
Preoperative preparation of patient skin	X	X	
Surgical hand scrub	X	X	

Source: Larson, E. 1988. Guideline for use of topical antimicrobial agents. *American Journal of Infection Control* 16:253–266.
[a] If only this column is checked, plain soap is recommended.
[b] If this column is checked, antiseptics may be desirable.

Plain soap and water act to remove microorganisms from the hands. For general patient care, plain soap is acceptable. Antimicrobial soaps kill or inhibit microorganisms and may be indicated for use in high-risk patient areas (newborn nursery, intensive care unit) and before performing certain invasive procedures (Table 19–3).

According to the CDC, hands should be washed:

1.   Before performing invasive procedures (whether or not sterile gloves are worn).

2.   Before and after contact with wounds, whether surgical, traumatic, or associated with an invasive device.

3.   Before contact with particularly susceptible patients (such as patients who are severely immunocompromised and newborns).

4.   After contact with a source that is likely to be contaminated with virulent microorganisms, such as an infected patient or an object or device contaminated with secretions or excretions from patients.

5.   Between contacts with different patients in special-care units.

Barrier Precautions

In addition to hand washing, barrier precautions may be necessary to prevent the transmission of infectious agents to patients and personnel. Barrier precautions are the use of personal protective equipment (gloves, masks, eye protection, aprons and gowns) for contact with a patient's blood, any moist body substance, mucous membranes, or nonintact skin. Previously, barrier precautions were used only for patients with known or suspected infections; now they are recommended for all

TABLE 19-4. INDICATIONS FOR BARRIERS

BARRIER	INDICATION
Gloves	Anticipated contact with blood or any moist body substance, mucous membranes, or nonintact skin. Gloves should be changed between patients.
Aprons/gowns	Anticipated soiling of clothing with blood or moist body substances
Masks/eye protection	Anticipated splashing or aerosolization of blood or moist body substances
Masks	When caring for a patient with a disease known to be transmitted by the airborne route (e.g., tuberculosis, measles, influenza)

patients because clinically inapparent cases of infection and colonized patients are a major reservoir for infectious agents. Table 19-4 outlines the indications for specific types of barriers.

CASE STUDIES

Case Study 1

An 82-year-old female nursing home resident was admitted to the intensive care unit for hypoxemia and respiratory failure. Her temperature and white blood count were normal. She was intubated and placed on a mechanical ventilator. Two days after admission, the microbiology laboratory reported her sputum culture was growing methicillin-resistant *Staphylococcus aureus* (MRSA).

Antibiotic-resistant organisms are a major problem in hospitals and extended-care facilities. MRSA has been referred to as "supergerm" or a "modern plague." In many institutions, elaborate isolation precautions are implemented once the organism is identified. Unfortunately, MRSA and many other resistant organisms can colonize a patient and the patient have no clinical signs or symptoms of infection. Any mucous membrane or moist body substance has the potential to be colonized and should always be treated as such. Consistent barrier usage, especially gloves, for all patients decreases the risk of transmission from clinically inapparent colonized or infected patients and eliminates the need for ritualistic isolation precautions. Barriers should always be readily available to ensure proper usage.

Case Study 2

The head nurse of a surgical unit initiated a comprehensive campaign to increase hand washing among the staff. She used education, role modeling, and evaluation and feedback of performance as the means to change behavior. What data may be available from the infection control program to evaluate this campaign?

Prospective surveillance of nosocomial infections is a component of all infection prevention and control programs, but the data differ significantly among hospitals. The nurse needs to be aware of the limitations in using nosocomial infection data to evaluate practice. First, there is variation in the recognition of nosocomial infection due to the unavailability of standardized objective definitions, differential diagnostic practices, intensity of surveillance, and the skill of the infection control staff. Second, there is no generally accepted method to control for severity of underlying illness when determining nosocomial infection rates. Finally, there is no standardized method for the calculation of rates so the denominators used may not adequately define the population at risk.

Most institutions do not conduct comprehensive (total house) surveillance of nosocomial infections because of the tremendous cost. Instead, most use a more focused approach, such as surveillance of a particular high-risk area (intensive care, nursery, oncology unit) or a particular infection type (bacteremia, pneumonia). Hospitals frequently use a combination of focused methods designed for their particular case mix to obtain the greatest preventive impact at reasonable cost.

If nosocomial infection data are not already available to evaluate practice, the infection control nurses may be able to assist the nursing staff in identifying what data to collect and the methodology for analysis.

CONCLUSION

Infection Control is an important intervention for all patients. The intervention as presented here focuses on two key measures: hand washing and barrier precautions. Conscientious hand washing and the consistent use of protective barriers are but a part of an overall infection prevention and control program, but they are measures that any nurse can and should perform for all patients.

REFERENCES

Centers for Disease Control. 1970. *Isolation techniques for use in hospitals.* Atlanta, Ga.: CDC.

Centers for Disease Control. 1975. *Isolation techniques for use in hospitals* (2d ed.). Atlanta, Ga.: CDC.

Centers for Disease Control. 1987. Recommendations for prevention of HIV transmission in health care settings. *Morbidity and Mortality Weekly Report* (suppl. 2):1s–18s.

Centers for Disease Control. 1988. Update: Universal precautions for prevention of transmission of human immunodeficiency virus, hepatitis B virus and other bloodborne pathogens in health-care settings. *Morbidity and Mortality Weekly Report* 37:377–382, 387–388.

Garner, J.S., and Simmons, B.P. 1984. Guideline for isolation precautions in hospitals. *American Journal of Infection Control* 12:103–163.

Haley, R.W., Culver, D.H., White, J.W. et al. 1985a. The nationwide nosocomial infection rate: A new need for vital statistics. *American Journal of Epidemiology* 121:159–167.

Haley, R.W., Culver, D.H., White, J.W., et al. 1985b. The efficacy of infection surveillance and control programs in preventing nosocomial infections in U.S. hospitals. *American Journal of Epidemiology* 121:182–205.

Jackson, M.M., and Lynch, P. 1984. Infection control: Too much or too little? *American Journal of Nursing* 84:208–210.

Jackson, M.M., Lynch, P., McPherson, D.C. et al. 1987. Why not treat all body substances as infectious? *American Journal of Nursing* 87:1137–1139.

Larson, E. 1988. A causal link between handwashing and risk of infection? Examination of the evidence. *Infection Control and Hospital Epidemiology* 9:28–36.

Lynch, P., Jackson, M.M., Cummings, M.J., and Bond, W.E. 1987. Rethinking the role of isolation practices in the prevention of nosocomial infections. *Annals of Internal Medicine* 107:243–246.

Lynch, P., Cummings, M.J., Roberts, P.L., et al. 1990. Implementing and evaluating a system of generic infection precautions: Body substance isolation. *American Journal of Infection Control* 18:1–12.

Price, P.B. 1938. New studies in surgical bacteriology and surgical technique. *Journal of the American Medical Association* 111:1993–1996.

Schaberg, D.R., Haley, R.W., Highsmith, A.K., et al. 1980. Nosocomial bacteriuria: A prospective study of case clustering and antimicrobial resistance. *Annals of Internal Medicine* 93:420–424.

Schaberg, D.R., Weinstein, R.A., and Stamm, W.E. 1976. Epidemics of nosocomial urinary tract infection caused by multiply resistant gram-negative bacilli: Epidemiology and control. *Journal of Infectious Diseases* 363–366.

Shannon, R., McArthur, B.J., Weinstein, S., et al. 1984. A national task analysis of infection control practitioners, 1982. *American Journal of Infection Control* 12:187–196.

Weinstein, R.A, Nathan, C., Gruensfelder, R., and Kabins, S.A. 1980. Endemic aminoglycoside resistance in gram-negative bacilli: Epidemiology and mechanisms. *Journal of Infectious Diseases* 141:338–345.

Wenzel, R.P. 1985. Nosocomial infections, the diagnostic related groups and the study on the efficacy of nosocomial infection control: Economic implication for hospitals under the prospective payment system. *American Journal of Medicine* 78(6B):3–7.

20

ENVIRONMENTAL STRUCTURING

LORRAINE C. MION

DEFINITION AND DESCRIPTION

For the purposes of this chapter, environment is all the conditions that surround an individual. It is a broad multidimensional concept that includes physical aspects and properties, social factors, psychological factors, and cultural factors. The physical environment encompasses the space inhabited by the individual; it includes natural as well as built settings (Williams 1988)—for example, lighting, temperature, sound, aroma, color, and tools and objects used by the individual. The social environment refers to the interactions of the individual with others and the organizational policies that can affect or influence the individual's social climate (Moos and Igra 1980). The psychological environment refers to the individual's perceptions of the environment, preferences for specific features of the environment, and reactions to characteristics within the environment (Hiatt 1990). The cultural environment refers to the habits, traditions, codes, and mores that influence and affect the individual's behavior (Hiatt 1990).

The intervention Environmental Structuring is an assortment of nurses' actions that directly or indirectly affect environmental features and conditions. The purpose of this intervention is to facilitate healing, promote health and well-being, and protect patients from potential adverse effects. Environmental Structuring can range from simple one-time maneuvers to complex, intertwined constellations of ongoing activities. The nursing actions can focus on selected physical aspects of the individual's environment, nurse-patient interaction, and institutional policies and programs that may have a direct or influential impact on the individual's health and well-being. Examples of physical environmental structuring include the use of body prosthetics to promote functional independence (such as visual and hearing aids, ambulatory devices, and communicative devices), manipulating the environment to minimize adverse effects (such as noise reduction, temperature control, and minimizing glare), and manipulating the environment to promote psychological well-being (such as sensory diversity and stimulation and use of colors). Examples of Environmental Structuring as it pertains to nurse-patient interaction include those actions that enhance and respect the individual's personal space and need to control the immediate environment. Examples of organizational policies or programs include focus on primary care approaches as opposed to functional or team approaches, allowing choice of food items for meals, and promoting restorative rather than custodial nursing care.

The use of Environmental Structuring implies that the nurse recognizes the contribution of the environment to the well-being of the individual, identifies those aspects of the environment that are harmful to the individual, and is willing to focus attention on environmental features as they affect the individual.

LITERATURE REVIEW

The environment and its effects on individuals have been subjects of interest to nursing as well as to a variety of other disciplines, such as architecture, engineering, psychology, and anthropology. Since the time of Florence Nightingale, nurses have recognized the importance of the environment in the healing process. Indeed, Nightingale devoted whole chapters to the environmental topics of ventilation, lighting, temperature control, noise, and sanitation in her work, *Notes on Nursing: What It Is, and What It Is Not* (1859 [1946]). Later, nurse theorists and leaders incorporated the concept explicitly or implicitly within their models of nursing practice (Fitzpatrick and Whall 1989). Paradoxically, modification or enhancement of the environment has been a secondary issue to nurses (Williams 1990) and others in the health care field (Lawton 1990). Lawton postulated that health care professionals' minimization of the environment arises from the clinicians' difficulty to focus on every possible contextual feature that affects individuals. Nevertheless, evidence and interest of the environment's impact on physical and psychosocial health have been increasing.

Various disciplines have developed theoretical or conceptual models that attempt to explain the nature of the environment and its influence on the person. Gerontologists especially have been interested in the environment's effect on the functioning of elderly individuals. Lawton (1982) proposed a model of the transactions between a person and the environment in terms of personal competence and environmental press, or demand. There is a range of environmental demand within which a person can achieve a positive outcome in behavior or affect. The clinician can assist the person to improve or enhance the person's competence to meet the environmental demands. Alternatively, the clinician can alter the environment either to reduce or enhance the demands on the person. Personal limitations increase the individual's susceptibility to the influence of environmental demands. Hence, the frail elderly, the newborn, and immunocompromised individuals are at high risk for potentially adverse effects of the environment.

Kahana (1982) developed a model that emphasized the fit between the person and the environment. She proposed that the more congruent or better the fit between the person and environment, the greater is the contribution of the environment to the individual's well-being. Kahana's model emphasized the uniqueness of the person and his or her perceptions and preferences for specific physical and social environmental features.

Moos (1979) used a social ecological theory and postulated that the environment determines an individual's behavior. The environment consists of physical aspects, such as physical attractiveness and diversity, and social aspects, such as staff-patient interactions and organizational policies. In this model, the person's perception of the environment influences behavior in that particular environment. Topf (1984) proposed a model adapted from Moos's social ecological theory for nurses to guide their research efforts. Topf suggested that nurses examine not only personal and environmental factors but also the nursing actions related to Environmental Structuring, to examine the outcomes of the patient's health status.

Nursing research on environmental effects and interventions is limited. Most of it centers on the physical aspects of the environment. Rogers's (1970) model for nursing was a catalyst for her students to delineate the effects of particular environmental characteristics on patient outcomes (Williams 1988). For a thorough review of nursing research and the environment, see Williams (1988). The following review highlights selected nursing studies and is not intended to be exhaustive.

Institutional Design

Nurses have examined the effects of institutional design on patients and staff in both acute-care and long-term-care settings. Kayser-Jones (1982) compared patients' satisfaction with specific environmental aspects and quality of care in two long-term-care settings, one in Scotland and one in the United States. One aspect of her study was environmental features pertaining to meals. The Scottish facility featured selective menus, small table arrangements in a variety of areas, and table decorations. The American facility had no menu selection, used long tables covered in plastic, and had one dining room, which resulted in a high noise level. The Scottish residents overwhelmingly rated mealtime as a pleasant experience, while the American residents rated it as unpleasant.

Porter and Watson (1985) assessed the environment for all units in an acute-care setting on five separate occasions spanning 2½ years. The authors rated the units on physical attractiveness, patient functioning, staff functioning, and environmental diversity. The information proved to be useful in evaluating the implementation of a career ladder program, providing feedback to the hospital director after major renovations took place, and assisting nursing directors in matching employees to specific units.

Wood (1977) compared the effect of single- and two-bed rooms in an acute-care setting on patients' sensory stimulation. Patients in the single-bed rooms had more sensory and cognitive disturbances as compared to patients in the two-bed rooms. Interestingly, visual and hearing acuity and patient age had no relationship with the disturbances. The degree of immobility, however, was a significant factor in developing sensory or cognitive disturbances. Thus, lack of sensory stimulation and diversity appears to have a significant adverse effect on patients.

Davies and Peters (1983) examined patients' and nurses' views of patient stresses in a short-stay (mean length of stay was 1 month) geriatric unit at 1 week and 3 weeks of hospitalization. They found that the nurses' ratings were incongruent with the patients' ratings; nurses either underestimated or overestimated the level of patient stress. Moreover, patients had increased stress ratings from 1 week to 3 weeks regarding the hospital environment and routines, while the nurses rated the patients' stress as decreasing over time. From these findings, it appears that patients may not habituate or adapt to a stressful environment, and nurses make erroneous assumptions of patients' views of stress.

Space

A number of disciplines have examined human behavior within the context of space related to privacy, crowding, and territoriality. Kerr (1982) thoroughly reviewed the concepts and various theoretical frameworks of personal space and territoriality. Allekian (1973) surveyed hospitalized patients on their levels of anxiety regarding staff intrusion into the patients' territory (patient's room) and personal space (an area extending 4 feet from the patient's body). Patients expressed anxious feelings with staff intrusions of territory but not of personal space.

Louis's (1981) examination of the personal space boundaries of independently functioning elderly individuals yielded several findings of interest. Elderly subjects approached the interviewer more closely than they would allow themselves to be approached. There was a wide variation in the amount of preferred personal space among the subjects, with distances ranging from 1 inch to more than 3 feet. The angle of the interviewer's approach also elicited varying distances for each subject. The face-to-face approach had smaller distances than lateral or side approaches, a finding that implies that an individual's sense of personal space is asymmetrical.

Geden and Begeman (1981) examined hospitalized adults' personal space preferences for the home setting and for the hospital setting by type of approaching individual (family, doctor, nurse, stranger). Preferred personal space was smaller in the hospital than in the home. Subjects placed family members closest to self, followed by doctor, nurse, and stranger.

Sound

Nursing research on sound has focused primarily on noise levels within care settings and the adverse effects of sound on patients. Noise levels exceeding recommended levels have been reported in acute- and long-term-care settings (Hilton 1985; Topf 1983; Walgenbach 1990). Up to 46% of interviewed patients reported disturbed sleep because of high noise levels within hospitals and nursing homes (Davies and Peters 1983; Hilton 1985; Walgenbach 1990). Besides impaired sleep, other adverse effects from noise include impaired nutritional intake (Kayser-Jones 1982, 1989), altered blood pressure and heart rates (Topf 1984), infant agitation (Catlett and Holditch-Davis 1990; Gordin 1990), and subjective feelings of stress or anxiety (Davies and Peters 1983; Hilton 1985). Young, Muir-Nash, and Ninos (1988) examined whether noise had a beneficial effect on patients. The authors evaluated the effect of white noise—in this case the sound of a slow surf—on the occurrence of nocturnal wandering by elderly individuals with moderately advanced Alzheimer's disease. For two of the eight study patients, nocturnal restlessness decreased.

Light and Color

Williams (1988) noted that studies of changing light patterns showed little or no effect on human behavior. Continuous bright light, however, has been shown to have deleterious effects. Retinopathy, agitation, sleep deprivation, and endocrine changes have been reported in preterm infants exposed to continuous bright light (Catlett and Holditch-Davis 1990; Gordin 1990). Carefully designed studies of color and its effects on patient behavior are lacking (Williams 1988). Nevertheless, numerous articles are available in the gerontological literature on the use of color for safety and orientation purposes.

INTERVENTION TOOLS

Various tools are available for the nurse to assess or evaluate the environment. The tools vary in content depending on the focus of the evaluation. Moos and Lemke (1979) developed the Multiphasic Environmental Assessment Procedure (MEAP) to evaluate long-term-care settings in four areas: social climate, physical and architectural features, policies and programs, and patient and staff characteristics. The social environment subscale evaluates patients' and staff's perceptions of the social climate, such as the degree of perceived cohesion or conflict. The physical and architectural environment subscale assesses the presence of physical conveniences that add comfort and attractiveness, the presence of social-recreational aids, such as patient lounges, the extent that the patient has control over the physical environment, and space availability. The policy and program environment subscale assesses the degree of patient control over aspects of daily care. The patient and staff environment subscale assesses the staffing ratio and patient characteristics. Although MEAP has been used primarily in long-term-care institutions, Porter and Watson (1985) adapted it for use in the acute-care setting.

Chang (1978a) developed the Situational Control of Daily Activities Scale (SCDA) to assess patients' perceptions of source of control over their activities of daily living, such as grooming and toileting. Using this scale, Chang (1978b) found that situational control was a strong contributor to morale among nursing home patients. Ryden (1985) used the SCDA as part of a study to examine environmental aspects that have the potential for influencing the autonomy of nursing home residents. Ryden used the SCDA to obtain staff's perceptions as well as patients' perceptions regarding situational control.

A variety of assessment forms are available to examine environmental features that may contribute to the occurrence of a fall by an elderly individual. For example, Rubenstein and Robbins (1984) combined a situational environmental assessment with an assessment of symptomatology to assess elderly individuals who present with complaints of falling. Tideiksaar (1986) developed a checklist of environmental hazards common in the home setting, with simple suggestions for correcting the hazards—for example, replacing loose or slippery rugs (a hazard) with rugs with nonskid backs or tacking the rugs down to prevent curling and slipping (correction).

ASSOCIATED NURSING DIAGNOSES AND APPROPRIATE CLIENT GROUPS

A variety of nursing diagnoses are amenable to environmental structuring since the interventions can affect or modify physical aspects, social aspects, and/or psychological aspects of the environment. Table 20–1 lists the nursing diagnoses that might be treated with Environmental Structuring.

All patients or clients might benefit from the intervention of Environmental Structuring. Some groups, however, are especially vulnerable to the effects of the environment: the frail or institutionalized elderly, comatose individuals, infants, and immunocompromised individuals. Another group of patients commonly considered for Environmental Structuring are those with cognitive and/or physical impairments. Rehabilitation nurses are especially cognizant of environmental prosthetics to assist disabled individuals to meet environmental demands.

TABLE 20–1. NURSING DIAGNOSES SUITABLE FOR TREATMENT WITH ENVIRONMENTAL STRUCTURING

Activity Intolerance	Pain
Altered Thought Processes	Potential Altered Body Temperature
Diversional Activity Deficit	Potential for Infection
Hyperthermia	Potential for Injury
Hypothermia	Powerlessness
Impaired Home Maintenance Management	Self-care Deficits
Impaired Physical Mobility	Sensory/Perceptual Alterations
Impaired Skin Integrity	Sleep Pattern Disturbance
Impaired Verbal Communication	Social Isolation

IMPLEMENTATION

The function of Environmental Structuring must be performed with specific and well thought-out goals of therapy. Williams (1988) stated that difficulties arise in implementing Environmental Structuring when therapeutic goals are ambiguous or when a setting must serve many users and functions. Hiatt (1990) also listed a variety of barriers to improving the environment, such as clinicians' assumed expertise or deferred involvement and responsibility. Because of the enormous variety of conditions and phenomena that could be treated with Environmental Structuring, only three therapeutic goals for the use of this intervention will be described.

Enhance Safety

The very young and the very old are especially prone to injury from accidents or traumatic events in the community as well as in institutional settings. In the elderly, falls are one of the most common accidents and the leading cause of injury-related deaths for this age group (Baker and Harvey 1985). Elderly individuals who are at greatest risk of falling in all settings are those with cognitive impairments, physical impairments, or both (Fos and McLin 1990; Morse, Tylko, and Dixon 1987; Robbins, Rubenstein, Josephson, Schulman, Osterweil, and Fine 1989; Tinetti, Speechley, and Gintner 1988). Environmental Structuring to prevent falls consists of a combination of approaches that address the physical environment, institutional programs and policies, and personal competencies. Physical environmental structuring includes use of color to improve visual clarity, selection of furniture to facilitate rising from a sitting or lying position, elimination of hazards or obstacles from pathways, use of assistive devices at the macro level, such as handrails or grab bars, use of assistive devices at the micro level, such as walkers, eyeglasses, or braces, and attention to footwear and clothing (Andreasen 1985; Cooper 1985; Hayter 1983; Hindmarsh and Estes 1989; Lawton 1990; Morton 1989; Tideiksaar 1986). Organizational policies and programs aimed at preventing falls include careful assessment and identification of high-risk patients, facility-wide staff approaches and interactions with the identified patients, reorganization of nursing personnel's functions and duties to maximize available staff on wards, and planned daily physical activities that can be as simple as walking to enhance the patient's strength and balance (Mion, Gregor, Buettner, Chwirchak, Lee, and Paras 1989; Morton 1989; Suprock 1990).

Organizational programs and policies in acute- and long-term-care settings have also been recommended for elderly demented patients who wander. Physical measures combined with policies and programs aimed at maintaining the safety of these individuals include careful assessment and subsequent identification with visual cues of at-risk patients, use of electronic sensors at exits with specified staff actions when an alarm sounds, visual barriers in front of exits, and in-depth educational programs for staff in approaching and managing patients who wander (Blackburn 1988; Gaffney 1986; Namazi, Rosner, and Calkins 1989; Negley, Molla, and Obenchain 1990; Rader 1987).

Enhance Orientation

Manipulating the environment to enhance orientation for the cognitively impaired has been used in combination with reality orientation programs in nursing homes. (See Chapter 9 on Confusion Management.) Burton (1982) and Campos

(1984) reviewed studies of reality orientation programs and reported ambiguous and even negative effects of such programs. The term, reality orientation, refers to those therapeutic programs that emphasize consistent orientation over a 24-hour period from all staff members who come into contact with the patient combined with small group classes aimed at reducing social isolation. For mildly demented individuals, reality orientation programs may temporarily improve orientation to the environment, but they do not lead to changes in other behaviors. Nevertheless, use of this program as a way to enrich the environment and increase opportunities for social interaction may very well enhance the morale of residents and staff (Campos 1984). Indeed, environmental modifications for dementia patients have been reported to minimize agitation, reduce wandering, stimulate resident interaction, and maximize function (Maas 1988; Roberts and Algase 1988). Minimizing agitation can be attained through control of sensory stimulation from sound (radios, televisions, visitors), light (glare or poor illumination), and color (brightness, boldness, diversity). Maximizing function for dementia patients can be attained by assessing and addressing the cues available in the setting, as well as the degree of stability within the setting (Roberts and Algase 1988). For example, a chime can be sounded at mealtime (cue) to direct the patient to a room specifically defined as the dining room (stability).

Williams, Campbell, Raynor, Mlynarczyk, and Ward (1985) examined the efficacy of environmental activities on the incidence of acute confusional states among hospitalized elderly patients. They found that the most effective actions were those that provided orientation, such as clocks, corrected sensory deficits, and increased continuity of care. Brigman, Dickey, and Zegeer (1983) reported on environmental actions to deal with head injury patients who are in the agitated phase of recovery. As with dementia patients, many of the activities are geared toward orientation and controlling stimuli.

Improve Physical and Social Function

In the rehabilitation field, environmental prosthetics are well recognized as an appropriate route to the successful attainment of activity goals. Environmental prosthetics bring environmental demands within the person's competence (Lawton 1990). Frequently, clinicians consider prosthetics only in terms of body aids that enhance sensory or motor function, such as hearing aids and ambulatory devices. Environmental prosthetics encompass much more than body prostheses, however (Hiatt 1990; Lawton 1990). Prostheses can range from the simple prosthetics of eyeglasses to the high technology of computer-regulated life functions. For nurses to utilize an environmental prosthetic effectively, several steps are necessary. Initially, the nurse is more likely to consider the need for a particular prosthetic if the patient's physical or social functional impairment is clearly specified. To decide on the level and type of technological prosthesis to meet the specified need, one considers the environmental change(s) that would compensate for the identified functional impairment.

Sensory impairments have traditionally been approached with recommendations limited to eyeglasses or hearing aids. A large number of devices are available, however, from centers for the blind and deaf and from private companies, such as Sears Roebuck. These devices can assist the person to continue to function independently in the community and to enhance the persons' ability to socialize. Some examples of sensory prosthetics are closed-circuit television reading devices, talking typewriters and computers, talking clocks, speech amplifiers, and microprocessor-based communication systems for nonspeaking individuals.

Motor impairments can severely limit a person's ability to move freely. Prosthetics to enhance the individual's ability to move range from canes to highly complex electronic devices that are activated by gross upper body movements, such as brow wrinkling or blowing air.

Cognitive impairments have been primarily addressed by prosthetics that enhance an individual's safety, such as body-carried devices to track an individual who wanders. Memory enhancers are used for those with mild to moderate impairments. Nurses are familiar with the various medication reminders to elderly patients. Other memory enhancers are being devised and tested to assist persons in performing daily activities, such as sweeping the floor and dressing.

Impairments of activities of daily living include any of the self-care deficits. Various prosthetics are available to assist the person with eating, bathing, dressing, and toileting. Indeed, occupational therapists focus on the individual's manual dexterity and are excellent resources for the nurse. Examples of prosthetics designed to enhance self-care capabilities are dinnerware designed to protect from spills, silverware with various grips, long-handled reachers and sponges, raised toilet seats with grab bars, tub seats, and clothes with Velcro fasteners.

In conclusion, a wide variety of diagnoses can be treated appropriately with Environmental Structuring. The nurse needs to consider the environment within his or her repertoire of nursing care approaches. Creative thinking and use of objects within the environment will enhance patient outcomes. It is as timely now as when Nightingale (1859) first penned these words: "Put the patient in the best possible condition for nature to act upon him" (p. 75).

CASE STUDY

Mrs. M is a 76-year-old married woman who recently fell at home. She is admitted with a subtrochanteric fracture of the right femur to an acute medical-surgical unit at the local community hospital. Her past medical history includes hypertension and a cerebrovascular accident with left-sided hemiparesis. In spite of the hemiparesis, Mrs. M is able to ambulate independently with the use of a cane. She is alert and oriented at the time of admission.

Mrs. M undergoes surgery the next morning. Upon her return to the unit from the recovery room, she is restless and disoriented to time and place. The evening shift nurse does a careful assessment of Mrs. M and determines that the restlessness and disorientation are most likely a result of the anesthesia, pain, and unfamiliar surroundings. Mrs. M is medicated for pain. The nurse clearly introduces herself each time she enters the room and gives unobtrusive repetition of important facts to Mrs. M. She attaches the signal cord to Mrs. M's hospital gown and watches while Mrs. M returns a demonstration of how to summon help. A large clock and calendar are on the wall opposite of the head of the bed, and the nurse points them out to Mrs. M. Mrs. M is easily reoriented each time the nurse enters the room.

Mr. M, who has been at his wife's side for most of the evening, is concerned over her restlessness and confusion. The nurse reassures him that the confusion is temporary and asks him to bring in several of Mrs. M's personal articles to help make the environment more familiar.

At the change of shifts, Mrs. M is still awake. The evening nurse introduces the night nurse to Mrs. M. Mrs. M falls asleep and awakens the next day much more alert and oriented. By the end of the second day, Mrs. M exhibits no further disorientation or confusion.

When the surgeon clears Mrs. M for progressive ambulation commencing with non–weight bearing toe touch, it becomes apparent that she will have difficulty because of her hemiparesis. Physical and occupational therapists become involved with her care. The occupational therapist (OT) issues a long-handled sponge and reachers and teaches Mrs. M how to use these tools for bathing and dressing independently. The physical therapist decides that a walker with front wheels rather than a standard walker will be more effective for Mrs. M. The primary nurses on the day and evening shifts work closely with the therapists to reinforce the techniques with Mrs. M in her daily care. Since Mrs. M is not allowed to flex her hip less than a 90-degree angle, a raised toilet seat and chair cushion are recommended. Mr. M expresses concern about obtaining the items and caring for Mrs. M at home.

A home health nurse who has been contacted makes a home visit prior to Mrs. M's discharge. The couple lives in a two-story home, and their bedroom is on the second floor. The home health nurse suggests that Mr. M temporarily convert a first-floor den into a bedroom until Mrs. M can safely manage stairs. Fortunately, there is a bathroom on the first floor. The nurse makes other environmental recommendations to enhance Mrs. M's safety: a nonslip grab bar installed in the bathroom, nonslip adhesive strips along the sink top to provide Mrs. M with a nonslip surface for grasping, a raised toilet seat, and removal of throw rugs until Mrs. M no longer requires a walker.

On the tenth day following surgery, Mrs. M is discharged home. She is able to bathe independently and requires help only with donning her shoes. She is able to transfer independently. She requires standby assistance and cuing for walking 30 feet. Because of the home health nurse's involvement, the home environment has been adapted prior to Mrs. M's discharge.

The home health nurse continues to monitor Mrs. M's functioning in the home, and a physical therapist sees Mrs. M in the home three times a week for therapy. In 2 months, Mrs. M is again able to ambulate independently with a cane and negotiate stairs.

REFERENCES

Allekian, C.I. 1973. Intrusions of territory and personal space: An anxiety-inducing factor for hospitalized persons. An exploratory study. *Nursing Research* 22:236–241.

Andreasen, M.E.K. 1985. Make a safe environment by design. *Journal of Gerontological Nursing* 11:18–22.

Baker, S.P., and Harvey, A.H. 1985. Fall injuries in the elderly. *Clinics in Geriatric Medicine* 1:501–511.

Birren, F. 1979. Human response to color and light. *Hospitals* 53:93–96.

Blackburn, P. 1988. Freedom to wander. *Nursing Times* 84:54–55.

Bonk, J.R. 1979. Don't pass the buck: The full moon is not responsible for an increase in the occurrence of untoward events in a hospital setting. *Journal of Psychiatric Nursing and Mental Health Services* 17:33–36.

Brigman, C., Dickey, C., and Zegeer, L.J. 1983. The agitated aggressive patient. *American Journal of Nursing* 83:1409–1412.

Burton, M. 1982. Reality orientation for the elderly: A critique. *Journal of Advanced Nursing* 7:427–433.

Campos, R.G. 1984. Does reality orientation work? *Journal of Gerontological Nursing* 10:53–61,64.

Catlett, A.T., and Holditch-Davis, D. 1990. Environmental stimulation of the acutely ill premature infant: Physiological effects and nursing implications. *Neonatal Network* 8:19–26.

Chang, B.L. 1978a. Perceived situational control of daily activities: A new tool. *Research in Nursing and Health* 1:181–188.

Chang, B.L. 1978b. Generalized expectancy, situational perception of control and morale among institutionalized aged. *Nursing Research* 27:316–324.

Cooper, B.A. 1985. A model for implementing color contrast in the environment of the elderly. *American Journal of Occupational Therapy* 39:253–258.

Davies, A.D.M., and Peters, M. 1983. Stresses of hospitalization in the elderly: Nurses' and patients' perceptions. *Journal of Advanced Nursing* 8:99–105.

Fitzpatrick, J.J., and Whall, A.L. 1989. *Conceptual models of nursing: Analysis and application.* Norwalk: Appleton & Lange.

Fos, P.J., and McLin, C. 1990. The risk of falling in the elderly: A subjective approach. *Medical Decision Making* 10:195–200.

Gaffney, J. 1986. Toward a less restrictive environment. *Geriatric Nursing* 7:94–95.

Geden, E.A., and Begeman, A.V. 1981. Personal space preferences of hospitalized adults. *Research in Nursing and Health* 4:237–241.

Gordin, P.C. 1990. Assessing and managing agitation in a critically ill infant. *Maternal Child Nursing* 15:26–32.

Hayter, J. 1983. Modifying the environment to help older persons. *Nursing and Health Care* 4:265–269.

Hiatt, L.G. 1990. Environmental factors in rehabilitation of disabled elderly people. In S.J. Brody and L.G. Pawlson (eds.), *Aging and rehabilitation II.* New York: Springer.

Hilton, B.A. 1985. Noise in acute patient care areas. *Research in Nursing and Health* 8:283–291.

Hindmarsh, J.J., and Estes, E.H. 1989. Falls in older persons: Causes and interventions. *Archives of Internal Medicine* 149:2217–2222.

Kahana, E. 1982. A congruent model of person-environment interaction. In M.P. Lawton, P.G. Windley, and T.O. Byerts (eds.), *Aging and the environment: Theoretical approaches.* New York: Springer.

Kayser-Jones, J.S. 1982. Institutional structures: Catalysts of or barriers to quality care for the institutionalized aged in Scotland and the U.S. *Social Science and Medicine* 16:935–944.

Kayser-Jones, J. 1989. The environment and quality of care in long-term care institutions. In *Indices of quality in long-term care: Research and practice* (pp. 87–107). (New York: National League for Nursing No. 20-2292).

Kerr, J.A. 1982. An overview of theory and research related to space use in hospitals. *Western Journal of Nursing Research* 4:395–405.

Lawton, M.P. 1982. Competence, environmental press, and the adaptation of older people. In M.P. Lawton, P.G. Windley, and T.O. Byerts (eds.), *Aging and the environment: Theoretical approaches.* New York: Springer.

Lawton, M.P. 1990. Environments of rehabilitation. In J.D. Frengley, P. Murray, and M.L. Wykle (eds.), *Practicing rehabilitation with geriatric clients.* New York: Springer.

Lawton, M.P., Brody, E.M., and Saperstein, A.R. 1990. Social, behavioral, and environmental issues. In S.J. Brody and L.G. Pawlson (eds.), *Aging and rehabilitation. II. The state of the practice.* New York: Springer.

Louis, M. 1981. Personal space boundary needs of elderly persons: An empirical study. *Journal of Gerontological Nursing* 7:395–400.

Maas, M. 1988. Management of patients with Alzheimer's disease in long-term care facilities. *Nursing Clinics of North America* 23:57–68.

Miller, A. 1984. Nurse/patient dependency: A review of different approaches with particular reference to studies of the dependency of elderly patients. *Journal of Advanced Nursing* 9:479–486.

Mion, L.C., Gregor, S., Buettner, M., Chwirchak, D., Lee, O., and Paras, W. 1989. Falls in the rehabilitation setting: Incidence and characteristics. *Rehabilitation Nursing* 14:17–22.

Moos, R. 1979. Social-ecological perspectives on health. In G. Stone, F. Cohen, N. Adler, and Associates (eds.), *Health psychology.* San Francisco: Jossey-Bass.

Moos, R.H. 1981. Environmental choice and control in community care settings for older people. *Journal of Applied Social Psychology* 11:23–43.

Moos, R., and Igra, A. 1980. Determinants of the social environments of sheltered care settings. *Journal of Health and Social Behavior* 21:88–98.

Moos, R.H., and Lemke, S. 1979. *Multiphasic environmental assessment procedure (MEAP): Preliminary manual.* Palo Alto, Calif.: Social Ecology Laboratory, Stanford University and Veterans Administration.

Morse, J.M., Tylko, S.J., and Dixon, H.A. 1987. Characteristics of the fall-prone patient. *Gerontologist* 27:516–522.

Morton, D. 1989. Five years of fewer falls. *American Journal of Nursing* 89:204–205.

Namazi, K.H., Rosner, T.T., and Calkins, M.P. 1989. Visual barriers to prevent ambulatory Alzheimer's patients from exiting through an emergency door. *Gerontologist* 29:699–702.

Negley, E.N., Molla, P.M., and Obenchain, J. 1990. No exit: The effects of an electronic security system on confused patients. *Journal of Gerontological Nursing* 16:21–24.

Netten, A. 1989. The effect of design of residential homes in creating dependency among confused elderly residents: A study of elderly demented residents and their ability to find their way around homes for the elderly. *International Journal of Geriatric Psychiatry* 4:143–153.

Nightingale, F. 1946 (1859). *Notes on nursing: What it is, and what it is not.* Philadelphia: J. B. Lippincott.

Porter, R., and Watson, P. 1985. Environment: The healing difference. *Nursing Management* 16:19–24.

Rader, J. 1987. A comprehensive staff approach to problem wandering. *Gerontologist* 27:756–760.

Roberts, B.L., and Algase, D.L. 1988. Victims of Alzheimer's disease and the environment. *Nursing Clinics of North America* 23:83–93.

Robbins, A.S., Rubenstein, L.Z., Josephson, K.R., Schulman, B.L., Osterweil, D., and Fine, G. 1989. Predictors of falls among elderly people: Results of two population-based studies. *Archives of Internal Medicine* 149:1628–1633.

Rogers, M.E. 1970. *The theoretical basis of nursing.* Philadelpha: F.A. Davis.

Rubenstein, L.Z., and Robbins, A.S. 1984. Falls in the elderly: A clinical perspective. *Geriatrics* 39:67–71, 75–78.

Ryden, M.B. 1985. Environmental support for autonomy in the institutionalized elderly. *Research in Nursing and Health* 8:363–371.

Suprock, L.A. 1990. Changing the rules. *Geriatric Nursing* 11:288–289.

Tideiksaar, R. 1986. Preventing falls: Home hazard checklists to help older patients protect themselves. *Geriatrics* 41:26–28.

Tinetti, M.E., Speechley, J., and Gintner, S.F. 1988. Risk factors for falls among elderly persons living in the community. *New England Journal of Medicine* 319:1701–1707.

Topf, M. 1983. Noise pollution in the hospital. *New England Journal of Medicine* 309:53–54.

Topf, M. 1984. A framework for research on aversive physical aspects of the environment. *Research in Nursing and Health* 7:35–42.

Walgenbach, J.C. 1990. Lullabye and not a good night? *Geriatric Nursing* 11:278–279.

Williams, M.A. 1988. The physical environment and patient care. *Annual Review Nursing Research* 6:61–84.

Williams, M.A. 1990, October 5. *The physical environment and patient care: Can theories be developed?* Paper presented at the Third Annual Rosemary Ellis Scholars' Retreat: Concepts of the significance for nursing, Case Western Reserve University, Cleveland.

Williams, M.A., Campbell, E.B., Raynor, W.J., Mlynarczyk, S.M., and Ward, S.E. 1985. Reducing acute confusional states in elderly patients with hip fractures. *Research in Nursing and Health* 8:329–337.

Wood, M. 1977. Clinical sensory deprivation: A comparative study of patients in single care and two-bed rooms. *Journal of Nursing Administration* 7:28–32.

Young, S.H., Muir-Nash, J., and Ninos, M. 1988. Managing nocturnal wandering behavior. *Journal of Gerontological Nursing* 14:6–12.

DISCHARGE PLANNING

KATHLEEN C. KELLY
ELEANOR McCLELLAND
JEANETTE M. DALY

Nursing interventions are moving to the forefront in nursing practice, education, and research. Perhaps there are few other nursing interventions receiving the degree of attention that health care policymakers and funders are focusing on Discharge Planning. As an intervention, Discharge Planning is defined as the "preparation for moving a patient from one level of care to another within or outside the current health care agency" (Iowa Intervention Project 1992 forthcoming). With the current emphasis on health care access, quality, and cost, Discharge Planning is represented in recent literature as an intervention that can address all three issues (Naylor 1990b). Such outcomes of Discharge Planning are feasible but require certain qualities and behaviors within and among health care organizations and professions if they are to be achieved. They also require evaluation of existing methods of providing continuity of care in varied care settings and testing of new Discharge Planning strategies. This chapter addresses current forces driving Discharge Planning and the responses from health care providers, describes the research-based practices reported in the literature, and raises issues for nursing practice, education, and research.

DRIVING FORCES

The forces that are driving current interest in Discharge Planning come primarily from outside the health care delivery system. These include the cost of health care delivery, the aging population, discharge planning–specific regulations, and payment for care. Most prominent among these is the cost of health care delivery, resulting in the search for mechanisms that preserve client safety and satisfaction while controlling the cost of delivery. The introduction of the prospective payment system based on diagnosis-related groups (DRGs) was the impetus for many Medicare-certified institutions to take seriously the long-standing discharge planning accreditation criteria of the Joint Commission on Accreditation of Health Care Organizations (JCAHO). This new payment system ultimately led to patients' leaving hospitals at unprecedented levels of acuity and using alternative services at a level previously unknown in the privatized health care system of the United States (Naylor 1986; Rogers, Draper, Kahn, Keeler, Rubenstein, Kosecoff, and Brook 1990; Van Gelder and Bernstein 1986).

In an investigation of the DRGs influence on health care delivery at eight midwestern hospitals, Bull (1988) reported Discharge Planning to be one of the areas of practice critically affected. Specifically, subjects reported increased routinization, communication, and collaboration. Examples of strategies used after DRG implementation were Discharge Planning rounds, high-risk screening protocols, and documentation requirements aimed at communication and collaboration between nurses and physicians. Another major change related to physicians' control over this activity. Four of eight hospitals reported that a physician's order for Discharge Planning was required prior to DRGs. At the time of Bull's data collection, all institutions reported that nurses and social workers were encouraged to initiate Discharge Planning without physician orders. Bull also reported a perceived increase in collaboration among nurses, social workers, and clients but described no specific actions.

Another major force driving the concern for continuity of care and an investment in Discharge Planning as the means to achieve it is the aging population, with the concomitant increase in chronicity and the related use of health care resources. The projections for the twenty-first century regarding the numbers of very old and other populations with self-care deficits suggest that current health care delivery models are unprepared to handle the impact of this demographic shift.

In the United States the population aged 65 years to 74 years will grow by 87% between 2005 and 2025, compared with a 5% growth from the mid-1980s to 2005. By 2025 nearly 9% of the population will be aged 75 years or older, compared with 5% today (Bureau of Census 1987). The fastest growing component of the aging population is the very old (persons aged 80 years and older), who now number more than 6 million (22% of all elderly) in the United States. By 2005, 31% of elderly persons in this country will be aged 80 years or older (Bureau of Census 1987).

With this increase in the elderly population, the number of people eligible for Medicare will escalate. This growth, coupled with the fact that nearly one-third of elderly Americans live alone (Bureau of Census 1987), will influence the number of persons needing long-term care from resources beyond their personal and/or family capability or availability. The need for long-term care, while commonly associated with health problems, is frequently related to an inability to perform necessary activities of daily living rather than to a medical condition and its treatment (Congressional Clearinghouse for the Future 1984; Jessee and Doyle 1984; McClelland and Kelly 1980). The recognition of functional status and client well-being as key outcome variables is evident in current medical effectiveness research efforts (Ellwood 1988).

Societal views of long-term care, focused on medical treatment and institutional care, are not economically feasible in the light of the demographic shifts that lie ahead. It is imperative that the keys to containing health care costs for a population requiring interventions for acute, chronic, and self-care deficit problems be identified in this century (Congressional Clearinghouse on the Future 1984). Effective discharge planning in every care setting can be one of these keys.

Recent nursing research testing Discharge Planning strategies has focused on elderly clients (Naylor 1990a; Neidlinger, Scroggins, and Kennedy 1987). Other homogeneous study populations at risk due to health care or developmental characteristics are reflected in contemporary Discharge Planning research (Brooten, Kumar, Brown, Butts, Finkler, Bakewell-Sachs, Gibbons, and Delivoria-Papadopoulos 1986; McCorkle 1987; Quay and Alexander 1983).

The last two driving forces to be discussed in this chapter relate to incentives being offered to health care providers. The first is the proliferation of Discharge Planning–specific regulations, credentialing criteria, and review guidelines. Health Care Financing Administration (HCFA) Conditions of Participation (1986) make clear the continuity of care responsibilities for any provider certified for payment by Medicare and Medicaid. More recently the American Medical Peer Review Association published *Guidelines for PRO Use to Assess the Adequacy of Hospital Discharge Planning* (1990). The latest edition of the JCAHO *Accreditation Manual for Hospitals* (1990) reflects a clear expansion of standards and criteria specific to Discharge Planning. This is most pronounced in the standards for nursing care and documentation. These developments serve as a stick driving nursing and health care toward a rational approach to Discharge Planning.

The final force driving health care to a rational system of continuity of care to be reviewed is payment for services. The nature of the health care system's funding dictates that providers must demonstrate compliance with regulations or specified credentialing standards to be paid prospectively or retrospectively for services rendered. Therefore, providers must comply with HCFA regulations, PRO standards, and/or accrediting criteria specified by HCFA to receive national health insurance payment. Blue Cross and virtually every other private insurance company have used proof of such compliance as their criterion for eligible provider status. The intensified interest in Discharge Planning may be associated with the threat of losing certification and/or accreditation and the resulting loss of payment by most third-party sources. Whether the interest in this intervention is driven by threat or opportunity, nursing is in a position to take leadership in developing and testing continuity of care mechanisms across the continuum of care that serve clients and meet the demands placed on the provider organization and practicing professionals.

ORGANIZATIONAL TRENDS

Feather and Nichols (1984), based on the results of a nationwide survey of subjects in discharge planner positions, reported evidence that the discharge planner role was not institutionalized. The evidence ranged from lack of job descriptions to lack of role identity within the staff.

Since that time, there has been a general trend of incorporating Discharge Planning into care planning by members of the health care team. To achieve this, those in designated Discharge Planning positions act as consultants, screening and addressing organizational concerns regarding Discharge Planning and utilization. The assignment of discharge planners within the organization reflects this trend toward broad responsibilities of the discharge planner position. Findings in a 1986 national survey (Kelly 1986) supported this as reflected in Table 21–1. The same survey indicated that hospital discharge planner positions were being assigned to a wide variety of departments, including the finance and risk management

TABLE 21–1. DISCHARGE PLANNER ORGANIZATIONAL ACTIVITIES

ACTIVITY	NUMBER INVOLVED	PERCENTAGE
Utilization review	77	63.6
Quality assurance	70	57.8
Patient education program	57	47.1
Patient advocacy	32	26.4
Professional review	23	19
Other	15	12.4

TABLE 21–2.   DEPARTMENTAL ASSIGNMENT AND SUPERVISION OF
DISCHARGE PLANNER POSITIONS

SUPERVISION BY		DEPARTMENTAL ASSIGNMENT	
Title	Frequency	Department	Frequency
Nursing director/assistant	34	Nursing	23
Social service director	29	Social services	54
Central administrative representative	21	Patient services	11
Quality assurance/quality review director	10	Discharge Planning	7
Patient/support service/human service director	9	Quality management/ utilization review	6
Continuing care/discharge planner director	3	Other	12
Other	8		

departments (Kelly 1986) (Table 21–2). The survey reported six organizational models of Discharge Planning with the models differentiated by the extent to which the discharge planner provided direct services related to moving the patient to the next care setting.

In a 1989 pilot survey of nurse managers in a midwestern hospital with more than 500 beds, the primary nursing model of Discharge Planning was reported to be used by more than 60% of the unit managers and division directors (Kelly and McClelland 1989). This may demonstrate a trend toward incorporating Discharge Planning into the general delivery of care.

PRACTICE-BASED RESEARCH

Very little testing of practice-based strategies for Discharge Planning has been reported in the health care literature. In the 1980s, there was a focus on protocols and, to some extent, client and cost outcomes. Populations targeted in individual studies have been defined by age and generally by discrete medical diagnoses or conditions. Examples include very low-birth-weight infants (Brooten et al. 1986), chronically ill elderly (Falcone 1983; Kennedy, Neidlinger, and Scroggins 1987; Naylor 1990a; Neidlinger, Scroggins, and Kennedy 1987; Saltz, McVey, Becker, Feussner, and Cohen 1988), children with burns (Quay and Alexander 1983), and early hospital discharge of patients with cancer (McCorkle 1987). This literature demonstrates some lack of differentiation between Discharge Planning as an intervention and the specific strategies used.

As the preparation for discharge from a care setting becomes more integral to the client's total care plan, specialized practice roles and protocols are being tested and reported. These include nurses with advanced clinical preparation assuming responsibility for complex cases, organization-wide screening for at-risk clients, protocols for Discharge Planning with discrete populations, home follow-up by specialized staff for defined at-risk populations, and combinations of these. Table 21–3 summarizes selected research using specific Discharge Planning strategies as the treatment for experimental groups.

Table 21–3 demonstrates the trend toward using age grouping and specific medical parameters to define the target population. Additionally, it reflects trends toward Discharge Planning's being provided by staff with advanced clinical prepa-

TABLE 21–3.   SUMMARY OF SELECTED DISCHARGE PLANNING INTERVENTION RESEARCH

INVESTIGATOR	YEAR REPORTED	METHOD	POPULATION	SAMPLE SIZE	EXPERIMENTAL TREATMENT	FINDINGS
Brooten et al	1986	Clinical trial	Very low birth weight	79	Clinical nurse specialist (CNS) provided predischarge preparation and home follow-up	Reduced Length of Stay; 27% cost savings for first hospitalization; no difference in rehospitalization or number of acute care-visits
Kennedy et al.	1986	Double-blind experiment	Chronically ill elderly	80	Geriatric CNS used discharge planning protocol and home follow-up	Reduced Length of Stay, increased time between readmits
McCorkle	1987	Clinical trial (3 groups)	Early discharge of lung cancer patients	166	Oncology CNS provided home follow-up Referred for home care	CNS group had fewest rehospitalizations Fewer rehospitalizations than control group
Naylor	1990	Clinical trial	Chronically ill elderly	40	Combined Kennedy protocol and Brooten cost model	Decreased rehospitalization
Quay and Alexander	1983	Experimental	Children with burns	48	Long-term discharge preparation protocol on patient teaching and self-care	Decreased anxiety demonstrated at first outpatient visit
Saltz et al.	1988	Clinical trial	Elderly	185	Multidisciplinary evaluation within 48 hours of admission and staff consultation by team	No statistically significant difference in rehospitalization or posthospital placement

ration and the use of specialized staff to follow the individual out of the care setting, as opposed to collaboration and referral with other provider entities.

There are mixed findings regarding reduced rehospitalizations. Initial costs of care were positively affected by experimental treatment in studies reporting cost as the dependent variable. In no case was the experimental treatment reported to be associated with increased patient problems or increased cost.

To provide some insight into the rigor of these investigations, design, method, and sample descriptions reported by the researchers are provided also. While the sample sizes of those reported tend to be small, it must be recognized that these studies are testing methodologies, with ongoing research based on these findings. The most important features of these studies is their experimental nature. While exploratory and descriptive research is still appropriate for investigating some Discharge Planning phenomena, testing the intervention is timely and has implications for future effectiveness research in terms of client and organizational outcomes.

CONSIDERATIONS FOR CLINICAL PRACTICE AND MANAGEMENT

The implications of selecting a Discharge Planning strategy for practice can be viewed from the position of the clinical practitioner and the nurse manager. Since the efficiency and effectiveness of preparing the client to move quickly and safely through the continuum of care is a growing quality and risk management issue, staff and management must collaborate on developing a Discharge Planning model appropriate to their client population and the organization. The strategies used must fit the organization and must address individual client needs.

As some of the earlier descriptive research has suggested, organizations have been slow to use discharge planners and to integrate them into the delivery system. Since staff hired in these positions come from a variety of disciplines, no one professional group is guiding the development of the role. In fact, turf issues regarding responsibilities in this area have been reported (Bailis 1985).

Complicating the management is the proliferation of regulatory and accreditation criteria that specify Discharge Planning responsibilities of the organization and clinical staff. The history of Discharge Planning in the U.S. health care delivery system, combined with the need for rapid change imposed by regulatory and economic forces, produce new challenges in communication and staffing throughout organizations. Although JCAHO is assigning major responsibility for Discharge Planning activities and documentation to nurses involved directly in patient care, there is evidence that baccalaureate-prepared nurses are the only group in the profession who perceive Discharge Planning as a nursing responsibility (Caldera, Colangelo, DiBlasi, Garman, Kowalczyk, Mason, Murphy, Olson, Orr and Ouellette 1980). The influence of education on knowledge and sense of responsibility for Discharge Planning is supported in a recent study (Fritsch-deBruyn and Cunningham 1990). This may suggest that the majority of staff nurses do not recognize Discharge Planning as an appropriate nursing intervention.

The efforts to develop greater role clarity and reduce role conflict are not the work of management and clinical staff alone. Educators in all health fields must recognize that the role socialization they provide sets the stage for future practice. This should include remediation for current practitioners that defines Discharge Planning and the role of various providers in ensuring continuity of care that crosses organizational and professional boundaries. The case study at the end of this chapter demonstrates the attitude, knowledge, and behaviors that would be developed to facilitate continuity of care through the primary nurse providing the Discharge Planning intervention. Students need to understand there are discharge planner positions but that Discharge Planning also permeates many other roles and prescribed positions in an organization. Staff development departments need to provide the same role clarification to current employees so energy is used to institute effective Discharge Planning and is not spent on duplication, conflict, and confusion.

What new issues are raised by the reported research (Table 21–3) testing specific discharge strategies? No doubt most strategies had a desired effect from a quality of care and, in some cases, an economic perspective. The most common intervention strategy noted is the use of clinical nurse specialists prepared in the clinical area specific to the target population (oncology, gerontology, and maternal-child health). The use of this strategy was reported to be effective and to save money when compared to routine protocols in an acute inpatient setting (Brooten et al. 1986; Kennedy, Neidlinger, and Scroggins 1987). Following are some questions that arise from these findings:

- Can the health care system afford a clinical nurse specialist for each at-risk population identified?
- If clinical specialists were affordable, how available are they in most service areas with high numbers of at-risk clients?

- Would there be additional savings and effectiveness if the clinical trials included a group receiving early discharge and referral to a community-based agency with clinically competent community health–prepared staff?
- How would geographic and demographic variables influence the outcomes?

These and many other questions need to be addressed as successful techniques are considered for implementation in a given setting. The ideal research method for addressing these questions would be clinical trials.

An important caveat to add here is the striking similarity between Discharge Planning strategies being tested and case management models being reported in the literature. It is not the purpose of this chapter to compare and contrast the concepts of Discharge Planning, case management, and managed care, but it is relevant to identify the similarities in the forces driving their development and the target populations addressed. These similarities could lead to confusion, duplication, wasted resources, and the inevitable gaps in delivery that occur when terms, roles, and responsibilities are not clear.

CASE STUDY

Ann was a 42-year-old Caucasian who had a total abdominal hysterectomy with bilateral salpingoopherectomy as treatment for endometriosis. She was admitted to the hospital the day of surgery and had an uneventful postoperative recovery. Discharge Planning for Ann began on the day of admission to the hospital, since no contact was made with her during her outpatient appointment for preoperative tests. In addition to providing demographic information she was asked the following questions:

Will you live alone after discharge from the hospital?
Do you need a ride home from the hospital?
Who will care for you after you are discharged from the hospital?

Ann reported that she was single and lived alone. She was a high school graduate and had an annual income of $12,000. After discharge from the hospital, a friend would stay with her for a week. Thus, she would not have to worry about household duties or self-care deficits during that time.

On the third postoperative day, teaching and home management preparation was completed. Teaching content consisted of a guide to understanding hysterectomies, guidelines for incision healing, pain control, use of antibiotics, home activities, sexual activity, hormone therapy, prevention of osteoporosis, cancer facts, breast self-examination, and menopausal facts. A bibliography was provided.

During home management preparation, the nurse and patient assessed problems that might occur at home — for example, the physical layout of the home environment; the availability of someone in the home to assist as needed; mobility, such as climbing stairs, driving, taking a bath, and shopping; household tasks, such as meal preparation, cleaning, and laundry; and care for dependent others (friends, relatives, pets). For problems identified, alternate solutions were discussed with the patient. Ann anticipated no problems since a friend was staying in her home after the hospitalization.

Ann was discharged on the fourth postoperative day. The first day after discharge, when the staff nurse telephoned her at home, Ann's friend reported that Ann was in the bathroom vomiting. Her friend was concerned about the vomiting and reported that Ann had had no bowel elimination since shortly after surgery. The staff nurse advised Ann's friend to telephone the physician immediately. The nurse would telephone again later that evening to monitor Ann's condition. That evening, the staff nurse learned that Ann had taken a suppository and milk of magnesia as the physician had prescribed. When the staff nurse telephoned the following day, Ann's friend had several questions about the food Ann should be eating. Ann was now experiencing abdominal cramping.

In addition to responding to the immediate questions, the staff nurse explained that health promotion home visits from a community health nurse would be helpful and were part of county health promotion/prevention services. With Ann's consent, the staff nurse initiated a referral to a local community health nursing agency, explaining the medical and surgical history and that the major needs at this time were teaching, reassurance, and encouraging continued independence in monitoring recovery and seeking assistance as needed. If complications developed, the community nurse would follow up with the surgeon and personal physician.

The telephone referral was followed with a written summary, requesting feedback on the outcome of the community health nurse's activity.

SUMMARY

A variety of organizational models for providing continuity of care have been established in which nursing plays a prominent role. Discharge Planning has gained recognition as a nursing intervention, and research testing appropriate strategies has moved forward rapidly, with major funding sources giving higher priority to this practice area. As existing research is utilized and further research is implemented, practicing nurses, educators, and researchers are encouraged to build on this excellent beginning.

Eventually Discharge Planning may need to be integrated into the practice roles of all health care providers, with specialists acting as consultants and providing direct care in complex cases, much as case managers are described currently. Since planning a continuum of care is not the isolated responsibility of one health discipline, systems for crossing professional and organizational boundaries must be designed and tested. More focus on cost and alternatives based on using existing resources will be needed. Without these, the strategies tested in the past decade may fail, not because they are ineffective in themselves but because of communication and financial barriers encountered.

As research-based Discharge Planning evolves, the goal should be an integration that reflects the clients' movement through a continuum of care crossing organizational and professional boundaries. The product should be a continuum of care matching needs mutually identified by provider and client. Finally, Discharge Planning should be evaluated in terms of patient outcomes and the ability to contribute to the control of health care costs.

REFERENCES

American Medical Peer Review Association. 1990. *Guidelines for PRO use to assess the adequacy of hospital discharge planning.* Washington, D.C.: AMPRA.

Bailis, S. 1985, May–June. A case for generic social work in health settings. *Social Work,* 209–212.

Bakewell-Sachs, S., Gibbons, A., and Delivoria-Papadopoulos, M. 1986. A randomized clinical trial of early hospital discharge and home follow-up of very low birth weight infants. *New England Journal of Medicine* 315:934–938.

Brooten, D., Kumar, S., Brown, L., Butts, P., Finkler, S., Bakewell-Sachs, S., Gibbons, A., and Delivoria-Papadopoulos, M. 1986. A randomized clinical trial of early hospital discharge and home follow-up of very low birth weight infants. *New England Journal of Medicine* 315:934–938.

Bull, M. 1988. Influence of diagnosis-related groups on discharge planning, professional practice, and patient care. *Journal of Professional Nursing* 4(6):415–421.

Bureau of Census. 1987. An aging world. *International Population Reports,* Series P-95, No. 78. Washington, D.C.: U.S. Government Printing Office.

Caldera, K., Calangelo, R., DiBlasi, M., Garman, D., Kowalczyk, S., Mason, S., Murphy, M., Olson, A., Orr, C., and Ouellette, F. 1980. Exploration of the effect of educational level on the nurse's attitude toward discharge teaching. *Journal of Nursing Education* 19(8):24–32.

Congressional Clearinghouse on the Future. 1984. *Tomorrow's elderly: Issues for Congress.* Washington, D.C.: Congressional Institute for the Future.

Ellwood, P. 1988. Outcomes management, A technology of patient experience. *New England Journal of Medicine* 318(23):1549–1556.

Falcone, A. 1983. Comprehensive functional assessment as an administrative tool. *Journal of the American Geriatrics Society* 32(11):542–649.

Feather, J., and Nichols, L. 1984. Hospital discharge planning: The other side of continuity of care. *Caring* 2(10):37–38.

Fritsch-deBruyn, R., and Cunningham, H. 1990, July–August. A check on knowledge and sense of responsibility for discharge planning. The *Journal of Nursing Staff Development.* 173–176, 185.

Health Care Financing Administration. 1986, June 17. Conditions of participation. *Federal Register* 51(116):22042–22052.

Iowa Intervention Project (1992 forthcoming) *Nursing Intervention Classification.* St. Louis, M.D. C.V. Mosby Co.

Jessee, W., and Doyle, B. 1984, December. Discharge planning: Using audit to identify areas that need improvement. *Quality Review Bulletin,* 552–555.

Joint Commission of Accreditation of Health Care Organizations. 1990. *The 1991 Joint Commission Accreditation Manual for Hospitals.* Oakbrook Terrace, Ill.: JCAHO.

Kelly, K. 1986. *Discharge planner role: A study of factors related to bureaucratic, professional, and service role conceptions.* Doctoral Dissertation, University of Iowa. 87-21414, University Microfilms.

Kelly, K., and McClelland, E. 1989. *Individual and organizational factors associated with discharge planning structure, process, and outcomes.* Unpublished research report funded by USPHS Teaching Nursing Home grant (5P01 AG 07094-02), University of Iowa College of Nursing, Iowa City.

Kennedy, L., Neidlinger, S., and Scroggins, K. 1987. Effective comprehensive discharge planning for hospitalized elderly. *Gerontologist* 27(5):577–580.

McClelland, E. and Kelly, K. 1980. Characteristics of clients referred for posthospital health care. *Home Health Review* 3(3):11–22.

McCorkle, R. 1987. Complications of early discharge from hospital. *Proceedings of the Fifth National Conference — Human Values and Concerns.* New York: American Cancer Society.

Naylor, M. 1986. *The health status and health care needs of older Americans* (Serial No. 99-L). Washington, D.C.: U.S. Senate Special Committee on Aging.

Naylor, M. 1990a. Comprehensive discharge planning for hospitalized elderly: A pilot study. *Nursing Research* 39(3):156–161.

Naylor, M. 1990b. Comprehensive discharge planning for the elderly. *Research in Nursing and Health* 13(5):327–347.

Neidlinger, S., Scroggins, K., and Kennedy, L. 1987. Cost evaluation of discharge planning for hospitalized elderly. *Nursing Economics* 5(5):225–230.

Quay, N., and Alexander, L. 1983. Preparation of burned children and their families for discharge. *Journal of Burn Care and Rehabilitation* 4(4):288–290.

Rogers, W., Draper, D., Kahn, K., Keeler, E., Rubenstein, L., Kosecoff, J., and Brook, R. 1990. Quality of care before and after implementation of the DRG-based prospective payment system. *Journal of the American Medical Association* 264(15):1989–1994.

Saltz, C., McVey, L., Beeler, P., Feussner, J., and Cohen, H. 1988. Impact of a geriatric consultation team on discharge placement and repeat hospitalization. *Gerontologist* 28(3):344–350.

Van Gelder, A., and Bernstein, J. 1986. Home health care in an era of hospital prospective payment: Some early evidence and thoughts about the future. *Pride Institute Journal of Long Term Home Health Care* 5:3–11.

SECTION III

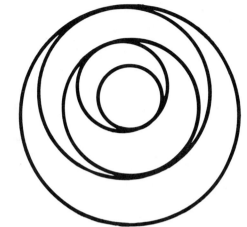

LIFE-STYLE ALTERATION

Overview: Assisting with Changes in Behavior

GLORIA M. BULECHEK
JOANNE C. McCLOSKEY

Nurses routinely work with clients who desire or need to alter their life-styles. Most people find security and comfort in their daily routines, and altering health behavior means changing familiar habits. The need for change often comes coupled with the grief and stress associated with catastrophic illness or injury. Changing behavior, especially long-term patterns, is never easy for the clients.

Psychologists continue the debate about what produces individual behavioral change. Cognitive theorists believe that a change in behavior is preceded by an internal change in attitudes, values, or beliefs. Rosenstock's Health Belief Model is a cognitive model that focuses on decisions that clients make based on their perceived susceptibility to disease or illness and the likelihood of goal attainment. On the other side of the debate are the behaviorists, who argue that behavior is shaped externally through reinforcement. Operant conditioning research has demonstrated that positive reinforcement rather than negative reinforcement or punishment is accompanied by behavioral change.

The professional practitioner is forced to conclude that the theory to explain life-style change is inadequate. The challenge for nurses is to develop skills that will facilitate self-directed change in clients. Life-style alteration can be viewed as a three-step process: (1) goal setting, (2) goal achievement, and (3) goal maintenance. This section of the book presents 10 interventions designed to assist with this process. The chapter authors draw from both cognitive and behaviorist theories to formulate treatments to assist clients with changes in behavior.

Counseling, presented in Chapter 22, involves a series of interactions over time in which the counselor helps the client to focus on feelings and behaviors that have interfered with usual adoptive behavior. Linda Jo Banks looks at the numerous approaches to Counseling, which fall into two major camps: cognitive, which emphasizes factual knowledge and increased awareness of the client, and affective, which focuses on exploration of the client's attitudes, emotions, and feelings. Banks favors an elective approach, and her definition of Counseling reflects this. Banks differentiates Counseling from Psychotherapy. Counseling is useful in helping the client focus resources to cope; Psychotherapy is needed to change pathologic behavior. Nurses must be able to distinguish these patient needs and refer to other health professionals when unable to perform the needed intervention skill. Counseling can be used with a multitude of nursing diagnoses in a variety of settings. Banks describes its application with a number of client groups. She provides techniques and strategies for implementing the intervention and discusses a number of ethical considerations in use of Counseling. The case study illustrates how Counseling can be coordinated with physical care. Implementation of Counseling in conjunction with physical interventions is a unique opportunity that nurses have over other helping professionals.

Reminiscence Therapy, the subject of Chapter 23, has developed to take advantage of the aged individual's normal developmental tendency to think about and relate personally significant past experiences. The aim is to enhance wellness in the aged client who is lonely, depressed, and withdrawn. Diane Hamilton indicates that Reminiscence Therapy can be used with individual clients or in small groups. The social sciences have studied reminiscence as a phenomenon, merely trying to describe it. Nursing is interested in Reminiscence Therapy as an intervention, and nursing research has focused on the outcome of the intervention. Favorable outcomes demonstrated through research include decreases in depression and in the amount of required medication and increases in socialization and self-care activities. Hamilton gives many suggestions for implementing the intervention; presents topics, objects, and activities to stimulate reminiscence; and discusses related nursing diagnoses and possible outcomes of Reminiscence Therapy. Hamilton suggests that Reminiscence Therapy might be appropriate for age groups other than the elderly, as relating past events tends to occur after the age of 10 years. The chapter concludes with a case study of a middle-aged woman with Alzheimer's disease who showed improved ability to carry out activities of daily living following Reminiscence Therapy.

Barbara Redman and Sue Ann Thomas define Patient Teaching (Chapter 24) as an intervention that uses a stimulus to help the patient develop a new thought, skill, or attitude that is permanent enough to be useful in behavioral change. They state that Patient Teaching is used in situations in which a combination of cognitive, affective, and psychomotor skills are to be developed and that the nurse's role in Patient Teaching requires counseling skills, but they distinguish between the counseling and teaching interventions. They believe the primary focus of the Counseling intervention is the affective domain. The body of literature for Patient Teaching is larger than for any other intervention in the book. Redman and Thomas synthesize the various reports on Patient Teaching from the health care field and present a state-of-the-art report on Patient Teaching, giving direction for future practice and research development. There are more intervention tools available for Patient Teaching than for any of the other interventions described in the book. Nurses use computers and assessment scales as teaching tools, as well as the more traditional written and audiovisual materials. Well-developed standard protocols are available for many common teaching situations. Application of the Patient Teaching intervention is illustrated through two case studies.

Values Clarification (Chapter 25) can assist clients in making important decisions about personal life-style. Many clients are ambivalent about changing their behavior to deal effectively with health promotion or chronic illness. Self-understanding of the personal value system may be a first step in helping to establish realistic goals. James Z. Wilberding defines values, describes the process of valuing, and outlines the use of Values Clarification in nursing. Nurses have tested the use of the intervention with clients with heart disease and adolescents in a public school. The literature relating to the field of education contains a number of intervention tools. Wilberding recommends two of these that are applicable in nursing. The chapter concludes with a case study in which Wilberding implemented Values Clarification in helping a young man with leukemia decide whether to have a bone marrow transplant.

Newspapers and other publications are filled with announcements for meetings of various self-help groups. These groups form around some common theme, such as a handicapping condition or a stressful life experience. In Chapter 26, Carolyn K. Kinney, Rebecca Mannetter, and Martha Carpenter present a framework that professional nurses can use to determine the type of Support Group most appropriate for a client. The framework is based on social support needs, and these authors give guidance in assessing the needs of individual clients. The framework also describes the characteristics of groups that are effective in providing social support. These authors present a unique model that demonstrates how nursing diagnoses result from a social support need and how group benefits can assist in treating the diagnoses. The model should help readers see how much of the nursing literature that is organized around needs can be utilized in deriving and treating nursing diagnoses. The recommendations for practice can assist both the nurse who is assessing a client for possible referral to an appropriate support group and the nurse who will be serving as a leader for a group. Matching of client and group and timing of the intervention appear to be crucial to a successful outcome. The authors present recommendations for research and conclude with a case study example of a Support Group for individuals who were recent widows.

The purpose of Group Psychotherapy (Chapter 27) is to help the client develop abilities and strengths that can be used in interpersonal relationships both within and outside the group. Veronica Wieland and Sandra Cummings outline a five-step intervention for which the nurse provides group members with an experience that allows them to develop new skills and abilities in understanding themselves in relating to others. This intervention is based on the stages of group development. The authors describe two interaction tools that the nurse can utilize to help the group progress through the developmental stages. Clinical examples of each of the five stages of the intervention are given, along with illustrations of application of the two tools.

Mutual Goal Setting is based on the premise that nurses and patients are equal partners in a relationship, each with different but equal responsibilities for reaching common health goals. Michele S. Maves describes Mutual Goal Setting as a process whereby nurses and patients collaboratively define a set of patient goals and agree on the goals to be attained. The process is facilitated by using Goal Attainment Scaling (GAS) to define, weight, rate, and score a set of goals. The expected outcome is specified at various levels of accomplishment. The patient's behavior is scored at the appropriate level at a predetermined target line. A formula is available for calculating a standardized score so that improvement can be compared across patients and settings. GAS is recommended for use with three to five goals at a time. Thus, it is suitable to use with a cluster of related nursing diagnoses. GAS is a ready-made evaluation tool for use in program evaluation or research. A nurse must be skilled in problem identification and goal setting to use it. The scoring process is quite easy, although the formula looks formidable on first glance. We have assisted graduate students in using it in both inpatient and clinic settings.

A holistic approach to dealing with persons who are dying is taken by Gail Ardery in Chapter 29, Terminal Care. Her first-hand experience with the approach in her practice in a hospice is reflected. She describes, reviews, and critiques four frameworks for describing the components of terminal care; explains the implementation of the intervention in application to particular nursing diagnoses; identifies nine nursing diagnoses that are prevalent in dying patients; and presents treatment approaches for each diagnosis. Ardery emphasizes the importance of bringing meaning to the experience of dying for the patient, the family, and the nurse. The case study provides an example of successful accomplishment of this goal.

Wendy L. Watson describes Family Therapy (Chapter 30) from a philosophical framework rather than as a treatment modality. A systemic view looks for connections and reciprocal influences among systems of ideas, people, and events. This approach focuses on relationships, effects of behavioral patterns of events, and information about the present. The three guidelines of hypothesizing, circularity, and neutrality are used to create a context for a family interview to become a therapeutic conversation. The goal is to enable family members to develop solutions to their problems. This approach is utilized by nurse family therapists at the University of Calgary's family nursing unit. Watson presents a list of belief statements to guide the practice of this group of nurses and outlines a series of skills that these nurse therapists use to provide systemic Family Therapy. A detailed case study of a suicide survivor illustrates the approach.

Robert J. Kus and Mary Ann Miller have incorporated Art Therapy (Chapter 31) in their practice of nursing with chemically dependent clients. They define this unique intervention as the creation of visual artwork for the purpose of healing and personal growth by individuals and the visual and verbal sharing of the resultant artwork in a group setting. Thus, they use art as a treatment, a purpose distinct from the usual use of art for diversion and recreation. The intervention has both benefits and limitations and can be used in association with a number of nursing diagnoses. The authors illustrate the use of the intervention through the description of five art projects they have implemented. A case study shows application of the intervention to help a young adult male admit cocaine abuse and begin the road to recovery.

The 10 interventions presented in Section 3 can be used by nurses to facilitate self-directed change in their clients. The need for life-style alteration is great among the escalating numbers of chronically ill. Several of the interventions can also be used in conjunction with the interventions by clients who wish to emphasize health promotion activities in order to prevent chronic illness. Nurses are key professionals in assisting with the changes in behavior that will foster healthy life-styles in clients.

22

Counseling

LINDA JO BANKS

There is no single, inclusive definition of Counseling. Meier (1989), citing Karasu (1986), estimates the number of different Counseling approaches at more than 400. Neither is there a clear delineation between Counseling and psychotherapy. Corsini (1968) points out that both share the processes of listening, questioning, evaluating, interpreting, supporting, explaining, informing, advising, and ordering, but they differ in the amount of time the therapist denotes to each of these processes. I agree with the broader statement by Corsini and Wedding (1989) that no clear definition exists that includes all psychotherapy methods and excludes all Counseling methods.

Counseling approaches have also been grouped as those having either a predominantly cognitive or an affective approach (Shertzer and Stone 1980). It is more useful, however, to think of all psychotherapies and Counseling approaches as methods of learning intended to help people change. These changes may serve to help the client think differently (cognition), feel differently (affection), or act differently (behavior). These changes may be new learning, remembering something forgotten, learning how to learn, unlearning something, or even learning what one already knows (Corsini and Wedding 1989, p. 5). All psychotherapies are essentially combinations of these three modalities.

Another approach to examining Counseling is that of the helping model and the professional helper (Carkhuff 1969, 1973; Egan 1986; Avila, Combs, and Purkey 1974; Hames and Joseph, 1986). The concept of helping involves both relationship and interaction. Relationship refers to the emotional experience or affective component between the helper (counselor) and the helpee (client). There is general agreement that the core elements of the Counseling relationship are acceptance (sometimes referred to as unconditional positive regard), empathy, congruency, and genuineness. A message of caring is communicated as the counselor affirms the client's personhood and self-worth. Helping also involves facilitating interaction not only between the client and counselor but also with the client and his or her environment (Rogers 1951, 1961; Carkhuff 1969; Truax and Carkhuff 1967).

It is important to differentiate between social and professional helping relationships. In social relationships, both parties share a mutuality related to self-disclosure and communication. The interaction is often casual, and friendship and enjoyment are often the key goals. In contrast, professional helping relationships are therapeutic in nature. The focus is centered and directed toward client self-disclosure and growth. Although the components of caring and concern are important, the professional helping relationship is one in which the client's true needs are uncovered and addressed (Hames and Joseph 1986). Carkhuff and Berenson (1977) identify the four goals of this type of helping: client exploration, client understanding, client action, and client learning. Professional helping relations

TABLE 22–1.   COUNSELING AND PSYCHOTHERAPY APPROACHES

APPROACH	KEY FIGURES
Psychoanalytic psychotherapy	Sigmund Freud
Ego psychology	Anna Freud
	Heing Hartmann
	Gertrude Blanch, Rubin Blanch
Interpersonal theory	Harry Stack Sullivan
Adlerian therapy	Alfred Adler
Person (client)-centered therapy	Carl Rogers
Gestalt therapy	Frederick Perls
Transactional analysis	Eric Berne
Existential therapy	Viktor Frankl
	Rollo May
	Irvin Yalom
Behavioral therapy	Arnold Lazarus
	Albert Bandura
	Joseph Wolpe
	Alan Kazdin
	B. F. Skinner
Cognitive therapy	Aaron Beck
Reality therapy	William Glasser
Rational-emotive therapy	Albert Ellis
Eclectic therapy	Frederick Thorne
	Lawrence Brammer
	C. H. Patterson
Object relations therapy	Sandor Ferenczi
	Melanie Klein
	Margaret Mahler
	Donald Winnicoth
	Althea Horner

usually do not occur spontaneously. They have time constraints and often involve a fee.

Building on the concept of helping as a formal professional activity and the problem-solving model, Egan (1986) developed a problem-management model, described as a cognitive-behavioral approach to Counseling and psychotherapy, which, he states, has been favorably received by both behaviorists and humanists. Although Egan's model supports an interdisciplinary approach to helping, he cautions that helping is a powerful process and in the hands of unskilled or unprincipled helpers can actually cause harm to the client (p. 5). Egan categorizes four types of helpers. First-level helpers (counselors, psychiatrists, psychologists, social workers) and second-level helpers (nurses, doctors, dentists, lawyers, ministers, teachers, parents, police officers) are specialists in their own professions who also help their clients manage problem situations in a holistic way. Egan's last two categories include managers, supervisors, relatives, friends, acquaintances, and other laypeople.

Egan purports that his problem-management model can be used to make sense of the vast literature in Counseling and psychotherapy. The model allows users to select techniques and methods that fit their own style and the needs of each client. He suggests that these techniques can be organized under the various steps of his three-stage model: (1) problem definition, (2) goal development, and (3) action. Egan offers use of his model as a way to counteract the criticism of the eclectic approach to counseling as lacking an organizing system and random use of counseling strategies and techniques.

The nurse counselor needs to be familiar with a wide variety of Counseling and psychotherapy approaches. Table 22–1 lists some of these therapies and the key figures associated with each approach. In this way, the nurse can incorporate knowledge of the nurse-patient relationship and nursing theories in beginning to develop a workable, personal Counseling approach. Review texts by Corey (1991), Corsini and Wedding (1989), Patterson (1986), Hansen, Stevic, and Warner (1986), Osipow, Walsh, and Tosi (1984), Shertzer and Stone (1980), as well as others that compare the key concepts, therapeutic process, and application of various techniques and procedures of each approach, may be particularly helpful to novice nurse counselors. In addition, the chapter on Counseling in the first edition of this text (Bulechek and McCloskey 1985) discussed four Counseling approaches: client centered, existential, behavioral, and eclectic approaches. Beginning counselors should become familiar with the client (person)-centered approach of Carl Rogers.

DEFINITION

The following definition of Counseling is compatible with my eclectic approach and draws heavily from works by Rogers, Carkhuff, and Egan:

> Counseling is an interactive helping process between a counselor and a client characterized by the core elements of acceptance, empathy, genuineness, and congruency. This relationship consists of a series of interactions over time in which the counselor through a variety of active and passive techniques, focuses on the needs, problems, or feelings of the client which have interfered with the client's usual adoptive behavior.

According to this definition, the counselor is a nurse functioning in a professional helper role, and the client is either one individual or a group of individuals with a common need or concern, such as family members or significant others. The term *client* is generally used in a community setting or home environment, while *patient* is used in the hospital setting.

ETHICAL CONSIDERATIONS

Ethical issues must always be considered when engaging in a counselor role. Confidentiality is imperative. All information shared in the Counseling session is appropriately discussed only within that relationship and, when necessary, with other health professionals who are directly involved in the client's care. In an emergency or crisis situation, the counselor's responsibility is to explain to the client as soon as feasible both the reason for and nature of the information shared.

The nurse's responsibility is to avoid engaging in conflicting roles with a given client. It is just as important to know when not to counsel as when to counsel. The nurse should avoid circumventing accountability for direct, hands-on patient care when this care is the nurse's specific responsibility. However, with a shortage of nurses in today's complex health care environment, in both hospital and nonhospital settings, the expertise of the professional nurse is often a limited commodity. More and more frequently, it is necessary for the nurse to evaluate carefully and then delegate those patient care measures to other members of the nursing team — licensed practical nurses (LPN) and nursing assistants (NA). When carefully and appropriately made, such prioritizing can free up time for the registered nurse (RN) to engage in patient/family teaching, problem-solving, and counseling activities.

One final consideration remains: appropriate and timely referral. No one individual, no matter how caring or committed, can meet the needs of all clients.

Neither will the nurse have the specific knowledge, academic training, or background necessary to work with a specific client effectively. In practicality, a working distinction does need to be made between Counseling and psychotherapy. When the nurse acts as a counselor, the goal is usually focused on helping the client regain or increase coping behavior. In contrast, psychotherapy is indicated when the client exhibits severe personality disorder or pathological behavior. Therapy in this type of situation requires a highly skilled practitioner who has both the legal right and educational preparation to intervene. When the nurse counselor is knowledgeable of local and community, public and private resources, referral may be the most helpful and valuable action the nurse can take for a client. The nurse is always ethically and morally responsible to make a referral when the client's needs are beyond the nurse's scope of practice, training, or expertise.

The issues of fee and length of counseling session need to be determined. In the hospital or clinic setting, the fee is often indirect and a part of the hospital or clinic service—for example, counseling by the enterostomal nurse (ET) with a new ostomy patient. In this type of setting, the duration of Counseling is usually limited by the length of hospital stay or the number of clinic visits. In the community setting, the considerations of fee and length are usually discussed by the public health or visiting nurse, parish nurse, or hospice nurse at the time of the initial visit.

APPLICATION

The use of Counseling has a wide range of applications in many nurse client situations. Hildegard Peplau, Orlando, and others made major contributions in the 1950s and 1960s in defining and clarifying the nurse-client relationship and the importance of communication skills, such as empathy and congruency. However, it has only been in the last few years that a variety of nursing publications have focused on Counseling as a specific intervention and that the term *counseling* can be found in the title, abstract, or opening paragraphs of nursing articles.

The intervention of Counseling is appropriate for many of the NANDA (North American Nursing Diagnosis Association) diagnostic categories, including the following:

Altered Family Processes
Anxiety
Body Image Disturbance
Decisional Conflict
Defensive Coping
Ineffective Denial
Family Coping: Compromised
Family Coping: Disabling
Family Coping: Potential for Growth
Fear
Anticipatory Grieving
Dysfunctional Grieving
Hopelessness
Ineffective Individual Coping
Knowledge Deficit
Noncompliance
Parental Role Conflict

Altered Parenting
Potential Altered Parenting
Personal Identity Disturbance
Post-Trauma Response
Powerlessness
Rape—Trauma Syndrome
Altered Role Performance
Chronic Low Self Esteem
Self Esteem Disturbance
Situational Low Self Esteem
Sexual Dysfunction
Altered Sexuality Patterns
Impaired Social Interaction
Social Isolation
Spiritual Distress
Potential for Violence: Self-Directed or
    Directed at Others

Nurses might use Counseling for any of the following purposes:

- Managing specific disease entities and disease processes.
- Coping with chronic or terminal illness.
- Adjustment to changes in self-esteem, body image, or self-care deficit.
- Adjustment to alterations in family coping or parenting.
- Dealing with feelings of anxiety, fear, denial, anger, or grief often associated with crisis or trauma situations.

Various authors have examined the special needs of cardiac patients and their spouses. Breu and Dracup (1978) developed a nursing care plan focused on helping the spouses of coronary care unit patients who were experiencing anticipatory grief. Specifically, they identified the spouses' needs for support and ventilation. Consistent with a Counseling approach, one of the key interventions used was the establishment of a consistent one-to-one relationship with a primary nurse. Sivarajan, Almes, and Mansfield (1983) studied how best to help cardiac rehabilitation patients modify their life-style and decrease their risk factors. A dual approach of teaching and Counseling was used with the primary focus on providing education. In analyzing their study findings, the authors reported that they felt the emphasis should have been on Counseling to promote behavioral change.

Various other authors (Boykoff 1989; Whipple 1987–1988; Baggs and Karch 1987; Scalzi 1982; Moore, Folk-Lighty, and Nolen 1984) looked at the psychological factors associated with sexual dysfunction after myocardial infarction (MI). There was general agreement that insufficient sexual counseling or none at all contributed greatly to their clients' feelings of anxiety, fear, embarrassment, frustration, rejection, withdrawal, and even shame. The spouses frequently reported feelings of isolation and aloneness once the threat of death was no longer imminent for their loved one. Boykoff stressed the important role that nurses, especially critical care nurses, play in not only providing information but also the environment that allowed the patients and their partners to explore their questions and concerns. Whipple emphasizes that nurses first must be aware of their own sexuality and value system before interacting with others in the sensitive area of sexuality. It is not only of limited help but also unethical for nurse counselors to impose their own value judgments, beliefs, or practices on others.

Numerous articles can be found regarding acquired immune deficiency syndrome (AIDS) and human immune deficiency virus (HIV). Holman, Sunderland, Berthaud, Moroso, and Cancellier (1989) developed pre- and posttesting counseling schedules addressing what they felt were the essential components of HIV counseling and testing of pregnant women. Key issues they included were informed consent, confidentiality, documentation of test results, and counseling the women regarding negative or positive test results. They emphasized the importance of assessing the individual's coping mechanisms, support systems, potential suicide risk, and previous psychiatric problems when reporting a seropositive test result. It was suggested that, when feasible, two staff people be present when having to report positive test results and that referral for additional counseling be discussed.

Nelson and Hellman (1989), from the perspective of occupational health nursing, discussed the role of the nurse in counseling employees at risk for HIV. They too discussed the importance of pre- and posttest counseling in accordance with Centers for Disease Control (CDC) recommendations. The communication strategies they used were open-ended questions, terminology (common or street language) easily understood and meaningful to the client, and recognition of cultural, ethnic, and religious beliefs. Nurses can play a key role in providing accurate information and counseling regarding this major public health crisis.

The role of nurses in providing holistic care for individuals and their families who are coping with chronic or terminal illness has long been recognized. In an effort to support and intervene in these situations even more effectively, nurses have been helping other nurses learn how to teach, counsel, and coordinate this care more effectively.

Anderson (1989) provides an extensive review of the literature related to the nurse's role in cancer rehabilitation. Frank-Stromborg and Wright (1984), Byrne, Stockwell, and Gudelis (1984), and Kaufman, Fox, and Swearengen (1990), examine how nurses can assist cancer and other chronically ill patients in adapting to disease and body image changes using structured support groups. Kaufman, Fox, and Swearengen (1990) identified three stages of adaptation: shock and disbelief; recognition and becoming aware of physical, mental, and emotional changes; and resolution. They identified common feelings associated with each stage and communication strategies effective in helping the person work through each stage. From a developmental approach, Byrne, Stockwell, and Gudelis (1984) studied the effect of adolescent suppport groups in oncology. Maguire and Faulkner described a short, intensive (4-day) workshop they developed to help doctors and nurses improve their skills in interviewing, assessing, and counseling.

Wilson (1989) conducted a qualitative study of the experiences of 20 caregivers who had assumed primary responsibility for home care for a relative with Alzheimer's disease. Conceptualization of an eight-stage model was developed reflecting the progressive course of the disease and the increasing and changing demands placed on the family members as the disease progressed. The model can be used to help plan an educational and supportive program for affected family members.

Engelking (1987) discussed a Counseling approach applicable for cancer patients faced with making choices regarding chemotherapy and other treatment modalities. Engelking emphasized the importance of being an effective listener and asking questions that help patients feel comfortable with their own decisions.

Parish nursing or health ministry offers nurses a unique opportunity to develop their counseling skills while practicing holistic health care. Granger Westberg (1989), credited as the pioneer of parish nursing, describes the role as health educator and health counselor. Parish nurses McDermott and Mullins (1989) and Smucker (1989) identified the need for a committed, caring, nonjudgmental attitude and communication skills of listening, enabling, facilitating, supporting, and promoting.

Numerous authors have addressed the importance of Counseling for ostomy patients. Watson (1983) determined that short-term supportive Counseling during the postoperative period resulted in improvement of patients' self-concept. Klopp (1990) and Gawron (1989) discussed the special role of enterostomal nurses in helping the ostomates deal with body image changes. Landmann (1989) addressed the developmental needs of adolescent ostomy patients. Using a Q-sort methodology, Coe and Kluka (1990) compared the priority concerns of ostomy patients and their spouses. Nurses can use these data in helping patients and spouses verbalize their key concerns.

Nurses also engage in Counseling activities with other nurses. Casey (1989) discussed an innovative practice in one hospital in which all new nurse managers were provided with Counseling by psychiatric nurse clinicians. The program was successful in helping new managers cope with the stress of first-line manager jobs, as well as increasing job satisfaction.

A few articles discuss nurses' use of a particular Counseling approach. Stockdale

(1989) described how she used Rogers's person-centered model in interacting with critical care patients and their families. Rogers's core concepts of empathy, genuineness, and positive regard provided the framework she needed to help her interact effectively with families and patients experiencing feelings of anxiety, fear, shock, and grief. Rogers's strategies for communicating both verbal and nonverbal empathy were also helpful. Stockdale cautioned that providing person-centered Counseling as part of nursing care in the intensive care unit setting is often more an ideal than a reality.

Burnard (1989) evaluated the advantages and disadvantages in the psychiatric setting of Rogers's nondirective approach compared to an existentialist approach to Counseling. She concluded that a key advantage of existentialism is that both the nurse and client can differ in how they view the world but with neither viewpoint seen as right or wrong. Both parties are left free to grow and change. Burnard referred to this as "counseling through negotiation." The author cautioned that this approach may not be suitable for all clients, especially psychotic patients.

TECHNIQUES AND STRATEGIES

The process of Counseling is generally considered to consist of three overlapping stages: initial phase, working or maintenance phase, and closure and termination. During the initial phase, counselor and client establish a therapeutic relationship, determine the length of the relationship, and begin goal setting. In the working or maintenance phase, the counselor helps the client move toward greater self-understanding and self-regulation, supporting and challenging the client in self-exploration; verbalizing, clarifying, and prioritizing concerns; sharing feelings and risking greater self-disclosure; and experimenting with new or alternative thoughts and behaviors. Counseling activity in this phase frequently involves a variety of active and passive techniques. It may appear that the process is moving both forward and backward as the client experiences and is helped to understand what are often uncomfortable feelings of fear, anger, mistrust, sadness, and even hopelessness or despair. Counseling activities in this phase are focused on helping the client develop new coping skills. In the third and last phase, closure and termination, the client begins to internalize new ways of thinking and use new behaviors of coping. The counselor helps the client look at the consequences and potential pitfalls regarding choices and identify possible contingency plans. Plans for termination are discussed, and Counseling activities are summarized. Ideally, counselor and client mutually agree on the appropriateness and time of termination.

Egan (1986) proposes a somewhat different approach to the stages and identifies several steps underneath each stage of his problem-management model: (1) problem definition, (2) goal development, and (3) action. In stage 1, the client is helped to identify problem situations that are not manageable and to explore opportunities to resolve these problems. In stage 2, the counselor helps the client set goals to bring about the desired change. The client develops a "preferred scenario"—a conceptualization of the desired situation if changes were made. The third stage is that of identifying strategies for action to achieve the desired change. The client is assisted in formulating and implementing a plan of action.

The stages of Counseling are never exact or rigid, rather, they are overlapping and fluid. The client may move in and out of the stages several times and still remain an active, working member of the counselor-client relationship.

The initial phase involves the establishment of a trusting relationship between the counselor and client. Rogers (1951) refers to this as establishing a "therapeutic relationship," which he sees as the most significant element in determining Counseling effectiveness. The core elements of this relationship have been well described by Rogers (1951), Carkhuff (1969), and Truax and Carkhuff (1967) as congruence or genuineness, acceptance or unconditional positive regard, and empathy.

Congruency or genuineness implies that the counselor is authentic and real and without a false front. To be genuine, counselors first need to be in touch with their own feelings and behaviors, positive or negative, and be integrated within the self before trying to interact in a meaningful way with another.

Acceptance or unconditional positive regard exists when the counselor has a deep and genuine caring for the client as a human being with intrinsic worth and dignity. This caring, accepting, and prizing is nonjudgmental of the client's feelings, thoughts, or behaviors as good or bad, right or wrong. Words such as *should* or *ought* are avoided. This does not mean that the counselor necessarily approves of all client behavior, but it does acknowledge and respect the client's right to have feelings and experiences without risking loss of the counselor's acceptance. It is also important that the counselor's caring be nonpossessive and not stem from the counselor's own need to be liked or appreciated. Caring that becomes possessive can thwart the process and decrease or negate the client's opportunity to gain new insights and achieve self-growth.

Empathy, the third core element, involves experiencing or sensing the client's feelings and behaviors sensitively and accurately as if they were one's own. Being empathetic reflects an attitude of deep interest in the client's world, particularly in the here and now. The counselor endeavors to communicate back to the client these understandings in a warm and sensitive manner. As this exchange between counselor and client moves back and forth, the client feels acceptance and the freedom and risks of disclosing still more. Sometimes the client confirms this by making comments such as, "You really do understand what I mean."

Goal setting is an important part of the initial phase of Counseling. The client may have very specific or vague and confusing ideas of what to expect. The counselor's perspective of goal setting is reflective of the Counseling approach used. Goals can be seen as existing on a continuum from those that are long term, general, and global to those that are short term, specific, and concrete. Humanistic or relationship-oriented counselors tend to stress the former and behavioral-oriented counselors the latter (Corey 1991, p. 431). Although it is generally seen as the client's responsibility to decide the objectives of counseling, the actual process of goal setting is shared between client and counselor. Goals are clarified as the therapeutic relationship evolves between the client and counselor.

Attending and listening skills are essential in all phases of the Counseling process. The counselor is perceived as empathetic when the client feels understood. Attending and listening require the counselor to be fully present to what the client is trying to say. It is important that the counselor's manner and eye contact indicate openness and attentiveness. There needs to be congruency between the counselor's verbal and nonverbal messages.

Helpful communication strategies include questioning, reflecting, clarifying or interpreting, and summarizing (Table 22–2). However skillful the counselor may be in using these strategies, the essential element is that the counselor be perceived as genuine and attentive. A technique that is sometimes useful is to help the client find words that reflect the degree of meaning the client wants to express. Various word lists can be used that provide synonyms for feelings that are often hard to express, such as anger, sadness, fear, and even joy. Taking the time to help the

TABLE 22-2. COMMON COUNSELING STRATEGIES

STRATEGIES	DESCRIPTION	USES
Active listening	An attitude of total attentiveness focusing on the client's expression of verbal and nonverbal behavior	Most effective tool to communicate counselor empathy with the client To provide cues to the client's inner experience To minimize the counselor's tendency to make premature judgment
Questioning	Inquiring or asking for more information in the form of a question	To clarify a matter open to discussion; to minimize doubt or uncertainty To facilitate client exploration of a problem or situation
Reflecting	Restating or rephrasing the content or feeling of a client's statement (one type of active listening)	To understand the meaning of what the client is trying to express in behavior or speech
Clarifying or interpreting	Stating the client's message with additional feedback or explanation	To increase the clearness of communication between counselor and client
Providing information or feedback	Using professional expertise to transmit pertinent information into facts, data, and responses	To add to current knowledge or relate new knowledge to prior understanding
Selecting or weighing alternatives	Assisting the client to list and prioritize all possible alternatives to a problem	To aid in expanding options and narrowing choices May facilitate the client's experimentation with unfamiliar options in a nonthreatening setting
Confrontation	Verbalizing the discrepancy between the client's feelings and behaviors (between real and ideal self)	To focus the client's awareness on actions that are incongruent with self-image and actual behavior
Tests and appraisal tools	Using psychological paper-and-pencil tests or other appraisal tools, which the counselor can administer and interpret	To help increase client self-awareness; to add to the counselor's data base about the client (examples: self-inventory of cardiac risk factors or the Holmes and Rahe Social Readjustment Rating Scales)
Self-disclosure	Revealing selected aspects of one's own experiences or personality	To foster genuineness and trust in the counseling situation when used appropriately.

client find the most meaningful words also portrays the counselor's genuine interest. It is important that the counselor be aware of any personal biases so as not to listen in an evaluative or judgmental way. Neither should sympathetic listening on the part of the counselor be allowed to move the focus away from the story that is being shared by the client. A good rule to remember in Counseling is that sympathy does not take the place of empathy.

Egan (1986) describes basic empathy as "listening carefully to the client and then communicating understanding of what the client is feeling and of the experiences and behaviors underlying these feelings" (p. 99). Basic empathy focuses on relevant surface feelings and meanings; advanced empathy deals with "feelings and meanings that are buried, hidden, or beyond the immediate reach of the client" (p. 213). Egan suggests several ways to help communicate advanced empathy. One way is to express back to the client what was implied but not said. The counselor can help the client identify and explore behavioral and emotional themes in problem situations. These themes are described as self-defeating behavioral and emotional patterns, such as poor self-image or dominance. Advanced empathy can be helping the client pull together pieces of data that were presented separately but are actually related to each other. Still another way is for the counselor to help the client draw conclusions or a greater level of understanding from that which the client presented as just a premise.

As the working phase of Counseling progresses, the client may experience blocks to self-disclosure — fear of intensity of the work, concerns about confidentiality, fear of finding out "too much" about oneself, feelings of shame, or fear of change (Egan 1986, pp. 140–142).

Challenging is the technique of helping the client examine the discrepancies between the client's experiences of self and the world and the way things really are (Egan 1986). Challenging also helps the client focus on the actions needed to manage problems and then take appropriate action. Challenging should be undertaken carefully as probable hunches, not as accusations. When challenging is used accurately and carefully, the client has the opportunity to reexamine experiences, behaviors, and feelings for greater self-awareness and growth.

The last major activity in the working phase of Counseling is helping the client to identify, prioritize, and evaluate possible actions to increase coping and/or solve problems. Egan (1986) refers to this as helping the client choose "best-fit" strategies. The client is encouraged to brainstorm possible actions and examine each. The following questions can aid the client in this process:

- Is the strategy specific and measurable?
- Is the course of action realistic (within the client's control)?
- Is the strategy adequate to achieve the desired goal?
- Is the action owned by the client and consistent with the client's own values?
- Can the strategy be completed within a reasonable time frame?

The final phase of the Counseling process, closure and termination, actually begins during the first stage as goal setting occurs and the time framework is established. Potential pitfalls of selected actions are discussed, as well as ways to avoid or minimize future risks. Together the counselor and client talk about the client's readiness to end counseling and how the client can best maintain self-growth and new learning. Possible actions and support systems are discussed should the client experience regression to old or ineffective coping behaviors. Generally, the counselor indicates that should the client feel the need for a follow-up visit that this can be arranged. Occasionally, referral may be indicated because the counselor or counselor client agree that they have not reached a workable solution to identified problems or concerns.

Some basic guidelines facilitate Counseling (Meier 1989). Several are related to the amount and type of counselor feedback. Generally, it is better for the counselor to respond to the client in one- or two-sentence replies. The focus needs to remain on what the client has to say. In the therapeutic setting, silence can be golden. When in doubt about what to say, saying nothing is a choice. Periods of silence may seem awkward to the counselor, but the client may need this time for internal processing of thoughts and feelings and thus gain new insights. A nurse in doubt as to what would be the most helpful feedback to the client can focus on the client's feelings. Apart from the initial interview and when making summary comments, it is largely the client's, not the counselor's, responsibility to talk.

Just as there are strategies that help the client's self-exploration, there are also pitfalls to avoid. One is to offer advice indiscriminately. Another is not to fall into the habit of just asking the client questions, particularly "why" questions, which can put the client on the defense and thwart the process.

CASE STUDY

Carol, a 51-year-old woman with severe debilitating multiple sclerosis, lived with her mother, who was her primary caregiver. Carol was hospitalized for treatment of an infected, draining wound. I was consulted to "pouch" the site and devise a skin care treatment program that consisted of a 45-minute dressing change every other day.

During my initial visits, I recognized the value of using the nursing intervention of Counseling. Not only did Carol have total self-care needs, she also experienced psychosocial limitations related to being hospitalized, away from the home environment, and with limited control of how and when her daily cares were given. In addition, Carol had neurological impairment that made her speech sound almost garbled. The Counseling goal was to provide a supportive, caring relationship in which Carol would experience an increased sense of control. During this initial stage, I established with Carol the length and duration of visits. I told Carol that I would come three times a week to do her dressing changes and that we could also use this time to "just talk" about whatever was of interest or concern to her at the time.

The working phase of Counseling focused on establishing a relationship based on congruency, acceptance, and empathy. It was important for Carol to believe that I did want to hear what she had to say and that I would take the time to clarify and listen even when her speech was difficult to understand. Carol's trust in the relationship grew as I encouraged and allowed her to talk about herself as a person, her special interests, favorite television programs, and visits from her two granddaughters. It also allowed me as counselor to identify major issues of concern. Carol began to share her fear that the doctor might suggest she be discharged to a skilled care facility rather than return home. This was a realistic concern since Carol's mother also took care of her own frail, elderly mother.

It was important that my manner and actions reflect a sensitivity to Carol's fears and how important it was for her to retain as much control of her own life as possible. I used both passive and active strategies. Often I remained silent while sitting attentively by Carol's bed and allowed her to talk about her fears. Other times, I took a more active role by providing Carol information related to possible nursing home care as well as follow-up by a visiting–home care nurse.

Transition to the third and last phase of Counseling (closure and termination) was initiated as the wound began to show signs of definite healing. As counselor, I worked in collaboration with Carol and social services to continue discharge planning and explore all possible options. I arranged to have Carol's mother come to visit during a dressing change so that she could observe the procedure. Twelve weeks after her admission to the hospital, arrangements were completed for Carol to return home but with increased weekly visits by the public health nurse, who would do the dressing changes.

This case study is in no way unique, but it does illustrate an important point: the bedside nurse frequently has the opportunity to support, guide, teach, and counsel patients and families while also providing necessary physical cares.

SUMMARY

Counseling as an intervention has only recently been addressed in the nursing literature. This is true despite a widely accepted assumption that nursing is a helping, caring process based on a personal relationship between a nurse and a patient. This chapter has provided an overview of terminology surrounding this intervention and a definition that is applicable in nursing. Strategies for application of the intervention with different client groups with diverse diagnoses, along with ethical considerations, have been presented.

REFERENCES

Anderson, J. 1989. The nurse's role in cancer rehabilitation. *Cancer Nursing* 12(2):85–94.

Avila, D., Combs, A., and Purkey W. 1974. *The helping relationship sourcebook.* Boston: Allyn and Bacon.

Baggs, J., and Karch, A. 1987. Sexual counseling of women with coronary heart disease. *Heart Lung* 16:154–159.

Banks, L. Counseling. 1985. In G. Bulechek and J. McCloskey (eds.), *Nursing interventions — treatments for nursing diagnoses.* Philadelphia: W.B. Saunders.

Boykoff, S. 1989, November–December. Strategies for sexual counseling of patients following a myocardial infarction. *Dimensions of Critical Care Nursing* 8(6):368–373.

Breu, C., and Dracup, K. 1978. Helping the spouses of critically ill patients. *American Journal of Nursing* 78:51–53.

Burnard, P. 1989. Existentialism as a theoretical basis for counseling in psychiatric nursing. *Archives of Psychiatric Nursing* 3(3): 142–147.

Byrne, C., Stockwell, M., and Gudelis, S. 1984. Adolescent support groups in oncology. *Oncology Nursing Forum* 11:36–40.

Carkhuff, R. 1969. *Helping and human relations.* New York: Holt, Rinehart, and Winston.

Carkhuff, R. 1973. *The art of helping.* Amherst, Mass.: Human Resource Development Press.

Carkhuff, R., and Berenson, B. 1977. *Beyond counseling and therapy* (2d ed.). New York: Holt, Rinehart, and Winston.

Casey J. 1989. Counseling nurse managers. *Nursing Management* 20(9):52–53.

Coe, M., and Kluka, S. 1990. Comparison of concerns of clients and spouses regarding ostomy surgery for treatment of cancer: Phase II. *Journal of Enterostomal Therapy* 17(3):106–111.

Corey, G. 1991. *Theory and practice of counseling and psychotherapy* (4th ed.). Pacific Grove, Calif.: Brooks/Cole Publishing Company.

Corsini, R. 1968. Counseling and psychotherapy. In E.F. Borgotta and W.W. Lambert (eds.), *Handbook of personality theory and research.* Chicago: Rand McNally.

Corsini, R., and Wedding, D. 1989. *Current psychotherapies* (4th ed.). Itasca, Ill.: F.E. Peacock Publishers.

Egan G. 1986. *The skilled helper* (3d ed.). Monterey, Calif.: Brooks/Cole Publishing Company.

Engelking, C. 1987. Teaching, counseling, and caring. *American Journal of Nursing* 11:1439–1450.

Frank-Stromborg, M., and Wright, P. 1984. Ambulatory cancer patients' perceptions of the physical and psychosocial changes in their lives since the diagnosis of cancer. *Cancer Nursing* 7:117–130.

Gawron, C. 1989. Body image changes in the patient requiring ostomy revision. *Journal of Enterostomal Therapy* 16(5):199–200.

Hames, C., and Joseph, D. 1986. *Basic concepts of helping — a holistic approach* (2d ed.). Norwalk, Conn.: Appleton-Century-Crofts.

Hansen, J., Stevic, R., and Warner, R. 1986. *Counseling: Theory and Process.* Boston: Allyn and Bacon.

Holman, S., Sunderland, A., Berthaud, M., Moroso, G., and Cancellieri, F. 1989. Prenatal HIV counseling and testing. *Clinical Obstetrics and Gynecology* 32(3):445–455.

Karasu, T. 1986. The specificity versus nonspecificity dilemma: Toward identifying therapeutic change agents. *American Journal of Psychiatry* 143:687–695.

Kaufman, J., Fox, R., and Swearengen, P. 1990. How a support group can help your chronically ill patient. *Nursing 90* 20(10):65–66.

Keane, E. 1989. Listening and the counseling process. *Nursing Standard* 4(12):34–36.

Klopp, A. 1990. Body image and self-concept among individuals with stomas. *Journal of Enterostomal Therapy* 17(3):98–105.

Landmann, L. 1989. When your ostomy patient is an adolescent. *Journal of Enterostomal Therapy* 16(2):87–88.

McDermott, M., and Mullins, E. 1989, Winter. Profile of a young movement. *Journal of Christian Nursing.* 29–30.

Maguire, P., and Faulkner, A. 1988. Improve the counselling skills of doctors and nurses in cancer care. *British Medical Journal* 297(6651):847–849.

Meier, S. 1989. *The elements of counseling.* Pacific Grove, Calif.: Brooks/Cole Publishing Company.

Moore, K., Folk-Lighty, M., and Nolen, M.J. 1984. The joy of sex after a heart attack: Counseling the cardiac patient. *Nursing 84* 14:104–113.

Nelson, L., and Hellman, S. 1989. Counseling employees at risk for HIV. *American Association of Occupational Health Nurses Journal* 37(10):404–411.

Osipow, W., Walsh, W.B., and Tose, D. 1984. *A survey of counseling methods.* Homewood, Ill.: Dorsey Press.

Patterson, C. 1986. *Theories of counseling and psychology* (4th ed.). New York: Harper and Row.

Rogers, C. 1951. *Client-centered therapy—implications and theory.* Boston: Houghton Mifflin.

Rogers, C. 1961. *On becoming a person.* Boston: Houghton Mifflin.

Scalzi, C. 1982. Sexual counseling and sexual therapy for patients after myocardial infarction. *Cardiovascular Nursing* 18:13–17.

Shertzer, B., and Stone, S. 1980. *Fundamentals of counseling* (3d ed.). Boston: Houghton Mifflin.

Sivarajan, E., Almes, M.J., and Mansfield, L. 1983. Limited effects of outpatient teaching and counseling after myocardial infarction: A controlled study. *Heart and Lung* 12(1):65–73.

Smucker, C. 1989, Winter. Church nurse—caring for a congregation. *Journal of Christian Nursing,* 32–33.

Stockdale, L. 1989. Person-centered counseling: Application in an intensive care setting. *Heart and Lung* 18(2):139–143.

Truax, C., and Carkhuff, R. 1967. *Toward effective counseling and psychotherapy.* Chicago: Aldine.

Watson, P. 1983. The effects of short-term postoperative counseling on cancer/ostomy patients. *Cancer Nursing* 6(1):21–29.

Westberg, G. 1989, Winter. Parish nursing pioneer. *Journal of Christian Nursing,* 26–29.

Whipple, B. 1987–1988. Sexual counseling of couples after a mastectomy or myocardial infarction. *Nursing Forum* 23(3): 85–91.

Wilson, H. 1989. Family caregivers: The experience of Alzheimer's disease. *Applied Nursing Research* 2(1):40–45.

23

REMINISCENCE THERAPY

DIANE BRONKEMA HAMILTON

Reminiscence, or reviewing one's past life, is an independent nursing intervention that therapists have used in multiple settings since World War I (Martin 1944). Using a psychoanalytic perspective, Martin asked an aged patient to relate the details of his earliest memories. After analyzing the patient's cognitive pattern, she provided him with a series of "correctable verbal slogans" to assist him in altering his perception of his life. In addition to this early clinical report, psychologists studying memory discussed reminiscence within the context of behavioral theory (Ballard 1913; Hull 1943).

More recently, a profusion of scholarly inquiry regarding Reminiscence Therapy was stimulated by Butler (1960, 1963, 1974), who provided concepts of reminiscence and life review as a healthy psychological adaptation of the last phase of life. Butler (1960) maintained that mental reconstruction and relating one's past assists the aged in attaining a positive understanding of their lives, accomplishments, and ultimate value to others. For Butler, life review is a universal mental process that includes but is not synonymous with reminiscence.

While Butler's seminal work precipitated scholarly inquiry into the phenomenon of reminiscence, more recent work has revealed conceptual diversity regarding its definition. Lieberman and Falk (1971) defined reminiscence as the remembered past, while Lewis (1971) conceptualized it as an evolving process of memory combined with an action property of reaching out to infuse others with their memories. Others have defined reminiscence as dwelling on the past, both purposive and spontaneous, oral and silent (Havighurst and Glasser 1972); the recall of long-forgotten experiences (Merriam 1980); or the process of recalling one's past (Oleson 1989). Burnside (1990, p. 35) captured the complexity of the concept: "Reminiscence is the act or process of recalling the remote past in a silent, spoken, solitary, interactional, spontaneous, or structured way."

Theoretical speculations regarding the structure of reminiscence support the notion that the phenomenon is quite complex. Meacham (1977) argued that while reminiscence is not identical to the process of memory, it may include a type of memory construction that provides the individual with integrity and purpose within the person's current life context. Hamilton (1985) observed that the structure of reminiscence includes memory, experiencing, and social interaction. Remembrances occur within the individual and are affected by current experiences, hopes, values, and social context. As the memories are triggered, individuals engage in experiencing, a type of introspective examination of feelings (Gendlin 1962). With the memory chosen and felt, the person's reminiscences unfold before another person. This social interaction may enhance the therapeutic value of Reminiscence Therapy. In contrast, Merriam (1989) formulated four components of reminiscence structure: selection, immersion, withdrawal, and closure. Merriam observed that memory selection occurs when people search their memory bank for a particular memory. The selection of a memory is related to certain emotional or environmental triggers. Once selection is completed, reminiscers immerse themselves into the remembered event, expressing vivid descriptions and emotionality. As affect and details fade, the reminiscer withdraws from the memory and briefly reflects on the event, closing out the experience with a short summary, often in the form of a succinct piece of wisdom (e.g., "I learned to live one day at a time").

Merriam (1989) suggested that the four components of reminiscence differ from the components of life review. Life review and reminiscence both begin with recall or memory; but during the life review, the person evaluates, analyzes, interprets, and gains insight into the meaning of the memory and then synthesizes the insight into his or her self-concept (Webster and Young 1988). Although novice nurses may perceive the two processes as similar, Burnside (1990) clearly differentiated life review and reminiscence. She suggested that life review is insight oriented, has a psychoanalytical theory base, elicits defense mechanisms, and is focused on reworking conflicts. This description suggests that life review is a type of psychotherapy conducted by advanced practitioners. In contrast, Reminiscence Therapy is supportive in nature. It is an independent nursing activity whereby the nurse stimulates or taps into the ongoing process of reminiscence. As the reminiscer selects a memory, immerses into the experience, withdraws, and closes out the reminiscence, the nurse responds with the supportive communication skills. A nurse conducting Reminiscence Therapy identifies a therapeutic goal (such as increased sociability, self-care, or self-esteem) and determines the nursing strategies (caring, presence, action listening, attending behaviors) designed to realize the stated goal. Thus, Reminiscence Therapy is a nursing intervention in which the normal process of reminiscence combines with nursing knowledge and communication skills to support the patient's life situation.

REVIEW OF LITERATURE

The reminiscence literature has been discussed through developmental, adaptation, psychoanalytic, and existential frameworks. Often authors use one or more of these perspectives to argue that reminiscence is a normal developmental process that assists the aged to adapt to losses by expressing feelings regarding their life state so as to find meaning in life.

Authors such as Erikson (1950), Butler (1963), and Neugarten (1966) proposed that human psychological development progresses in stages. Life culminates in the eighth stage (ego integrity versus despair) whereby individuals begin to weigh their past life and failures. Thus, old age is a time to resolve and reconciliate life conflicts prior to death. Reconsideration of past experiences, missed opportunities, and mistakes allows the aged to find meaning in their lives, integrate their life experiences, reach ego integrity, and face death without fear. Successful resolution of conflict is considered adaptive; the inability to resolve and accept the vicissitudes of one's past is judged as maladaptive (David 1990). Over a decade of descriptive research supports the notion that reminiscence is a component of the normal developmental process. Boylin et al. (1976) found that reminiscence increases ego integrity, and Miller and Lieberman (1965), Havighurst and Glasser (1972), Grunes (1980), and Lieberman and Tobin (1983) linked it to life satisfaction of the aged. Chiriboga and Gigy (1975) reported that reminiscence is associated with effective coping during life transitions. Several authors, including McMahon and Rhudick (1967), Pincus (1970), Coleman (1974) and Myerhoff (1980), suggested that reminiscence promotes social exchanges, adaptation, and ego interaction. The inability to reminisce has been linked to depression by McMahon and Rhudick (1961, 1967) and to poor adaptation to relocation by Miller and Lieberman (1965). Other authors have searched for a relationship between self-esteem and reminiscence. Researchers discovered that reminiscence favorably affects the aged's self-esteem, allowing positive adaptation to occur (Lewis 1970; Castenuevo-Tedesco 1980; Grunes 1980; Revere and Tobin, 1980–1981; Lieberman and Falk 1971, 1983).

Several authors have qualified the finding that reminiscence increases self-esteem, arguing that an increase in self-esteem and successful adaptation to aging depend on the quality or type of reminiscence (Butler 1963; Postema 1970; Lo Gerfo 1980–1981; Molinari and Reichlin 1984–1985). Authors of review articles (McCarthy 1977; Romaniuk 1981; Merriam 1989; Thorton and Brotchie 1987; David 1990) note that while studies suggest that reminiscence may increase self-esteem; sociability; affective, cognitive, and behavioral function; ego integrity, and life satisfaction; problems with both definition and methodologies make the empirical evidence to support the therapeutic adaptive value of reminiscence questionable.

In addition to exploring the function of reminiscence, researchers have considered the types of reminiscence. Thorton and Brotchie (1987) observed that while conversational or interpersonal reminiscence are most frequently researched, the aged may experience cognitive (or intrapersonal) reminiscence. Several authors speculate that there are more than these two types of reminiscence. Coleman (1974, 1986) differentiated among simple reminiscence, defined as recall of past experiences; life review, insight-oriented conflict resolution; and informative reminiscence, similar to storytelling. Other authors (McMahon and Rhudick 1964; Lewis 1971) argued that positive reminiscence is a fourth type of reminiscence and grief work a fifth type (Walker 1984). Lo Gerfo (1980–1981) defined three types of reminiscence: informative reminiscence, recreation for the pleasure of telling a story; valuative reminiscence, equivalent to life review; and obsessive reminiscence, a function of unresolved guilt and grief. In contrast, Bliwise (1982) identified five types of reminiscence; informative, ruminative, idealized, integrative, and flight from the past. Finally, Clements (1982) referred to recreational reminiscence, which is entertaining in nature, and therapeutic reminiscence, which is emotional work and may involve pain. As Perotta and Meacham (1981–1982) pointed out, these types of reminiscence have not been validated, lack conceptual clarity, and overlap in function and description.

Despite the multiple opinions regarding types of reminiscence, patterns that are useful to nursing practice emerge from the typologies. There seems to be some agreement that reminiscence may be oral (interpersonal, conversational) or silent (intrapersonal, reflective). In addition, it appears that some aged engage in a type of reminiscence that may be characterized as simple, recreational, or informative in nature. This type of reminiscence helps the aged review the past, relays history to the young, and has few negative sequelae. A second pattern of reminiscence includes the therapeutic, life review, integrative, or evaluative reminiscences, which are similar to insight-oriented psychotherapy in which conflicts are resolved. A third category appears more negative, with labels such as "obsessional," "ruminative," and "flight from the past." This pattern describes an aged person who feels despair, depression, pain, or an ungratifying past. A fourth category, which has received little attention, is the absence of reminiscence. The patterns of reminiscence, although varied, support the notion that the functions, styles, and triggers of reminiscence vary considerably.

Romaniuk and Romaniuk (1981) questioned earlier theoretical views that death, dissatisfaction, and simple pleasure trigger reminiscence. The results of their investigations suggest that mortality of others and one's own biological decline stimulate intrapersonal reminiscence, while accomplishments of self or family trigger interpersonal reminiscence. This conclusion suggests that reminiscence is not simply a component of a fixed developmental process but rather a strategy of self-presentation within a social context (Goffman 1959; Tarman 1988). That is, humans, by their very nature, analyze and critique their past and their place in the world so as to present themselves in a positive way.

While sociologists have explored the function, types, and triggers of reminiscence, nurses have focused on the effects of reminiscence. Nurses have reported clinical accounts regarding the effects of reminiscence with acutely ill patients (Beadleson-Baird and Lara 1984, 1988) and with groups of aged (Hala 1975; Ebersole 1976; Blackman 1980; Hogan 1982; King 1986). Clinical observations suggest that reminiscence positively affects the cognitive, affective, and behavioral function of the elderly. Nursing research has linked the effects of reminiscence to self-esteem (Gibson 1980; Hamilton 1985; Baker 1983; Moore 1984; Lappe 1987), depression (Hibel 1971; Matteson 1978; Michelson 1981; Burnside 1989), confusion (Witchita 1974), life satisfaction (Mace 1979; Haight 1988), and social interaction (Wilkinson 1978). Reviewing the nursing research, Kovach (1990) noted that reminiscence studies vary considerably in degree of methodological sophistication and limit the ability to make direct comparison of results. The lack of conceptual and operational definitions, measurement tool validity, and inadequate sample size limit the generalizability of the research findings. Despite the problems, Kovach suggested that a pattern emerged that lends support to the idea that some persons use reminiscence to evaluate their lives, that there are multiple types of reminiscence, and that reminiscence may have positive effects on mood, self-esteem, cognitive function, and life satisfaction. Because clinical reports and nursing research consistently suggest a positive effect of reminiscence on the aged, Kovach urged nurses to continue research efforts in order to develop a body of knowledge from which to practice.

IDENTIFICATION OF NURSING DIAGNOSES AND APPROPRIATE CLIENT GROUPS

The nursing assessment determines the appropriateness of Reminiscence Therapy. As the nurse listens, observes, and collects data, a pattern illuminating the patient's problems, issues, conflicts, and strengths will emerge. This pattern is a synthesis of information, which is then transformed into a nursing diagnosis and includes the problem, its risk factors, and the defining characteristics. The nurse considers the elements of the nursing diagnosis and the subsequent goals when designing Reminiscence Therapy as an intervention.

The following nursing diagnoses may be amenable with Reminiscence Therapy:

Impaired Adjustment
Anxiety
Family Coping: Potential for Growth
Ineffective Family Coping
Ineffective Individual Coping

Decisional Conflict
Ineffective Denial
Diversional Activity Deficit
Fear
Anticipatory Grieving
Dysfunctional Grieving
Altered Growth and Development
Health-Seeking Behaviors
Hopelessness
Powerlessness
Self Esteem Disturbance
Social Interaction Impaired
Social Isolation
Spiritual Distress

Generally authors believe that reminiscence may be useful in periods of crises, transition, loss, or stress (Preifer and Gambert 1984; Lewis 1980). Thus, the nursing diagnoses are those associated with chronic, situational, and developmental change or loss. Reminiscence is a component of one's lived autobiography. Because of life's inconsistencies, losses, and shifting realities, reminiscence allows one to remove oneself mentally from the present and create meaning of the losses.

Although reminiscence is often described in terms of the aged, the phenomenon is not distinctive to this population. Clements (1986) utilized Reminiscence Therapy to help families interpret traumatic events in a way that enhanced problem solving, while Borden (1989) observed that reminiscence assisted patients with acquired immune deficiency syndrome (AIDS) to gain a cohesive sense of self and relative health. Demented, confused, and psychotic aged benefit from reminiscence by integrating the past into a familiar structure that satisfies intrapsychic needs (Orten et al. 1989, Lesser et al. 1981; Goldwasser et al. 1987; Hughston and Merriam 1982). And homebound and nursing home elderly respond to reminiscence and gain comfort and familiarity (Sherman 1987; Haight 1988; Osborn 1989; Taft and Nehrke 1990).

Despite the use of Reminiscence Therapy with multiple patient groups, not all patients respond favorably to reminiscence. Alcoholic patients (Gibson 1980) and paranoid patients (Burnside 1990) seem to resist and fear the past. Because reminiscence is a powerful intervention, the nurse must use judgment when using Reminiscence Therapy and reassess the situation if the patient's response is negative.

INTERVENTION ACTIVITIES

Reminiscence Therapy can be conducted with individuals or groups. The nurse's decision will be guided by the setting, the nursing diagnoses, and the goal established with the patient. In acute-care settings, individual reminiscence may be combined with bathing, feeding, and mobility activities. Patients who are eager to reminisce need only encouragement from health care providers in order to elicit a stream of thought and conversation about the past. The nurse responds with empathy and active listening, with few interruptions. Often patients need only a leading question, for example, "When you remember the past, what occurs to you?" to stimulate a catharsis of memories. At times, objects stimulate reminis-

TABLE 23 – 1. TOPICS TO STIMULATE REMINISCENCE

"Firsts" (car, telephone, date, dress, house)
"Favorites" (Christmas, birthday)
Significant events (wedding, birth, graduation)
Transportation
Weather
Occupation, skills, hobbies
Travel
Fashion
Presidents, politics, elections
Relationships (pets, relatives)
Food preparation
Entertainment (movies, books)
Music
School days
Romance
Ethnic cultural or family tradition
Gardens
Child-raising customs
Medical care and practices
Home health customs

cence. For example, a nurse may observe a patient with flowers and ask, "Have you always liked flowers?"

When a nurse stimulates reminiscence, she begins where the patient is emotionally and proceeds sensibly. A judgmental attitude, poor timing, inappropriate interpretations, or confrontations will be met with defenses such as anger or denial. Drawing the patient out in a supportive manner and using basic therapeutic communication skills such as attending, focusing, reflecting, and validation allow the reminiscence to proceed. By reinforcing memories, the patient will feel supported and cared for.

Individual reminiscence is also conducted in a structured manner. The nurse begins by explaining the principles of Reminiscence Therapy to the patient. If the patient agrees to participate, the nurse establishes a schedule of sessions to provide structure and consistency. Short, frequent visits are most useful. Three sessions weekly of 30 minutes each will assist the nurse to maintain continuity without exhausting the patient. While the topics of reminiscence may be predetermined by the nurse (Table 23 – 1), the sessions often evolve into a pattern of topics significant to the patient. It is common for specific topics to reoccur as the aged weigh, analyze, and reflect on their past. As the patient moves between the space and time of the past, the themes of conflict, pleasure, or feeling provide the nurse with data that generate a clear picture of the essence of the human being cared for. Occasionally fatigue, pain, or suspiciousness thwarts the Reminiscence Therapy. The nurse can refocus the patient, substitute silence and presence for reminiscence, or end the therapy session. The decision depends on the context of the situation and the status of the patient.

About 5 minutes before the end of each visit, the nurse begins to terminate the session by refocusing the patient to present time and place. As the nurse leaves the session, she should remind the patient when she will return. Reminders of scheduled sessions can be marked on a calendar to reinforce the consistency of reminiscence sessions. As a rule of thumb, a series of Reminiscence Therapy continues for 6 to 12 sessions. At the end of the series, the nurse discusses the overall experience with the patient and compares the patient's status at the beginning of Reminiscence

Therapy to the status at the conclusion. In long-term facilities, Reminiscence Therapy may be ongoing. The life story can be compiled and documented to assist the staff in gaining useful insight into the patient.

Group reminiscence is effective in inpatient, outpatient, and community settings. It offers the advantage of helping a greater number of patients, as well as strengthening cohort identification, socialization, memory stimulation, and self-growth (Butler 1974; McMordie and Blom 1979; Ebersole 1976; Beaton 1980; Ellison 1981; Matteson and Munsat 1982; King 1982, 1986; Huber and Miller 1984; Baker 1985; Parsons 1986; Sherman 1987; Tourangeau 1988; Osborn 1989; Rattenberg and Stones 1989). Groups of 6 to 10 members are most effective for Reminiscence Therapy groups. The small group allows for group stages to proceed but allows each member enough time to interact.

Although the group members are chosen using criteria consistent with the group goals, generally members should be able to sit still, be silent, hear, and listen; be interested in attending a reminiscence group; and have nursing diagnoses amenable to Reminiscence Therapy. Despite these guidelines, exceptions may be successful. For example, group stimulation and communication about the past could prove an effective intervention for a repressed patient.

The environment for the group should be comfortable and large enough to accommodate disabilities (walkers and wheelchairs). A consistent meeting time and place should be chosen, with reminders posted in patient rooms or on wall calendars. Enough time must be allowed for the group to arrive and settle (clean glasses, lock wheelchairs, store purses).

The group leader sets the tone for the group. Often the aged respond to a warm and patient but structured leadership style. Nonetheless, the leadership style chosen somewhat depends upon the group's characteristics. Severely depressed groups may need a highly structured and direct leadership style; a group of high-functioning aged may respond to a more informal but supportive leader.

As the group progresses through the stages of development (form, norm, storm, perform, terminate; Tuckman 1967), the leader will sense the group's distinctive style and group norms. In most groups, members will adopt specific roles, such as clarifier, initiator, or monopolizer. The leader should be aware of the roles and balance acceptance with redirection. Occasionally, a member who tends to monopolize needs to be refocused gently, without stifling self-reliance or spirit.

The group leader usually introduces various activities and topics to stimulate memory and interaction (Tables 23 – 1 and 23 – 2). As the group sessions continue, members may have their own preference for activities and topics. Music, food, or more creative activities may be added to the group. Berger (1978) used brief body exercises to stimulate a reminiscence group. She had the members raise their arms and asked them to share what they were reaching for. Imagery may stimulate memories by asking members to close their eyes and imagine the past. Objects such as antique clothes or household objects usually bring a spark of recognition to the eyes of the aged. High-button shoes and gas-rationing stamps remind the elderly of their rich past. At times, the present will trigger memories of the past. In one group, the 1989 San Francisco earthquake stimulated a host of stories of natural disasters, survival, and strength. The group was able to share both the humor and sadness associated with human disaster with the wisdom of age.

Silent periods may occur in reminiscence groups. Time seems to expand and contract in the aged's minds' eye as stories leap from 1990 to 1946. As the aged move through their time, they often reflect quietly or rehearse their thoughts before sharing them with the group. The nurse can wait and honor their private thoughts or comment, "You seem to be in a special time and space."

TABLE 23 – 2. ACTIVITIES TO STIMULATE REMINISCENCE

Family reunions
Family slides, photographs, scrapbooks
Writing stories, poems
Reminiscence diaries
Storytelling
Fashion shows
Taped sounds (machinery, rain)
Exercise
Structured interview
Flash cards
Music of golden era
Advertisements (Pear's Soap, Dutch Boy paint)
Sears catalog (mock ordering)
Visualization or focused experiencing
Old newspaper reading
Genealogy work
Touch
Historical documentary films
Map reading

At times group members become uncomfortable with a topic. They may frankly state that they do not wish to discuss a topic, but more often, they ignore the topic or create a stream of conversation that seems safer. It is usually wise for the nurse to neither confront nor judge the resistance but reinforce the group's topic of interest. Often the uncomfortable topic will resurface when the group is ready to remember and feel safe with those memories.

Principles of termination guide the nurse in terminating with a group of reminiscers. The group's beginning and working stages are reviewed. Group roles are discussed, and the members share their perceptions of the experience. Members may recount their favorite topic within the group or express their view of the meaning of the experience. It is important that the nurse acknowledge and appreciate each member's expenditure of energy and contributions to the group. At times, the nurse will choose to share with the group the feelings and insights gained from the group experience. Sharing a lifetime of events, meaning, and accomplishments can be a rewarding and enlightening experience for group leaders.

The aged are living novels who have written and acted out their past. Their personal sense and meaning of their lives clearly unfolds as they review and transcend their individual existences. The aged have moved through changing social contexts and create a link between generations. While the literature suggests that the interest in Reminiscence Therapy is for the purpose of helping the aged find meaning in their lives, the caretakers may also gain hope that individual lives are unique and worthwhile. The unexpected recoveries from illness, the escapes from danger, the managed losses, and deserved accomplishments may provide both the aged and the caretaker with an opportunity to preserve the wish that throughout time humans have contributed in a meaningful way to the universe.

CASE STUDY

Jane Alex, a 46-year-old white female, was admitted to a psychiatric hospital with the chief complaint of anxiety. Her mother reported that Jane was a college graduate who had worked as a pediatric nurse for 20 years. Seven years prior to admission, Jane had been fired from her position as nurse manager. After losing her home, car, and other possessions, she moved to her parents' home. Her mother reported that her behavior had deteriorated severely over the past 7 years. Her average day consisted of rising at 4:00 P.M., being fed and bathed by her mother, and watching television until 3:00 A.M. Jane had frequent complaints of vertigo, displayed anger outbursts, and had limited mobility. She spoke with no one, ritualistically cleaned her face, and had blurred vision.

Jane's primary nurse, Ms. Sawyer, was puzzled by the complex of symptoms. Her initial assessment revealed nuring diagnoses of Impaired Physical Mobility, Activity Intolerance, Fatigue, Sleep Pattern Disturbance, Defensive Coping, Chronic Low Self Esteem, Impaired Skin Integrity, Altered Thought Processes, Altered Growth and Development, and Perceived Constipation. The initial care plan included group therapy, occupational therapy, and music therapy, but after the first treatment day, Jane refused all therapies and displayed frequent outbursts of swearing, crying, and screaming. Moreover, she demanded to eat only prunes, began to hoard toilet paper, and had ritualistic cleaning patterns.

The clinical nurse specialist (CNS) was consulted. Dr. White noted that Jane's unusual complex of behavior seemed organic in nature. The physician suspected a brain tumor. Nonetheless, the nurses were in need of a strategy to manage Jane on the unit. During a case conference, the nurses agreed to initiate individual Reminiscence Therapy in order to decrease anxiety, to validate the patient's sense of self, and to establish rapport.

Dr. White, the CNS, met with Jane daily for 30 minutes. They discussed memories of college, nursing, and a discarded traumatic marriage. From the onset, Jane's outbursts decreased, and gradually she acknowledged her fear regarding her diminished capacity. Within 2 weeks, Jane was able to contract for small activities of daily living. She began to make her bed, bathe, and eat a relatively balanced diet. Although Jane was medically diagnosed with Alzheimer's disease and transferred to a nursing home, the nursing staff had successfully used reminiscence as an intervention to enhance her well-being.

CONCLUSION

The tendency of older persons to reminisce has often been viewed as senility or somewhat more empathetically as an expression of loneliness. Scholarly inquiry has confirmed, however, that Reminiscence Therapy can help people deal with crises and loss. While conceptual clarification and research regarding Reminiscence Therapy is not yet complete, positive outcomes have been reported from clinicians and researchers. Old age need not be a stage of alienation from society or one's self; instead it can be a continuation of the process of life, growth, and experience.

REFERENCES

Babb-de Ramon, R. 1983. Life review for the dying patient. *Nursing* 83(2):44–48.

Ballard, P. 1913. Oblivescence and reminiscence. *British Journal of Psychiatry* 1(Suppl.):1–82.

Baker, J. 1983. *Change in morale and self-esteem among institutionalized elderly using touch and reminiscence.* Unpublished master's thesis, San Jose State University, San Jose, California.

Baker, N. 1985. Reminiscing in group therapy for self-worth. *Journal of Gerontological Nursing* 11(7):21–24.

Beadleson-Baird, M., and Lara, L. 1984. Verbal reminiscing and the mood, ego-integration and socialization of the institutionalized elderly. Proceedings of Octoberquest Research Conference, 99–104.

Beadleson-Baird, M., and Lara, L. 1988. Reminiscing: Nursing actions for the acutely ill geriatric patient. *Issues in Mental Health Nursing* 9(1):83–94.

Beaton S. 1980. Reminiscence in old age. *Nursing Forum* 19(3):271–283.

Berger, L. 1978. Activating a psychogeriatric group. *Psychiatric Quarterly* 50(1):63–67.

Blackman, J.C. 1980. Group work in the community: Experience with reminiscence. In I. Burnside (ed.), *Psychosocial nursing care* (pp. 126–144). St. Louis: C.V. Mosby.

Bliwise, N. 1982. *Reminiscence: Presentation of the personal past in middle and late life.* Unpublished doctoral dissertation, University of Chicago, Chicago.

Borden, W. 1989. Life review as a therapeutic frame in the treatment of young adults with AIDS. *Health and Social Work* 9:253–259.

Boylin, W., et al. 1976. Reminiscing and ego-integrity in institutionalized elderly males. *Gerontologist* 16(2):118–124.

Bramwell, L. 1984. Use of the life history pattern identification and health promotion. *Advances in Nursing Science* 7(1):37–44.

Burnside, I. 1989. Group work with elder women: A modality to improve the quality of life. *Journal of Women and Aging* 1(1,2,3):265–290.

Burnside, I. 1990. Reminiscence: An independent nursing intervention for the elderly. *Issues in Mental Health Nursing* 11(1):33–48.

Butler R.N. 1960. Intensive psychotherapy for the hospitalized aged. *Geriatrics* 15(9):644–653.

Butler, R.N. 1963. A life review. *Psychiatry* 26(2):65–76.

Butler, R.N. 1974. Mental health and aging. *Geriatrics* 29:53–54.

Castenuevo-Tedesco, P. 1980. Reminiscence and nostalgia: The pleasure and pain of remembering. In S. Greenspan et al. (eds.), *The course of life: Psychoanalytic contribution toward understanding personality development.* Washington, D.C.: U.S. Government Printing Office.

Chiriboga, D., and Gigy, L. 1975. Perspectives on the life cycle. In M.F. Lowenthal et al. (eds.), *Four stages of transitions* (pp. 122–145). San Francisco: Jossey-Bass.

Chubon, S. 1980. A novel approach to the process of life review. *Journal of Gerontological Nursing* 6:543–553.

Clements, D. 1986. Reminiscence: A tool for aiding families under stress. *Maternal Child Nursing* 11(2):114–117.

Clements, W. 1982. Therapeutic functions of recreation in reminiscence with aging persons. In M.L. Teague (ed.), *Perspectives on leisure and aging.* Columbia, Mo: University of Missouri Press.

Coleman, P. 1974. Measuring reminiscence characteristics from conversations as adaptive features of old age. *International Journal of Aging and Human Development* 5(4):281–294.

Coleman, P. 1986. *Aging and reminiscence processes: Social and clinical implications.* New York: Wiley.

Cora, V.L. 1989. *Recollection of our past.* Unpublished paper, Third Annual Southern Research Conference, Austin, Texas.

David D. 1990. Reminiscence, adaptation, and social context in old age. *International Journal of Aging and Human Development* 30(3):175–188.

Ebersole, P. 1976. Reminiscing. *American Journal of Nursing* 76(8):1304–1305.

Ellison, K. 1981. Working with the elderly in life review groups. *Journal of Gerontological Nursing* 7(9):537–540.

Erikson, E. 1950. *Childhood and society.* New York: W.W. Norton.

Fry, P. 1983. Structured and unstructured reminiscence training and depression among the elderly. *Clinical Gerontologist* 1:15–37.

Gendlin, E.T. 1962. *Experiencing and the creation of meaning.* Glencoe, Ill.: Free Press.

Gibson, D. 1980. Reminiscence, self-esteem and self-other satisfaction in adult male alcoholics. *Journal of Psychiatric Nursing and Mental Health Services* 18(3):7–11.

Goffman, E. 1959. *The presentation of self in everyday life.* New York: Doubleday.

Goldwasser, A., Auerbach, S., and Harkins, S. 1987. Cognitive, affective and behavioral effects of reminiscence group therapy on demented elderly. *International Journal of Aging and Human Development* 25(3):209–223.

Grunes, J. 1980. Reminiscences, regression and empathy. In S. Greenspan et al. (eds.), *The course of life.* Washington, D.C.: U.S. Government Printing Office.

Haight, B. 1988. The therapeutic role of a structured life review process in homebound elderly subjects. *Journal of Gerontology* 43(2):40–44.

Hala, M. 1975. Reminiscence group therapy project. *Journal of Gerontological Nursing* 1(3):34–41.

Hamilton, D. 1985. Reminiscence therapy. In G. Bulechek and J. McCloskey (eds.), *Nursing intervention: Treatments for nursing diagnoses.* Philadelphia: W.B. Saunders.

Havighurst, R., and Glasser, R. 1972. An explanatory study of reminiscence. *Journal of Gerontology* 27(2):245–253.

Hibel, D. 1971. *The relationships between reminiscence and depression among 30 selected institutionalized aged males.* Unpublished doctoral dissertation, Boston University, Boston.

Hogan, J. 1982. *The use of nonprofessional leaders in reminiscing groups for the institutionalized elderly.* Unpublished master's thesis, San Jose State University, San Jose, California.

Huber, K., and Miller T. 1984. Reminiscence with the elderly—do it! *Geriatric Nursing* 5(2):84–89.

Hull, C.I. 1943. *Principles of behavior.* New York: Appleton-Century.

Hughston, G., and Merriam, S., 1982. Reminiscence: a nonformal technique for improving cognitive functioning in the aged. *International Journal of Aging and Human Development* 15(2):139–149.

Ingersoll, B., and Silverman, A. 1978. Comparative group psychotherapy for the aged. *Gerontologist* 18:201–296.

Jessup, L. 1984. The health history. In B. Steff (ed.), *Handbook of gerontological nursing.* New York: Van Nostrand.

Kaminsky, M. 1984. *The uses of reminiscence.* New York: Hawork.

King, K. 1982. Reminiscing Psychotherapy with aging people. *Journal of Psychiatric-Mental Health Nursing* 20(2):21–25.

King, K. 1986. Reminiscing, dying and counseling: A contextual approach. In I. Burnside (ed.), *Working with the Elderly: Group process and techniques* (2d ed., pp. 272–286). Boston: Jones & Bartlett.

Kovach, C. 1990. Promise and problems in reminiscence research. *Journal of Gerontological Nursing* 16(4):10–14.

Kvale, S. 1974. The temporality of memory. *Journal of Phenomenological Psychology* 5:7–31.

Lappe, J. 1987. Reminiscing: The life review therapy. *Journal of Gerontological Nursing* 13(4):12–16.

Lesser, J., Lazarus, L., Frankel, R., and Havasy, S. 1981. Reminiscence group therapy with psychotic geriatric inpatients. *Gerontologist* 21(3)291–296.

Lewis, C. 1970. *Reminiscence and self-concept in old age.* Unpublished doctoral dissertation, Boston University, Boston, Massachusetts.

Lewis, C. 1971. Reminiscing and self-concept in old age. *Journal of Gerontology* 26(2):240–243.

Lewis, C. 1973. The adoptive value of reminiscing in old age. *Journal of Geriatric Psychiatry* 7(1):112–121.

Lewis, C. 1980. Memory adaptation to psychological trauma. *American Journal of Psychoanalysis* 40:319–323.

Lieberman, M., and Falk, J. 1971. The remembered past as a source of data for research on the life cycle. *Human Development* 14(2):132–141.

Lieberman, M.A., and Tobin, S.S. 1983. *The experience of old age.* New York: Basic Books.

Lindeman, E. 1944. Symptomatology and management of acute grief. *American Journal of Psychiatry* 101:141–148.

Lo Gerfo, M. 1980–1981. Three ways of reminiscence in theory and practice. *International Journal of Aging and Human Development* 12(1):29–48.

McCarthy, H. 1977. Time perspective and aged persons' attribution of their life experiences. *Gerontologist* 17:97.

Mace, M. 1979. *Reminiscence and life satisfaction in older persons.* Unpublished master's thesis, Texas Women's University, Denton, Texas.

McMahon, A., and Rhudick, P. 1964. Reminiscing. *Archives of General Psychiatry* 10(3):292–298.

McMahon, A., and Rhudick, P. 1967. Reminiscing in the aged. In S. Levin et al. (eds.), *Psychodynamic studies in aging: Creativity, reminiscing and dying* (pp. 182–192). New York: International University Press.

McRae, I. 1982. Reminiscence: An underused nursing resource. *Perspectives in Nursing* 14:52–54.

Martin, L.A. 1944. *A handbook for old age counselors.* San Francisco: Geertz Printing.

Matteson, M.A. 1978. *Treatment for the depressed institutionalized elderly.* Unpublished master's thesis, Duke University, Durham, North Carolina.

Matteson, M., and Munsat, E. 1982. Group reminiscence therapy with elderly clients. *Issues in Mental Health Nursing* 4(3):177–189.

McMordie, W., and Blom, S. 1979. Life review therapy: psychotherapy for the elderly. *Perspectives in Psychiatric Care* 17(4):292–298.

Meacham, J. 1977. A transactional model of remembering. In N. Datan et al. (eds.), *Life span developmental perspectives in experimental research.* New York: Academic Press.

Meacham, J. 1984. The social bias of intentional action. *Human Development* 27:119–124.

Merriam, S. 1980. The concept and function of reminiscence: A review of the research. *Gerontologist* 20(5):604–609.

Merriam, S. 1989. The structure of simple reminiscence. *Gerontologist* 29(6):761–767.

Michelson, L. 1981. *Reminiscence as a means of decreasing depression in the aged.* Unpublished master's thesis, Boston University, Boston.

Miller, D., and Lieberman, M. 1965. The relationship of affect state and adaptive capacity to reactions of stress. *Journal of Gerontology* 20:492–497.

Molinari, V., and Reichlin, R. 1984–1985. Life review of reminiscence in the elderly: A review of the literature. *International Journal of Aging and Human Development* 20:81–92.

Moore, M. 1984. *Effects of reminiscing and touch in group therapy on self esteem and morale of institutionalized elderly.* Unpublished master's thesis, San Jose State University, San Jose, California.

Myerhoff, B. 1980. Life history among the elderly. In K. Black (ed.), *Life course: Integrative theory and exemplary populations.* Boulder, Colo.: Westview Press.

Neugarten, B. 1966. Adult personality: A development view. *Human Development* 2:61–73.

Norris, A. 1982. Reminiscence groups. *Nursing times* 78(30):1368–1369.

Oleson, M. 1989. Legacies, reminiscence and ego integrity. *Nurse Educator* 14(6):6–7.

Oliveria, O.H. 1977. *Understanding old people: Patterns of reminiscing in elderly people and their relationship to life satisfaction,* Unpublished doctoral dissertation, University of Tennessee, Knoxville, Tennessee.

Orten, J.D., Allen, M., and Cook, J. 1989. Reminiscence groups with confused nursing center residents: an experimental study. *Social Work Health Care* 14(1):73–86.

Osborn, C.L. 1989. Reminiscence—when the past eases the present. *Journal of Gerontological Nursing* 15(10):6–12.

Parsons, C. 1982. Group reminiscence therapy and levels of depression in the elderly. *Nurse Practitioner* 11(3):68–70.

Perotta, P., and Meacham, J. 1981–1982. Can reminiscing intervention alter depression and self-esteem? *International Journal of Aging and Human Development* 14(1):23–30.

Pincus, A. 1970. Reminiscence in aging and its implications for social work practice. *Social Work* 15:47–53.

Postema, L. 1970. *Reminiscing, time orientation and self-concept in old men.* Unpublished doctoral dissertation, Michigan State University, Ann Arbor.

Priefer, B., and Gambert, S. 1984. Reminiscence and life review. *Psychiatric Medicine* 2(1):91–99.

Poulton, J., and Strassberg, D. 1986. The therapeutic use of reminiscence. *International Journal of Group Psychotherapy* 36(3):381–399.

Rattenburg, C., and Stones, M. 1989. A controlled evaluation of reminiscence and current topics discussion groups in nursing homes. *Gerontologist* 29(6):768–771.

Revere, V., and Tobin, S. 1980–1981. Myth and reality: The older person's relationship to his past. *International Journal of Aging and Human Development* 12:15–25.

Romaniuk, M. 1981. Reminiscence and the second half of life. *Experimental Aging Research* 7(3):315–335.

Romaniuk, M., and Romaniuk, J.G. 1981. Looking back: An analysis of reminiscence functions and triggers. *Experimental Aging Research* 7(4):477–489

Sherman, E. 1987. A phenomenological approach to reminiscence and life review. *Clinical Gerontologist* 3(4):3–16.

Taft, L., and Nehrke, M. 1990. Reminiscence: Life review ego integrity in nursing home residents. *International Journal of Aging and Human Development* 30(3):189–196.

Tarman, V. 1988. Autobiography: The negotiation of a life time. *International Journal of Aging and Human Development* 27(3):171–191.

Thornton, S., and Brotchie, J. 1987. Reminiscence: A critical review of the empirical literature. *British Journal of Clinical Psychology* 26:93–111.

Tourangeau, A. 1988. Group reminiscence therapy. *American Association RN Newsletter* 44(8):17–18.

Tuckman, B. 1967. Developmental sequences of small groups. *Psychological Bulletin* 63:384–399.

Walker, L.I. 1984. *The relationships between reminiscing, health state, physical functioning and depression in older adults.* Unpublished doctoral dissertation, Catholic University, Washington, D.C.

Webster J., and Young, R. 1988. Process variables of the life review: Counseling implications. *International Journal of Aging and Human Development* 26(4):315–323.

Wilkinson, C. 1978. *A descriptive study of increased social interaction through reminiscing.* Unpublished master's thesis, Tulane University, New Orleans.

Witchita C. 1974. *Reminiscing as a therapy for apathetic and confused residents of nursing homes.* Unpublished master's thesis, University of Arizona, Tucson.

24

PATIENT TEACHING

BARBARA K. REDMAN
SUE ANN THOMAS

Patient Teaching is an interpersonal intervention that uses stimuli already in the environment or creates new ones to help the patient develop new thoughts, skills, attitudes, intentions, and feelings of self-efficacy, usually in combination, that are permanent enough to be useful in behavioral change. Patients are people under the care of a health care provider, either intermittently or at a particular time. Patient education may be thought of as the process of helping someone to learn through planned sequences of teaching, supportive activity, and directed practice and reinforcement.

Although historically centered on a rather rigidly defined goal of compliance with the medical regimen, Patient Teaching today is more focused on self-care skills and on making informed choices. Examples include self-management of asthma, choice among options for surgery for breast cancer, self-care skills in management of diabetes mellitus, including self-monitoring of blood glucose, and cognitive control by family members of their experiences in dealing with a loved one with cancer. All of these outcomes require not only knowledge but thinking, problem-solving, and performance skills in real situations, undergirded by a sense of self-efficacy.

Stimuli used to create a new skill may be presented in a wide variety of ways: through written materials, in support groups, through observation of someone performing the skill, and through carrying out an action under direction in a real situation. The initial stimulus used in teaching must be simple enough for the patient to comprehend. Eventually teaching stimuli must be like those to which patients will need to respond, practiced to a level of mastery and maintained. While teaching frequently occurs within a relationship with a provider, it can occur through a mass media campaign such as those used to decrease risk factors for heart disease or through other information systems, such as computer-based health information on acquired immune deficiency syndrome (AIDS), anonymously provided on a college campus.

In most cases, the special issues of motivation surrounding health learning are important. Management of fear and anxiety is almost always important. As people adapt to illness, they frequently move through phases of denial and acceptance, sometimes oscillating between the two. Frequently it is important to have acknowledged and built on the patient's and family's view of the health situation. And it is always necessary to factor in how the patient is feeling: whether there are symptoms, what they mean to the patient, and how all of this motivates or does not motivate and reinforce learning.

The nurse's task is to orchestrate conditions for learning and motivation so that they match what the patient needs to build skills. The research base for this activity consists primarily of principles and strategies that must be combined to fit each patient. Teaching is perhaps best managed within a relationship between a provider and a patient, over the time necessary to complete a teaching-learning episode.

LITERATURE RELATED TO PATIENT TEACHING

The literature instructive for Patient Teaching encompasses theory and research on general conditions of learning and teaching, results of a growing number of research studies on teaching of and learning in patients, and summaries of these studies; reports on patient education practice thought to be exemplary; and delivery and management of patient education services, including legal and ethical aspects. This is clearly an interdisciplinary literature, much of it focused on patient conditions or special areas of practice, including prenatal and postnatal, parenting, rehabilitation, cancer, hypertension, diabetes, arthritis, dialysis, transplant, mental health, preoperative or preprocedure, and compliance with drug regimens.

General Conditions of Learning

There are well-established conditions of learning, including how to support normal and abnormal limitations of memory, need for the learner to see a model and practice skills, and direction provided by the developmental stage of the learner (Redman 1988). Currently used learning theory includes behavioral (reinforcement of desired behavior), cognitive (cognitive schema direct thinking and actions), and social learning theory, which combines these two perspectives and emphasizes the usefulness of modeling and development of self-efficacy.

Learning theory implies certain actions. In addition, there is other work about teaching forms and process that is instructive. The many studies of readability of written materials quantify one element important in judging how well these materials will be understood. There are entire fields of instruction in which materials are written at a much higher level than most patients can understand.

There are additional general principles of teaching and learning useful in patient teaching situations. Concrete, pictorial instructional modes are frequently superior to those that are abstract and verbal. Breaking a complex skill into component parts and teaching each part to mastery, gradually combining them into larger chunks, is useful. Teaching is best directed through a process of learner assessment, clear definition of behavioral goals, opportunity for directed learning until mastery, and evaluation.

Research and Research Summaries in Patient Education

A broad range of research reports available in the patient education field addresses the variety of clinical problems, content, and behaviors for which Patient Teaching is used. There are more than 40 published summaries of research in various areas of patient education, some of which use the more sophisticated statistical methods of meta-analysis. A number review preoperative teaching or coping with health care procedures or hospitalization. Others focus on health promotion and still others on teaching in particular disease entities, such as arthritis, cardiac rehabilitation, management of diabetes mellitus, self-help in persons with cancer, and childbirth education. A very few focus on particular instructional procedures, such as contingency contracting to improve patient compliance and television as a teaching tool.

Most reviews have found Patient Teaching to be efficacious and clearly better than outcomes for patients who had no teaching. Teaching has also been found to have consistent effects on such variables as length of hospital stay and pain and disability. What is also clear is that for behaviors considered to be clinically important, purely informational approaches are not the most effective option. The addition of teaching approaches that developed self-management skills and emotional support has improved outcomes.

Complicating research and clinical practice in patient education is the lack of a standardized language by which to describe teaching activities. Perhaps this in part explains why it is common to find activities called teaching that are totally inadequate for the task at hand. If a teaching activity seems to be failing, the first step is to look at how it has been defined.

Finally, there is interesting new work ongoing in areas that undergird patient education. For example, in every phase of health, patients are instructed by how their body feels, how symptoms are controlled, and how they interpret these signals. Yet symptoms of organic disease vary widely among patients with the same tissue abnormality. For example, the relationship between pain and cardiac ischemia is variable, the presence of a peptic ulcer as documented endoscopically or radiologically is only weakly related to the presence of symptoms, arthritic pain cannot be predicted by lumbar spine X-rays, and symptoms of diabetes correlate better with depression levels than with glycosylated hemoglobin levels. Are some patients hyposensitive to pain, or do their thoughts, expectations, and beliefs about symptoms cause them to ignore or dismiss sensory input that contradicts their beliefs (Barsky et al. 1990)? Another area deserving of more investigation is the quality of the unintended learning that occurs in health care settings. Clearly the environment teaches all the time, and it is necessary to manage it so that it is therapeutic.

Practice and Management of Patient Teaching

Standards for patient education exist in many fields, most notably in diabetes, in oncology, and for childbirth education. Generally these standards represent consensus on good practice and include patient education process and content standards. The former include documented ongoing assessment of learning needs developed with the patient's participation, suggested teaching-learning strategies, and the need for evaluation.

There are also many case studies of excellent Patient Teaching, hopefully based on documented learning outcomes. Some examples creatively use multiple principles of effective learning. For example, Crowe and Billingsley (1990) describe a camp-based support group for teenagers with diabetes, using active learning by doing, feeling in control, peer group discussion of daily experiences with diabetes, including role playing, use of outdoor activities and T-shirts to build group cohesion, sessions on experiences in development of self-reliant behavior, and an award ceremony rewarding success. Other programs are excellent because they restructure an environment to be optimally supportive of learning. In these special units, patients and families have responsibility for much of the care delivery and educational resources are readily available to help them, including learning centers for supervised practice of self-care skills. Still other programs are excellent because they deliver educational principles in a creative new way to a population greatly in need. An example is psychoeducation for patients with schizophrenia or those who are depressed and their families. The psychological knowledge and skill taught in these sessions includes learning community living skills, awareness of environmental stress and its relationship to relapse, and networking among families to lessen isolation and stigma.

Still other practice is exemplary because it integrates new, more potent learning elements. A good example is self-efficacy: an individual's perceptions, beliefs, and confidence about how capable one is of performing a specific activity or task. Relevant tasks post–myocardial infarction include climbing stairs, walking distance and time, and overall ability to tolerate physical exertion.

The small literature on management of Patient Teaching generally shows that providers must have teaching skills, must be rewarded for teaching, and are helped by structural expectations such as patient education protocols and chart forms. Studies also frequently show that patients who get care in the health care system believe that they have not been taught.

INTERVENTION TOOLS

Perhaps the most basic intervention tool is an ongoing relationship with a provider, one that is educative and supportive and undergirds development over time of self-management skills. This teacher can use a wide range of interpersonal skills, such as storytelling, role playing, a written contract, and puppets (Redman 1988). In addition, there is a wide range of physician and conceptual tools that assist with learner assessment, teaching activities, and evaluation of outcome.

The Health Belief Model says that people are not likely to take a health action unless they believe they are susceptible, the health problem would have serious effects, they know what to do to avoid the problem, and they believe that this action is beneficial to them. This model has been used to assess a patient's readiness to learn and to build elements of the model into the teaching activities.

Written and audiovisual instructional materials are available from commercial sources and voluntary health organizations and most frequently are developed within an institution to support its specific programs. An example is a videotape of how the most common cognitive dysfunctions post–brain injury affect life after discharge, developed for families who are taking such a patient home (Sanguinetti and Catanzaro 1987). Another example is written instructions in the form of decision trees—a series of steps in the decisions parents must make as they care for a child's tracheostomy, such as: "Is my child breathing OK?" "How are my child's secretions?" "The tracheostomy tube won't go in; what do I do?" (Kennelly 1987).

Computers provide anonymous access to information and practice in decision-making skills, including storing and analyzing information on which the decisions can be based and decision tools (for example, for diabetes management). They can also generate teaching materials tailored to a particular regimen, such as a daily medication schedule to be used as a teaching tool. Computers simultaneously provide opportunity to try new actions, such as for teenagers learning sexual, contraceptive, and parenting decisions, modeling, and desensitization to difficult topics. They are also motivating and help to establish self-esteem (Starn and Paperny 1990).

Observation and assessment scales can be used as both teaching and as evaluation tools. Beal (1986) reports use of the Brazelton Neonatal Behavioral Assessment Scale to demonstrate to parents the infant's behavioral repertoire and how to enhance parent-infant interaction. In another instance, mothers were taught to make clinical judgments about the degree of illness of febrile children by means of a six-item observational scale, including evaluation of color and hydration. The educational intervention involved showing mothers videotapes of children that best illustrated the scale points and giving them practice in jointly rating the behavior with experts. The usual tendency of parents to overstate the degree of illness lessened (McCarthy et al. 1990).

Other evaluation tools such as self-efficacy scales and knowledge tests are also useful.

ASSOCIATED NURSING DIAGNOSES AND APPROPRIATE PATIENT GROUPS

Patient Teaching is relevant for most groups of patients, including many with psychiatric disorders and those with learning disabilities, and for families and communities.

For a number of the nursing diagnoses approved at the Eighth Conference of the North American Nursing Diagnosis Association (Carroll-Johnson 1988) patient education is a central or a useful tool. One of the most directly relevant is Knowledge Deficit, which can come from lack of exposure, lack of recall, information misinterpretation, lack of interest in learning, or unfamiliarity with information resources. Ineffective Individual Coping and Ineffective Family Coping: Compromised can be due to lack of skill in problem solving or lack of knowledge of how to use skills and thus be amenable to teaching intervention, as can Family Coping: Potential for Growth and Impaired Home Maintenance Management. There are teaching actions that can be preventive for patients with a diagnosis of Altered Protection. Teaching may be effective for the subgroup of those diagnosed with Noncompliance who lack knowledge, skills, and motivation, but it may be only a component of the treatment for others with more complex problems; the same may be said for Altered Parenting and Sexual Dysfunction. Clients with Self-Care Deficits often require retraining.

So, also, Impaired Social Interaction can come from a knowledge or skill deficit about ways to enhance mutuality; Altered Role Performance can come from lack of knowledge of the role; Decisional Conflict can result from a lack of relevant information or multiple and confusing sources of information; Health Seeking Behaviors usually involve learning; and Ineffective Breastfeeding can involve knowledge and skill deficit.

SUGGESTED PROTOCOLS FOR USING PATIENT TEACHING

General Protocol

The most general protocol is to use a teaching process of assessment of need and readiness to learn, goal setting, teaching-learning, and evaluation. This process is embedded within the nursing process in that assessment of need to learn is part of the general nursing assessment, and if learning is necessary, goals to accomplish it become part of the overall set of goals and activities planned for the patient. This use of process is necessary because teaching is not an exact science, and it is important to catch imperfect learning through the evaluation process and correct it.

Assessment

Does the patient have the skills, knowledge, and belief in self-efficacy to meet his or her health care goals and/or those necessary to meet self-care requirements? The answer to this question will change as people age, as they incorporate a health problem into their lives, and as treatment changes. Appropriate points of reassessment are important.

Goals

What are the patient's goals? To what extent are they congruent with those of caregivers? Is the desired goal amenable to teaching, is the behavioral change impossible for the patient to reach, or is the need for learning simply covering basic societal problems like poverty? Goals provide direction.

Teaching-Learning

What is the basic kind of learning needed: new knowledge, high-level problem solving for independent self-care, or a range of skills and attitudes for a new life-style? Each of these needs requires particular kinds and amounts of teaching activities. Are these resources available? What combination of cognitive-behavioral strategies is best?

Evaluation

What evidence have the patient and caregiver collected about whether the goal has been met? To be valid, the evidence must be accurate and convincing to the patient.

Have the goals or the patient's ability to learn changed part way through the teaching process, reflecting change in health status or the patient's perception of his situation or treatment plans? If the desired level of learning is not being achieved, is it clear how to redirect teaching, and can that care be delivered?

System questions are also appropriate. Is appropriate education available to patients? Have legal and ethical standards been met? Availability of education is especially important as the patient crosses sectors of the health care system: office and clinic, long-term care, home care, hospital. Will the patient's own environment support and reinforce the new learning? In many instances, interventions to maintain the new learning are necessary.

More Specific Patient Teaching Protocols

Well-developed standard protocols are available for particular common teaching goals or approaches to induce learning. Several will be described here: self-management for a chronic disease, teaching supporting health regimens, and group- or population-based educational programs.

Self-management of a chronic condition at home is a common situation. It generally includes a sequence of learning: basic information, negotiating readiness to change, building skills for dealing with the health problem (including problem solving, coping in high-risk situations, and dealing with setbacks), and developing social support. For example, regarding AIDS, people need sound information about how the disease is transmitted, guidance on how to regulate their behavior, and a firm belief in their personal efficacy to turn concerns into effective preventive actions. People with a low sense of efficacy that they could manage their behavioral and sexual relationships were unable to act on their knowledge. Teaching by videotaped model, imaginal rehearsal of prototypical troublesome situations, and strong social supports for personal change, including alteration of subcommunity norms, were important (Bandura 1990).

Managing asthma at home is a complex problem for most families, requiring appropriate responses in the face of a wheezing episode, efforts to prevent the onset of attacks, and attempts to decrease psychologic and social burdens that asthma imposes. In less than a decade, 14 asthma self-management programs have been developed and rigorously evaluated, showing that these educational efforts can improve self-management, reduce wheezing, help families adjust to the demands the disease imposes on family life, improve school attendance and performance, and change the use of health services, especially decreasing emergency visits and hospitalizations. These asthma self-management programs share three basic premises: doctors and patients are partners in management of asthma; patient situations, medical treatment, and home environment continually change; and at-home management tasks must fit the family's life-style. The programs cover recognizing signs and symptoms of asthma, administering prescribed medicine correctly and managing side effects, remaining calm and avoiding panic, recognizing and responding to symptoms that require emergency care, decreasing exposure to known triggers, normalizing the child's physical and social activities, and communicating effectively with physicians and other health care personnel (Clark 1989). It is of concern that these programs may not be widely available.

Assisting a patient to adhere to a regimen is a common requirement. Research shows much nonadherence. The patient may believe that some regimens may deserve not to be followed because they protect against an eventuality that the patient views not to be immediately important, because the condition gets worse even if the patient does comply, because it does not treat what the patient believes to be the problem, or because it makes the patient feel terrible or out of control. Adherence education requires elements of knowledge building, motivation, memory aids such as cuing, and frequently decision-making skills about how to adjust the regimen. Compliance with short-term medication treatments (less than 2 weeks) can be improved by clear instructions, by special-reminder pill containers and calendars, and by simplified drug regimens. For long-term regimens, multiple additional strategies are required, such as rewards that help sustain behavioral change (although when rewards are removed, the behavior tapers off and eventually becomes extinguished), counseling, group discussions, social support, self-monitoring, and telephone reminders from the provider that serve as motivational as well as memory aids. Relapse prevention is also important. In general, provider compliance with strategies designed to increase patient adherence to regimens is low (Green 1987).

Mass media behavioral change campaigns are aimed at large audiences and operate within defined time limits and an organized set of communication activities that seek to influence individuals. Generally multiple media are used, combined with community, small group, and individual action options, with careful targeting or segmenting of the audience the campaign is intended to affect. The campaign uses a simple, clear message with repetition, the message having been field-tested for its effectiveness. It emphasizes positive behavioral change more than negative consequences of current behavior and builds on a perception of current rewards rather than avoidance of distant negative consequences. Such campaigns have been carried out for substance abuse, AIDS, smoking, and heart disease (Bacher 1990).

Campaigns change as they achieve success or when the behavior has changed. For example, when the high blood pressure media campaign was begun in 1972, its focus was on making people aware of the connection between high blood pressure and stroke and heart disease. Now much of the target population is aware and knowledgeable, and the focus of the campaign is on staying on the prescribed treatment regimen and understanding its benefits. The most credible source is known to be another hypertensive person. The cholesterol mass media campaign, initiated in 1986, is building audience awareness but must now contend with widespread consumer confusion (Bellicha and McGrath 1990).

In Patient Teaching, these examples of specific, standardized protocols have an increasing presence. Yet the more usual situation is that the provider faces a patient situation with a particular constellation of concerns and strengths and must fashion teaching using whatever programs, materials, and expert resources are available, guided by her own reasoning in use of the teaching process.

CASE STUDIES

The following case studies illustrate the use of a consistent process. The first step is assessment. The nurse must assess if the patient has the necessary knowledge and skills to meet his or her health care goals. Simultaneously, the nurse must assess the patient's motivation to learn. The patient needs to relate specific factors involved with his or her health care problems, and then can begin to identify concerns and goals of therapy. The second step begins by determining the nursing diagnosis and negotiation of a plan with active patient involvement. The nurse must determine the particular kinds and amount of teaching that will be necessary and assemble the appropriate resources and tools to accomplish the task. The third step is carrying through the plan with an ongoing evaluation of its effectiveness. The evidence that the goals are being met should be as tangible as possible. The evaluation should involve active participation of the patient.

While the nurse's role in Patient Teaching requires counseling skills, there are differences between counseling and teaching. Counseling is used when the primary focus is on emotions (see Chapter 22), whereas teaching is used in situations where cognitive, affective, and psychomotor skills are to be developed. Generally, in counseling the therapist encourages the patient to set his or her own goals. In Patient Teaching, the nurse has specific goals for the teaching-learning process, negotiated with the patient, since there are definite areas of content that each patient needs to learn for self-care.

The cases also illustrate that in clinical situations, patient education methodology includes not only the traditional instructional approaches and aids but also demonstration, counseling, peer group and family discussions, behavioral modification, simplifying regimens, community organizing, and other approaches that serve to stimulate learning and help make environments supportive to learning.

Case Study 1

Mrs. R. is a 74-year-old female seen in the outpatient department by a clinical nurse specialist. Her chief complaint is uncontrolled blood pressure and weight gain. She is 5 feet, 4 inches tall and weighs 206 pounds. She is a widow and lives with her son, daughter-in-law, and 3-year-old granddaughter in a large, single-family home. The daughter-in-law is a legal secretary, and the son works as a salesman in a local retail store.

To assess the factors that may be contributing to Mrs. R's elevated blood pressure and weight gain, the nurse uses open-ended questions about Mrs. R's usual day and her family. The nurse finds out that Mrs. R has just moved from her own apartment to live with her son.

The nurse measures Mrs. R's blood pressure and finds it to be 160/104, an increase from 150/96 2 months ago. Mrs. R has gained 6 pounds. The nurse carefully reviews with Mrs. R her current health status. Mrs. R clearly understands the relationships among her blood pressure, medications, diet, and weight. The nurse then asks Mrs. R what she thinks has happened to her blood pressure and weight. Mrs. R softly replies, "I don't know. I watch what I eat, take my pills, and I have been walking with my granddaughter." The nurse asks if Mrs. R is satisfied with her recent move. Mrs. R emphatically states, "Yes; the house is new and clean. My son and daughter-in-law are wonderful." The nurse takes Mrs. R's blood pressure again. It is now 186/110. The nurse has Mrs. R lie down on the examining table for 30 minutes and do deep breathing.

The nurse returns and takes Mrs. R's blood pressure again. It is now 146/90. The nurse gives Mrs. R a diet and activity diary and explains that she should eat as usual but write down the time of day she eats and her daily exercise patterns for 2 weeks and return. The patient thanks the nurse for spending so much time with her and agrees to do the diary.

The first step of patient education is assessment; the nurse must elicit the patient's story. Each patient must trust the nurse enough to describe the specific facts in his or her life that relate to the health care goals and must become involved in identifying needs and strengths.

Mrs. R demonstrates the nursing diagnosis of Ineffective Individual Coping. She lacks the skill to evaluate her own blood pressure changes and weight gain. She has the correct knowledge of blood pressure, medications, and diet but is not using her skills effectively. The plan of having the patient keep a diet diary will help both the nurse and Mrs. R uncover areas in her life that may contribute to her blood pressure and weight gain.

Two weeks later, Mrs. R returns to clinic. Her blood pressure is 154/92, and her weight remains the same. The nurse congratulates Mrs. R on not gaining any weight and reviews the activity and diet diary with the patient. She calculates Mrs. R's calorie intake from the food lists and finds her daily calories to be only 1500 per day. Mrs. R has also charted two 30-minute walks per day. The nurse senses a discrepancy between Mrs. R's weight and her diary and asks Mrs. R what other foods she ate. The patient laughs and answers: "These were the only meals I ate." The nurse coaxes Mrs. R to explain, and she says, "My granddaughter eats poorly—only eggs, sausage, and sweets. She also needs a snack in the morning and afternoon, so I fix her what she will eat. She never finishes it, so I finish what the child won't." The nurse then calculates with Mrs. R her actual calorie intake: over 3000 calories per day. Mrs. R exclaims, "That's too much. I'll never lose weight." The nurse asks Mrs. R about her walks and explains that walking at the granddaughter's pace will not burn up many calories.

Mrs. R has shown her involvement with her health care goals by doing the diary. Upon continued assessment, the original diagnosis of Ineffectual Individual Coping is supported. The nurse and patient then negotiate a plan to change Mrs. R's eating habits and increase her activity. The patient agrees to increase fruits, vegetables, and fiber in both her own and her granddaughter's diet, walk for 30 minutes alone once a day, and return to clinic in a month.

The next month when Mrs. R returns to clinic, she has lost 4 pounds, and her blood pressure is 146/86. She reports enjoying her walks alone and thinks she is helping the whole family improve their diets with more fruits and vegetables. The nurse has successfully negotiated with Mrs. R significant changes in diet and activity. Evaluation of the success of the plan is based on Mrs. R's blood pressure, weight, and satisfaction with the results.

Case Study 2

Ms. N, a 35-year-old single female, has been diagnosed with ovarian cancer. After surgery, she begins a course of chemotherapy in the hospital and experiences extreme vomiting for 2 days after discharge. She starts vomiting on the way to the hospital for her second treatment and again does not stop for 2 days postdischarge. The patient admits that both times she was "scared to death" but refused to take Compazine before coming to the hospital.

After the second episode, the nurses caring for Ms. N hold a care plan conference and identify several factors that might be contributing to her vomiting: she is extremely frightened of the chemotherapy, she has been alone during the treatment, and she had not taken Compazine to help control the nausea and vomiting. The nurses decide on the nursing diagnoses of Knowledge Deficit and Ineffective Individual Coping. A primary nurse is assigned to Ms. N and calls her to discuss her next chemotherapy treatment. The patient indicates she will gladly discuss the situation with the nurse because she wants to stop vomiting and is "very upset over her lack of control."

The nurse meets Ms. N in another area of the hospital to decrease her association with the chemotherapy treatment. The nurse asks Ms. N what she is doing to help herself during the chemotherapy, and the patient replies, "Nothing. I try not to think about it. I hate it. It makes me sick. If I think about it, I will vomit. Everyone is disgusted with me, and I don't blame them." The nurse tells Ms. N that everyone responds differently to chemotherapy and no one is angry with her. The patient replies, "So this is hopeless. There is nothing I can do!" The nurse explains there are quite a few strategies that work well with vomiting and asks if Ms. N would like to try some deep breathing, relaxation, and imagery. The patient says she has tried meditation in the past and it has helped her with anxiety. The nurse then leads Ms. N through a deep breathing and relaxation routine. The patient relaxes and is able to do the deep breathing and relaxation quite well for about 10 minutes. Ms. N then opens her eyes and says, "This won't work. I can't stay like this for hours." The nurse gives Ms. N an audiotape to practice at home twice a day for a half-hour, which the patient gratefully says she will listen to daily. The nurse then inquires about the nonadherence to Ms. N's Compazine prescription. The patient replies, "I can't drive when I take it. I get so drowsy, and I feel so frightened and alone." The nurse asks Ms. N if she can take the Compazine and get a ride to the hospital, and the patient acknowledges that one of her friends has offered to drive her to the hospital for the treatment. Ms. N agrees to try Compazine and have her friend drive her to the hospital. The nurse assures Ms. N that she will meet her on arrival at the hospital and stay with her throughout the chemotherapy treatment.

This plan is carried out for the patient's next treatment. The Compazine makes her feel drowsy, and she needs a wheelchair. Once in the treatment area, Ms. N begins to feel nauseated. The nurse has her deep breathe and sit up in bed with the audiotape. The chemotherapy proceeds uneventfully. Ms. N vomits during the treatment but is about to stop once the drugs are finished.

Throughout this case, the nurse provides the support and encouragement that Ms. N needs. Realistic goals are negotiated with the patient and evaluated for effectiveness. The nurse combines innovative nursing activities with appropriate medical treatment to help Ms. N complete her therapy.

REFERENCES

Bacher, T.E. 1990. Comparative synthesis of mass media health behavior campaigns. *Knowledge* 11:315–329.

Bandura, A. 1990. Perceived self efficacy in the exercise of control over AIDS infection. *Evaluation and Program Planning* 13:9–17.

Barsky, A.J., et al. 1990. Silent myocardial ischemia; is the person or the event silent? *Journal of the American Medical Association* 264:132–136.

Beal, J.A. 1986. The Brazelton Neonatal Behavioral Assessment Scale: A tool to enhance parental attachment. 1:170–176.

Bellicha, T., and McGrath, J. 1990. Mass media approaches to reducing cardiovascular disease risk. *Public Health Report* 105:245–252.

Carroll-Johnson, R.M. (ed.). 1988. *Classification of nursing diagnoses; Proceedings of the Eighth Conference.* Philadelphia: J.B. Lippincott.

Clark, N.M. 1989. Asthma self management education. *Chest* 95:1110–1112.

Crowe, L., and Billingsley, J.I. 1990. The Rowdy Reactors; maintaining a support group for teenagers with diabetes. *Diabetes Educator* 16:39–43.

Green, C.A. 1987. What can patient health education coordinators learn from ten years of compliance research? *Patient Education and Counseling* 10:167–174.

Green, L.W., et al. 1980. *Health education planning; A diagnostic approach.* Palo Alto, Calif.: Mayfield Publications.

Kennelly, C. 1987. Tracheostomy care: Parents as learners. MCN 12:264–267.

McCarthy, P.L., et al. 1990. Mothers' clinical judgment; a randomized trial of the Acute Illness Observation Scales. *Journal of Pediatrics* 116:200–206.

Redman, B.K. 1988. *The process of patient education.* St. Louis: C.V. Mosby.

Sanguinetti, M. and Catanzaro, M. 1987. A comparison of discharge teaching on the consequences of brain injury. *Journal of Neuroscience Nursing* 19:271–274.

Starn, J., and Paperny, D.M. 1990. Computer games to enhance adolescent sex education. *Maternal Child Nursing* 15:250–253.

25

VALUES CLARIFICATION

JAMES Z. WILBERDING

Values Clarification is designed to assist people to learn the process of valuing and thereby be clearer about their own values. Because values are one basis for decision making, Values Clarification is relevant in nursing as clients assume more responsibility for decisions about their care. Since the nurse's goal is to assist and support the client, the nurse should understand the Values Clarification process. In some instances, the nurse may choose to initiate the process.

LITERATURE REVIEW

Raths, Harmin, and Simon (1966) assert that there is no consensus on the definition of value, although they state that "a value represents something important in human existence" and that values are "those elements that show how a person has decided to use his life" (pp. 6, 9). An important function of values, according to Simon, Howe, and Kirschenbaum (1972), is to serve as a basis for decisions and choices. According to these authors, health is an area of potential value conflict. Health, of course, is a major concern of the nurse, and thus the nurse is appropriately concerned with value conflicts about health. At least one nursing theory states that "the humanistic nursing effort is directed toward increasing the possibilities of making responsible choices" (Paterson and Zderad 1976, p. 17). If choice involves value decisions, the nurse will be interested in a client's valuing ability. In the realm of health care decisions, Curtin (1979) puts the case for concern for values more strongly:

> Insofar as patients' values are ignored, or replaced with others' values, patients cease to exist as unique human beings. Depersonalization may be partial or complete, but those individuals will die as the persons they were. If the depersonalization is complete, those individuals will not be able to create new values and goals in their life and they will lose a sense of meaning or purpose in their existence. (p. 7)

Thus, nurses committed to the well-being of the whole person must be interested in supporting the unique wholeness of each client with appropriate intervention in the area of values and at the same time avoid the imposition of their own values.

In 1966 Raths, Harmin, and Simon proposed that changes in family relationships, exposure to violence in the media, diminished religious influence, mobility, and more choices impinged on children's values. They postulated that children do not learn well because of lack of clarity about the purpose of life. These children were likely to be apathetic, flighty, uncertain, inconsistent, and possibly drifters, overconformers, overdissenters, role players, and underachievers. A common problem of children so affected is confusion in values.

315

There are three traditional ways of helping children acquire values (Kirschenbaum 1977; Simon, Howe, and Kirschenbaum 1972). Moralizing, one of them, basically consists of telling the child what is right or wrong. Modeling, which seeks to set an example for others to follow, is another traditional way (Kirschenbaum 1977). That there are many different sources of moralizing and modeling, such as parents, religion, entertainment, and peers, adds to the confusion; nevertheless, moralizing and modeling have been traditional parental prerogatives. A third approach is the laissez-faire attitude, which consists of letting children do what they want in the belief that things will turn out all right. It is quite likely that this approach will lead the child to confusion (Simon, Howe, and Kirschenbaum 1972). A different but nontraditional approach is Values Clarification (Kirschenbaum 1977; Raths, Harmin, and Simon 1966, 1978; Simon, Howe, and Kirschenbaum 1972). The process described by Raths and colleagues will be discussed from this point as applying to both children and adults, although the focus of their writings was on children.

Raths, Harmin, and Simon (1966) call Values Clarification a theory. The theory applies critical thinking techniques to matters that are in the affective domain. Values Clarification is a method whereby persons are encouraged to undertake the process of valuing, and there is emphasis on the human "capacity for intelligent, self-directed behavior" (p. 46). The point seems to be that valuing is more than an affective process; it requires intellectual activity in the form of critical thought to be brought to completion.

There are seven essential steps in the valuing process as described by Raths, Harmin, and Simon (1966):

1. Choosing freely.
2. Choosing from among alternatives.
3. Choosing after thoughtful consideration of the consequences of each alternative.
4. Prizing and cherishing.
5. Affirming.
6. Acting upon choices.
7. Repeating. (pp. 28–29)

Steps 4 and 5 involve feeling happy about the choice made in the first three steps and being willing to affirm this choice publicly. Step 7 means that we act repeatedly on our choices in life. The seven steps can be summarized as choosing, prizing, and acting.

According to the theory, these steps function as criteria for what is and what is not a value. A true value meets all seven of the criteria. The steps have been listed in the order in which they are usually placed in the literature, but they do not always occur in this order. For example, someone may perform an act repeatedly, such as visiting with an elderly neighbor. Perhaps only later, after some reflection, does he discover that he prizes this experience and that this contact with an aging person represents a value for him. These "expressions which approach values, but which do not meet all of the criteria" are value indicators; examples of these are goals, aspirations, interests, feelings, and worries. These value indicators may become values as the valuing process is applied to them (Raths, Harmin, and Simon 1966, pp. 30–33).

According to Raths, Harmin, and Simon (1978), there are three sources of content for clarification: value indicators, personal issues, and social issues. In nursing, all three of these sources may need to be considered.

In initiating Values Clarification, the helper and client focus on a life issue, the helper communicates acceptance of the client, and the helper invites the client to progress through the seven steps of valuing. During this intervention, the nurse remains nonjudgmental, accepting the client's decisions and never coercing him or her (Raths, Harmin, and Simon 1978, p. 48).

Kirschenbaum (1977) has criticized the seven criteria, primarily on the grounds that they are not operational. In addressing the criteria of prizing and cherishing, he asks, "How proud must someone be of a belief before it may be considered a 'value'?" (p. 9). He is also careful to point out that Values Clarification does not simply mean clarity about one's own values without consideration of others' values. The personal and social consequences of an individual's position are important in the clarification process. Kirschenbaum's criticisms and ethical commentary are an important element in the literature on this topic. Prior to Kirschenbaum's affirming that the consequences of values are important, the major ethical emphasis of values clarification literature was on the individual's right to choose values autonomously.

The better-defined ethical position of Kirschenbaum is evident in his definition of the valuing process: "a process by which we increase the likelihood that our living in general or a decision in particular will, first, have positive value for us, and second, be constructive in the social context" (Kirschenbaum 1977, pp. 9–10). Values Clarification aims to teach this. According to Kirschenbaum, "Values clarification can be defined as an approach that utilizes questions and activities designed to teach the valuing process and that helps people to skillfully apply the valuing processes to value-rich areas in their lives" (p. 12). Kirschenbaum views the valuing process as consisting of five dimensions: thinking, feeling, choosing, communicating, and acting. Kirschenbaum formulated three hypotheses based on the theory, which relate to children. The nursing profession has not yet tested formal hypotheses from the theory, although it is evident from the literature that nurses are predicting outcomes for persons who undergo Values Clarification—for example, "The end result is a person with more awareness, empathy, and insight than a person who has not had this experience" (Steele and Harmon 1979, p. 9).

The most serious development of a rationale for Values Clarification is by Gadow (1979, 1980a, 1980b, 1981). She believes that self-care is a philosophical basis of nursing. By self-care, Gadow means a type of care that respects the client's autonomy, a fundamental human right. Self-determination is an expression of this right, and self-determination calls for decisions to be made that express the client's values (Gadow 1980a). Thus, throughout her writings, Gadow proposes that the nurse act as an advocate for this type of care by assisting the client in clarifying his or her values. Gadow does not offer an elaborate methodology for this clarification but does propose discussions between nurse and client (Gadow 1981). There is no mention of the methods used by Raths and colleagues in Gadow's work; she has conceptualized Values Clarification independently on the basis of her dual background as nurse and philosopher.

Other nurses who write on Values Clarification have drawn from the work of Raths and associates (Berger, Hopp, and Raettig 1975; Coletta 1978; Rheinscheld 1980; Rosner 1975; Steele and Harmon 1979; Uustal 1977, 1978, 1980). Thus, we have the rather odd situation of nurses' basing an intervention on a theoretical framework from another discipline when one of their own colleagues, Gadow, has independently developed a nursing-based framework for it. The appeal of the Raths and co-workers' theory may lie in the fact that there are numerous published collections of tools for Values Clarification based on this theory.

Uustal's writing focuses on using Values Clarification as a tool for personal growth and ethical reflection by nurses. She touches on Values Clarification as useful in client teaching. She believes that Values Clarification could be a way of finding out what the client wants to learn so that this could be taught first (Uustal 1978). Neither Raths and colleagues nor Gadow views Values Clarification as stimulating an individual to adopt any value. Rather, the person is supposed to engage in valuing. Choice of values is up to the client. Nurses who use Values Clarification have to reflect on whether they could accept a client's values that differ greatly from their own or those of other professionals. The ultimate question is whether the nurse can accept the client as an autonomous agent. Recognition of the validity of the client's values is important according to Carey (1989) in situations where the nurse is attempting to engage in mutual goal setting. In a cross-cultural setting it is also important to avoid the imposition of the professional's values (Nolde and Smillie 1987).

RESEARCH ON VALUES CLARIFICATION

There is a great need for research on Values Clarification as a nursing intervention. Rheinscheld (1980) hypothesizes that the client who is noncompliant with a prescription for reduced activity after a myocardial infarction might become more compliant following Values Clarification. She believes that once his values become clearer, he will see the dissonance between his values and behavior, and, if he values health, he will change his behavior. The assumption here is that the client will value health more than the forbidden activities. Rheinscheld goes on to recount a case report of such a client and describes a method for allowing him to prioritize his values. She does not report whether the person's behavior changed. Thus, Rheinscheld offers a testable hypothesis but no case data to support it, much less experimental evidence.

Rosner reports on "action research" (1975, p. 410) on Values Clarification done by school nurses. According to Rosner, "While this type of research lacks the rigid control of laboratory research, it is of value to educators since it provides an orderly, disciplined base for change" (p. 410). Action research is also described as "a type of research in which one of the purposes is to change the behavior of the researchers themselves, and in which they themselves are the consumers of the research" (p. 410). The study involved five nurses in a school district using Values Clarification with students in various areas, such as drug education, teenage pregnancy counseling, and Red Cross work. Rosner reports that one of the nurses believed the Values Clarification project strengthened students' sense of self-worth about service to others, and all nurses had positive feelings about the experience. Student response to the techniques was neither analyzed descriptively nor measured.

Berger, Hopp, and Raettig (1975) conducted an exploratory study of Values Clarification as an aid in assisting chronic heart clients to examine their life-styles, set priorities, and make changes necessitated by their disease conditions. Values-clarifying strategies were used on a one-to-one basis with a convenience sample of 20 cardiac clients. Some of these exercises were adapted from the book *Values Clarification* (Simon, Howe, and Kirschenbaum 1972). After a baseline assessment of history and life-style, each client participated in eight clarifying strategies: four in the hospital and four at home after discharge. The strategies were designed to help them set goals regarding their life-styles. They were then asked to rate themselves in their progress toward the goals they themselves set and were interviewed about their reactions to the Values Clarification approach. After reviewing their life-styles, 15 of 20 clients were able to set behavioral objectives to deal with an area of conflict. In their self-evaluation, 13 of the 20 clients said they had acted on their goals. The investigators believed that conducting strategies in the home was helpful because it was a quieter environment and afforded family involvement. Use of strategies on a one-to-one basis was believed to permit a safe way of discussing topics that would be difficult to handle in a group. Chi-square analysis demonstrated "a close relationship between age and the patient's willingness to engage in decision making as it related to changes in life style ($p < .05$)" (p. 198). All clients in the age range of 51 years to 60 years in the study acted on self-set goals, but this was not true of other age groups. According to these findings, Values Clarification may help cardiac clients cope with their illness.

The bulk of research on Values Clarification is found in education. Raths, Harmin, and Simon (1966, 1978) published reports of research on the subject. An example of these studies is one by Klevan, who looked at college students' responses to Values Clarification in an education course. There were two unmatched control groups. Effect of the treatment was measured according to "(1) changes in consistency of attitudes, (2) expressions of purposefulness, and (3) expressions of friendliness among class members." The treatments consisted of values-clarifying discussions with the type of issues in education applying critical thinking. Students in the experimental group were found to have developed more consistent attitudes and personal purposes. Friendliness was unchanged. The results cannot be attributed to the experimental treatment alone because of uncontrolled variables.

Governali and Sechrist (1980) criticize the weak research that has been done on Values Clarification. In their study, they hypothesized that college students would change their ranking on Rokeach's Value Survey after one experience with a values-clarifying technique. The subjects were divided into a directive group in which the instructor focused discussion on six focus values after subjects read a values-oriented story, a nondirective group in which open discussion of the story ensued but without calling attention to focus values, a group in which subjects read the story and answered questions about it in writing without discussion, and a nontreatment control group. Before and after the Values Clarification experience, the subjects ranked 18 values of Rokeach's Value Survey. Nonparametric statistical analysis was done. Little shifting in value rankings was found after the treatment. From this, we may conclude that Values Clarification has little effect on value ranking. But we must remember that the subjects were exposed to only a single Values Clarification period using one type of exercise. Perhaps a longer treatment period would yield different results. It might also be asked how the hypothesis of the study came about. Raths, Harmin, and Simon (1966) view Values Clarification not as a way to change values rankings but as a way to teach valuing.

Other educational studies have shown Values Clarification to have some effect. Salzano (1975) evaluated the effects of Values Clarification on self-image using the Tennessee Self-Concept Scale. Although he found no significant difference between his control (no Values Clarification) and experimental (received Values Clarification) groups, he believed that Values Clarification had some impact on the experimental subjects because the total positive subscores of the Tennessee Scale showed dramatic increases or decreases from one individual to another. Graham (1976) found that persons who had undergone Values Clarification made more value-based choices than those who had not been so exposed.

The effectiveness of Values Clarification as a nursing intervention is not yet evident in nursing research. Educational research leads us to believe that the technique has some effect, but better studies are needed. We cannot be certain that effects demonstrated in educational settings will translate to the nursing setting.

CASE REPORTS

Levinger and Toomey (1982) have provided a case report of a Values Clarification group with adolescents. They were aiming to foster interaction, increase self-awareness, and provide for discussion of adolescent identity issues. The counselor and teacher of the adolescents involved evaluated the experience positively, finding the students more cohesive and caring. The students responded positively as well. Toohey and Valenzuela (1983) reported on their use of Values Clarification in family planning education. They believed that Values Clarification reduced hostility and suspicion of those whom they were teaching.

INTERVENTION TOOLS

There is a wealth of intervention tools described in the Values Clarification literature (Raths, Harmin, and Simon 1966, 1978; Simon and Clark 1975; Simon, Howe, and Kirschenbaum 1972). Two techniques are applicable in the nursing situation: the clarifying response and the value sheet. A number of the other techniques described in the literature are for classroom use. They might have some applicability for nurses working in a school or community group but probably not for nurses working in acute care. The clarifying response is useful for work with individuals, and the value sheet is useful for group endeavors.

The clarifying response is a technique devised by Raths, Harmin, and Simon whereby questions are asked of clients with the aim of getting them to reflect on their situations and what is important to them. The interaction is usually brief because the objective is to get the client to think on his or her own, and this can only be done quietly and often when the client is alone (Raths, Harmin, and Simon 1978). Brevity also prevents the client from feeling "cross-examined" (p. 57). Thus, the nurse does not expect the client to solve immediately whatever problem he or she is dealing with at the end of a clarifying dialogue. Rather, the nurse expects that the client will be more able to think through the situation. As an example, consider a nurse who finds a post – myocardial infarction client with the oxygen turned off, smoking a cigarette while eating potato chips brought into the hospital by a friend. The patient has been advised to stop smoking and maintain a low-sodium, low-fat diet:

Client: Don't lecture me. I know I'm not supposed to do this.
Nurse: Is this what you want to do?
Client: I've been dying to all the while I've been here.
Nurse: How do you feel about your diet?
Client: I hate it. You know I love to cook . . . rich things with creamy sauces. I love giving dinner parties, and I love good food.
Nurse: What other things are important to you?
Client: My children and grandchildren. My oldest granddaughter stays with me while attending college to save money.
Nurse: You hate your diet and smoking restrictions but love your social life and family. Given your condition, can you have all your favorite foods, smoke, and expect a lot of time with your friends and family? Think about it.

TABLE 25-1. VALUE SHEET ON CHILD DISCIPLINE

Situation

Four-year-old Marty recently saw chicks hatch from eggs at a museum. He was delighted and fascinated and asked endless questions about the process. A water leak in the basement preoccupies Marty's parent, and Marty slips into the kitchen, climbs onto a chair, opens the refrigerator door, and retrieves a full carton of eggs. Marty has been forbidden by his parents in the past to open the refrigerator. In closing the door, Marty loses his balance and falls from the chair. He is unhurt but crying with fright, the eggs lying broken around him.

Questions

1. Name as many forms of child discipline as you can think of.
2. In a two-parent family, is it sometimes preferable for one parent to deal with disciplinary matters rather than the other? Why?
3. In what ways can parents deal with their anger at a child? How would you? How would you like to?
4. How do you feel about your disciplinary methods? Do you feel good about the way you manage discipline? Explain.
5. Imagine yourself to be Marty's parent. Does this situation call for disciplinary measures? Why? Which of the techniques you mentioned in question 1 would you use in the situation? Why?

This brief exchange attempts to get the client to assess what she prizes and what the consequences of her behavior will be. The nurse's last remark encourages the client to think about possible consequences of her behavior. The nurse avoids judgment and coercion and merely encourages consideration of the issues, maintaining an accepting attitude toward the client (Raths, Harmin, and Simon 1978).

The value sheet is used in a more structured situation, such as a parenting class for families with preschool children. At the top of the value sheet is a statement that the nurse believes will have value implications for the group members. The statement is followed by a series of questions that lead the clients through the values-clarifying process with regard to the issue raised by the statement. Each client writes out his or her answers to the questions. These may be used as discussion material later (Raths, Harmin, and Simon 1978). Table 25-1 provides an example of a values sheet for use in a parenting class. The questions on the value sheet encompass all three aspects of the valuing process: choosing, prizing, and acting. Questions 1 through 3 explore alternative choices, question 4 examines prizing, and question 5 covers acting.

Whatever technique the nurse uses, he or she must maintain an accepting attitude toward the client. The client's individuality should be kept in mind, and in particular the clarifying response should be tailored to the client's needs (Raths, Harmin, and Simon 1978). The nurse should also be permissive. If the client chooses not to participate, that choice is respected. Many other clarifying techniques are described elsewhere (Pender 1982; Raths, Harmin, and Simon 1966, 1978; Simon, Howe, and Kirschenbaum 1972; Steel and Harmon 1979).

APPROPRIATE CLIENTS

Before choosing a nursing intervention, it is necessary to determine the nursing diagnosis. Inadequate Decision Making is a nursing diagnosis to which Values Clarification is suited.

Most nursing literature views decision making in the light of how nurses make decisions (Bailey and Claus 1975; Gill 1979; Grier 1976, 1977; Grier and Schnitzler 1979; McDonald and Harms 1966; Sculco 1978; Taylor 1979). It is possible to summarize a definition of decision making based on the nursing literature and impose it on the client. Following this approach, we could conclude that the antecedent conditions of decision making are the existence of a discrepancy between what is and what could or ought to be in the life of a person (Bailey and Claus 1975) and the existence of alternative actions for dealing with that discrepancy (Grier 1976, 1977; McDonald and Harms 1966). The behaviors of decision making consist of acknowledging preferences for alternatives available (Grier 1976), assigning probabilities to outcomes of alternative actions (Grier 1976; McDonald and Harms 1966), and awareness of and ranking of the value of the possible outcomes of the alternative actions (Grier 1976; Shontz 1974). Taking risks may also be involved in some decisions (Grier and Schnitzler 1979).

Descriptive studies of clients involved in decision making are much needed. The summary of decision making provided here should be considered tentative until it is validated by research. It is evident that awareness of and ranking of values are part of decision making. Therefore, we may hypothesize that Values Clarification would facilitate a client's decision making. Decisional Conflict would result from lack of clarity about values.

Clients sometimes have important decisions to make, such as a cancer patient who has a choice about treatment modalities. All such clients need to be assessed in terms of the antecedent conditions and behaviors of decision making before initiating Values Clarification. Their permission to participate in Values Clarification should also be sought. Values Clarification should not be used with persons with serious emotional problems (Raths, Harmin, and Simon 1966).

Two other nursing diagnoses for which Values Clarification is appropriate are Spiritual Distress and Spiritual Despair (Kim and Moritz 1982).

PROTOCOLS

The use of Values Clarification in nursing practice is likely to fall into one of two categories: individual client teaching and counseling, and group teaching and counseling. In both cases, the intervention should be planned and based on a nursing assessment. We frequently think of the nursing process as a stepwise progression from assessment through goal setting, intervention, and evaluation. Values Clarification may prove helpful with any of the first three elements of the nursing process. For example, a nurse working with a client who is newly diagnosed with a chronic illness may wish to use Values Clarification as part of her assessment of the patient's response to the illness and any indicated behavioral changes.

In the goal-setting stage, she would be able to use Values Clarification techniques as a way of helping the client formulate goals reflective of his values. The goals so formulated would become more realistic and more achievable.

Values Clarification is most likely to be effective in assisting with decision making regarding treatment. There are a number of techniques available for using Values Clarification, so there is no single protocol. What is important is for the nurse to be creative in tailoring these techniques to meet the need of the client at the time. It is important to note that it is the client's need, not the nurse's, that is to be met. The nurse is clarifying the client's values rather than aiming to force her values on the client. As a moral agent, the nurse has a right to make her views known to the client—for example, in the case of a diabetic patient unwilling to change his diet. This could be viewed as an attempted imposition of her values, but she has a professional duty to uphold that which promotes health. This said, she can still maintain a frame of reference in which the client's decision is final.

CASE STUDY

DL, a 23-year-old mechanic from a small midwestern town, developed a persistent headache and shortness of breath in December. A chiropractor advised him to eat a regular diet of three balanced meals per day rather than the one meal per day he had been accustomed to eat. The headache was unrelieved. DL began to experience fatigue and malaise and went to see a medical doctor. After blood counts and a bone marrow biopsy were done, DL was admitted to a teaching hospital in early January. There, blood counts and a bone marrow biopsy were repeated, and DL was told that he had acute lymphocytic leukemia.

DL was begun on a course of chemotherapy consisting of a combination of vincristine, doxorubicin, L-asparaginase, and prednisone.

The medical team offered DL the possibility of having a bone marrow transplant for his leukemia when he obtained a remission. Chemotherapy effected a remission, and so a bone marrow transplant was possible. It was up to DL to decide whether to have it.

The existence of a discrepancy and alternative courses of action are antecedent conditions for decision making. Both were present in this case. The discrepancy was that DL was now very ill, whereas he had been healthy prior to December. His alternatives consisted of continuing with chemotherapy for three to four years until a cure was achieved, having the transplant during the present remission, or having the transplant after obtaining a second remission. He was told the probabilities of survival for each of the alternatives: a 60% chance of survival with the transplant and a 10% chance of getting leukemia again after the transplant. An important consideration in the matter was that with his type of leukemia, he had a 73% chance of surviving 48 months and longer with chemotherapy alone.

Because DL was confronted with a difficult decision and was uncertain, I decided to use Values Clarification with him. I believed his uncertainty may have led to inadequate decision making. Using clarifying responses, I listened for DL's value-oriented statements with regard to the bone marrow transplant, such as "I think I'll wait until next winter to have it so I'll have another summer to enjoy." I would then reflect the value part back to DL with a statement like, "You want to enjoy another summer?" to promote further consideration and thinking on this. I also asked, "What do you think you want to do about the bone marrow?" This was done in brief dialogues over several visits. Direct questions drew DL out more than did reflective questions.

DL eventually decided against having the bone marrow transplant. From our discussion, it was evident that his decision was based on the probabilities of survival associated with his alternatives. Survival is a value, and the probability of survival is what DL based his decision on. The difficulty here is evaluating to what degree our values-clarifying interactions affected his decision making. It is certain that they caused him to think about what he wanted. After making his choice, DL's affect indicated a feeling of peace with his decision. He seemed comfortable, and comfort is a basic nursing goal.

Follow-up interviews with patients like DL might be useful in determining the amount of help that Values Clarification provides in decision making. Such interviews would allow for exploration of the decision-making process. In DL's case, time and distance made such interviews impossible.

SUMMARY

The health care professions are increasingly recognizing client autonomy as a central feature of the client-provider relationship. The client becomes the ultimate decision maker in his care. Nurses recognize and support this and yet realize that it is necessary to assist clients in decision making. To do so without undermining the client's autonomy by subtly imposing one's own values is a challenge. Values Clarification is a systematic intervention which provides assistance in making authentic decisions consonant with the client's values.

REFERENCES

Bailey, J.T., and Claus, K.E. 1975. *Decision making in nursing.* St. Louis: C.V. Mosby.

Beauchamp, T.L., and Childress, J.F. 1979. *Principles of biomedical ethics.* New York: Oxford University Press.

Berger, B., Hopp J.W., and Raettig, V. 1975. Values clarification and the cardiac patient. *Health Education Monographs* 3:191–199.

Carey, R. 1989. How values affect the mutual goal setting process with multiproblem families. *Journal of Community Health Nursing* 6:7–14.

Coletta, S.S. 1978. Values clarification in nursing: Why? *American Journal of Nursing* 78:2057.

Curtin, L.L. 1979, April. The nurse as advocate: A philosophical foundation for nursing. *Advances in Nursing Science,* 1–10.

Gadow, S. 1979. Advocacy nursing and new meanings of aging. *Nursing Clinics of North America* 14:81–91.

Gadow, S. 1980a, October. Toward a new philosophy of nursing. *Nursing Law and Ethics,* 1–2, 6.

Gadow, S. 1980b. Existential advocacy: Philosophical foundation of nursing. In S.F. Spicker and S. Gadow (eds.), *Nursing: Images and ideals.* New York: Springer-Verlag.

Gadow, S. 1981. Advocacy: An ethical model for assisting patients with treatment decisions. In C.B.Wong and J.P. Swazey (eds.), *Dilemmas of dying: Policies and procedures for decisions not to treat.* Boston: G.K. Hall Medical Publishers.

Gill, S. 1979, September. Leadership guidelines for decision-making. *Imprint,* 29–31, 44.

Gordon, L.V. 1975. *The measurement of inter-personal values.* Chicago: Science Research Associates.

Governali, J.F., and Sechrist, W.C. 1980. Clarifying values in a health education setting: An experimental analysis. *Journal of School Health* 50:151–154.

Graham, M.D. 1976. The process of teaching decision-making through values clarification and its effects on students' future choices as measured by changes in the self-concept. *Dissertation Abstracts International, 37,* 1885-A. (University Microfilms No. 76-22,540)

Greenberg, J.S. 1975. Behavior modification and values clarification and their research implications. *Journal of School Health* 45:91–95.

Grier, M.R. 1976. Decision making about patient care. *Nursing Research* 25:105–110.

Grier, M.R. 1977. Choosing living arrangements for the elderly. *International Journal of Nursing Studies* 14:69–76.

Grier, M.R., and Schnitzler, C.P. 1979. Nurses' propensity to risk. *Nursing Research* 28:186–191.

Kim, M.J., and Moritz, D.A. (eds.). 1982. *Classification of nursing diagnoses.* New York: McGraw-Hill.

Kirschenbaum, H. 1977. *Advanced value clarification.* LaJolla, Calif.: University Associates.

Kohnke, M.F. 1982. Advocacy: *Risk and reality.* St. Louis: C.V. Mosby.

Levinger, L., and Toomey, B. 1982. A values clarification group with adolescents. *Social Work in Health Care* 8:95–98.

McDonald, F.J., and Harms, T.A. 1966, August. A theoretical model for an experimental curriculum. *Nursing Outlook,* 48–51.

Moore, M.L. 1976. Effects of value clarification on dogmatism, critical thinking, and self-actualization. *Dissertation Abstracts International, 37,* 907-A. (University Microfilms No. 76-18,586)

Nolde, T., and Smillie, C. 1987. Planning and evaluation of cross-cultural health education activities. *Journal of Advanced Nursing* 12:159–165.

Osman, J.D. 1973. A rationale for using value clarification in health education. *Journal of School Health* 43:621–623.

Osman, J.D. 1974. The use of selected value-clarifying strategies in health education. *Journal of School Health* 44:21–25.

Paterson, J.G., and Zderad, L.T. 1976. *Humanistic nursing.* New York: John Wiley & Sons.

Pender, N.J. 1982. *Health promotion in nursing practice.* Norwalk, Conn.: Appleton-Century-Crofts.

Raths, L.E., Harmin, M., and Simon, S.B. 1966. *Values and teaching: Working with values in the classroom.* Columbus, Ohio: Charles E. Merrill Books.

Raths, L.E., Harmin, M., and Simon, S.B. 1978. *Values and teaching: Working with values in the classroom* (2d ed.). Columbus, Ohio: Charles E. Merrill Publishing Company.

Rheinscheld, M.J. 1980. Values clarification and the post-myocardial infarction patient. *Aviation, Space, and Environmental Medicine* 51:521–523.

Rosner, A.C. 1975. Values clarification and the school nurse. *Journal of School Health* 45:410–413.

Salzano, M.A. 1975. The effects of a values clarification program on the self-image of capable continuation high school students. *Dissertation Abstracts International, 36,* 1418-B (University Microfilms No. 75-20,258)

Sculco, C.D. 1978, June. Development of a taxonomy for the nursing process. *Journal of Nursing Education*, 40–48.

Shontz, F.C. 1974. Forces influencing the decision to seek medical care. *Rehabilitation Psychology* 21:86–94.

Simon, S.B., and Clark, J. 1975. *Beginning values clarification*. San Diego: Pennant Press.

Simon, S.B., Howe, L.W., and Kirschenbaum, H. 1972. *Values clarification: A handbook of practical strategies for teachers and students*. New York: Hart Publishing Company.

Steele, S.M., and Harmon, V.M. 1979. *Values clarification in nursing*. New York: Appleton-Century-Crofts.

Taylor, A.G. 1979, September. Decision making in nursing. *Imprint*, 32–35.

Toohey, J.V., and Valenzuela, G.J. 1983. Values clarification as a technique for family planning education. *Journal of School Health* 53:21–125.

Uustal, D. 1977, May–June. The use of values clarification in nursing practice. *Journal of Continuing Education in Nursing*, 8–13.

Uustal, D. 1978. Values clarification in nursing: Application to practice. *American Journal of Nursing* 78:2058–2063.

Uustal, D. 1980. Exploring values in nursing. *AORN Journal* 31:183–193.

26

SUPPORT GROUPS

CAROLYN K. KINNEY
REBECCA MANNETTER
MARTHA A. CARPENTER

Use of groups as a means of providing support for identified segments of the general population has a relatively long history. Self-help organizations such as Alcoholics Anonymous (AA), which began in the 1930s, reflect a group approach well established as a viable method of effecting change in the behaviors and attitudes of their members. The structure of an AA group provides an intensive support system not only in the regularly scheduled meetings but on an individual basis, whenever a member is in need (Lieberman, Borman et al. 1979). Many populations benefit from support groups, including individuals with acquired immune deficiency syndrome (AIDS), multiple sclerosis, and other chronic illnesses; families of individuals who have mental health problems, who are handicapped, or hospitalized with a critical illness; and survivors of stressful or traumatic events or disasters.

Theoretical examination of Support Groups, particularly those of a self-help nature, has been a recent development. Research relative to the efficacy of small groups has most often focused on those groups that could be controlled and studied in laboratory or clinical setting. Professionals are now becoming more interested in exploring the use of small groups to reach many client populations. In addition, the study of informal social networks and their role in both the mitigation of stress and handling of life's dilemmas has also become more widespread. Such study has increased our understanding of how professionals can enhance adaptive capabilities of the people they serve.

A Support Group as a mode of intervention represents a merging of two theoretical perspectives: social support and small groups. Social support is defined as the feeling of being sustained through need gratification (Weiss 1974), as well as the gaining of knowledge that allows individuals to recognize that others care for and love them and that they belong to a "network of mutual obligations" (Cobb 1976, p. 300). A small group is a planned gathering of individuals in a face-to-face encounter, which meets with some regularity over time, and is designed to accomplish some common compatible goal (Lago and Hoffman 1977–1978). Thus, a support group provides some measure of social support for its members through the use of the group environment.

Attempts to classify and characterize the different types of support groups are numerous, and a wide variety of descriptive labels have been used, such as self-help groups, mutual aid groups, integrity groups, and information-educational groups. In general, Support Groups take some common theme related to a handicapping condition or stressful life experience. Each group tends to develop its own purpose, depending on the makeup of the group and the structure imposed on it by the group members or initiators. In this chapter, a framework will be presented to help professional nurses determine the type of Support Group most appropriate for a client. This framework is based on the social support needs of the client and will provide direction for the formulation of nursing diagnoses.

LITERATURE REVIEW

Social Support

Social support has been discussed in the social and behavioral sciences as a construct that assists an individual in coping with stressful events and maintaining health. Several investigators have shown relationships between psychosocial events and illness or poor recovery from illness (Cassel 1974, 1976; Cobb 1976; Hogue 1977; Kaplan, Cassell, and Gore 1977). It also has been found that some individuals who are exposed to stressful life events and subsequently do not become ill "may be protected by coping resources, social assets, or social integration" (Hogue 1977, p. 66).

Assessment of social support as adequate or inadequate has been described as a way to decide whether intervention is needed. If social support is readily available to an individual in time of need and the individual utilizes the support, intervention is not necessary. Intervention is indicated, however, when the availability of social support or the utilization of social support by an individual is assessed as inadequate. Assessing social support has been proposed by Murawski, Penman, and Schmitt (1978) to include the following (pp. 370–371):

1. An inventory of persons or institutions believed to constitute an interpersonal support system, including some measure of the nature, strength, and availability of support in health and in time of illness.
2. An assessment of background characteristics that define the individual's social obligations (roles) within the primary support group.
3. An assessment of the beliefs about the sources of support available to meet role obligations during a time of illness.
4. A measure of a pattern of social affiliation.
5. A measure of need for social affiliation.

Brandt and Weinert (1981) and Weinert (1987) have developed the Personal Resources Questionnaire (PRQ and PRQ85) to measure a variety of social support sources. Part 1 of the questionnaire provides "descriptive information about the person's resources, the satisfaction with these resources, and whether or not there is a confidant" (Brandt and Weiner 1981, p. 277). The second part of the PRQ provides a measure of perceived social support. The tool is intended for research, although the authors plan to develop it for use in clinical assessment concerning the kind and amount of social support needed to buffer life stressors. Further psychometric evaluation of the most refined measure, the PRQ85, has been delineated (Weinert 1987).

The Norbeck Social Support Questionnaire (NSSQ) (Norbeck, Lindsay, and Carrieri 1981, 1983) is another self-report tool; it measures multiple dimensions of social support and has been applied to a variety of populations and conceptual variables. The authors have studied its psychometric properties as have Byers and Mullis (1987).

Several other instruments for measurement of social support have been recently developed: the Duke-UNC Functional Social Support Questionnaire (Broadhead, Behleck de Gruy, and Kaplan 1988); the Social Support Questionnaire (Sarason, Levine, Basham, and Sarason 1983); the Interpersonal Support Evaluation List (Brookings and Bolton 1988); the Interpersonal Network Questionnaire (Pearson 1987); the Social Network Questionnaire (Nair and Jason 1985); the Questionnaire on Resources and Stress — Short Form (Salisbury 1986); and the Brief Social Support Questionnaire (Siegert, Patten, and Walkey 1987). Methodological variance is found in the development refinement of these measures. Specific psychometric properties need to be reviewed before implementation of these measures in the clinical setting.

Weiss (1974) has categorized social support into six needs, which correspond to six relationship provisions. Each provision is normally a part of different relationships, but in combination these form a supportive network. These six needs are:

1. *Attachment*, being secure and comfortable and having a sense of place in an intimate relationship.
2. *Social integration*, being able to share common concerns and experience a network of relationships in which the individual has the opportunity for companionship, participation in social events, and exchange of services.
3. *Opportunity for nurturance*, being responsible for the well-being of another, wherein the person providing the nurturance has a sense of commitment and being depended on.
4. *Reassurance of worth*, being competent in a social role and respected or admired and valued in a colleague relationship.
5. *Sense of reliable alliance*, being counted on for continued asistance, whether or not there is mutual affection or reciprocation.
6. *Obtaining of guidance*, being able to have access to a trustworthy and authoritative person who can furnish support and assistance in formulating a plan of action during a stressful time.

Each of these social support needs can be met to some extent in a Support Group, depending on the original intent of the group and the progress and growth of the members as the group evolves. Support Groups can be organized or recommended by the nurse on the basis of the client's perceived support need or the needs that are assessed and diagnosed by the nurse. It must be recognized that a group may have one area of need as the major focus, but other needs of members may be met through the group process during the life of the group. For example, a group designed to function as a means of providing information related to coping with a disease condition common to all its members falls under the category of meeting the need for obtaining guidance. However, this educational group may also meet the members' needs for social integration through social interactions required for group maintenance, such as transportation to meetings and determination of meeting times and places. The primary focus of the group structure would be on providing guidance, with the sharing and companionship aspect developing on an incidental basis.

Conversely, a group could be initiated solely to meet the social integration needs of its members, which is the case in many self-help groups. Then, through the course of the group meetings, the member might determine they are in need of information from a knowledgeable expert and decide to devote some group sessions to a more structured educational format.

A group for a small gathering of professionals, such as hospital staff nurses, is an example of a group primarily designed to meet the need for reassurance of worth; however, in the process of the group's discussions, the younger and less experienced nurses could learn new skills from the more knowledgeable members, thus meeting their need for guidance from an authoritative person.

Group Dynamics

The study of small group dynamics has provided an increasing understanding of why a group is an effective way of providing social support and meeting relational needs. A group environment has unique therapeutic elements that are not as readily available in other relationships. Yalom (1985) has identified 11 curative factors that are evident in group processes. Five of these factors are described by Loomis (1979) as being relevant to Support Groups:

1. *Imparting of information*, the teaching or sharing of information and knowledge. This has been an implicit, if not explicit, objective of support groups. Boisvert (1976) states that one of the major objectives for a group of coronary patients following surgery was to provide health information. Information seeking regarding a disease process has been a mechanism used by medical patients to improve their coping through discussion groups and information-sharing groups (Pavlou, Hartings, and Davis 1978).

2. *Universality*, the sharing of common experiences and recognition that others have similar concerns and problems. The use of discussion in group meetings for patients following coronary surgery allowed participants to share common experiences, thus facilitating the successful rehabilitation and transition from the hospital to the home (Boisvert 1976). Discussion groups have also provided a means of improving coping skills of individuals with chronic illnesses, specifically multiple sclerosis (Pavlou, Hartings, and Davis 1978). Groups can be used as a way to promote adaptive coping through affiliation with others who share the same illness or who have loved ones with similar medical conditions.

3. *Group cohesiveness*, the sense of belonging and acceptance, a "necessary condition for the therapeutic functioning and outcomes of most, if not all, health care groups" (Loomis 1979, p. 35). Gaining a sense of hope that the future will be better and that internal and external resources are available to contend with stressors in life can come from the sense of belonging and acceptance. Sharing, learning, and identification are more likely to occur when the group is cohesive. Support groups will be less able to meet their specific objectives if participants do not feel a sense of commitment and attraction to the group.

4. *Altruism*, or helping others in an unselfish manner, which occurs in support groups when individuals realize they have something to offer other group members, as Spiegel and Yalom (1978) found for individuals with metastatic breast cancer.

5. *Interpersonal learning*, interacting effectively with others. As new coping skills, problem-solving techniques, viewpoints, and attitudes are experienced and incorporated into an individual's behavior, interpersonal learning occurs (Loomis 1979). Such group objectives as learning stress management (Webster, Kelly, Johst, Weber, and Wickes 1982), improving coping skills (Pavlou, Hartings, and Davis 1978; Whitman, Gustafson, and Coleman 1979), facilitating rehabilitation (Kerstein 1980), providing health teaching (Boisvert 1976), and fostering grief work (Speigel and Yalom 1978) enable interpersonal learning to take place.

NURSING DIAGNOSES

Nursing has long recognized that identification of patient needs can provide a method of organizing nursing care. Maslow's hierarchy of needs (1970) has been used extensively as a way of determining which needs, based on the perception and condition of the individual, are addressed most effectively by nurses. Various nursing models and grand theories have been developed that provide overarching frameworks for assessment, diagnosis, implementation, and evaluation of nursing care. For example, Orem (1980) has identified the individual's capacity for self-care as the appropriate focus of nursing activities. When the self-care capacity does not meet health care demands, a deficit occurs. In this context, needs related to social support reflect deficits in the individual's capacity to meet the demands of daily living. A Support Group becomes the vehicle used by the nurse to assist individuals in meeting their needs for social support.

Another nursing theory and paradigm, Modeling and Role-Modeling (Erickson, Tomlin, and Swain 1988), provides a comprehensive perspective for understanding an individual's need for support. From this theoretical approach, the nurse can systematically assess what internal and external resources are or are not available to the client and then identify whether additional social support through interventions such as Support Groups can be recommended.

A framework that aligns the social support needs described by Weiss (1974) with the potential benefits of support groups identified by Yalom (1985) and Loomis (1979) can be used to identify helpful nursing diagnoses (Table 26–1). Those diagnoses recognized by the North American Nursing Diagnosis Association (NANDA) and that have a direct association with social support needs and group benefits are addressed specifically in the following section. Many other nursing diagnoses may be identified that are not mentioned here. This discussion merely

TABLE 26–1.   RELATIONSHIP OF SOCIAL SUPPORT NEED AND GROUP BENEFITS TO NURSING DIAGNOSES

SOCIAL SUPPORT NEED	NURSING DIAGNOSES	GROUP BENEFITS
Obtaining guidance	Knowledge Deficit	Imparting information
Reassurance of worth	Self Esteem Disturbance	Altruism Interpersonal learning
Reliable alliance	Social Isolation Noncompliance Potential for Violence Potential for Injury Altered Protection	Cohesion Interpersonal learning Universality
Opportunities for nurturance	Spiritual Distress Powerlessness Hopelessness	Instillation of hope Altruism Cohesion
Attachment	Fear Anxiety Anticipatory Grieving Normal Grieving	Universality Cohesion Instillation of hope
Social integration	Diversional Activity Deficit Altered Family Processes Altered Parenting Ineffective Individual Coping Impaired Adjustment	Interpersonal learning Cohesion

provides examples of diagnoses that readily come to mind. Further, additional nursing diagnoses that identify strengths and positive health processes are especially worth considering given the primary focus of care falling under the provision of support is directed at tapping clients' healthy components and enhancing their coping abilities.

In addition to the framework presented here, nurses use a broader overarching theoretical perspective consistent with their own view of nursing as a basis for data collection, diagnosis, and implementation of nursing care. Nursing diagnoses derived through an inductive process alone do not provide sufficient information for understanding complex human beings, their needs, and their behaviors. When nurses use a theory as a basis for practice, all aspects of the nursing process can be more systematic and purposeful (Erickson 1990).

The Need for Obtaining Guidance

The diagnosis of Knowledge Deficit is clearly related to the need for obtaining guidance. By imparting information, Support Groups clarify and expand material that is new to the client — for example, an unfamiliar medical diagnosis and the resultant impact on the individual and family.

Knowledge may serve to supplement what is already known or offer alternatives to a client's mythlike or inaccurate beliefs. Realistic problem solving and the formulation of a feasible line of action are based on obtaining accurate information (Gussow and Tracy 1976; Powell 1975). Through the imparting of information, the professional supports the belief that respect for the client's own best choice is a basic health care principle. Shared power through the exchange of information is vital to the concept of self-care (Gussow and Tracy 1976; Orem 1980).

The Need for Reassurance of Worth

Lack of self-worth is a concomitant of Self Esteem Disturbance. The mutual aid afforded by Support Group interactions creates an arena for the display and recognition of altruistic behavior (Loomis 1979). The client gives of his or her own experience. Self-worth is defined, and esteem develops as individuals recognize and are recognized as being able to give (Lago and Hoffman 1977–1978). The sharing of what one is counters the idea that one is nothing. It is in this area that the group may give a type of support not often found in the client's family (Dimond and Jones 1983). Family membership presupposes roles in a hierarchical structure, but the group affords mutual interaction with equals. Familial dependency and its secondary gains may be examined in the group, where self-reliance is valued. Group members learn from each other how to handle family relationships and can begin to imitate the coping skills demonstrated and reported in group sessions.

The Need for a Sense of Reliable Alliance

The diagnosis of Social Isolation identifies a lack of dependable and supportive relationships. The benefit of group cohesion implies the formation of reliable and trusted alliances (Loomis 1979). Relationships build as group members identify more closely with each other and their common purpose.

The reciprocity inherent in a viable alliance, associated with the desire to belong and interact, encourages adherence to the rules (Cole, O'Connor, and Bennett, 1979). The support of rational behavior may also prove beneficial in cases of Noncompliance, Potential for Violence: Self Directed or Directed at Others,

Potential for Injury, and Altered Protection. Cohesive group ties may represent an alternative to long-term relationships that have been lost (Dimond and Jones 1983). Affirmation by the group of the client's real and potential capacities serves to refocus the client's behaviors (Cassel 1976; Cole, O'Connor, and Bennett 1979; Powell 1975). Belonging presents responsibilities outside the self and may lead to the formation of reliable relationships, which then enable the individual to discard self-recriminating and destructive behavior.

The Need for Opportunities for Nurturance

Through the instillation of hope, support group participants nurture each other. Inherent in the human condition is a sense of the future and expectation that it will be better than the present, which may appear unbearable. Hopelessness, Spiritual Distress, and Powerlessness may reflect the inability to project oneself into the future (Erickson, Tomlin, and Swain 1988). Alone, the individual has no choice but to endure without joy or even choose to end it all. Group sharing and cohesion present alternative courses of action to the client. Mutual sharing allows the client to draw on the strengths of others. The strength of others nurtures those adjusting to new demands on spirituality. Clients thus nurture each other's hopes for the future and are encouraged to hold a more optimistic view (Spiegel and Yalom 1978).

The Need for Attachment

Although each individual is unique in his or her own being, many experiences are shared. Attachment needs and the related grief associated with situational and developmental losses are common experiences of human beings across the life span. Fear, Anxiety, Loss, and Grieving are diagnoses that reflect universal emotional reactions. Individuals identified as having these diagnoses may tend to feel that no one can understand the loss and grief they are experiencing. The discovery through a group that others are concerned and even share such feelings is reported as having a therapeutic effect (Powell 1975; Spiegel and Yalom 1978). Simply knowing that one is not alone with this emotional pain serves to encourage adaptive recovery and promote the ability to establish new attachments and form new roles, images, and ideas about oneself. Perceiving that one is supported provides the security for exploring new ways of being, trying out new behaviors, and developing new problem-solving approaches (Sarason, Sarason, and Pierce, 1990).

The Need for Social Integration

Appropriate and productive interaction is one result of interpersonal learning. Alternative ways of thinking, acting, and problem solving are possible outcomes of experience sharing. Diagnoses identifying problems in coping are most closely related to the need for social integration. Coping is defined by Cobb (1976) as the "manipulation of the environment in the service of self" (p. 311). Sharing of experiences within the group expands the client's options for productive manipulation of the environment. The client is bolstered by evidence that others have coped (Cole, O'Connor, and Bennett 1979; Gussow and Tracy 1976).

Sharing experiences increases knowledge about activities available, thus benefiting those with Diversional Activity Deficit (Lago and Hoffman 1977–1978). This sharing may also preclude the client's failing as others share a learning experience rather than total devastation. The client learns to use new knowledge as it is shared with group members.

Parenting and Family Process Alterations are diagnoses in which interpersonal learning in support groups has direct benefit. Group members serve as role models and supportive fellows through stages of adjustment (Powell 1975). Individual behaviors are reflected in group interactions. Clients are supported in the difficult task of looking at themselves, as well as their life events, from a more distant and perhaps more objective viewpoint (Ross, Collen, and Soghikian 1977; Pavlou, Hartings, and Davis 1978). Social integration is enhanced as personal social space is defined in relationship with others in the environment. Therefore, the diagnoses of Impaired Adjustment and Ineffective Individual Coping are also benefited through interpersonal learning. As new information is integrated into an individual's repertoire of coping skills, functional adjustment will be enhanced.

RECOMMENDATIONS FOR PRACTICE

Many factors must be considered before setting up or referring a client to a support group: who the leaders are, what approach is utilized, and what group process model is followed. The structure of the group needs to be determined as well, including the duration, frequency, and timing of group meetings. The location of the meetings is an additional consideration, especially when there are mobility or transportation problems for some participants.

Client Selection

A primary consideration when suggesting Support Groups is the client's perception of the need(s) to be met (Norbeck, Lindsey, and Carrieri 1981). This perception may be revealed through a discussion of the structure and interactions of the client's existing support system. An intact system is to be fostered and protected. Such intervening variables as the client's stage of development, resources, ability to use those resources, and existing and past means of need gratification should be considered if the Support Group is to be a viable and productive intervention (Hogue, 1977; Norbeck, Lindsey, and Carrieri 1981).

The PRQ, PRQ85, and NSSQ are structured methods of obtaining information about the client's resources and perceived social support. Another method of determining a client's resource potential and social support needs is to follow the line of inquiry recommended by Erickson, Tomlin, and Swain (1988). The client's network of social support can be determined by such questions as, "Where do you get your support?" "With whom do you talk things over?" "How do you keep going?" "Is there anyone who provides you with reinforcement and helps you solve problems?" "Do you have family members or friends nearby and available?"

It is also important to obtain information related to how the client perceives the social support obtained from this network. Families may "at first sight seem very reinforcing but when the client's perspective is asked are revealed to be energy draining rather than energizing" (Erickson, Tomlin, and Swain 1988, p. 125). The nurse can help clients assess whether their dependency needs are being met by asking questions such as, "Do you feel you are being supported by your family or friends, or are you the one doing the supporting?" Determining the appropriateness of Support Groups can be a collaborative effort between the client and nurse once the client's support needs have been mutually examined and determined.

Timing

Support Groups appear to be most beneficial during transitional stages (Dimond and Jones 1983), periods of adjustment to a new life-style that is replacing one interrupted by crisis or loss. One-to-one relationships are most productive during acute crises or in deficit situations. When the crisis has passed or when the deficit is recognized as permanent, the adjustment process begins. It is during this period that Support Groups are most appropriate. Proper timing is an important aspect in assessment of the fit between the needs of the client and the benefits of the group.

Group Leadership

The leadership style can range from a nondirective to a more structured, directive approach. A nondirective technique appears to be the approach leaders employ when the structure of the supportive group meeting is for sharing experiences and feelings (social integration). A more directed and structured approach may be useful when the group has a predetermined format or schedule designed for education purposes (obtaining guidance).

Boisvert (1976) stated that in leading groups for patients following coronary surgery, a modified nondirective technique was used, with emphasis on support and clarification, information and correction of erroneous notions or perceptions, problem solving for current difficulties experienced by the patient, and reinforcement of feeling expression associated with heart disease and the rehabilitation.

Spiegel and Yalom (1978) relate that the role of the leader is to identify topic themes that occur in the group discussion. Keeping the group from becoming a nonproductive social gathering as well as clarifying group themes was seen as an important therapeutic tool in working with cancer patients (Whitman, Gustafson, and Coleman 1979).

When the leader is functioning as a group facilitator, the goal is to foster the emergence of a process that enables group members to be more effective in seeking help from and giving help to one another. The desire for the group to become an alternate care-providing system encourages each member to "maintain a higher standard of self-care" (Cole, O'Connor, and Bennett 1979, p. 332). Eight principles have been identified that may be utilized to facilitate the group process of new Support Groups:

1. Monitor and direct active involvement of group members.
2. Encourage the expression and sharing of experiential knowledge.
3. Encourage the expression of mutual aid.
4. Encourage appropriate referrals to professionals for information.
5. Emphasize personal responsibility and control.
6. Maintain positive pressure for behavior change.
7. Emphasize the importance of active coping.
8. Minimize leader input. (Cole, O'Connor, and Bennett 1979)

Biegel and Yamatani (1987) found that nondirective and nonthreatening activities of catharsis, explanation, and normalization within the group correlated with group satisfaction. These activities also occurred more frequently. The least frequent activities were perceived as more threatening and focused on behavioral change. Examples of these activities are confrontation and adherence to group norms.

The leader or facilitator of a group may be a professional, a paraprofessional, or a layperson. One or more individuals may initiate and lead groups. When two or more individuals lead a group, it is sometimes beneficial to have a man and a woman lead together. Leadership of groups can also rotate when different sessions of the group have different leaders.

Group Process

Awareness of the group process is an important responsibility of the leader or facilitator. If there is a relaxed, accepting atmosphere, group members have opportunities to clarify group themes, share personal feelings and experiences, and interact with other members.

Two models of group process were identified in the literature relevant to the development of Support Groups. Yalom's group stages (1985) were used to identify the group process occurring in discussion groups for individuals with multiple sclerosis (Pavlou, Hartings, and Davis 1978). The first stage is the orientation phase, wherein individuals are looking for approval and acceptance within the group. Next, the members are preoccupied with finding who is dominant in the group, who has control in the group, and who has power within the group. The third stage of the formative group is the occurrence of group cohesiveness. After the formative stages have been completed, the working phase of the group occurs, with the final stages of termination occurring after the work phase is completed.

Stages of group development identified by Garland, Jones, and Kolodney (1973) were used when discussing the activities of support groups for nurses (Webster, Kelly, Johst, Weber, and Wickes 1982). Again, five stages of group development were identified: (1) preaffiliation, wherein individuals decide whether they will participate or belong to the group; (2) the power and control stage, in which the autonomy of each member is developed (as in Yalom's second stage, conflicts for control occur at this stage); (3) intimacy, when interpersonal sharing, concern, and dependency occur within the group; (4) differentiation, as the group becomes cohesive and mutual support occurs; and (5) separation, when the group comes to an end. The progression of a group through the identified stages has an effect on how well the group benefits are operating. (Chapter 27, Group Psychotherapy, contains further discussion of group stages and processes.)

Structure of the Group

The structure of Support Groups varies depending on the desires of facilitators and group members. No concrete guidelines for the structure or formation of such groups are found in the literature. Most authors agree that homogeneity of group members regarding their specific illness or situation is mandatory. Examples of some populations that have benefited from Support Groups include alcoholics (AA), dying patients (Spiegel and Yalom 1978), drug-dependent individuals (Synanon), patients with cancer (Whitman, Gustafson, and Coleman 1979), vascular disease amputees (Kerstein 1980), patients following coronary surgery (Boisvert 1976), individuals with multiple sclerosis (Pavlou, Hartings, and Davis 1978), and nurses on an intensive-care burn unit (Webster, Kelly, Johst, Weber, and Wickes 1982).

The specific characteristics of individuals who participate in groups have not been determined. Aiken (1982) reported a pilot study designed to examine whether individuals with cancer who utilized psychological support groups were from nuclear or extended family structures. She hypothesized that the greater proportion of individuals would be from nuclear families. Her pilot study did not significantly uphold her hypothesis but did indicate the need to determine the characteristics of individuals who participate in Support Groups.

Membership of Support Groups may consist of individuals with common problems, family members, friends, or interested visitors. Support Group membership may be limited or open, depending on the desires of the members and the leaders or facilitators and the purpose of the group.

Participants of the groups may be required to sign a contract at the beginning of their involvement in the group as a way of formally showing commitment to the Support Group. The literature reveals that few groups require contracts unless the structure of the group is well defined and there is need for the experience to be directive in nature.

RECOMMENDATIONS FOR RESEARCH

The literature about Support Groups primarily includes thoughts, feelings, and experiences that collectively underscore the therapeutic value of the group approach. Scientifically designed studies collecting empirical data to support the relationship between individual needs and group benefits are warranted. Future studies might focus on the development of tools to measure the success or failure of Support Groups. Empirical measures are needed in the following areas:

1.   Psychological mechanisms through which social support operates (Cobb 1976).
2.   Specific needs met through social support: grieving (Spiegel and Yalom 1978), chronic illness (Dimond and Jones 1983), anxiety reduction in families with a critically ill member (Halmi 1990), mental distress (Loomis 1979), and worried but well persons (Ross, Collen, and Soghikian 1977).
3.   Individuals most likely to use and benefit from Support Groups (Aiken 1982).
4.   Specific leadership types most effective in Support Groups (Yalom 1985).
5.   Relationship of internal versus group focus to therapeutic value (Lusky and Ingman 1979).

Longitudinal studies concerned with the effects of Support Groups over time are needed to evaluate their derived benefits. Studies involving Support Groups are difficult to design because of the extremely sensitive and diverse nature of each individual's concerns, as well as the highly complex structure of social support.

CASE STUDY

A Support Group for recent widows offered through a community agency for the elderly is an example of how a small group can be used to meet the members' needs for social support. The structure of and focus for the group was drawn from theoretical principles derived from the Modeling and Role-Modeling theory and paradigm (Erickson, Tomlin, and Swain 1988). The group was offered by placing an announcement in the local newspaper emphasizing that the group would provide support for women going through the grieving process by helping the participants tap into their strengths, regain a healthy perspective, and focus on adjustment related to losses, including role changes and decision making.

The introductory meeting was attended by six women ranging in age from 58 years to 83 years. It was explained that the group sessions would be held for a minimum of 6 weeks and would be developed to meet the expressed needs of the members. The facilitators for the group were a nursing professor and a graduate nursing student. Several topics and activities were suggested, and the group members chose what they felt would be most beneficial to them. It was decided that the first two meetings would be led by the facilitators and would be used to cover two topics: (1) loss and grief process and (2) problem-solving or decision-making process. The activities for subsequent meetings would be decided later and would possibly be led by group members on topics of mutual interest to the group. The group members, including the facilitators, introduced themselves briefly, and all indicated a hopeful anticipation of what was to follow.

The session on the topic of loss and grief covered the stages of the grief process and emphasized the importance of individualization of the stages and a wide range of normal responses for individuals experiencing loss and grief. Members were supported in moving at their own pace and in their self-care knowledge (Erickson, Tomlin, and Swain 1988), that is, they know for themselves what will help them resolve the loss and move forward with their life.

The members then shared their reactions to the material presented and the meaning it had for them. One point that seemed especially helpful for several group members was the idea that it was appropriate to continue to keep objects that represent the deceased loved one; they themselves would know when it was time to move on and attach to new objects, people, and personal ideas of who they are and want to be. One member was very relieved to learn it was acceptable to feel a special comfort from and attachment to her husband's old work shirt. She had given away most of his clothes but could not let go of that shirt and, moreover, had not told anyone she had kept this treasured item. She said, "I was beginning to think I might never be able to get over his death, but now I understand it is okay to keep a part of him alive in me by keeping his shirt with me." She was supported in this idea by the co-facilitators and reinforced by several members who also indicated they had similar concerns about their own inability to "get over" their grief and had secretly hung on to something belonging to their deceased husband. A supportive discussion followed, with several members taking turns expressing emotions and comforting each other. Before departing at the end of the session, hugs were shared all around, and each member indicated how she already was feeling much better. They indicated that listening to how others were handling their grief, sharing their own experiences, and feeling connected to and supported by the group had helped them.

The decision-making session presented the steps of the problem-solving approach and introduced the idea of expanding one's image about self, the roles one assumes in life, and how one can think differently about how to make decisions and handle problems as they arise. It was emphasized that it is appropriate to seek help from others for tasks and decisions that were handled previously by the spouse. At the same time, it was proposed that new roles and responsibilities could be assumed gradually. The members indicated that an understanding of how to break down the decision-making process into stages was new to them and they could see how this approach would be helpful in the future.

The topics for the subsequent meetings were selected and then led by the members as they felt ready to assume such responsibility. At the last of the six originally scheduled meetings, the group decided to meet for at least two more sessions; they were not sure they were ready to end their scheduled contact as a group. By the end of the eighth meeting, all group members indicated an interest in keeping in touch on a casual basis. The members were beginning to get involved in other activities and they did not think time would be available to attend the Support Group meetings. Further, all felt they were ready "to get on with things."

While it is likely that all the social support needs were met to some extent for these individuals through their involvement in this Support Group, the need for opportunities for nurturance and need for attachment were focused on most directly. Providing the group members with a supportive atmosphere where these two needs could be mutually shared and addressed facilitated the grieving process and the individuals were able to gain the strengths needed to begin seeing themselves in the future (Erickson, Tomlin, and Swain 1988). The members gained a sense of hope rather than hopelessness and were empowered to begin seeing themselves in new ways and begin making new attachments rather than continue to feel powerless and lonely.

SUMMARY

The use of Support Groups continues to challenge professional practice and investigation. Although they are not a panacea, Support Groups present fertile ground for research. Much has yet to be discovered about the curative and preventive mechanisms of group interaction (Cobb 1976). It is hoped that the framework presented here will be used as a guide for development and implementation of Support Groups, as well as a basis for research examinations of the efficacy of Support Groups as a nursing intervention.

REFERENCES

Aiken, S. 1982. Family structure and utilization of cancer support groups. *Oncology Nursing Forum* 9(1):22–26.

Biegel, D.E. and Yamatani, H. 1987. Help-giving in self-help groups. *Hospital Community Psychiatry* 38:1195–1197.

Boisvert, C. 1976, November. Convalescence following coronary surgery: A group experience. *Canadian Nurse*, 26–27.

Brandt, P.A., and Weinet, C. 1981. The PRQ—a social support measure. *Nursing Research* 30:277–280.

Broadhead, W.E., Gehlback, S.H., de Gruy, F.V., and Kaplan, B.H. 1988. The Duke-UNC Functional Social Support Questionnaire: Measurement of social support in family medicine patients. *Medical Care* 26:709–723.

Brookings, J.B., and Bolton, B. 1988. Confirmatory factor analysis of the Interpersonal Support Evaluation List. *American Journal of Community Psychology* 16:137–147.

Byers, P.H., and Mullis, M.R. 1987. Reliability and validity of the Norbeck Social Support Questionnaire in psychiatric inpatients. *Educational and Psychological Measurement* 47:445–448.

Caplan, G. 1974. *Support systems and community mental health.* New York: Behavioral Publications.

Cassel, J. 1974. An epidemiological perspective of psychosocial factors in disease etiology. *American Journal of Public Health* 64:1040–1043.

Cassel, J. 1976. The contribution of the social environment to lost resistance. *American Journal of Epidemiology,* 104–123.

Cobb, S. 1976. Social support as a moderator of life stress. *Psychosomatic Medicine* 38:300–314.

Cole, S., O'Connor, S., and Bennett, L. 1979. Self-help groups for clinic patients with chronic illness. *Primary Care* 6(2):325–340.

Dimond, M. 1979. Social support and adaptation to chronic illness: The case of maintenance hemodialysis. *Research in Nursing and Health* 2:101–108.

Dimond, M., and Jones, S. 1983. *Chronic illness across the life span.* Norwalk, Conn.: Appleton-Century-Crofts.

Erickson, H. 1990. Theory based practice. In H. Erickson and C. Kinney (eds.), *Modeling and Role-Modeling: Theory, practice and research,* (vol. 1, pp. 1–27). Austin, Tex.: Society for the Advancement of Modeling and Role-Modeling.

Erickson, H., Tomlin, E., and Swain, M. 1988. *Modeling and Role-Modeling: A theory and paradigm for nursing* (2d printing) Lexington, SC: Pine Press.

Garland, J., Jones, H., and Kolodney, R. 1976. A model for stages of development in social work groups. In J. Bernstein (ed.), *Explorations in group work: Essays in theory and practice.* Boston: Charles Rivers Books.

Gussow Z., and Tracy C. 1976. The role of self-help club in adaptation to chronic illness and disability. *Social Science and Medicine* 10:407–414.

Halmi, M. 1990. Effects of support groups on anxiety of family members during critical illness. *Heart and Lung* 19:62–72.

Hogue, C.C. 1977. Support systems for health promotion. In J.E. Hall and Weaver B.R. (eds) *Distributive nursing practice. A systems approach to community health.* Philadelphia: J.B. Lippincott.

Kaplan, B., Cassel, J., and Gore, D. 1977. Social support and health. *Medical Care,* 15 (Suppl.): 47–58.

Kerstein, M.D. 1980. Group rehabilitation for vascular-disease amputee. *Journal of the American Geriatrics Society* 28:38–41.

Lago, D., and Hoffman, S. 1977–1978. Structured group interaction: An intervention strategy for the continued development of elderly populations. *International Journal of Aging and Human Development* 8:311–324.

Lieberman, M., Borman, L., and associates. 1979. *Self-help groups for coping with crisis.* San Francisco: Jossey-Bass.

Loomis, M.E. 1979. Group process for nurses. St. Louis: C.V. Mosby.

Lusky, R., and Ingman, S. 1979. The pros, cons and pitfalls of self-help rehabilitation programs. *Social Science and Medicine* 13A:113–121.

Maslow, A.H. 1970. *Motivation and personality* (2d ed.). New York: Harper and Row.

Murawski, B.J., Penman, D., and Schmitt, M. 1978, October. Social support in health and illness: The concept and its measurement. *Cancer Nursing,* 365–371.

Nair, D., and Jason, L.A. 1985. An investigation and analysis of social networks among children. *Special Services in the Schools* 1:43–52.

Norbeck, J.S. 1981, July. Social support: A model for clinical research and application. *Advances in Nursing Science,* 43–59.

Norbeck, J.S., Lindsey, A.M., and Carrieri, V.L. 1981. The development of an instrument to measure social support. *Nursing Research* 30:264–269.

Norbeck, J.S., Lindsey, A.M., and Carrieri, V.L. 1983. Further development of the Norbeck Social Support Questionnaire: Normative data and validity testing. *Nursing Research* 32:4–9.

Orem, D.E. 1980. *Nursing: Concepts of practice* (2d ed.). New York, McGraw-Hill.

Pavlou, M., Hartings, M., and Davis, F.A. 1978. Discussion groups for medical patients: A vehicle for improved coping. *Psychotherapy and Psychosomatics* 30:105–115.

Pearson, J. 1987. The Interpersonal Network Questionnaire: A tool for social support network assessment. *Measurement and Evaluation in Counseling and Development* 20:99–105.

Powell, T.J. 1975. The use of self-help groups as supportive reference communities. *American Journal of Orthopsychiatry* 45:756–764.

Ross, H.S., Collen, F.B., and Soghikian, K. 1977. Pilot study of discussion groups for "worried well" patients in an ambulatory care setting. *Health Educaton Monographs* 5:51–61.

Salisbury, C.L. 1986. Adaptation of the Questionnaire on Resources and Stress—Short Form. *American Journal of Mental Deficiency* 90:456–459.

Sarason, I.G., Levine, H.M., Basham, R.B., and Sarason, B.R. 1983. Assessing social support: The Social Support Questionnaire. *Journal of Personality and Social Psychology* 44:127–139.

Sarason, I.G., Sarason, B.R., and Pierce, G.R. 1990. Social support: The search for theory. *Journal of Social and Clinical Psychology* 9:133–147.

Siegert, R.J., Patten, M.D., and Walkey, F.H. 1987. Development of a Brief Social Support Questionnaire. *New Zealand Journal of Psychology* 16:79–83.

Spiegel, D., and Yalom, I.D. 1978. A support group for dying patients. *International Journal of Group Psychotherapy* 28:233–245.

Webster, S., Kelly, L.A., Johst, B., Weber, R., and Wickes, L. 1982. The support group: A method of stress management. *Nursing Management* 13:26–30.

Weinert, C. 1987. A social support measure: PRQ85. *Nursing Research* 36:273–277.

Weiss, R. 1974. The provision of social relationships. In X. Rabin (ed.), *Doing unto others* (pp. 17–26). Englewood Cliffs, N.J.: Prentice-Hall.

Weiss, R. 1976. Transition states and other stressful situations: Their nature and programs for their management. In G. Caplan and Killiea, M. (eds.), *Support systems and mutual help: Multidisciplinary explorations* (pp. 213–232). New York: Grune & Stratton.

Whitman, H.H., Gustafson, J.P., and Coleman, F.W., 1979. Group approaches for cancer patients: Leaders and members. *American Journal of Nursing* 79:910–916.

Yalom, I.D. 1985. *The theory and practice of group psychotherapy* (3d ed.). New York: Basic Books.

27

GROUP PSYCHOTHERAPY

VERONICA WIELAND
SANDRA CUMMINGS

Group Psychotherapy has been defined as a method of psychotherapy in which the emotional reactions of members of the group are understood as being reflections of their interpersonal conflicts (Smith 1970). In this modality of treatment, the clients' relationship abilities, their interpersonal conflicts, and their problematical communicative patterns become the focus and concern of the leader. These issues are both cognitively and affectively explored in a group whose purpose is to provide the clients with the opportunity not only to verbalize their concerns and problems but also to experience them in the here and now of the group. A psychotherapy group replicates the interpersonal world of the clients. Significance is given to the relevance of their interpersonal history as a major determinant in why they behave as they do (Yalom 1975).

The nursing intervention of Group Psychotherapy is illustrated in this chapter through the application of the five stages of group development. Groups go through actual observable stages, and these stages can be classified into Me Centeredness; the Awful Me; the Very Good Me; the Union of the Awful and Very Good Me; and Me Letting Go. These titles are descriptive of the overall behavioral themes in the development of the group. These stages are fluid and in a constant state of change; they go forward and backward. The nurse may see a group in the Very Good Me stage one week, and the next week the group may be in the Me Centeredness stage. A number of factors influence this fluidity, such as member termination, introduction of new members into the group, the credibility of the therapist, the resistance to change, and unclear norms and expectations (Misel 1975).

The conceptualization of these titles resulted from our extensive work with inpatient and outpatient psychotherapy groups. Frequently these groups were supervised by experts in Group Psychotherapy. These groups consistently were videotaped or audiotaped. We also utilized a process recorder, who wrote verbatim the communications occurring in the group. By reviewing these data, we were able to determine the stages of group development and to develop the intervention.

Although the descriptive language varies according to author, there is considerable consistency regarding the basic stages of group development (Yalom 1975). Tuckman (1965) describes four developmental sequences in small groups; Martin and Hill (1957) describe six phases; Nudelman (1986) describes three phases. Whitaker and Liebeman (1964) talk about the brief, formative stage and the extended, established phase of Group Psychotherapy. An analysis of the orientation phase is discussed by Sweeney and Drage (1968). The termination process of groups and its relationship to the separation-individuation process is described by

Kauff (1977). The development stages of 18 sessions of Group Psychotherapy are described by Heckel, Holmes, and Salzberg (1967).

There is little in the literature, however, dealing with how the leader applies the knowledge of Group Psychotherapy developmental stages. Misel (1975) discusses five stages of group development and emphasizes the importance of the leader's role in each of these stages. A credible leader can move the group into the working stage. The quicker the group moves into this stage, the better the leader is as a therapist. Smith (1970) describes three stages of group development and discusses the nurse's role in each stage.

Lacoursiere (1980) focuses on the significance of the leader's being able to understand the similarity between the stages of group and individual development. A nurse who understands this sameness will be able to help clients develop a level of insight about their interpersonal behaviors, identify each stage of group development with their individual developmental stages, and maintain a separate identity while joining with others.

Yalom (1975) stresses the importance of the group leader's knowing the developmental stages of the group. This knowledge enables the leader to guide with a sense of direction, to assist the group in forming therapeutic norms, to prevent the group from establishing norms that hinder therapy, to diagnose group blockage, and to intervene in such a way as to allow the group to proceed. In order for nurses to intervene with their knowledge of the five stages of group development, they need the tools of process illumination and here-and-now activation (Yalom, 1975).

The term *process illumination* refers to relationship implications of interpersonal transactions. It is concerned not only with the verbal content but also with the how and why, especially if it illuminates some aspects of the client's relationship with others and those with whom he or she is interacting. The leader considers the meta-communication aspect of the message, or the communication about the communication (Cathart and Samouar 1979). For example, when a client in a group begins to talk about missing an old childhood friend, it may be important to consider how and why he is discussing the topic. Is his affect congruent with the content? To whom is he addressing the comment? How are his responses being received by other clients? Is he talking about a member of the group who is absent or about someone he has felt has been supportive and caring? It becomes the leader's responsibility to raise questions and make comments that encourage exploration so the significant meaning of the message is understood.

Here-and-now activation is another important tool used by the leader to facilitate the group movement through the stages of development. The members then begin to create their own interpersonal world within the group experience. The leader needs to think in terms of here and now (Moreno 1964). When he or she does so long enough, the group is reflexively steered into the here and now. Whenever an issue is raised in the group, it becomes important to think, "How can I relate this content to the group's life in the here and now?" The leader moves the focus from outside to inside, from the abstract to the specific, from the generic to the personal (Yalom 1975). For example, if a client describes a hostile confrontation with a friend, the leader may inquire, "If you were to be angry like that with anyone in the group, with whom would it be?" Additionally the leader must help members discuss their feelings about the group itself, as well as toward individual members (Yalom 1975). Often it is therapeutic to ask how members are viewing the group's movement; for example, do they feel the group is moving too quickly or too slowly?

In addition to group development knowledge, the nurse needs to have an understanding of individual psychodynamics, stages of the human life cycle, and

TABLE 27–1. GROUP PSYCHOTHERAPY: KNOWLEDGE AND APPLICATION OF THE FIVE STAGES OF GROUP DEVELOPMENT

Goals
1. To help clients achieve insight about their interpersonal behavior.
2. To help clients develop a separate identity and increase their ability to join with others.

Tools (process illumination, here-and-now activation)
1. Allow the group to form therapeutic norms.
2. Help the group to work through their ambivalence about change.
3. Give the group a sense of direction that enables them to identify and resolve each step of development.

Outcomes
1. Clients develop a level of insight about their interpersonal behaviors.
2. Clients can identify each stage of group development with their individual development stages.
3. Clients are able to maintain a separate identity while joining with others.
4. Clients develop new skills and abilities in relating to others.

psychotherapy (Smith 1970). This foundation helps the nurse determine the genesis of the clients' interpersonal problems and their resistances and blockages to achieving change.

Priority is given to the nurse's knowledge and application of the stages of group development. This intervention helps her to continue to focus on group process rather than on individual problems. The tools of process illumination and here-and-now activation help achieve the goals of Group Psychotherapy. Table 27–1 summarizes the goals, the tools, and the outcome of Group Psychotherapy.

SELECTION OF CLIENTS

The most important criterion for inclusion in Group Psychotherapy is the client's level of motivation. Motivation is required not only when relief of symptoms and discomfort is desired but also when the situation requires a willingness to change by working hard to find other ways of dealing with problems (Mann 1973).

In our experience, a client's willingness to participate actively in the group sessions and to take responsibility and ownership for his or her problems are the two major criteria for inclusion. These criteria are supported by Yalom (1975), Nash, Gludman, Imber, and Stone (1957), and Grotjahn (1972). Inclusion in the group need not be based on age, sex, marital status, sexual preference, socioeconomic class, or educational background.

Mann (1973) has identified seven factors that are helpful in evaluating a client's level of motivation. A client who has fewer than three of the following characteristics may be a poor risk for Group Psychotherapy:

1.   An ability to recognize that the symptoms are psychological.
2.   A tendency to be introspective and to attempt to give an honest account of emotional difficulties.
3.   A willingness to participate actively in the treatment situation.
4.   A curiosity to understand oneself.
5.   A willingness to change, explore, or experiment.
6.   A realistic expectation of the results of psychotherapy.
7.   A willingness to make reasonable sacrifices.

STAGES OF GROUP DEVELOPMENT

Stage 1: Me Centeredness

The purpose of this stage is for each client to find a sense of security, trust, and safety as a member of the group. The focus of the nurse's interactions with the members is the establishment of norms and expectations for behavior in the group. She verbally encourages members to share their commonalities with each other.

The first stage is characterized by members' groping for the meaning of Group Psychotherapy. There is confusion about the purpose of the group. Statements may emerge such as, "I don't really know how this will help me," or "I wish I knew how this was supposed to work."

Members are me centered and self-involved, absorbed with their personal struggles and their image in the group. They are doubtful and skeptical as to how talking with others can help them. Because of their feelings of helplessness in solving their personal problems, they have difficulty believing that they can be helpful to others.

At the same time, members are sizing up one another and the group as a whole. They are searching for a role for themselves, often worrying about whether they will be liked and respected or ignored and rejected. This search and testing of one another is done through discussing topics in a rational, cognitive manner. In this way, clients surmise which members have common viewpoints, ideas, and values. They are intrigued that they are not unique in their distress and may invest much time in sharing their similarities. Responses to each other might be, "Yes, I know exactly what you mean," "I thought I was the only one who felt that way," and "I've done that too."

Giving and asking for advice is another characteristic of the stage. Members present to the group low-risk problems, such as dealing with employees, children, and neighbors. The group attempts to provide a practical solution. The solution usually has been tried, does not work, or possibly will be tried in the future. The helpfulness is rarely of any functional value, but it is a safe way for members to express mutual concern, interest, and acceptance.

In this stage, group members look to the nurse for structure, guidance, answers, approval, and acceptance. Many of the interactions in the group are directed at or through her. Members will watch the nurse for nonverbal approval, such as eye contact, head nods, and smiles. Her comments are examined carefully for directives about desirable and undesirable behavior. Members attempt to discover the leader's expectations, thinking that if they make this discovery, they can be cured. Each member unrealistically expects the leader to exhibit special caring toward him or her, to guard each one from being emotionally hurt by other members, to protect from uncomfortable feelings, and to provide an instant cure.

Stage 2: Awful Me

The purpose of stage 2 is to find a place in the group by aggressively seeking approval or establishing individual territory. The focus of the nurse's interactions with the members is verbal acceptance of their anger toward and confrontation of her. The nurse also assists members in the process of exploration and acceptance of their anger toward others.

This second stage of Group Psychotherapy is characterized by frustration, conflict, competition, and preoccupation with dominance, power, and control. The conflict and competition occur between members or between members and the leader. Members attempt to establish boundaries for themselves and the group. Through power and control, a social pecking order is established.

Members are more critical of each other than during stage 1. They feel that they have the right to judge and analyze problems of other group members. As in the Me-Centered stage, advice is given but in a less caring manner. The intent is not to get to know or to help but to establish territory and position in the group. Social conventions are abandoned. There is increased personal criticism about members' behaviors, values, attitudes, and life-styles. Advice is given using the words *should* and *ought,* indicating judgment. Issues between members become polarized with an absence of choices and an intolerance of a middle ground.

The emergence of hostility and resentment toward the nurse is an inevitable occurrence in the Awful Me stage. The sources of hostility are obvious. They are linked to the unrealistic expectations that group members placed on the leader in the Me-Centered stage. Expectations are too high. Regardless of the nurse's competence, the clients will view her as a failure.

Gradually, as the members recognize these limitations, they view the nurse as less magical and powerful. This recognition creates doubts as to the nurse's ability to take care of them and guide them in the proper direction. Other members realize that they never will discover the leader's expectations of them. They will never know what to do to be cured. This is a frustrating time for members whose experiences have allowed them to get special treatment from authority figures. They no longer know what expectations to meet.

Resentment toward the nurse grows as each member realizes that he or she will not be the special, favored one. This realization started in the Me-Centered stage, but now it is more keenly experienced because of the increased rivalry among members.

Group members demonstrate hostility toward the nurse in varied ways. Some members complain that she is too authoritarian and say they want more permissiveness. Other members declare that they want more structure. They request specific group exercises and structuring of time. Or members may directly attack the leader's leadership style, a personality trait, a speech mannerism, or nonverbal behavior.

Indirect attacks are manifested by tardiness or absence of members. A change in seating order may occur. The group sits together, distancing themselves from the nurse, or a member may sit in the nurse's chair. Discussion in the group might focus on past useless therapies and hospitalizations. Scapegoating of a group member also may occur.

Stage 3: Very Good Me

The purpose of stage 3 is to sacrifice one's own needs for safety and individuality in service of group harmony. The focus of the nurse's interactions with the members is validation of their support and caring toward each other. She encourages this process through acknowledgment.

This third stage is characterized by the group's gradual development into a cohesive unit, with maintenance of group harmony at any cost. This stage is the opposite of the Awful Me stage, in which group members vied for territory. Now cohesiveness is more important than individual boundaries or working through group issues. The group suppresses all expressions of negative affect in order to maintain group amity. Individual differences are minimized or not discussed. Members enjoy the group's newly discovered unity. Silent members are encouraged to talk. It is important for all members to feel satisfied. Attendance improves, and there is considerable concern for missing members. Members may meet after the group session.

The main concern of the group is with intimacy, closeness, and acceptance. Members worry about being liked, getting too close, or not getting close enough. It is important for them to show this Very Good Me after having previously demonstrated the Awful Me. They need to give and receive acceptance and approval from each other and the leader. Eventually this harmony and unity seem ritualistic and unrealistic. This necessitates finding a balance between the Awful Me and the Very Good Me.

Stage 4: Union of the Awful Me and the Very Good Me

The purpose of stage 4 is to integrate both senses of me in the group by going through the process of legitimizing conflict. The focus of the nurse's interactions with members is the identification of a range of conflictual feelings. She encourages members to share their anger, sadness, humor, mistrust, and other feelings with each other. The emphasis is on the nurse's ability to help members provide feedback to each other so that they develop insights into their own behaviors.

In this stage, it has become apparent to the members that the methods of stage 3 are not proving to be effective. The Good Me of stage 3 has achieved a sense of security and of being liked and nurtured. These are not sufficient goals in themselves, but they are a condition for more effective action to take place. The members who are more willing to compromise recognize the self-defeating behaviors of stage 3: its focus limits the members to one aspect of who they are — the Good Me — and negates the more conflicted, ambivalent, angry side — the Awful Me. In stage 4, the members begin to talk about this conflict. They attempt to legitimize the feelings and the thoughts that were not positive. This focus creates conflict or forces the group to consider alternative approaches. Stage 4 has intense periods of conflict, but it also tends to be more effective without being destructive to the individual. Members grow in their ability to participate and to formulate perceptions about group process. They feel less judged by each other. Rapport is experienced by knowing what to expect from others.

The overall focus in this stage is on the here and now, for members are talking directly to one another about their feelings and thoughts. A sense of trust is experienced by their being more open about expressing their lack of trust. There is a willingness to take risks by sharing meaningful here-and-now reactions. Most members feel a sense of inclusion, and excluded members are invited to become more active.

Leadership is more shared. Members feel free to initiate exploration of specific areas. Interactions tend to be honest and spontaneous. An emotional bond is present because of the identification with each other's problems and areas of concern. This helps to promote a willingness of members to risk experimental behaviors. Conflict among members and the leader is recognized, discussed, and often resolved.

Previously when members were confronted or offered feedback, they frequently interpreted it as an attack or gave a defensive response. In stage 4 members accept the responsibility for whatever actions they will take to solve their problems. Feedback is given freely and accepted with less defensiveness. Each member seriously reflects on the accuracy of the feedback. Confrontation is viewed as an opportunity to examine one's behavior, not as an uncaring attack.

There is an emphasis on combining feeling and thinking functions. Catharsis and expression of feeling occur, but so does thinking about the meaning of various emotional experiences. This combination of both cognitive and affective components in evaluating themselves helps the members utilize nongroup time to work on problems. It will become apparent to the leader that the continuity of work from one session to the next will not be fragmented and lost. The leader will not need to do all the initiation to help the members address unfinished business or leftover concerns from a previous session. There is a strong commitment to work. This attitude has resulted from the unification of the Good Me and the Awful Me. The legitimization of the Awful Me provides a more objective and realistic basis from which to begin the process of change.

Stage 5: Me Letting Go

The purpose of the last stage is to achieve a sense of separation that promotes self-reliance and a joining with others. The focus of the nursing interaction is termination. The nurse helps the members to review the group history and each member's relationship with the leaving members and to share their anger, disappointments, frustration, sadness, joy, jealousy, and fears of leaving the group.

This final stage of Group Psychotherapy is characterized by members' feeling and acknowledging that they have or have not achieved their personal goals. These goals may have changed since the group's beginning. As members gained a more objective perspective of their interpersonal behaviors, their goals may have expanded or become more realistic.

Members have learned how they are viewed by other people. They know with whom they might demonstrate particular behaviors and why. They have increased their understanding of their need to protect themselves emotionally. Aloof, wary group members have begun to examine their fears of intimacy. Aggressive, vindictive members understand their need to control in order to protect themselves from feeling vulnerable or rejected. Group members have learned that they can behave in different ways without being destroyed, rejected, or abandoned. They feel less locked into one position because they have learned not to fear their feelings. They have expanded their behavioral choices. Members are talking about these changes. "I never thought I could feel like this when I started the group." "You have helped me a lot." "Did I really act like that?" "Now I know why I react this way." Clients also talk about healthier behavior occurring outside the group.

Because members leave at different times, they can experience how others leave before they decide to let go of the group. This will be experienced differently by each client, depending on the relationship of each with the separating member. Experiencing this letting go of individual members assists remaining clients in their preparation for their own termination with the group. Reactions from each other and the leader are watched closely. Members feel ambivalent about leaving the group and show this in varied ways. Some clients exhibit anger in having to let go of the group's security. Others minimize or deny the group's importance to them. Still others think of reasons to remain in the group.

Through the process of Group Psychotherapy, members have learned to cherish and respect their individual feelings, thoughts, and values. They accept themselves as an important, separate identity from others. This self-reliance is strong enough not to be lost when joined with another person. It enables them to develop relationships without sacrificing their identity.

An important outcome of Group Psychotherapy is the client's achievement of a level of insight about self: about his or her behavior, motivational system, fantasy life, or unconscious. Clients may obtain insight on at least three different levels. Yalom (1975) describes these levels:

1.   Insight about interpersonal behavior. Clients learn how they are seen by other people and how they manifest themselves interpersonally. Are they tense, warm, aloof, seductive, bitter? Clients learn about their dealings with others over a longer time span. Are they exploiting others, rejecting others, courting constant admiration from others, so needy of others that their effacing behavior elicits the opposite response from others?

2.   Insight about motivations. Clients learn why they do what they do to and with other people. Aloof, detached clients may begin to learn why they have so much fear about intimacy. Competitive, vindictive, controlling clients may learn about their needs to be taken care of, to be nurtured.

3.   Insight about genesis of behavior. Clients understand the genesis of present patterns of behavior through an exploration of their developmental history.

CASE STUDY

The group described is composed of eight members. (Identifying information for each member is contained in Table 27 – 2.) This case study contains one example from each developmental stage. Each has two components: (1) group process, which comprises the client's discussion and the nurse's inter-action, and (2) rationale for the nurse's interaction.

Stage 1: Me Centeredness

Bill: (looking at nurse) I can't stand reading the paper anymore. Society is unfair. How are people supposed to be creative in society today?
Paula: It's not just society; it's even right at home.
Marge: Yeah, I have problems at home, too.
Ed: (to Bill) Maybe if you didn't read the paper you wouldn't get so upset.
Nurse: It seems like people feel that society and home don't always treat them fairly. What concerns come to mind when people think about being treated unfairly in the group.'' [here-and-now activation]
Mike: Ha! Maybe we need a referee.
Ed: I hope he will be more fair than the one at the Hawks game last night.
Jean: I don't know much about sports, but sometimes my art teacher doesn't appreciate my work.
Nurse: It seems that it is more comfortable for members to talk about unfairness outside the group. Are people not knowing what to expect from each other in this group? [process illumination]

The nurse recognized that the discussion of unfairness and lack of appreciation reflected the members' concerns for safety and security in the group. She used the tool of here-and-now activation and moved the focus from outside to inside the group. Her second interaction recognized the members' concerns about needing approval and acceptance. She also addressed the issues of structure and expectations. She used the tool of process illumination to focus on the members' relationships to each other.

Stage 2: Awful Me

When group members come into the room, Elaine rushes over to a chair that Paula has occupied since the beginning of the group.

Bill: I am so sick of being a househusband. I can never do the things I really want to do. Everything keeps piling up.
Ed: It doesn't sound too bad to me. I would love to stay home and not work. If you want to do something different, you should get a real job.
Bill: I can't find a job where I can be creative. I like being my own boss.
Ed: I think you enjoy being a bum.

Nurse: As soon as the session began, Elaine took Paula's chair, and Ed told Bill what he should do to solve his problems. [process illumination] Are people concerned about their position in the group? [here-and-now activation]

Elaine: Paula doesn't need to have the most comfortable chair each week.

Ed: I'm not that concerned about position. I'm just expressing my feelings like you're always telling us to do.

Marge: (To nurse) Why aren't you helping us with this? Why isn't the group working on more important issues?

Nurse: It seems that members are feeling frustrated and angry because all your expectations are not being met in the group. [process illumination]

The nurse recognized that the members' aggressive behavior indicated their need to establish their own territory in the group. She used process illumination and here-and-now activation to bring this need to the group's attention. In her second interaction, she identified the issue of power and feelings of anger and frustration. This focus on group process reflected the significant meaning of the members' communication.

Stage 3: Very Good Me

(Marge appears sullen and sad.)

Jean: Marge, what's wrong? Are things going badly?

Kathy: You're much quieter.

Marge: Last week I had lots of problems to talk about, but there wasn't enough time. Everyone else was doing all the talking.

Bill: Why don't you tell us what's bothering you now? Maybe we can make you feel better.

Marge: Well, that's all right. It doesn't matter so much this week.

Mike: Come on now, we don't bite. I really want to hear what you have to say.

Marge: Well, two weeks ago I was at this party . . . (Marge describes her problem)

Nurse: People seem very caring and concerned about each other. Are people overlooking other feelings or concerns that they are having? [process illumination]

The nurse recognized the members' need for group harmony and their willingness to sacrifice their own concerns and feelings for group amity. She used process illumination by identifying the members' concern for others and by recognizing their minimizing of individual differences. She gave them the opportunity to explore these issues, a necessary step in order to move into the next group stage of development.

Stage 4: Union of the Awful Me and Very Good Me

Paula: I'm feeling nervous about going home. Everyone will be there — brothers, sisters, mother.

Kathy: What is it that you don't like about going home?

Paula: I always seem to do all the cooking and cleaning. I get so sick of it.

Mike: What is it you want us to do?

Paula: I don't know. I just needed to tell you that.

Elaine: It's hard for me to tell what you're really thinking about your problems. You don't show much feeling here. You're always so controlled.

Paula: (starts crying) I'm afraid to tell people what I want. No one understands me.

Jean: At least when you start to cry I know how painful this is for you. I don't know why you always feel that you must take care of everything by yourself.

TABLE 27-2. CHARACTERISTICS OF GROUP MEMBERS

NAME	IDENTIFYING DATA	CLIENT'S DESCRIPTION OF PROBLEM	CLIENT'S HISTORY OF INTERPERSONAL RELATIONSHIPS AND NURSING DIAGNOSES
Kathy	38: married, 2 children, homemaker	Nonassertive, unable to make decisions, procrastinates, lacks self-confidence	Passivity, dependency, low self-esteem. Nursing diagnosis: Self Esteem Disturbance
Ed	44: divorced, no children, head of hospital department	Drinks alcohol under stress, uncontrollable temper, doesn't get along with other people	Alcoholism, uses aggression to protect dependency needs; projection of problems onto others. Nursing diagnosis: Ineffective Individual Coping
Elaine	24: single, student	Wants to know why she can't form a relationship with a man: "No one understands me or gives me what I need"	Narcissistic, unrealistic sense of entitlement, lack of differentiation of self. Nursing diagnosis: Self Esteem Disturbance
Bill	42: married, 4 children, househusband	Anxiety, panic attacks, lack of motivation, psychosomatic complaints	Avoidant behavior, intellectualizes and rationalizes problems. Nursing diagnosis: Ineffective Individual Coping.
Paula	39: divorced 3 times, 1 child, part-time employment food service	Problems with marriage, difficulty getting along with people on the job and with roommate	Aggressive behavior, minimization of problems, compulsivity and rigidity as a way of maintaining control. Nursing diagnosis: Impaired Social Interaction
Marge	28: married, no children graduate student	Feels isolated, not cared for, cries a lot, has self-doubt about her work and studies	Passive-aggressive behavior, self-absorption, problems with boundaries, inability to negotiate her needs with the needs of others. Nursing diagnosis: Body Image Disturbance
Jean	25: divorced, no children, student	Feels misunderstood, lacks friends, wants to know why relationships with men don't work	Tangential and circumstantial verbal communication as protection for her confusion around sexual identity and early childhood trauma. Nursing diagnosis: Self Esteem Disturbance
Mike	21: single, full-time clerk	Unhappy with life, uncertain about future plans regarding work, school	Use of sarcastic humor as way to deflect his difficulty with issues of separation and individuation. Nursing diagnosis: Impaired Social Interaction

Nurse: (remains silent; the group continues to work).
(Next session)

Paula: I went home, and for the first time I asked for help with cooking and cleaning. I let the family plan their own activities. I didn't feel I had to do it all.

Nurse: Between this and the last session, Paula has struggled with some of the feedback that was given to her by group members. She was able to test out some new responses with her family. [process illumination]

Stage 5: Me Letting Go

(This is the first of the three sessions dealing with Paula's terminating from the group.)

Paula: Every time I think about leaving the group, I have so many feelings.

Nurse: Can you try and identify what you're feeling now? [here-and-now activation]

Paula: (becomes teary-eyed) I just feel confused.

Nurse: How do members feel about Paula's leaving the group? She has been a member of the group for a year. [here-and-now activation]

Jean: Oh, I feel sad and I'm going to miss her. I also feel happy for her (starts to cry).

Mike: (flippantly) Look at it this way. You won't have to sit with a bunch of maladjusted people every week.

Kathy: I would be afraid to leave this security.

Nurse: It seems that Paula's leaving the group has caused members to express a variety of feelings. Jean talked about feeling sad and missing Paula. Mike seemed angry. And Kathy expressed her fear of leaving the group. [process illumination]

Paula: Well, I guess I have some mixed feelings about leaving the group also.

Elaine: How do you think the group has helped you?

Paula: Well, I'm not as afraid of people. I don't need to control them anymore, and I understand more why I had to do that.

Nurse: Could people share with Paula how they experience her changes in the group? [here-and-now activation]

The nurse's use of here-and-now activation and process illumination made explicit the ambivalent feelings involved with the termination. She helped members focus on the components involved in the termination process. She acknowledged the importance of reviewing the client's change and development of insight. This process allows for the client and the remaining members to experience a successful separation that promotes self-reliance and a joining of others.

In this group, the nurse applied her knowledge of group development in each stage. By utilizing the tools of process illumination and here-and-now activation, she enabled the group to form therapeutic norms, to work through their ambivalence about change, and to identify and resolve each stage of development. The effects of this intervention resulted in the clients' developing a level of insight about their interpersonal behaviors and maintaining a separate identity while joining with others.

CONCLUSION

Psychiatric nurses increasingly are being encouraged and challenged to expand their traditional roles to include Group Psychotherapy. Armstrong and Rouslin (1963) recommended that this training be restricted to nurses with a master's degree in psychiatric nursing. Other qualifications that enable a nurse to practice Group Psychotherapy are a basic foundation in individual and group dynamics, observation and process recording of an ongoing psychotherapy group for a minimun of 6 months, and supervised experience for a minimum of 1 year.

Psychiatric nurses can extend their practice of Group Psychotherapy to include a variety of populations: clients with chronic disease; clients and families dealing with death; clients with substance abuse problems and prolonged mental illness; children of divorce and school-aged children with problems of aggression and peer relationships; those who have been abused; survivors of incest; and those with phobias or eating disorders. The focus of these groups would be the application of the knowledge of the five stages of group development. For example, clients with chronic diseases may have regressed to the individual developmental stage of autonomy versus shame (Erikson 1968). The major issues in this stage are control, aggressiveness, independence, and self-discipline. This regression can be resolved by the patient's identifying with and experiencing the stage of the Awful Me. This process allows the client to work through the remaining stages so that he or she is no longer resistive to the physical and emotional changes accompanying the chronic disease.

A current challenge for nurses is how to include research in their clinical practice. Areas for possible research projects are how to use this intervention in a time-limited group; how to correlate the stages of group development with Erikson's developmental stages; how to test the effectiveness of this intervention; how to judge if the effectiveness of the intervention depends on the selection of clients; and determining if the intervention is more effective when all the clients are in the same stage of human development.

The main objective of Group Psychotherapy is not to see how well the nurse can proceed through these five states; rather, it is to provide the clients with abilities and strengths they can use in interpersonal relationships both within the group and outside it. By using Group Psychotherapy, the nurse provides the group members with an experience that allows them to develop new skills and abilities in understanding themselves in relation to others. It also provides them with the opportunity to explore and to test out new behaviors.

REFERENCES

Armstrong, S.W., and Rouslin, S. 1963. *Group psychotherapy in nursing practice.* New York: Macmillan.

Cathcart, R.S., and Samouar, L.A. 1979. *Small group communication.* Dubuque, Iowa: Wm. C. Brown Company.

Corey, G., and Corey, M.S. 1977. *Groups: Process and practice.* Monterey, Calif.: Brooks/Cole Publishing Company.

Erikson, E.H. 1968. *Identity: Youth and crisis.* New York: W.W. Norton Company.

Grotjahn, M. 1972. Learning from dropout patients; A clinical view of patients who discontinued group psychotherapy. *International Journal of Group Psychotherapy* 22:306–319.

Heckel, R.V., Holmes, G., and Salzberg, H. 1967. Emergence of distinct verbal phrases in group therapy. *Psychological Reports* 21:630–632.

Kauff, P.F. 1977. The termination process: Its relationship to the separation-individuation phase of development. *International Journal of Group Psychotherapy* 27:3–18.

Lacousiere, R. 1980. *The life cycle of groups.* New York: Human Sciences Press.

Laube, J., and Wieland, V. 1989. Developing prescriptions to accelerate group process in incest and bulimia treatment. *Journal of Independent Social Work* 4:95–112.

Mann, J. 1973. *Time-limited psychotherapy.* Cambridge, Mass.: Harvard University Press.

Martin, E.A., Jr., and Hill, W.F. 1957. Toward a theory of group development. *International Journal of Group Psychotherapy* 7:20–30.

Misel, L.T. 1975. Stages of group treatment. *Transactional Analysis Journal* 5:385–391.

Moreno, J.L. 1964. *Psychodrama* (vol 1 rev. ed.). Beacon, N.Y.: Beacon House.

Nash, E., Gludman, L., Imber, S., and Stone, A. 1957. Some factors related to patients remaining in group psychotherapy. *International Journal of Group Psychotherapy* 7:264–275.

Nudelman, E.S. 1986. Group psychotherapy. *Nursing Clinics of North America* 2:505–514.

Smith, A.J. 1970. A manual for the training of psychiatric nursing personnel in group psychotherapy. *Perspectives in Psychiatric Care* 8:106–126.

Sweeney, A., and Drage, E. 1968. Group therapy: An analysis of the orientation phase. *Journal of Psychiatric Nursing and Mental Health Nursing* 6:20–26.

Tuckman, B.W. 1965. Developmental sequence in small groups. *Psychological Bulletin* 63:384–399.

Whitaker, D.S., and Lieberman, M.A. 1964. *Psychotherapy through the group process.* New York: Atherton Press.

Yalom, I.D. 1975. *The theory and practice of group psychotherapy.* New York: Basic Books.

28

MUTUAL GOAL SETTING

MICHELE S. MAVES

Mutual Goal Setting as an intervention concept first appeared in the nursing literature in the late 1970s but had been in development since the late 1960s. Mutual Goal Setting is a process whereby nurses and patients collaboratively define a set of patient goals and agree on the goals to be attained. The goal-setting process can be facilitated by using Goal Attainment Scaling, a method developed by Kiresuk and Sherman (1968) to evaluate the effectiveness of community health programs. Goal Attainment Scaling (GAS) involves the construction of a Goal Attainment Follow-up Guide (GAFG), which includes a set of goals that are mutually defined, weighted, rated, and scored for each patient. Research evidence on Mutual Goal Setting has shown that patient involvement in the goal-setting process can result in more effective goal achievement and greater patient satisfaction with health care.

DEVELOPMENT OF THE CONCEPT

Recent health care trends have fostered changes in the traditional nurse-patient relationship: increased health care provider and consumer accountability and responsibility, the development and promotion of the self-care concept, and decreasing government reimbursements for care delivery. Nurses have always played a prominent role in the patient's health care planning. In 1859, Florence Nightingale defined nursing as taking charge of an individual's personal health and putting the patient in the best possible condition for nature to act upon him or her (Eck, Meehan, Zigmund, and Pierro 1988). As of the early 1970s, a majority of hospitalized patients were still given little opportunity to exercise autonomy in self-care activities. Patient input into health planning was seldom solicited, although the patient was expected to assume primary responsibility for carrying out the plan (Alexy 1985).

Accountability and responsibility among health care providers has increased over the last several decades as evidenced by peer review committees, professional certification requirements (Fine 1988), and a gradual shift in the nursing literature from a "military metaphor" to a "legal metaphor" (Winslow 1984). Nurses are no longer bound by a code of obedience to physicians but rather to a code of ethics to which they are legally responsible for the care they deliver (Loomis 1985). Nurses are now governed by a need to be accountable to and responsible for their patients' becoming better equipped to care for themselves after discharge and to inform and educate consumers about their own responsibility for health maintenance and disease prevention (Zangari and Duffy 1980). Nursing theorists such as Orem

(1980) and Orlando (1972) have emphasized the development of patient self-care activities that will help in maintaining their life, health, and well-being. The underlying principle of self-care is that the patient is not viewed as a helpless victim of disease but rather as a client capable of negotiating his or her own health care (Loomis 1985).

The self-care concept has been gaining tremendous support. Reimbursement cutbacks and restrictions are forcing hospitals to limit patients' length of stay (Fine 1988). Concomitantly, technological advancements in medicine have resulted in an increase in the number and diversity of chronic diseases being diagnosed (Brykcznski 1982). Consequently, patients are being discharged with health problems that require short- and long-term maintenance at home. Nursing is helping patients to improve their ability to cope with illness, hospitalization, and transition to home through patient involvement in care planning. Involvement assists patients to gain control over their situations and increase their satisfaction with care delivery (Fine 1988; Zangari and Duffy 1980).

Accountability and responsibility among health care consumers has occurred as a result of the patient rights movement, increased public knowledge of health care and medicine, and escalating health care costs. Patients are demanding a more active role in decision-making processes that affect their health and well-being (Carter and Mowad 1988). The underlying premise is that patients are individuals who make daily decisions involving risks and hazards that may result in major consequences in their lives. Thus, inclusion of patients in decisions about their health care is felt to be necessary and appropriate (Brykcznski 1982).

With health care costs rising, government reimbursements for care delivery decreasing, and restrictions on third-party reimbursements being mandated, hospitals are being forced to embrace a more competitive mode of operation with a marketplace orientation (Fine 1988). Patients are viewed as consumers who use products or services supplied by the health care institution (patient care). "To compete successfully for the consumer's dollars, a hospital must be able to offer a product that is perceived by the consumer as being of high quality and fairly priced" (Eck et al. 1988, p. 1). Customer satisfaction is a priority (Carter and Mowad 1988). Lemke (1987) conducted a study on patient-consumer satisfaction and found that patients' overall satisfaction with a hospital was directly related to their participation in the nursing care delivered. The satisfied consumer is perceived as "a major public relations advocate for hospitals and the nursing service" (Fine 1988, p. 70). Thus, by facilitating patient involvement in the planning and implementing of their care, nurses can increase patient satisfaction with nursing services and thereby promote the interests of the institution (Carter and Mowad 1988).

Mutual Goal Setting has evolved from the changing nurse-patient relationship. Identification of Mutual Goal Setting as a nursing intervention establishes negotiation as an inherent component of the nursing process and fosters a "relationship of mutual influence between the clinician and the patient to the benefit of both parties" (Lazare, Eisenthal, and Wasserman, 1975, p. 553). Negotiation is the dialogue between the patient, who has developed a certain set of needs and expectations, and the nurse, who has formulated a set of needs for the patient based on her evaluation of the situation (Lazare, Eisenthal, and Wasserman 1975). Initially, the needs and expectations identified by the nurse and the patient concerning the latter may not be congruent. Brill, Koegler, Epstein, and Forgy (1964) found a great disparity between goals identified by counselors for the patient and personal goals identified by the patient. Thompson and Zimmerman (1969) found that treatment outcomes from counseling were enhanced when goals were mutually determined by the counselor and the patient. Mutual Goal Setting can favorably affect treatment outcomes because the nurse is able to assist patients in setting more realistic goals for what can be expected with their illnesses and treatment regimens. The nurse can accomplish this by helping patients to reduce their expectations or facilitate the achievement of a different set of expectations. Thus, patients are more likely to achieve their goals.

Evidence of nursing's support for Mutual Goal Setting and patient involvement in care planning can be found in the literature. Several nursing theorists have emphasized a nursing process that includes Mutual Goal Setting (King 1981; Rogers 1970). Nursing's position on patient involvement in care is clearly stated in the American Nurses' Association's (1984) Standards of Practice: nursing actions should provide for patient participation in health promotion, maintenance, and restoration (Standard V), and the patient's progress or lack of progress toward goal achievement should be mutually determined between the patient and the nurse (Standard VII).

Goal setting is an essential part of problem solving and the nursing process. It gives direction for care delivery and the rationale for specific nursing actions, and it makes good evaluation possible (Shelagh 1985). Nurses' and patients' perceptions of the patient's problems, however, are not always congruent. Patients enter the health care setting with their own perceptions of and expectations for their health or illness, course of treatment, and recovery. The traditional role of the patient has been to have expectations that include the communication of relevant physical symptoms, limiting one's emotions and demands to reduce inconvenience to doctors and nurses, and to have the desire to get well (Roberts 1982). Consequently, nurses often are not made aware of patient problems that are "perceived as irrelevant, emotionally uncomfortable or unresolvable by nursing intervention" (Roberts 1982, p. 481). Expectations of the professional nurse include communicating "relevant information to patients about the medical plan of care, remain empathetic but emotionally intact, and have answers to health problems and the ability to resolve them" (Roberts 1982, p. 481). These role differences result in disparities between patient-identified and nurse-identified problems. Problems can be obvious—or expected, hidden, and uncommunicated. Problems that concern the nurse may not be the same as those that worry the patient. Roberts (1982) conducted a study involving 18 medical-surgical cardiovascular patients and their nurses to determine perception differences in patient problem identification. The results indicated a significant difference between problems identified by the patients and those identified for them by their nurses.

Goal discrepancies result when problem identification disparities exist between the patient and the nurse. When discrepancies exist, patient compliance with medical and nursing treatment regimens is threatened. Compliance is based on trust that is nurtured by the patient's feeling he or she is understood. A patient feels understood if what he or she says has been heard and considered (Lazare, Eisenthal, and Wasserman 1975). Feedback verifies perceptions to ensure accuracy of information. The lack of feedback contributes to noncompliance (Francis, Korsch, and Morris 1969). Steckel and Swain (1977) demonstrated that when the patient outcome was identified in measurable and realistic terms acceptable to both nurse and patient, compliance with therapy improved markedly when compared with a control group of patients who were routinely treated for hypertension.

Goal discrepancies can also threaten patient outcomes of care. Starfield, Wray, Hess, Gross, Birk, and D'Lugoff (1981) found that practitioner-patient agreement about problems was associated with better patient outcomes regardless of the severity of the problem. In another study, Leonard and Skipper (1965) found that increased collaboration between the nurse and patient resulted in more effective health care. Predelivery enemas were administered to two groups of obstetric patients. The patients who participated in goal setting and planning found the treatment to be more acceptable and more effective than the control group of patients who did not participate.

GOAL ATTAINMENT STUDIES

Goal achievement is the ultimate indicator of success. Kiresuk and Sherman (1968) developed a method for measuring goal attainment called Goal Attainment Scaling (GAS), which vastly expanded the research base for Mutual Goal Setting. They originally presented the GAS method as a tool to evaluate the effectiveness of community mental health programs. GAS requires the systematic establishment of individualized, specific, realistic, and futuristic goals, which are used to construct the Goal Attainment Follow-up Guide (GAFG). A rating of goal attainment is then obtained and a score computed for each client. The goal attainment score provides a quantifiable measurement of the success of the patient's achievement of his or her expectations for personal change and reflects, in general, the degree to which patient goal expectations have been realized. Kiresuk and Sherman's original formulation of GAS, however, did not include the mutual establishment of goals between the client and the therapist. Goals were established only by an intake worker within the institution. Many studies have attempted to demonstrate the potential usefulness of GAS as a therapeutic technique rather than an evaluative technique by using it in combination with Mutual Goal Setting. Used in this way, GAS resembles a form of therapeutic contracting. The beneficial aspects of this approach are that behavioral criteria are specified, goals are mutually defined, meaningful communication occurs, expectations are clear, and feedback is mutual and continuous (Smith 1976).

Jones and Garwick (1973) examined the effects of patient participation in goal setting on therapeutic outcomes using GAS. Fourteen patients were randomly assigned to two treatment modalities: group A patients mutually established therapy goals with the therapist to develop the GAFG; group B patients had their goals set by the intake interviewer. Group A patients who had been involved in the construction of their GAFG achieved significantly higher goal attainment scores and recorded a significantly higher degree of satisfaction than group B members. The results support the idea that goal setting involving patients leads to higher levels of goal attainment.

Willer and Miller (1976) explored the relationship between patient involvement in goal setting and various measures of treatment outcomes. Seventy-two patients from a psychiatric hospital were randomly assigned to a physician or therapist who was encouraged to involve the patient in the goal-setting process. Four groups were established based on the degree of patient involvement in goal setting: actively involved, not actively involved but informed, had no knowledge of goals set, and no goals set. The patients involved in goal setting had higher goal attainment scores than the other groups. These investigators also found that the greater was the patient involvement in goal setting, the greater was the level of patient satisfaction and goal attainment. They concluded that the relationship of patient involvement in goal setting with patient satisfaction and goal attainment warranted its use in therapy.

Galano (1977) conducted a study on 92 patients at a psychiatric outpatient facility to examine the effect of varying levels of patient participation in goal setting on the attainment of treatment goals and on patient satisfaction with treatment. The patients were randomly assigned to four treatment groups: goal-naive group (therapist constructed the GAFG), goal-aware group (patient viewed the goals constructed by the therapist), goal-setting group (goals were developed jointly between the patient and therapist, but involvement ceased after that), and goal-planning group (goals were constructed jointly between the patient and therapist and patients remained involved in the goal-planning process). Goal planning is a procedure developed by Houts and Scott (1975–1976) that involves mutually setting goals and subgoals, developing plans to achieve the goals, and use of the therapist's encouragement to maintain patient commitment and involvement in working toward those goals. The results of Galano's (1977) study indicated that treatment is more effective when collaborative goal setting is used. Galano concluded that patient participation in goal setting was more important for increasing goal attainment scores than goal setting itself or goal planning.

LaFerriere and Calsyn (1978) also conducted a study using GAS in combination with Mutual Goal Setting. Sixty-five patients in a short-term mental health outpatient center were randomly assigned to a GAS condition or a control condition in which members were not involved in the goal-setting process. When compared to the control group, patients receiving GAS with Mutual Goal Setting had significantly more positive therapeutic outcomes; they exhibited better adjustments on standardized measures of self-esteem, depression, and anxiety and higher ratings of their own outcomes. The results of the study indicated that levels of patient satisfaction were significantly higher for the experimental group as compared to the baseline and control groups, patients who participated in developing written health-goal-planning statements reached higher levels of goal attainment than those who did not develop such statements, and nurse satisfaction with their own patient care activities and responsibilities were higher when working with the patients to develop written health goal statements. This study supports the beneficial effects of Mutual Goal Setting and participation in health care planning.

One of the most recent nursing studies using GAS and Mutual Goal Setting was conducted by Ledray (1982) on a group of rape victims. The patients were randomly assigned to eight different treatment groups: the control group received medical attention only; the other seven received medical attention in combination with either counseling or counseling plus individual goal setting, family involvement with or without counseling, or family goal setting with or without counseling. GAFGs were mutually constructed between the counselor and the client or their families, depending on the group. The study was presented at a symposium before final results were available; thus, Ledray (1982) was unable to determine any meaningful differences in outcomes between the treatment groups. However, mean goal attainment scores for all cases in the study showed a steady, positive progression from the point of entry to the 6-month follow-up. Also, *t*-test results for goal setting versus no goal setting showed a significant difference in mean scores, with goal setting being higher. These early results led the researcher to conclude that goal setting could be an effective facilitator of treatment for rape victims.

The research on Mutual Goal Setting, although limited and inconsistent at times, does tend to support the contention that collaborative goal setting between the nurse and the patient leads to goal attainment. There has been some question raised in the health literature as to whether goal attainment is actually influenced by the mutual discussion about goals or the agreement on goals. Several studies have attempted to begin research into this complex concept (Alexy 1985; Kovner 1989).

NURSING DIAGNOSES AND APPROPRIATE PATIENT GROUPS

Goal setting is an important element in nursing intervention selection. Mutual Goal Setting should be considered as a way to facilitate collaborative goal setting. It also provides a quantifiable score to judge the progress toward meeting the goals.

The universality of Mutual Goal Setting should be obvious. It can be used for most nursing diagnoses as long as the patients are coherent and able to discuss their health goals. It is very useful in helping to increase health-seeking behaviors such as exercise, weight control, sound nutrition, and smoking cessation. It can be used with psychosocial problems such as Noncompliance, Social Isolation, and Self Esteem Disturbance, where a range of measurable behaviors can be identified. It is very helpful to use with a cluster of diagnoses because a number of goals can be worked on simultaneously.

Patients experiencing alteration in thought processes are not considered likely candidates for Mutual Goal Setting because of their inability to understand or remember. Very young children and the severely retarded are also poor candidates.

IMPLEMENTATION OF THE INTERVENTION

The implementation of Mutual Goal Setting requires that a set of goals be mutually defined between the nurse and the patient and agreed upon. The GAS format developed and tested for validity and reliability by Kiresuk and Sherman (1968) can be used as a clinical aid to facilitate the Mutual Goal Setting process and as an evaluation tool for measuring patient progress. The general characteristics of GAS are: "(1) futurism—expectations are set for future outcomes; (2) individualism—personal scales are built for each client; (3) specificity—specified measures, specific times; (4) realism—'what will be', not 'what should be'; (5) nondichotomy—there are 5 possible levels of outcome, not merely a 'success' or 'failure' indication; and (6) rating: an empirical score may be derived, if desired" (Garwick 1976, p. 67, 70). Several other studies have also tested GAS for validity and reliability (Garwick 1974a, 1974b; Sherman, Baxter, and Audette, 1974).

The success of GAS depends on several factors. The Mutual Goal Setting process and GAS can be implemented only with patients who are coherent and able to participate in a discussion concerning their health goals. To use the method with maximum reliability and validity, the nurse must be skilled in problem identification (nursing diagnosis), predicting levels of functioning, and goal plan development (Hefferin 1979). Staff collaboration on and commitment to the methodology are necessary to ensure success of the intervention. It is also necessary for the nurse to have adequate knowledge of the patient's medical diagnosis and medical regimen to facilitate goal setting and planning (Horsley 1982a).

Construction of the Goal Attainment Follow-Up Guide

The construction of GAFG is the core of GAS. The GAFG is a flexible instrument, and its open grid format "puts no restrictions on possible goals, helps to avoid measuring patients on irrelevant variables, and allows the freedom to assign relative weights appropriate to each patient" (Kiresuk and Sherman 1968, p. 452).

The GAFG is mutually developed between the nurse and the patient. Develop-

The Goal Attainment Follow-Up Guide

Levels of Predicted Attainments	Scale 1: (Weight$_1$ =)	Scale 2: (Weight$_2$ =)	Scale 3: (Weight$_3$ =)	Scale 4: (Weight$_4$ =)	Scale 5: (Weight$_5$ =)
Much Less Than the Expected Level of Outcome					
Somewhat Less Than the Expected Level of Outcome					
Expected Level of Outcome					
Somewhat More Than the Expected Level of Outcome					
Much More Than the Expected Level of Outcome					

Source: Reprinted with permission from Program Evaluation Resource Center, 501 Park Avenue South, Minneapolis, MN 55414.

FIGURE 28–1. Goal Attainment Follow-up Guide

ment of the guide should occur as soon as possible after admission of the patient or after the patient's initial contact with the health care setting (Horsley 1982a). Mutual Goal Setting is initiated in the nursing assessment phase of the nursing process. At this time, the nurse discusses with the patient his or her feelings, worries, and concerns; understanding of his or her own disease process; and any other observations made. Following a detailed assessment and physical examination, the nurse can discuss with the patient her observations and nursing diagnoses. Through this process of collaboration, patient goals can be identified and agreed upon. The goals must be specifically defined to ensure that the nurse and patient will be working toward achieving the same goals or the same desired changes.

Once the goals have been determined and the guide has been constructed, the nurse carries out her plan of action for care delivery and patient recovery. No alteration in the nursing care delivery is required between the time that the goals are set and when goal attainment is scored. However, the use of GAS requires that the nurse be flexible and creative when developing the written treatment plan for achievement of the patient's goals (Hefferin 1979). Goal attainment is not possible without a well-conceived and appropriate nursing care plan. Once the GAFG has been constructed, it is critical that the expected goals be communicated to the entire staff to ensure continuity of care (Horsley 1982a).

The GAFG consists of a five-point scale of observable outcomes: much less than expected, somewhat less than expected, expected, somewhat more than expected, and much more than expected (Figure 28–1). The guide can be constructed using the following steps identified by Garwick (1976):

1. Problem area identification: Each vertical column is called a scale and refers to a major concern or problem area of the patient. Describe the problem in a brief phrase, and place each separate problem in the box at the top of each vertical column (scale heading)—only one variable per column.

2.   Specify the target time on which the goals (or expectations) are focused—appropriate to the patient's needs.

3.   Assign weights to each problem area to reflect the relative importance of each scale. The higher the number designated as the "importance weight" of a problem area, the higher is the indicated importance.

4.   Select a specific, observable measurement indicator for the problem area (useful, relevant and easily rated—physiological or psychological tests, observations).

5.   Specify the period of time in which each variable is to be measured.

6.   Specify expected outcomes for each problem area (middle level of each scale). The outcomes should be realistic, pragmatic, what "will happen" not "what should" happen, and not reflective of the client's current behaviors. For most patients, a moderate amount of positive change would be the expected outcome; however, expected outcomes can also be no change or negative change.

7.   Fill in extreme levels (left margin) of each problem area's scale (at least three of five levels should be filled in for each scale).

8.   Fill in any of the other levels on the various scales (there should never be two blank levels adjacent to each other, and the expected levels should always be filled in).

9.   Indicate client's initial status level on each scale.*

Some key points to remember when constructing the follow-up guide are that the variables must be precise, all behaviors described on each level must be separate, no more than one gap should exist between levels, and there should be only one indicator for each scale (Garwick 1976). (Figure 28–2 contains a completed GAFG, based on the case study in this chapter.)

Scoring the GAFG

Success of goal setting and planning can be evaluated by calculating a score for goal attainment using the GAFG. The guide may be used without determining empirical results, but generally a numerical score is derived to show the degree of goal attainment (Garwick 1976). Scoring is conducted at the follow-up interview with the patient at the designated time. The GAFG may be scored by someone other than the person who constructed the guide. Therefore, it is important that the goals be described precisely and the levels be clearly discriminated for accurate follow-up and evaluation. After follow-up, the goal attainment guide can be renegotiated, with new goals, attainment levels, weights, and a follow-up date specified. In this manner, Mutual Goal Setting can provide a means to structure ongoing care planning with patients (Horsley 1982a).

Each of the outcome levels of attainment should be assigned a numerical value of −2 to +2, respectively, with 0 representing the expected level (Figure 28–1). Each scale is scored at the attainment level closest to the patient's behavior at the prespecified target time. The weights and outcome level scores are used to calculate the goal attainment score (Kiresuk and Sherman 1968).

---

* Rewritten and printed with permission from the Program Evaluation Resource Center, 501 Park Avenue South, Minneapolis, Minnesota 55414.

The formula for calculation (Kiresuk and Sherman 1968) is:[*]

$$\text{Goal Attainment Score} = 50 + \frac{10\Sigma w_1 x_1}{\sqrt{.7\ w_1{}^2 + .3(\Sigma\ w_1)^2}}$$

where x = raw score or outcome level
where Σ = sum
where w = weight of the scale

The final score is an adjusted standardized score that represents, in general, the degree to which a patient's goal expectations have been realized. Patient comparisons may be made using these adjusted scores, although each patient may have a different number of scales and different weightings. If all outcomes are scored at the expected level, the score is 50. An individual who scores greater than 50 has achieved greater than expected levels of goal attainment, whereas an individual who scores less than 50 has attained less than expected levels (Horsley 1982a).

Use of Goal Attainment Scaling

The use of GAS can have many beneficial effects for both nurses and their patients. Nurses can use the GAS methodology to increase their clinical effectiveness by structuring the therapy process or by increasing patient participation in therapy. Garwick (1976) reported that GAS had been used in over 200 settings since it was first developed, and it had been used in program evaluation, organizational goal setting, record keeping, and training in goal setting and therapy. Computing goal attainment scores in clinical situations provides a quantifiable means for measurement of outcomes for quality assurance. Goal information obtained from GAS can be entered into the patient's clinical record for use as a monitoring device for both the treatment and program progress (Hefferin 1979). The GAFG can be considered a written documentation of nursing's contribution to health care and can establish for nurses those areas in which they can demonstrate their accountability for independent nursing functions (Horsley 1982a).

The use of GAS in the clinical setting can be educative for patients. Realistic goal setting and planning requires patients to understand all aspects of their illness and treatment regimen. Mutual Goal Setting used with GAS provides a medium for information exchange, resulting in greater patient knowledge (Hefferin 1979). It also promotes patient acceptance of responsibility for care. When patients enter the health care setting, they often feel overwhelmed by routines, their diagnosis, and their feelings of loss of control. They tend to become more dependent on health care personnel and unresponsive to nursing efforts. Including patients in goal development and planning helps to minimize or prevent these negative patient role characteristics and promotes patient responsibility for self-care (Zangari and Duffy 1980). Striving toward health goals becomes more desirable to patients as a result of the control gained by having actively participated in establishing their own goals for treatment outcomes (Hefferin 1979).

In 1982, a series of research-based clinical protocols were published as a result of the Conduct and Utilization of Research in Nursing (CURN) Project, a joint effort between the University of Michigan, College of Nursing and the Michigan Nurses' Association. These protocols were developed in response to a growing desire

---

[*] Reprinted with permission from the Program Evaluation Resource Center, 501 Park Avenue South, Minneapolis, Minnesota 55414.

among nurses to use scientific nursing knowledge, generated by research studies, in the clinical setting. Research utilization is a process that results in new practices being defined, planned, implemented, and evaluated. The steps in this process are identification and synthesis of research studies in a common conceptual area, transformation of the knowledge into a clinical protocol (written documentation), and transformation of the clinical protocol into an innovation (Horsley 1982b). Mutual Goal Setting was among the 10 protocols developed in the CURN Project, a good resource for information on implementation of Mutual Goal Setting. It also describes how to conduct a research study to evaluate the effects of Mutual Goal Setting on goal attainment in any clinical setting. Any further testing of Mutual Goal Setting using this protocol should be reported, as it will help to strengthen the research base.

CASE STUDY

The setting is an outpatient Cardiac Rehabilitation Phase II program located in a major hospital in Cedar Rapids, Iowa. Patients attend this 6-week course to restore and/or build up stamina, both physically and mentally.

DH is a healthy-looking 45-year-old white male who was admitted with an acute inferior wall myocardial infarction (MI) in April. A cardiac catheterization showed complete distal occlusion of the right coronary artery. An angioplasty was performed that resulted in patency of the artery. His hospital course was unremarkable, and his 6-week follow-up physical assessment was negative.

Except for his MI, DH's general health has been good. There is a strong family history of heart disease. DH has a 23-year, two-pack-per-day smoking history. He has quit smoking since his admission to the hospital. DH's weight is 183 pounds, down 10 pounds since his MI (he is 5 feet, 6 inches).

DH considered himself to be in good physical shape prior to the MI. Since discharge from the hospital, he has been walking approximately 2 miles every day with his wife at a pace of 2 miles per hour. DH complains of general weakness, tiring easily, and some chest heaviness but no shortness of breath while exercising.

DH states that he has experienced some depression since his discharge. He is worried about his future health and the recurrence of heart trouble. He feels more vulnerable since his heart attack and, especially at night has fears of dying. These fears and anxieties initially resulted in loss of sleep. A prescription of 2 mg Ativan by mouth has somewhat improved his ability to sleep.

DH and I extensively discussed and mutually agreed on four major problem areas following my initial assessment and physical examination. We then rated the four problems in the order of importance and weighted them. Smoking (Smoking, weighted 4) was chosen as the most important problem area because of its connection to heart disease and because of the immediate beneficial effects on the body following cessation of smoking. The second most important problem we identified was DH's decreased strength and endurance, as evidenced by general fatigue, weakness, and slight chest heaviness with exercise (Strength & Endurance, weighted 3). The third most important problem area was his fears of dying and worries about his future health and life, which were interfering with his sleep (Fears & Worries, weighted 2). The fourth problem of importance mutually identified was DH's being overweight (Weight, weighted 1). DH and I then chose the indicators for the problem areas, set target dates for goal achievement and evaluation, and established the predicted levels of attainment. Figure 28–2 shows the fully constructed GAFG for the case study.

	STRENGTH & ENDURANCE (3)	SMOKING (4)	FEARS & WORRIES (2)	WEIGHT (1)
MOST UNFAVORABLE (−2)	# LESS THAN: 1.8 MET on exercise Treadmill (TM) 2.7 MET on exercise Bike (AD)	#5 CIGARETTES/ DAY OR MORE	USING MEDICATION TO HELP SLEEP EVERY NIGHT #	WEIGHT GAIN #
LESS THAN EXPECTED (−1)			USING MORE THAN 3 ATIVAN BUT LESS THAN 7 TO HELP WITH SLEEP	NO LOSS, OR LESS THAN 3 POUNDS LOST *
EXPECTED (0)	TM: 5 MET LEVEL AD: 4 MET LEVEL	1 CIGARETTES/ DAY	USING ATIVAN 3 TIMES/WEEK TO HELP WITH SLEEP	LOSS OF 3 POUNDS
MORE THAN EXPECTED (+1)			USING LESS THAN 3 ATIVAN/WEEK TO HELP WITH SLEEP	LOST MORE THAN 3 POUNDS BUT LESS THAN 6
MOST FAVORABLE (+2)	*TM: 7 MET LEVEL AD: 6 MET LEVEL	*NO SMOKING	FALLING ASLEEP WITHOUT ANY MEDICATION	LOST MORE THAN 6 POUNDS

**ALL GOALS TO BE ACCOMPLISHED &/OR EVALUATED ON 6/14 (IN 6 WEEKS)

*INDICATES LEVEL ATTAINED

#INDICATES INITIAL STATUS LEVEL

FIGURE 28–2. Case Study Goal Attainment Follow-up Guide

Using Houts and Scott's (1975–1976) study as a basis, I developed goal planning statements that indicated the specific actions to be taken by DH and the nurse. These were then placed in DH's chart. Information contained in the GAFG and the goal planning statements was shared with cardiac rehabilitation nursing staff to ensure continuity of care. DH's progress toward goal attainment was monitored during my weekly visits. The use of goal planning statements is not necessary; however, a well-conceived nursing care plan is essential for the recovery of any patient's health.

At DH's final visit in the rehabilitation program, goal attainment was evaluated (Figure 28–2). An asterisk indicates levels achieved. DH achieved his goal of no smoking and increasing strength and endurance to the most favorable level. He achieved less-than-expected levels for the problem areas of weight and fears. He did not lose any weight, but he did not gain any either. By the end of the 6 weeks, DH was taking the Ativan for sleep approximately five times per week.

DH's goal attainment score was 65.40; he achieved a greather than expected level of goal attainment. Figure 28–3 shows how the goal attainment score was computed.

$$\text{GOAL ATTAINMENT SCORE} = \quad 50 + \frac{10 \, \text{E} \, w_i \, X_i}{\sqrt{.7w_i + .3(\text{E}w_i)^2}}$$

Where X = raw score or outcome level
Where E = sum
Where W = weight of the scale

Case Study Example with 4 Goals: (See figure II)

$$50 + \frac{10[3(+2) + 4(2) + 2(-1) + 1(-1)]}{\sqrt{.7(3)^2 + (4)^2 + (2)^2 + (1)^2 + .3(3 + 4 + 2 + 1)^2}}$$

$$50 + \frac{10[6 + 8 - 2 - 1]}{\sqrt{.7[9 + 16 + 4 + 1] + .3(10)^2}}$$

$$50 + \frac{10[11]}{\sqrt{.7[30] + 30}}$$

FIGURE 28–3. Computing the Goal Attainment Score for the Case Study

$$50 + \frac{110}{\sqrt{21 + 30}}$$

$$50 + \frac{110}{\sqrt{51}}$$

$$50 + \frac{110}{7.14}$$

$$50 + \quad 15.5$$

Goal Attainment Score = 65.40

SUMMARY

Mutual Goal Setting as an intervention concept has emerged from changes in the traditional nurse-patient relationship whereby the patient is viewed more as a consumer of health care rather than a passive recipient of it. As consumers, patients have specific rights; one of which is to be an active participant in the decision-making processes that affect their health and well-being. Research evidence has shown that patient involvement in setting goals for their health and/or recovery results in more effective goal achievement and greater patient satisfaction with health care. This chapter presents a tool that can be used to facilitate mutual goal setting between the nurse and the patient.

REFERENCES

Alexy, B. 1985. Goal setting and health risk reduction. *Nursing Research* 34:283–288.

American Nurses' Association. 1984. *Standards of nursing practice.* Kansas City, Mo.: American Nurses' Association.

Brill, N., Koegler, R., Epstein, L., and Forgy, E. 1964. Controlled study of psychiatric outpatient treatment. *Archives of General Psychiatry* 10:581–595.

Brykcznski, K. 1982. Health contracting. *Nurse Practitioner* 7(5):27–31.

Carter, S., and Mowad, L. 1988. Is nursing ready for consumerism? *Nursing Administration Quarterly* 12(3):74–78.

Eck, S., Meehan, R., Zigmund, D., and Pierro, L. 1988. Consumerism, nursing, and the reality of the resources. *Nursing Administration Quarterly* 12(3):1–11.

Fine, R. 1988. Consumerism and information: Power and confusion. *Nursing Administration Quarterly* 12(3):66–73.

Francis, V., Korsch, B., and Morris, M. 1969. Gaps in doctor-patient communication: Patients' responses to medical advice. *New England Journal of Medicine* 280:535–540.

French, J., Kay, E., and Meyer, H. 1966. Participation and the appraisal system. *Human Relations* 19:3–19.

Galano, J. 1977. Treatment effectiveness as a function of client involvement in goal setting and goal planning. *Goal Attainment Review* 3:1–16.

Garwick, G. 1974a. *An introduction to reliability and the Goal Attainment Scaling Methodology* (pamphlet). Minneapolis: Program Evaluation Project Report.

Garwick, G. 1974b. *A construct validity overview of Goal Attainment Scaling* (pamphlet). Minneapolis: Program Evaluation Project Report.

Garwick, G. 1976. The Rudiments of Goal Attainment Scaling. In J. Brintall and G. Garwick (eds.), *Applications of Goal Attainment Scaling.* Minneapolis: Program Evaluation Resource Center.

Hefferin, E. 1979. Health goal setting: Patient-nurse collaboration at VA facilities. *Military Medicine* 12:814–822.

Horsley, J. 1982a. *Mutual goal setting in patient care: CURN project.* New York: Grune & Stratton.

Horsley, J. 1982b. *Using research to improve nursing practice: A guide.* New York: Grune & Stratton.

Houts, P., and Scott, R. 1975–1976. Goal planning in mental health rehabilitation: An evaluation of the effectiveness of achievement motivation training for mental patients being rehabilitated to the community. *Goal Attainment Review* 2:33–51.

Jones, S., and Garwick, G. 1973. Guide to quality study: Goal Attainment Scaling as therapy adjunct? *Program Evaluation Project Newsletter* 4(6):1–3.

King, I. 1981. *A theory for nursing.* New York: John Wiley & Sons.

Kiresuk, T., and Sherman, R. 1968. Goal Attainment Scaling: A general method of evaluating comprehensive community health programs. *Community Mental Health Journal* 4(6):443–453.

Kovner, C. 1989. Nurse-patient agreement and outcomes after surgery. *Western Journal of Nursing Research* 11(1):7–19.

LaFerriere, L., and Calsyn, R. 1978. Goal Attainment Scaling: An effective treatment technique in short-term therapy. *American Journal of Community Psychology* 6(3):271–282.

Latham, G., and Yukl, G. 1975a. Assigned versus participative goal setting with educated and uneducated wood workers. *Journal of Applied Psychology* 60(3):299–302.

Latham, G., and Yukl, G. 1975b. A review of research on the applications of goal setting in organizations. *Academy of Management Journal* 18:824–845.

Lazare, A., Eisenthal, S., and Wasserman, L. 1975. The customer approach to patienthood. *Archives of General Psychiatry* 32:553–558.

Ledray, L. 1982. Counseling victims of rape: Their needs and a new treatment approach. In H. J. Schneider (ed.), *The victim in international perspective—Third international symposium on victimology* (pp. 358–374). New York: Walter de Gruyter.

Lemke, R. 1987. Identifying consumer satisfaction through patient surveys. *Health Progress,* 56–58.

Leonard, R., and Skipper, J. 1965. *Social interaction and patient care.* Philadephia: J. B. Lippincott.

Likert, R. 1961. *New patterns of management.* New York: McGraw-Hill.

Locke, E. 1968. Toward a theory of task motivation and incentives. *Organizational Behavior and Human Performance* 3:157–189.

Loomis, M. 1985. Levels of contracting. *Journal of Psychosocial Nursing* 23(3):9–14.

McClelland, D., and Winter, D. 1969. *Motivating economic achievement.* New York: Free Press.

Maier, N. 1955. *Psychology in industry.* New York: Houghton.

Orem, D. 1980. *Nursing concepts of practice* (2nd ed.). New York: McGraw-Hill.

Orlando, I. 1972. *The discipline and teaching of nursing process.* New York: Putnam Publishing.

Reeder, L. 1972. The patient-client as a consumer: Some observations on the changing professional-client relationship. *Journal of Health and Social Behavior* 13(4):406 – 412.

Roberts, C. 1982. Identifying the real patient problems. *Nursing Clinics of North America* 17(3):481 – 489.

Rogers, M. 1970. *An introduction to the theoretical basis of nursing.* Philadelphia: F.A. Davis.

Sheglah, S. 1985, October. Teach yourself goal setting. *Nursing Times,* 24 – 25.

Sherman, R., Baxter, J., and Audette, D. 1974. *Analysis of the original reliability study of GAS* (pamphlet). Program Evaluation Project Report.

Smith, D. 1976. Goal Attainment Scaling as an adjunct to counseling. *Journal of Counseling Psychology* 23(1):22 – 27.

Starfield, B., Wray, C., Hess, K., Gross, R., Birk, P., and D'Lugoff, B. 1981. The influence of patient-practitioner agreement on outcomes of care. *American Journal of Public Health* 71(2):127 – 131.

Steckel, S., and Swain, M. 1977. Contracting with patients to improve compliance. *Hospitals* 51:81 – 83.

Thompson, A., and Zimmerman, R. 1969. Goals of counseling: Whose? When? *Journal of Counseling Psychology* 16:121 – 125.

Viteles, M. 1953. *Motivation and morale in industry.* New York: Norton.

Vroom, V. 1964. *Work and motivation.* New York: John Wiley & Sons.

Willer, B., and Miller, G. 1976. Client involvement in goal setting and its relationship to therapeutic outcome. *Journal of Clinical Psychology* 32(3):687 – 690.

Winslow, G. 1984. From loyalty to advocacy: A new metaphor. *Hastings Center Report* 14(3):32 – 40.

Zangari, M., and Duffy, P. 1980. Contracting with patients in day-to-day practice. *American Journal of Nursing* 80(3):451 – 455.

29

TERMINAL CARE

GAIL ARDERY

There is no reason to believe that death severs the quality of oneness in the universe. If we participate in this universal quality before our death, our survival after death is demanded. The oneness principle endures, and we with it.

L. Dossey

Care for persons who are dying and for their family members is rooted in a holistic approach to nursing. Assessments and interventions take into account the whole person: an individual's physical, psychological, social, emotional, and spiritual needs. Terminal Care focuses on the whole family as the unit of care: anyone who is important to an individual who is dying is also important to professionals providing Terminal Care. Terminal Care emphasizes living throughout the whole of one's life, even through the dying process. Finally, nurses and the families they assist can come to view themselves as parts of a larger universal whole — parts of an encompassing circle in which healing can occur.

Terminal Care extends so broadly that practitioners from various academic backgrounds are typically brought together by hospices in order to meet the varied needs of clients and families more completely. Although nurses themselves may not implement every facet of Terminal Care, they can intervene in many areas, even when other team members are involved. Therefore, understanding the many threads that are woven into a Terminal Care program will increase the degree to which a nurse can participate in holistic care.

COMPONENTS OF TERMINAL CARE

Terminal Care has been described in terms of a variety of different components. Petrosino (1986) has described six relatively concrete categories of activities undertaken by hospice nurses:

1. Individualization of care includes developing a detailed care plan that considers the family's values, characteristics, and environment.
2. Having nurses available around the clock gives families a greater sense of security.
3. Teaching families how to function in the illness situation increases their sense of control.
4. Preparing families for anticipated changes in the illness also enhances their self-control and self-esteem.
5. Symptom control through diverse activities such as relaxation, massage,

366

music, reminiscence, medication management, and positioning remains a central focus of hospice care.

6.   Getting involved with families quickly and interacting with other health care professionals make it possible to provide more comprehensive care.

This description of Terminal Care focuses on nursing roles and functions and neglects the more supportive types of activities typically included in a comprehensive approach to terminal care.

Hall and Kirschling (1990) have described eight basic goals in their conceptual framework for hospice care. Nurses foster (1) Adaptation through individualizing the environment and monitoring the flow of visitors. Families can increase their sense of (2) Integration through family counseling. Nurses can help families with (3) Processing Information and (4) Decision Making. By modeling and teaching (5) Communication techniques, nurses help family members to attain congruence among their thoughts, feelings, words, and nonverbal behaviors. Finally, counseling can assist families in (6) Coalition Formation, (7) Conflict Management, and developing a sense of (8) Commitment. This conceptualization of Terminal Care describes in detail many of the family interaction issues that arise but excludes physical, psychological, and spiritual issues.

Palliative care staff nurses participating in an exploratory study (Heslin 1989) identified numerous components of terminal care. Family care activities include facilitating expression of emotions, enabling conflict resolution, and teaching communication strategies. Personhood activities focus on promoting comfort measures, activity and rest, and nutrition but also include reaffirming one's personhood through life review and life preview. Symptom control entails implementation of a comprehensive regimen to relieve the varied discomforts resulting from an individual's illness. Life closure activities enable dying persons to recognize their own legacies and to find ways to say good-bye. Supporting an individual's spiritual belief system and providing bereavement follow-up are also important life closure activities. Heslin's description captures the breadth of activities implicit in a holistic approach to Terminal Care.

Davies and Oberle (1990), utilizing case study methodology, identified six interwoven but discrete dimensions of palliative care. First, valuing entails respecting other persons, both generally and because of their unique qualities. Connecting, the second dimension, is accomplished by getting to know the client and family in detail, being available, spending time, and giving of self. Third, empowering activities encompass five types of nursing behaviors: facilitating behaviors such as making suggestions, helping to plan strategies, and recognizing limitations; encouraging behaviors, specifically supporting client choices; defusing behaviors, which give persons permission to express negative feelings; mending behaviors, which enable individuals to see others' viewpoints; and giving information. The fourth dimension encompasses doing: for activities, which include controlling symptoms, making arrangements, negotiating the system on behalf of family, and sharing and consulting with other team members. Fifth, finding meaning entails helping clients to focus on living, retain hope, reflect on their own lives, and meet their spiritual needs while still acknowledging that death is approaching. Finally, preserving one's own integrity — valuing one's self and acknowledging one's own feelings — is critical if the nurse is to retain feelings of self-worth and self-esteem.

This conceptualization describes not only how the nurse helps family members to interact with one another but also how the nurse relates to family members and participates in self-care activities. By focusing on the interactions and exchanges that occur in nurse-family relationships, Davies and Oberle capture the reciprocal nature of Terminal Care: nurses foster family healing, and working with families, in turn, fosters healing in nurses. Holism attains a new meaning in such a circle of healing.

IMPLEMENTATION OF TERMINAL CARE

The holistic nature of Terminal Care is best characterized in terms of abstract dimensions of care as described above. However, the specific actions that nurses undertake in implementing Terminal Care can be described in much greater detail as they apply to particular nursing diagnoses. Although clients and families receiving Terminal Care potentially can have problems related to any of the diagnoses currently studied by the North American Nursing Diagnoses Association (Kim, McFarland, and Lane 1989), several of these diagnoses tend to occur with particular frequency.

Fatigue

Fatigue affects up to 75% of persons with terminal cancer. Weakness may be related to anemia, dehydration, pain and fever, infections, prolonged bed rest, psychotropic drugs, diuretics, oral hypoglycemic agents, and antihypertensives. A negative energy balance may result from reduced food intake. Muscle abnormalities may occur as a result of secreted substances. Finally, an increased rate of protein and fat breakdown to meet extra glucose demands can lead to muscle weakness and wasting (Bruera and MacDonald 1988; Lichter 1990).

Megestrol acetate (160 mg/day) can increase appetite and lead to gains in weight and strength in persons with advanced breast cancer, cancer of the prostate, and nonhormone-dependent tumors. Forty percent of persons with malignancies can benefit from corticosteroids such as methylprednisolone, which increase appetite, elevate mood, and decrease fever, sweating, and pain. The effect of steroids on weakness, however, is very short-lived (Bruera and MacDonald 1988). It is important, therefore, for nurses to teach clients how to pace their activities and how to set attainable goals.

Altered Nutrition: Less Than Body Requirements

The most common nutritional problems encountered in caring for persons with advanced disease result from increasing anorexia. Anorexia may be caused by medications, gastric stasis, extrinsic pressure on the stomach or bowel, discomfort, depression or anxiety, immobility, respiratory exhaustion, oral infections, or constipation. Malabsorption and nutritional losses due to vomiting and fistula formation can also contribute to malnutrition in persons with advanced malignancies. Finally, alterations in metabolism that result from "toxohormones" such as cachectin can result in profound weight loss. Undernourishment has widespread consequences for dying persons, leading to decreased mobility and independence, increased risk of infection and pressure sores, impaired wound healing, and mental and emotional changes (Taylor, Morgan, and Jackson 1989).

Administration of haloperidol, prochlorperazine, or metoclopramide can decrease nausea and vomiting due to morphine administration. Metoclopramide also is effective for decreasing the gastric stasis that can result from morphine. Extrinsic pressure on the stomach can be treated effectively by giving metoclopramide before meals, while haloperidol, chlorpromazine, and methotrimeprazine given by suppository or continuous infusion can decrease symptoms resulting from intestinal obstruction (Baines 1988). Administering corticosteroids can have a short-term positive effect on appetite (Taylor, Moran, and Jackson 1989).

Client diets can be fortified by adding eggs, grated cheese, cream, powdered milk, or powdered supplements to mashed potatoes, soups, sauces, or puddings. To stimulate poor appetites, 30 mL to 60mL of a complete, suitably flavored liquid supplement can be administered on an hourly basis when the client is awake. Alternatively, 1 L of supplemental nourishment can be administered via continuous nasogastric infusion overnight. Providing excess calories may lead to gains only in fat and water, however (Taylor, Moran, and Jackson 1989).

The environment around eating can be made more pleasing by having the client eat outside the bedroom if possible or by removing sickroom equipment. Serving small, appealing meals frequently will help clients from feeling overwhelmed by the task of eating. It is usually not possible for clients to eat a balanced diet, so setting attainable goals will decrease anxiety around eating times. Making the meal a social occasion also can make eating more appealing to some clients.

One of the most difficult decisions families face is whether to withold tube feedings. Nurses can facilitate family decision making by assessing whether, for a given client, lack of nutrition is likely to exacerbate other symptoms, such as skin breakdown, oral lesions, diarrhea, and vomiting (Taylor, Moran, and Jackson 1989).

Pain

Pain is experienced by 65% to 100% of persons having advanced cancer (Twycross 1984; Bonica 1984; Coyle, Adelhardt, Foley, and Portenoy 1990). Many clients exhibit a rapid increase in their analgesia requirements within the last week of life, and especially in the last 24 hours of life (Coyle et al. 1990). Pain and the therapies used to treat it can be significant factors contributing to other common symptoms experienced by persons with cancer: anorexia, weight loss, weakness, nausea, pressure sores, constipation, drowsiness, and insomnia (Levy 1988).

Levy (1988) has classified treatments directed at decreasing pain in the terminally ill into three major categories. First are measures designed to alter the source of pain, such as palliative surgery, radiation therapy, hormonal therapy, and chemotherapy. In addition, nonsteroidal anti-inflammatory drugs, such as aspirin, ibuprofen, and indomethacin can help reduce pain associated with bony metastases. Steroids such as prednisone and dexamethasone can reduce pain resulting from compressed nerves or from increased intracranial pressure.

Second, pain can be controlled by interfering with its transmission via the central nervous system. Transcutaneous electrical nerve stimulation, acupuncture, and tricyclic antidepressants are believed to work because of this mechanism. Injection of anesthetics or nerve toxins and surgical ablation of peripheral sensory fibers or ascending pain fibers also prevent transmission of pain messages within the central nervous system. Celiac plexus block with alcohol, for example, can be effective up to 14 months in relieving pain from carcinoma of the pancreas, especially when performed early in the disease process (Lebovits and Lefkowitz 1989).

Epidural administration of morphine has been shown to be effective in relieving pain during the advanced stages of cancer, particularly when pain results primarily from bone tumors (Kiss and Simini 1989). Chronic cancer pain has been successfully managed by once- or twice-daily injections of morphine into the intrathecal space (Gonzalez-Navarro, Molinero-Aparicio, and Manzo 1989). Intrathecal administration has been found to require lower daily volumes, though with higher concentrations and more frequent dose increases when compared to epidural administration (Nitescu, Appelgren, Linder, Sjoberg, Hultman, and Curelaru 1990).

Third, alteration of central pain perception is the most commonly used form of pain management for persons with advanced cancer. Steroids, benzodiazepines, phenothiazenes, and antidepressants can alter the central perception of pain. Morphine, the most effective analgesic used to treat moderate to severe pain, may be administered via oral, sublingual, rectal, continuous subcutaneous infusion, and continuous intravenous infusion routes. Controlled-release morphine products can yield satisfactory pain control with dosing required only every 12 hours or every 8 hours (Ventafridda, Saita, Barletta, Sbanotto, and De Conno, 1989). Subcutaneous morphine infusions are particularly effective in low doses when initiated before clients develop tolerance to morphine (Drexel, Dzien, Spiegel, Lang, Breier, Abbrederis, Patsch, and Braunsteiner 1989). Hydromorphone can be administered subcutaneously and has the advantage of being six times as soluble as morphine, making it desirable for low-dose subcutaneous infusions (Storey, Hill, St. Louis, and Tarver 1990). A promising new treatment for pain management rests in transdermal administration of narcotics such as fentanyl citrate, a synthetic narcotic that is 75 times as potent as morphine and readily absorbed through the skin (Enck 1990). Client adherence to an opioid regimen will be enhanced if nurses prepare them for and help them to manage such side effects as somnolence, nausea, impaired cognitive functioning, and constipation (Bruera, Macmillan, Hanson, and MacDonald 1989).

Cancer pain can result in hopelessness, anger, depression, and loneliness (Martin and Soja, 1989; Massie and Holland 1987). Cognitive-behavioral approaches can help clients cope with acute exacerbations of pain and maintain their functional abilities in spite of chronic pain (Fishman and Loscalzo 1987).

Behavioral techniques are designed to teach persons a new set of skills. Self-monitoring enables clients to acknowledge objectively their own behaviors, thoughts, and feelings, thereby decreasing anxiety associated with pain. Passive relaxation, progressive muscle relaxation, meditation, music therapy, biofeedback, and hypnosis can be used to reduce muscle tension, autonomic hyperarousal, and mental confusion (see also Chapter 34). Finally, systematic desensitization can extinguish anticipatory anxiety, especially anxiety related to specific medical procedures.

Cognitive coping techniques include distraction, focusing, and cognitive modification. Specific distraction techniques utilize imaginative inattention, mental distraction, behavioral task distraction, hypnosis, and music therapy. Focusing is based on imaginative transformation of pain, imaginative transformation of context, and dissociated somatization. Cognitive modification entails identifying dysfunctional automatic thoughts and images, recognizing how these thoughts or images are associated with emotions and behaviors, substituting more functional thoughts or images for the dysfunctional ones, and altering dysfunctional underlying beliefs and attitudes (Driscoll 1987; Fishman and Loscalzo 1987).

Touch can convey the message that someone is sharing the pain experience and is available to help. Touch also reduces muscle tension through gentle massage and produces a pleasant stimulus to oppose the experience of pain (Sims 1988).

Many people cannot achieve freedom from pain, especially with activity. Clients can gain some reassurance if nurses honestly share the pain patterns they observe and help clients to set realistic goals for pain management (Coyle, Adelhardt, Foley, and Portenoy, 1990).

Altered Thought Processes: Delirium

Delirium may occur in up to 85% of persons in the final stages of a malignant disease (Martin and Soja 1989). Elderly persons are at particularly high risk. Delirium may result from hypercalcemia, hypoglycemia, hyponatremia, infection, hematological or vascular complications, nutritional changes, and drugs (Zimberg and Berenson, 1990).

Symptoms of delirium include alterations in the processing of perception, such as perceptual distortions, illusions, or hallucinations. Thinking may become disorganized and fragmented, impairing decision making, problem solving, and self-care activities. Impaired memory, alterations in immediate orientation, inattentiveness or hypervigilance, disturbances of the sleep-wake cycle, alterations in psychomotor behavior, and changes in emotional state can create distress for those experiencing delirium and for their families (Zimberg and Berenson 1990).

Alterations in medications may reverse drug-induced delirium. Delirium related to hypercalcemia may be improved with hydration and steroids. Other pharmacological agents such as Haldol may generally be helpful in decreasing disturbing symptoms (Martin and Soja 1989).

Clients with delirium may need assistance with self-care activities and management of their medical regimen. Giving information in clear, concise terms and reinforcing it during specific pertinent situations can improve client understanding. Making sure the client has a telephone, important telephone numbers, a clock and calendar, paper and pencil, refreshments and reading material within sight and reach can increase the amount of time clients can be left alone. Providing disoriented clients with environmental clues, particularly light, and limiting extraneous stimulation can increase orientation. Restraints should be used judiciously and released regularly, allowing freedom of movement as tolerated (Zimberg and Berenson 1990).

Persons with acquired immune deficiency syndrome (AIDS) may develop a dementia complex that initially is characterized by memory problems and concentration difficulties. Ultimately, the deficits extend to cognitive, motor, and behavioral systems. Although some cognitive improvements have been demonstrated with Zidovudine (AZT), supportive services eventually become essential for persons who are living independently. Nurses need to assess carefully the client's ability to self-medicate, and can use pillboxes, alarms, and checklists to promote timed drug dosing. Reminder devices such as telephone calls, appointment books, and lists can increase client consistency in keeping appointments and managing household tasks. Buddy volunteer, day care, residential living, and respite care programs increase the numbers of support persons in a client's network. Finally, nurses can enhance client functioning and socialization by simplifying communications and by modeling interactive techniques (McMahon and Coyne 1989).

Constipation

Constipation can be one of the most distressing symptoms dying persons experience. Constipation may be due to direct compression of tumor on the large intestine or on the nerves innervating the large intestine, particularly in persons with malignancies in the bowel or pelvic organs. In advanced disease, immobility and decreased oral intake contribute to the development of constipation. Almost all persons taking opioids develop constipation. Antidepressants, neuroleptics, and antihistamines can contribute further to the problem. Finally, metabolic disorders such as hypercalcemia, hypokalemia, and uremia can result in constipation (Portenoy 1987).

The first therapy to consider in preventing constipation is increasing fluid and fiber in an individual's diet. Three to four grams of fiber may be added daily and then gradually increased to 6 to 10 g per day as tolerated. Fiber should not be increased for those with a structural blockage of the bowel. Bulk-forming laxatives such as bran, psyllium, and methylcellulose also are contraindicated in persons with bowel obstruction or decreased fluid intake. Mineral oil, suppositories, and enemas are useful primarily in the treatment of acute fecal impaction. Osmotic cathartics such as the magnesium and sodium salts and lactulose can cause cramping, bloating, and severe diarrhea.

The contact cathartics, including the docusates, cascara, senna, and bisacodyl, are the primary agents used to manage chronic constipation. Senna has been reported anecdotally to be particularly favorable in managing opioid-related constipation (Portenoy 1987). Docusate and Senokot are usually recommended whenever narcotics are started (Martin and Soja 1989).

Impaired Skin Integrity

Persons who are dying are at extremely great risk for skin breakdown, whether due to pressure sores, venous congestion, or lymphedema. An individual's mobility is the best indicator of risk for development of pressure sores. Persons experiencing pain, weakness, sedation, contractures, depression, or altered levels of awareness may have impaired mobility. Compromised circulation related to peripheral vascular disease, dehydration, surgical procedures, smoking, and anemia can cause hypoxia to tissues compressed under bony prominences. A compromised nutritional status, and in particular limited fat stores, increases risk. Skin maceration related to incontinence, heavy perspiration, or draining wounds increases risk. Movement is the key to prevention and treatment of skin breakdown, irrespective of the etiology (Low 1990).

Where pressure is a problem, foam, fluid, or alternating air support mattresses should be introduced. Clients should be turned at least every 2 hours, alternating 30 degrees oblique left, right, and supine. Clients should be turned more frequently if erythema develops over bony prominences in less than 2 hours. Foam, gel, or water cushions can be placed on wheelchairs. Doughnuts increase ischemia and should be avoided. Shearing forces can be decreased by using a footboard and placing sheepskin under the buttocks if the head is elevated more than 30 degrees. Using a drawsheet to move the client up in bed also decreases stress on the skin. Sheepskin heel protectors decrease the risk of skin breakdown on heels and ankles (Low 1990).

Emollient lotion applied to dry skin or edematous areas can prevent cracking of the skin (Badger and Regnard 1989). Bony prominences can be gently massaged unless the skin remains red after pressure is removed. Clients should not use soaps, which are drying, on fragile skin. Applying a protective skin barrier to moist or intertriginous areas will decrease risk of maceration. Assisting clients with active or passive range of motion will enhance mobility (Low 1990).

Clients experiencing venous stasis should have their lower extremities elevated and exercised regularly. Support bandaging applied after legs have been elevated can decrease pooling of fluid in the legs. For clients who experience lymphedema, massaging tissues and directing the edema into areas where the lymphatics can take the extra load can be helpful.

It is important in caring for dying persons that nurses make balanced decisions, taking into account both the risk for or degree of skin breakdown and other problems such as pain and dyspnea. Wound care regimes should not be painful, disturbing, expensive, or time-consuming where there is little probability of successful healing. Keeping wounds covered, and thus moist, prevents tissue dehydration and scab formation and facilitates epidermal migration and healing. They allow patients to be disturbed less frequently, as they need to be changed as seldom as every 7 days. They also have been reported to decrease pain, probably by keeping nerve endings moist and by decreasing the production of prostaglandin E in the hypoxic wound environment. Cavities may be filled with various paste, granular, or foam products that appear to facilitate healing (Gilchrist and Corner 1989).

Kaposi's sarcoma lesions that arise in persons with AIDS require special wound care. Nondraining, noninfected, open lesions should be cleansed with saline and covered lightly or left open to air and light. Open, draining, infected lesions should be cleansed daily with potassium permanganate or a solution of betadine with peroxide, followed by a normal saline rinse. Strips of medicated gauze can be used to pack deep wounds. Using Kerlix to secure dressings will prevent tape contact with skin and decrease the risk of further skin breakdown (McMahon and Coyne 1989).

Altered Oral Mucous Membrane

Persons who are dying can experience alterations in mucous membranes as a result of dehydration, decreased saliva production, and infection. Diligent oral care with normal saline rinses will promote comfort and healing. Drying agents such as alcohol, peroxide, and betadine should be avoided. Gentle suction or swabbing may be necessary to remove thickened secretions. Applying vitamins A and D ointment to the lips prevents drying and cracking. Persons with oral and esophageal lesions can obtain pain relief by sucking on popsicles (Keithley and Kohn 1990).

Spiritual Distress

Spiritual Distress permeates the lives of many dying persons. According to Conrad (1985), the spiritual needs of dying persons include searching for meaning and trying to attain or maintain forgiveness, hope, and love. For terminally ill persons, a positive association has been found between having a spiritual perspective and having a sense of well-being (Reed 1987). Similarly, terminally ill persons have demonstrated an inverse association between an index of spiritual well-being and measures of state and trait anxiety (Kaczorowski 1989).

Some clients and families may experience loneliness and isolation in anticipation of a death. Asking questions about family, children, and friends can decrease this sense of isolation. Persons often enjoy life review — discussing major events from their younger years. Reminiscing and sharing thoughts gives a sense of connectedness and that one's life has been fruitful and meaningful (Jeffery 1985). (See also Chapter 23, Reminiscence Therapy.)

A substantial number of persons who are terminally ill acknowledge suicidal ideation at some point in their illness, with a subportion of these also requesting euthanasia. Fatigue, pain, and depression may be related to suicidal ideation (Coyle et al. 1990). Clearly, management of physical symptoms is a key factor in supporting the spiritual lives of clients.

Spiritual healing can be enhanced through several nursing activities. First, nurses affect clients by being truly present — by accepting persons as they are and by listening to what they are trying to communicate. (See also Chapter 14, Presence.) Nurses exhibit compassion when they dare to share another person's pain and suffering rather than avoiding it. They provide hope by helping persons to focus on specific problems and develop solutions that improve their quality of life. Nurses can help families to resolve issues and to take advantage of time with family and friends. By doing so, they give families a sense that life remains fruitful despite illness and death (O'Connor 1986).

Finally, assisting clients to incorporate rituals and sacraments, reading, music, imagery, and meditation into their daily lives can enhance their spiritual health (Conrad 1985). Boerstler (1985) suggests that caregivers use a technique of co-meditation in which the client and caregiver engage in a shared breathing pattern. This experience helps dying persons to let go of the past, to stop rehearsing the future, and to experience the present fully.

Grieving

Nurses can assist clients and family members through the grieving process and protect them from depersonalization by fostering an environment in which authenticity, emotional closeness, belonging, and self-representation flourish (Martocchio 1987). Authenticity is fostered by helping families to identify the reality of the illness, its effect on choices they already have made and on choices they face, and the personhood changes that have arisen in response to the illness. Helping families plan for the future and anticipate possible situations decreases their sense of the unknown. Confirming a person's reality on both a factual and a feeling level additionally fosters authenticity.

Emotional closeness is based on trust, not exclusiveness. Bonding arises when families share hard truths — joys as well as suffering.

Belonging is the sense that one feels comfortable with certain people. Belonging is fostered when persons open themselves to sharing a common situation.

Nurses promote self-representation when they give clients permission to express what they want in their living, their dying, and their futures. Helping individuals to identify their own agendas and to share their agenda with others gives an added dimension of meaning to life.

Finally, dying persons need respect as living beings with unique personalities and future goals. There is always a future for dying persons, whether it is minutes, days, or years. Clients continue living up to the moment of death (Martocchio 1987).

Bereavement follow-up with families after a death has occurred may be provided in several ways. A hospice social worker or bereavement counselor may provide individual counseling to family members. A volunteer who grew close to the family during the course of the illness may continue to keep in touch for many months. Some hospices provide bereavement volunteers who step in after a death has occurred to offer support to family members. Finally, family members may be referred to a bereavement support group that is available through the hospice or another community organization.

Bereavement support groups can provide family members with affirmation, validation, education, and normalization — with a sense that it is possible to survive and to heal. It is important that survivors be given permission to explore and express their emotions and to find ways to manage their feelings. Encouraging persons to try to change their feelings or their behavior invalidates their grief. In contrast, affirming their need to continue to feel their current feelings decreases their fears that their grief is abnormal and relieves them of the responsibility for feeling better immediately (Buell and Bevis 1989).

HEALING AND TERMINAL CARE

Healing is "a process of bringing parts of oneself . . . together at deep levels of inner knowing, leading to an integration and balance, with each part having equal importance and value" (Dossey 1989, p. 38). Much healing can occur during the period in which an individual is dying. Some persons are able to become whole through their dying, bringing their physical bodies, their minds, their emotions, their spirits, their relationships, and their choices into harmony with each another. Life becomes perceived as a bountiful adventure, filled with ups and downs and with happiness and sadness but always rooted in goodness and in hope. Death becomes perceived as either an accepted ending or an exciting transition. Moreover, dying persons perceive themselves not as isolated, suffering individuals but rather as part of a larger scheme in which others have also found meaning in life and in death.

Clients hold the potential for healing within themselves. Nurses can facilitate healing by teaching clients ways to explore the purpose and meaning in their lives. One of the techniques clients can use to activate their healing powers is centering — moving to a state of inner being. When an individual is centered, the body and internal dialogue are both quieted, and one feels calm, integrated, and focused. Centering can be achieved by practicing relaxation exercises, meditation, or a combination of the two for at least 15 minutes to 20 minutes daily. Through centering, persons gain a greater understanding of the complexities and contradictions of life. They become better able to reach out to others nonjudgmentally, to resolve conflicts more readily, and to love others more openly (Dossey 1989). These outcomes can give both persons who are dying and their loved ones a great sense of wholeness — of healing.

Nurses will be able to facilitate their clients' healing processes only if they themselves have experienced the process. Nurses who strive for wholeness in their own lives, who have themselves experienced the quietude of being centered, can reflect the power of their own healing to others. They will have confidence that change is possible, and they will be able to share that confidence nonjudgmentally with their clients. Being centered also enables nurses to be fully present with their clients (Dossey 1989). Presence, in turn, enables nurses to utilize their knowledge and skills to their best abilities and thereby help clients achieve more positive outcomes. Finally, self-exploration of the meaning of one's life will help nurses to maintain their own integrity in the face of continual loss through death (Davies and Oberle 1990). Inner strength, born from self-exploration and nurtured through self-care, makes it possible for dying to result in healing.

CASE STUDY

Nathan, age 50, has had cancer for five years. Numerous surgeries, radiation, and chemotherapy have failed to prevent recurrences of the disease. The cancer has spread to his spine, leaving his lower extremities functionless. He experiences severe pain and weakness on moving and has decided not to get out of bed anymore. He is at high risk of skin breakdown due to his immobility and size (weighing 200 pounds). Nathan's appetite has been consistently good, and his nutritional status appears to be adequate. Constipation is an ongoing concern due to immobility and pain management with oral morphine. Nathan has had to resign his position as a research scientist due to his increasing debilitation.

Nathan's primary caregiver is his wife, Janette, who is available in the home most of the time. Nathan and Janette have two children, aged 14 years and 20 years, both living at home. The family has been active in their church and report a strong religious faith that has assisted them through their struggles with Nathan's illness.

A nurse makes a regularly scheduled visit to the family weekly and is available for more frequent visits when Nathan's condition changes. Nathan's pain is brought under better control by a combined regimen of intravenous morphine (administered via a central indwelling catheter and a portable pump), an oral nonsteroidal anti-inflammatory agent, and a tricyclic antidepressant. His wife is given a recipe for bars containing dried fruits and senna, which Nathan enjoys eating and which resolves his problems with constipation. A foam mattress is initiated to decrease his risk of skin breakdown. Nathan's wife is instructed in how to turn him just enough to ease the pressure off his sacral area without increasing his discomfort. She is also taught how to massage his back and gently perform range of motion to his legs to prevent discomfort from contractures.

The family is visited twice monthly by a counselor who assesses their level of coping and gives them each an opportunity to talk about how Nathan's illness is affecting their lives. The counselor assists Nathan in both life review and life preview, enabling him to identify the richness in his past, the meaning in his present, and his hopes for the future. The counselor arranges for young volunteers to meet with each of the children weekly and provide them either with a safe environment for talking or with some time away from the illness situation. These volunteers plan to continue seeing the children after their father's death. A nurse volunteer helps Janette with Nathan's bed bath three times per week. This nurse, whose own husband died 3 years ago, plans to provide bereavement support to Janette after Nathan's death.

Nathan's pastor is closely involved in his care, visiting the family weekly. He encourages Nathan to discuss his grief surrounding his many losses: loss of physical functions, loss of work, and anticipated loss of family and life. By praying regularly with Nathan, he reinforces Nathan's drawing upon a spiritual resource in difficult times. Nathan's pastor also spends a great deal of time helping Nathan to plan his own funeral. Nathan has specific messages he wishes to convey to others after he dies. The pastor notes these requests and talks with Nathan about how the eulogy plans to be structured. Church volunteers provide respite to Janette for several hours per week so that she has opportunities to step back from her caregiving role.

As Nathan grows closer to death, his nurse visits more frequently, eventually every day. She shares with Nathan and with his family information about how his illness is progressing. At Nathan's request, she helps him to complete a living will, stating that he does not wish to have his life prolonged artificially. When Nathan's paralysis spreads to his arms, the nurse talks with his family about options for further radiation treatment, which the family eventually decides not to pursue. As Nathan becomes weaker and his appetite decreases, the nurse talks with Janette about not encouraging Nathan to eat more than he feels comfortable eating.

The day before Nathan dies, the nurse shares with the family her perceptions regarding the closeness of his death. The children say their good-byes that evening and decide that they will go to school as usual the next day. Early the next morning, the nurse makes a visit and finds that Nathan appears to be comfortable and Janette is coping well. Janette and the nurse volunteer give Nathan his bath as usual. Janette takes a few minutes to sit quietly at Nathan's bedside after the volunteer leaves. She is ready, and she knows Nathan is ready. She wishes him well on his journey, knowing confidently that she will not lose touch with his spirit.

SUMMARY

Dying persons develop a variety of common problems, including fatigue, altered nutrition, pain, altered thought processes, constipation, impaired skin integrity, and altered oral mucous membranes. Spiritual distress and grieving can challenge dying persons and their family members. Terminal Care is a holistic nursing intervention. Care is directed at meeting the physical, psychosocial, spiritual, and emotional needs of dying persons and the support needs of family members. Through the intervention of terminal care, nurses can help clients make the time of dying a time of healing, resulting in feelings of integrity and wholeness.

REFERENCES

Badger, C. and Regnard, C. 1989. Oedema in advanced disease. *Palliative Medicine* 3:213–215.
Baines, M. 1988. Nausea and vomiting in the patient with advanced cancer. *Journal of Pain and Symptom Management* 3(2):81–85.
Boerstler, R.W. 1985. *Letting go: A holistic and meditative approach to living and dying.* Yarmouth, Massachusetts: Associates in Thanatology.
Bonica, J.J. 1984. Management of cancer pain. *Recent Results Cancer Research* 89:13–27.
Bruera, E., and MacDonald, R.N. 1988. Asthenia in patients with advanced cancer. *Journal of Pain and Symptom Management* 3(1):9–14.
Bruera, E., Macmillan, K., Hanson, J., and MacDonald, R.N. 1989. The cognitive effects of the administration of narcotic analgesics in patients with cancer pain. *Pain* 39:13–16.
Buell, J.J., and Bevis, J. 1989. Bereavement groups in the hospice program. *Hospice Journal* 5(1):107–118.
Conrad, N.L. 1985. Spiritual support for the dying. *Nursing Clinics of North America* 20(2):415–425.
Coyle, N., Adelhardt, J., Foley, K.M., and Portenoy, R.K. 1990. Character of terminal illness in the advanced cancer patient: Pain and other symptoms during the last four weeks of life. *Journal of Pain and Symptom Management* 5(2):83–93.
Davies, B., and Oberle, K. 1990. Dimensions of the supportive role of the nurse in palliative care. *Oncology Nursing Forum* 17(1):87–94.
Dossey, B.M. 1989. The healer and the inward journey. In B.M. Dossey, L. Keegan, L.G. Kolkmeier, and C.E. Guzzetta (eds.), *Holistic health promotion: A guide for practice* (pp. 37–50). Rockville, Md.: Aspen Publishers.
Dossey, L. 1982. *Space, time, and medicine.* Boulder, Colo.: Shambhala Publications.
Drexel, H., Dzien, A., Spiegel, R.W., Lang, A.H., Breier, C., Abbrederis, K., Patsch, J.R., and Braunsteiner, H. 1989. Treatment of severe cancer pain by low-dose continuous subcutaneous morphine. *Pain* 36:169–176.
Driscoll, C.E. 1987. Pain management. *Primary Care* 14(2):337–352.
Enck, R.E., 1990. Transdermal narcotics for pain control. *American Journal of Hospice and Palliative Care* 7(4):15–17.
Fishman, B., and Loscalzo, M. 1987. Cognitive-behavioral interventions in management of cancer pain: Principles and applications. *Medical Clinics of North America* 71(2):271–287.
Gilchrist, B., and Corner, J. 1989. Pressure sores: Prevention and management—a nursing perspective. *Palliative Medicine* 3:257–261.
Gonzalez-Navarro, A., Molinero-Aparicio, T., and Manzo, L. 1989. Cancer pain and intrathecal morphine. *Palliative Medicine* 3:287–292.
Hall, J.E., and Kirschling, J.M. 1990. A conceptual framework for caring for families of hospice patients. *Hospice Journal* 6(2):1–28.
Heslin, K. 1989. The supportive role of the staff nurse in the hospital palliative care situation. *Journal of Palliative Care* 5(3):20–26.
Jeffery, S. 1985. Nursing care plan for the terminally ill and his family. *Perspectives* 9(2):9–12.
Kaczorowski, J.M. 1989. Spiritual well-being and anxiety in adults diagnosed with cancer. *Hospice Journal* 5(3–4):105–116.
Keithley, J.K., and Kohn, C.L. 1990. Managing nutritional problems in people with AIDS. *Oncology Nursing Forum* 17(1):23–27.

Kim, M.J., McFarland, G.K., and Lane, A.M. 1989. *Pocket guide to nursing diagnoses.* St. Louis: C.V. Mosby.

Kiss, I.E., and Simini, B. 1989. Effect of epidural morphine on various kinds of cancer pain. *Palliative Medicine* 3:217–221.

Lebovits, A.H., and Lefkowitz, M. 1989. Pain management of pancreatic carcinoma: A review. *Pain* 36:1–11.

Levy, M.H. 1988. Pain control research in the terminally ill. *Omega* 18(4):165–179.

Lichter, I. 1990. Weakness in terminal illness. *Palliative Medicine* 4:73–80.

Low, A.W. 1990. Prevention of pressure sores in patients with cancer. *Oncology Nursing Forum* 17(2):179–184.

McMahon, K.M., and Coyne, N. 1989. Symptom management in patients with AIDS. *Seminars in Oncology Nursing* 5(4):289–301.

Martin, E.W., and Soja, W.D. 1989. Symptom management in the home-based terminal cancer patient. *Rhode Island Medical Journal* 7(72):243–252.

Martocchio, B.C. 1987. Authenticity, belonging, emotional closeness, and self-representation. *Oncology Nursing Forum* 14(4):23–27.

Massie, M.J., and Holland, J.C. 1987. The cancer patient with pain: Psychiatric complications and their management. *Medical Clinics of North America* 71(2):243–258.

Nitescu, P., Appelgren, L., Linder, L., Sjoberg, M., Hultman, E., and Curelaru, I. 1990. Epidural versus intrathecal morphine-bupivacaine: Assessment of consecutive treatments in advanced cancer pain. *Journal of Pain and Symptom Management* 5(1):18–26.

O'Connor, P.M. 1986. Spiritual elements of hospice care. *Hospice Journal* 2(2):99–108.

Petrosino, B.M. 1986. Research challenges in hospice nursing. *Hospice Journal* 2(1):1–10.

Portenoy, R.K. 1987. Constipation in the cancer patient: Causes and management. *Medical Clinics of North America* 71(2):303–311.

Reed, P. 1987. Spirituality and well-being in terminally ill hospitalized adults. *Research in Nursing and Health* 10:335–344.

Sims, S. 1988. The significance of touch in palliative care. *Palliative Medicine* 2:58–61.

Storey, P., Hill, H.H., St. Louis, R.H., and Tarver, E.E. 1990. Subcutaneous infusions for control of cancer symptoms. *Journal of Pain and Symptom Management* 5(1):33–41.

Taylor, M.B., Moran, B.J., and Jackson, A.A. 1989. Nutritional problems and care of patients with far-advanced disease. *Palliative Medicine* 3:31–38.

Twycross, R.G. 1984. Incidence of pain. *Clinical Oncology* 3:5–15.

Ventafridda, V., Saita, L., Barletta, L., Sbanotto, A, and De Conno, F. 1989. Clinical observations on controlled-release morphine in cancer pain. *Journal of Pain and Symptom Management* 4(3):124–129.

Zimberg, M., and Berenson, S. 1990. Delirium in patients with cancer: Nursing assessment and intervention. *Oncology Nursing Forum* 17(4):529–538.

FAMILY THERAPY

WENDY L. WATSON

Family Therapy requires a way of thinking and seeing that emphasizes the interrelatedness of a problem, the individual, the family and the social context. A family therapist views "behaviors as interconnected, mutually recursive, and part of a larger ecologically coherent system. For example, although one person may appear to cause harm to another, or to be resistant, or dysfunctional, such linear attributions may simply be flawed notions, false dualisms, when viewed from a holistic, mutually interactive philosophical framework" (Piercy and Sprenkle 1990, p. 1117).

Family Therapy requires an approach to human problems that is exquisitely curious about context. The interpersonal context of a problem and the interplay between this context and symptoms are of primary interest to a family therapist. "Non-family therapists often view family therapy as, a) a modality, that, b) usually involves the nuclear family. Family therapy is not simply a 'modality.' Nor is it necessarily a set of modalities. More fundamentally, it is a way of construing human problems that dictates certain actions for their alleviation" (Stanton 1988, pp. 7–8).

DESCRIPTION

Family Therapy is more than working with families. It is a worldview that involves a conceptual shift from linear to systems (systemic) thinking. The cause and effect thinking associated with a linear worldview is exchanged for a systemic worldview that looks for connections and reciprocal influences among systems of ideas, people, and events.

Linear versus Systems

The differences between a linear perspective and a systems perspective in conceptualizing human problems and solutions are outlined in Table 30–1 (Watson 1988a). A linear perspective focuses on the individual, while a systems perspective focuses on relationships. A linear perspective is interested in the intentions behind people's actions; a systems perspective seeks for the effects of one person's behavior on another and the effects of the effects. The content of what people say is a prime focus for the linearly oriented; process is foreground for the systems thinker.

Particular events are significant for the nurse who takes a linear view, while the systems thinking nurse–family therapist is drawn to discover patterns in a series of events. The nurse with a linear perspective becomes a historian mindful of details,

TABLE 30–1. LINEAR PERSPECTIVE VERSUS SYSTEMS PERSPECTIVE

LINEAR	SYSTEMS
Individual	Relationships
Intentions	Effects
Content	Process
Events	Patterns
History	Present
Linear causality	Circular effect

dates and data. A systems perspective invites a nurse to connect details and data to produce meaningful information about the present. The past is seen to be useful in its ability to illuminate the present.

A linear-thinking nurse adopts the linear causality model, which is intent on discovering the cause of the problem. The model proposes that A causes B. A systems-thinking nurse–family therapist uses a circular effect model to understand problems and to generate solutions. Her question is not, "Who is to blame" but rather, "How is each involved?" The circular effect model proposes that A affects B and B affects A. Connections are made with behavior seen as affecting the other rather than one causing the other. A systems perspective of problems and solutions involves a quest for connections, relationships, key patterns of interaction, redundancy, and reciprocity.

Tomm (1980) developed the circular pattern diagram to demonstrate interactions in problematic relationships; it illustrates the interaction and interconnectedness of two individuals' behaviors, thoughts, and feelings. Because the diagram is a circle, it is possible to begin anywhere — with a behavior, a cognition, or an affect — and to commence with either person. Person A's behavior (behavioral output) is perceptual input for person B. Person B makes sense of person A's behavior and generates a thought/cognition about person A, about self, or about their relationship. This thought or cognition draws forth a particular feeling. The cognition and affect of person B then elicit her behavior, which is perceptual input for person A. Person A makes sense of person B's behavior. His cognition and affect are generated which subsequently invites his behavior and the cycle continues! (See Figure

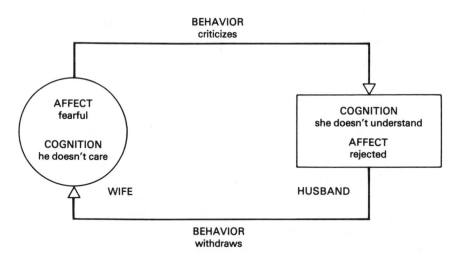

FIGURE 30–1. Circular Pattern Diagram

30–1 for an example of a vicious cycle.) Thus, a systems-thinking nurse–family therapist identifies the behaviors, thoughts, and feelings of family and systems members that co-evolve into vicious or virtuous cycles of communication.

Family Systems Approaches

There are variations within the systems approach to problems. Three systems approaches are strategic, structural and systemic. The strategic family therapist looks for ambiguous or inconsistent hierarchies within the family system, ferrets out power and control issues, and directs change by means of family assignments or paradoxical injunctions (Haley 1976; Madanes 1981). A structural family therapist assesses and intervenes into family structure, subsystems, and boundaries (Minuchin 1974). The structurally oriented family therapist has an ideal family structure in mind and therefore intervenes to realign boundaries so that the family is neither too enmeshed not too disengaged and supports the establishment of parental/executive coalition so that parents present a united front to their children.

The term *systemic* family therapy is frequently used to designate the work of the Milan Family Therapy team, whose approach has had a profound impact on the field (Selvini, Palazzoli, Boscolo, Cecchin, and Prata 1980; Boscolo, Cecchin, Hoffman, and Penn 1987). Throughout the 1980s, the family therapy field was energized and revolutionized by the Milan team's interviewing ideas. The three guidelines of hypothesizing, circularity, and neutrality/curiosity, create a useful context for a family interview to become therapeutic conversation. A therapeutic conversation enables family members to discover their own solutions to their problems.

Hypothesizing

Hypotheses are ideas about the possible connections between the system and the problem. Families have their own hypotheses about the problem. The families' ideas are usually linear in nature. To be useful to the family, the nurse–family therapist needs to generate hypotheses different from those of the family. Table 30–2 provides some questions a nurse can ask herself to generate hypotheses about the system and the problem.

Circularity

Circularity involves the cycle of questions and answers that is formed in the interview process. The nurse–family therapist's questions are based on information that the family gives in response to the questions the nurse asks, and thus the cycle continues. The family's reactions, responses, or answers to the questions provide information for the nurse and the family. It is important to note that the questions themselves may also provide new answers for the family. For example, the questions may invite family members to see their problems in a new way and subsequently to see new solutions. Thus, just as the family's answers provide information for the nurse, the nurse's questions may provide information for the family.

Circularity is operationalized by asking circular questions based on Bateson's (1979) idea that "information consists of differences that make a difference." Circular questions explore relationships or differences and are useful because they release new information into the family system. Circular questions invite family members to explore differences and make new connections between ideas, events, and behaviors.

Fleuridas, Nelson, and Rosenthal (1986) developed a taxonomy of circular

TABLE 30–2. QUESTIONS THAT INVITE HYPOTHESIZING ABOUT THE SYSTEM AND THE PROBLEM

Who
Who is in the system? Who are the key players?
Who first noticed the problem?
Who is concerned about the problem?
Who is affected by the problem? (most/least)
Who is interested in keeping things the same? (most/least)
Who referred the system?

What
What is the problem at this time?
What is the meaning that the problem has for the system/for different members of the system?
What solutions have been attempted?
What question(s) do I feel constrained to ask?
What positive function might the symptom serve in the system?
To what question could this symptom or problem be an answer?
What beliefs perpetuate the problem?
What beliefs are perpetuated by the problem?
What problems perpetuate the beliefs?
What problems are perpetuated by the beliefs?

Why
Why is the system presenting at this time?
Why this problem for this system?

Where
Where has the information about this problem come from?
Where does the system see the problem originating?
Where does the system see the problem and the system going if there is no change/if there is change?

When
When did the problem begin?
When did the problem occur in relation to another phenomenon of the system?
When does the problem occur?
When does the problem not occur?

How
How might a change in the problem affect other parts of the system (key players, relationships, beliefs)?
How does a change in one part of the system affect another part of the system? the problem?
How does the symptom maintain the system?
How does the system maintain the symptom?
How will I know when my work with this system is over?
How might my work with this system constrain the system from finding their solution?

questions to assist beginning family therapists. Loos and Bell (1990) applied circular questions to critical care nursing. Watson (1988a, 1988b, 1988c, 1989a, 1989b) demonstrated the therapeutic nature of circular questions with families coping with chronic illness, life-threatening illness, and psychosocial problems.

Four basic types of questions are described in Table 30-3. These were distinguished by Tomm (1988) when considering the intent of the therapist in asking a question as well as the assumptions (held by the therapist) about the nature of mental phenomena and the therapeutic process. Tomm determined that if a family therapist asked a question to orient herself (that is, to change her own perceptions) and viewed problems from a lineal/cause-effect perspective, she would ask lineal questions, such as problem-definition and problem-explanation questions. Lineal questions are predominantly investigative. If the same family therapist asked a question with the main intent to influence the family—that is, to "trigger a response that might alter the family's perceptions and understanding" (Tomm 1988, p. 5)—but maintained her lineal/cause-effect perspective, she would ask strategic

TABLE 30–3. FOUR TYPES OF QUESTIONS

Lineal (investigative)
Problem definition question: "What is the problem you would like to discuss today?"
Problem explanation question: "How do you explain his behavior?"

Strategic (corrective)
Confrontation question: "When you saw your son's tears and said nothing to him, did you realize you were making things worse?"
Leading question: "Is your habit of not answering questions something new?"

Circular (exploratory)
Difference question: "Are you more concerned or less concerned since your husband was hospitalized?"
Behavioral effect question: "How has your husband responded to your compliments?"

Reflexive (facilitative)
Observer perspective question: "When your sister gets angry what does your mother do?"
Hypothetical/future-oriented question: "If your relationship with your father were to improve by 10%, what do you think would be happening in the family 2 years from now?"

Source: Tomm (1988).

questions such as confrontation and leading questions. Strategic questions are corrective in intent.

If the intent were to orient herself but the family therapist operated from circular assumptions, she would ask circular questions, including difference and behavioral effect questions. Tomm (1988) notes that circular questions are exploratory and seek to "bring forth the patterns that connect persons, objects, actions, perceptions, ideas, feelings, events, beliefs, contexts and so on in recurrent or cybernetic circuits" (p. 7). Finally, if the primary intent of the therapist were to influence the family and a circular/cybernetic perspective were maintained, she would ask reflexive questions, including observer-perspective and hypothetical–future oriented questions. Reflexive questions are facilitating when offered with the intent of "triggering reflexive activity on the family's pre-existing belief systems" (p. 9), thus opening space for new solutions and options for the family.

Two other family therapists who have influenced the use and style of asking questions in a therapeutic conversation with a family are Michael White of Australia and Lorraine Wright, a nurse–family therapist in Canada. White's (1988–89) relative influence questions are a significant part of his approach to drawing a distinction between person and the problem. Through the use of questions such as, "What percentage of the time are you able to influence your anger?" and "What percentage of the time does your anger influence you?" the family therapist is able to objectify the problem instead of objectifying the person.

Wright (1989) offers a different approach to therapeutic questioning, suggesting that family therapists consider the usefulness of inviting family members to ask questions of the therapist. Her "one-question" question has proved to provide particularly potent information for the family and the therapist. Specifically, Wright asks families, "if you could have only one question answered in our work together, what question would that be?" Family members' responses assist in focusing the therapy process, give voice to previously unspoken or undetected fears, and provide the family with much to think about. The frequency with which families note the impact of the one-question question on their thinking is exciting. Wright also gives examples of other questions that can be asked to invite questions from families. She emphasizes that we can ask only what we know to ask; therefore, it is important to offer families an opportunity to ask questions.

Neutrality

Neutrality is present when the family perceives the nurse to be equally interested in and curious about each member's point of view. Neutrality also involves a therapeutic posture of being nonjudgmental, nonblaming, and noninvested in any particular solution or outcome that the family may choose.

Curiosity is the key to neutrality. There is a circular process that unfolds between curiosity and hypothesizing. The more curious a nurse is, the more hypotheses she generates. The more hypotheses she generates, the more curious she becomes to explore the hypotheses. Thus, a virtuous cycle of therapeutic curiosity and hypothesis generation evolves. Neutrality can be evidenced by asking questions of all family members. Neutrality helps the nurse maintain a therapeutic maneuverability with the family. When neutrality is present, the family does not see the nurse as being on only one person's side. Rather, the nurse is seen to be an advocate for all family members and for their relationships. In this way, the nurse maintains her meta-perspective and her ability to assist the family. A therapeutic conversation unfolds as the family experiences the family therapist's being neutral to persons, problems, pace, and direction of change and solutions.

RESEARCH

As Piercy and Sprenkle (1990) indicate, "a reasonable amount of evidence has been amassed to support the general efficacy of family therapy" (p. 1119). Their decade review of the field supports the following conclusion of Gurman, Kniskern, and Pinsof (1986):

> 1. Nonbehavioral marital and family therapies produce beneficial outcomes in about two-thirds of cases, and their effects are superior to no treatment.
> 2. When both spouses are involved in therapy conjointly for marital problems, there is a greater chance of positive outcome than when only one spouse is treated.
> 3. Positive results of both nonbehavioral and behavioral marital and family therapies typically occur in treatment of short duration; that is, from 1 to 20 sessions.
> 4. Family therapy is probably as effective and possibly more effective than any commonly offered individual treatments for problems attributed to family conflict. (p. 572)

Family therapy researchers have begun to address specificity issues: what approach to use with what problem under what circumstances. These issues will form the basis of family therapy inquiry in the future.

GUIDELINES FOR FAMILY THERAPY

Families that may benefit from Family Therapy are those that are experiencing difficulties with health problems: chronic illness (e.g., Alzheimer's disease, multiple sclerosis), life-threatening illness (e.g., cancer, cardiac conditions), or psychosocial problems (e.g., obesity, depression, temper tantrums). The family member with the difficulty may be either a child or an adult.

Family Therapy is a paradigm that does not specify any particular way of work-

TABLE 30-4. BELIEFS OF NURSE-FAMILY THERAPIST

- A part is best understood in the context of the whole. Depression is best understood in the context of a person's relationships. Noncompliance is best understood in the context of the relationship between the patient and the nurse.
- A change in one part of the system affects other parts of the system. A woman's stroke affects her daughter's concentration at work and her husband's commitment to his work.
- The whole is more than the sum of the parts. The relevant system is more than an accounting and description of its entities. With families, the family is more than an accounting and description of the members of the family. The family includes relationships, alliances, and coalitions.
- The family is able to create a balance between change and stability (Wright and Leahey 1984).
- The same results may spring from different causes.
- Disparate results may be produced by the same causes.
- Families/systems and their problems make sense and have strengths.
- Families' beliefs organize their behaviors (Wright, Watson, and Bell 1990).
- The family/system has the ability to solve its own problems.
- The family therapist is a participant in rather than a director of change.
- Things are not always the way they appear to be.
- Each member of a family/system has a unique and valid perspective.
- There are times when the system creates the problem and times when the problem creates the system.
- A family/system cannot be controlled or programmed from outside "but you can . . . perturb it and see how it compensates. Give it a bump and watch it jump" (Hoffmann 1985, p. 388).
- There is an interactional phenomenon occurring between the family/system and the problem. The family is affected by "the problem" and in turn influences the problem.
- The family therapist can be most useful to the family by inviting the family to consider an alternate view of the problem situation so that their solution-seeking and solution-finding ability is enhanced or otherwise opened up.
- The family therapist affects the system and also is affected by the system.

ing but contributes a set of guidelines for how methods used are put into practice. Thus, it tends to have the following characteristics:

1. An "observing system" stance and inclusion of the therapist's own context
2. A collaborative rather than a hierarchical structure
3. Goals that emphasize setting a context for change, not specifying a change
4. A circular assessment of the problem
5. A non pejorative, nonjudgmental view (Hoffman 1985, p. 393).

Still, the question persists, "How does a nurse 'do' family therapy?" To understand what prompts a nurse to do what she does in a family therapy interview, it is important to discuss what a nurse believes when she operates from a systemic orientation. Beliefs of a nurse—family therapist are outlined in Table 30-4.

Having considered some beliefs that invite a family systems perspective, the question can now be asked, "What does a nurse–family therapist *do* in her interactions with a family/system that requests help with a problem?"

Several family therapist clinicians and scholars have identified family therapy skills necessary for therapists to possess (Tomm and Wright 1979; Wright and Leahey 1984). The following is a list of some of the executive skills enacted by systems-oriented nurse–family therapists at the Family Nursing Unit, University of Calgary, Calgary, Alberta, Canada.

Executive Skills of Nurse–Family Therapists

A systemically oriented nurse–family therapist:

- Reviews literature relevant to the family problem presented.
- Hypothesizes about the connection between the family and the problem.
- Engages all family members.

- Takes as information about the system/problem those members who attend or do not attend therapy.
- Asks each family member, "What is the problem that is concerning you the most at this time?"
- Completes a genogram, not for the purpose of only finding out who is in the family but rather to discover the context of the problem and who is important to whom.
- Asks each family member to share his or her knowledge and understanding of the presenting problem or illness.
- Asks each family member what he or she believes or understands is the reason that a family member has a specific illness or problem.
- Seeks specifics about the problem by asking questions such as, "How does she show that she is angry?"
- Raises the problem to an interactional level by asking, "How is her anger a problem for you?"
- Explores attempted solutions.
- Identifies a vicious cycle of interaction that may be maintaining or maintained by the problem.
- Continually is open to new information.
- Listens and builds on what is said in the therapeutic conversation with an appreciation that she is being influenced by what the family says just as they are being influenced by what she says.
- Demonstrates neutrality to each person and his or her ideas by keeping curious.
- Asks questions in a manner that will introduce the family to a systemic view of itself by providing new information about their concerns, beliefs, behaviors, and relationships.
- Looks for the opportunity to commend. Commendations can gently nudge the system to draw forth more strengths.
- Refocuses and restates questions.
- Challenges constraining beliefs by asking, "If you were to believe [offer alternate facilitative belief], what would be different? What would you do differently?" "If you believed in what he was doing in an effort to [insert jeopardy question—for example, draw the family closer together], what would be different?" A jeopardy question might be, "To what possible benevolent-altruistic-system-sensitive question, is the symptom an answer?" (for example, "How can I draw our family closer together?").
- Draws forth and reinforces facilitative beliefs.
- Explores related cognition when affect is shown. Avoids the assumption trap of "I know how you feel" and shows respect for the unique experience of an individual by asking, "What are you thinking that is making you cry?"
- Prescribes a behavioral task as a way of introducing new information about the problem or about family members' reactions to the problem. New information may change the existing beliefs and perceptions the family holds about the illness and also their perceptions of other family members' behaviors, and motives. Thus a "new family reality" may emerge.
- Follows up on assignments by asking, What did the family learn by doing the assignment? What stood out or surprised them? How did they attempt to do it? She considers the doing or not doing of an assignment, with or without variations on the theme or what was initially suggested, more information about the family. This information is contrasted and compared with the previous assessment of the family.

- Systemically reframes a situation by positively connoting the connectedness between the system and other behaviors in the family. A positive connotation answers the questions, What positive function might the symptom serve in this family at this time? What positive, protective, or stabilizing effects could the problem's continuation have for members of the organized network? What new difficulties may emerge if the problem disappears?

- Listens for the family's metaphoric language. A metaphor is a statement about one thing that resembles something else. It is the analogous relationship of one thing to another. A family's metaphors add to our understanding of how a family experiences and views the world. The metaphors also communicate how they see their problems and themselves in relation to their problems.

- Offers a split-opinion that presents two or more opinions, views, or ideas about a situation. A split opinion serves to challenge the fixed beliefs of a family or an individual. Split opinions are useful when significant and rapid change has occurred and there is a need to maintain change, there is a difficulty resolving implicit conflictual issues, individuals hold rigidly fixed beliefs and there is a need to introduce complexity of thinking, or a symmetrical relationship is present (that is, a competition between equals is present, and there is a need to maintain engagement with both parties and show neutrality). A split opinion validates each party's divergent view and at the same time opens a possibility for considering an alternate view.

- Reframes a situation, not in a way of offering a more correct view to a misinformed person but rather as a way of opening up another possible perception, offering another lens, and then seeing if it fits for this family at this time. Reframing involves changing the entire meaning of a problem situation by altering the conceptual or emotional context in such a way that the entire situation is placed in a new framework. A problem, which was previously seen as negative by the family and the patient, is reframed and seen to be positive, functional, or benign.

- Externalizes the problem to allow the separation of the problem from the person. Instead of viewing the problem as residing in the person, the problem is externalized and viewed as being outside the person. Rather than a client's being objectified, a problem is objectified (White 1988–89). Externalizing the problem is accomplished during the session by questions that explore the relative influence of the family and the problem. The family is asked, "How much influence do you have over the problem?" and reciprocally, "How much influence does the problem have over you and your relationship?"

- Offers or participates in a reflecting team (Andersen 1987). During a reflecting team discussion, the family is invited to sit behind a one-way mirror with the interviewer to observe the team's discussion about the family's and therapist's previous conversation. The reflecting team's discussion invites the family to consider multiple and alternate views of the family situation. Team members wonder out loud about the problem, connections, and possible solutions. At the conclusion of the reflecting team discussion, the interviewer and family return to the interviewing room, and the team returns to its original position behind the mirror. At this point, the interviewer pursues the family's reactions to the reflecting team's ideas. Thus, the family and interviewer discuss the team's dialogue about the interviews and the family's previous dialogue.

- Writes letters to families. The use of the narrative mode has been highly developed by David Epston and Michael White (1989). Therapeutic letters assist with the reauthoring of people's lives and relationships and "can be considered a ritual through which persons reinsert themselves into, and reassert their place in, a familiar world" (p. 71).

● Offers rituals that require the family to engage in behaviors that are not or have not been part of their usual patterns of interaction. Rituals serve to introduce more clarity into the family system as in the Milan team's "odd day – even day" ritual, (Selvini Palazzoli, Boscolo, Cecchin, and Prata, 1978) which invites a family to do X behavior on Mondays, Wednesdays, and Fridays and Y behavior on Tuesdays, Thursdays and Saturdays. On Sundays the family is invited to be spontaneous.

● Offers the family an opportunity to view particular videotaped segments of a family session and/or an edited revision of highlights of the family sessions for the family's home videotape collection.

● Terminates family sessions in a manner that allows the family to acknowledge, take credit for, and maintain the changes that have occurred.

CASE STUDY

Jane, a 41-year-old woman, was referred to the Family Nursing Unit (FNU) for therapy because of her difficulty coping with the suicidal death of her common-law husband 6 weeks earlier, on New Year's Eve. Jane was seen for 10 sessions over a 12-month period. A team approach was utilized, with my providing live clinical supervision of all sessions by observing from behind a one-way mirror with graduate nursing students, while a student interviewed Jane. In the first session, Jane's understanding and explanation of John's death was explored. One predominant and problematic belief emerged from Jane's story: that she was responsible for John's death and could have prevented it.

Throughout the session, Jane's strengths were commended and her experiences were validated as normal grief reactions. A reflecting team was offered at the end of the first session. With Jane and the interviewer observing from behind the mirror, the team discussed their ideas about the family situation. The reflecting team offered the following ideas: Jane was experiencing a number of problems but was showing great strength, guilt of a survivor is a common response to a loved one's suicide, Jane could not have prevented John's actions, and John had made his own choice in the matter.

Sessions 2 and 3

Jane had three children from a previous marriage: Rob, aged 19 years; Megan, aged 17 years; and Kelly, aged 15 years. Jane was concerned about Kelly's escalating behavior of school truancy, staying overnight at her boyfriend's house, and "doing drugs." Jane believed that until Kelly obtained some help, she (Jane) would not be able to proceed with her own grieving. Kelly and Jane attended sessions 2 and 3 together. The therapist sought to get a better understanding of the effects of suicide on the entire family by asking: "How is Mom [Kelly, Megan, Rob] different since the suicide?" "Since the suicide, what is the biggest problem for Mom [Kelly, Megan, Rob]?"

Since letter writing was an important part of relationships in the family (Jane and John had always written letters to each other; John had left Jane a 14-page letter on the eve of his suicide), Kelly and Jane were invited to each write a love letter to herself to express what she was feeling at this time. The letters drew forth a different perspective of the situation and their own abilities.

Sessions 4 – 8

Jane came alone to the next five sessions, which took place over 11 weeks. During this time, Jane experienced several "anniversary" occasions. Exploration of her thoughts and actions drew forth her resourcefulness. The therapist asked questions that invited Jane to reflect on and solidify her strengths: "How has what you did on this anniversary been helpful to you?" "How will what you have learned about yourself on this occasion be helpful to you on upcoming anniversaries?"

Six months following John's suicide, John continued to be very present in Jane's life. Using John's presence as a way of enabling Jane to get on with her life, the following questions based on White's (1988) approach were asked: "What things do you see in yourself now that John would appreciate about you?" "How would thinking of these things be helpful to you today?" These questions drew forth several characteristics that Jane knew John would admire in her. The exploration assisted Jane in identifying strengths in herself that would be helpful in her new relationship with herself.

At the seventh session, Jane asked, "Am I on my way to recovering? Do I need more counseling?" She recounted a dream, which she interpreted as a sign of a new beginning for herself. To highlight and clarify the mixed feelings that Jane verbalized about continuing therapy, a reflecting team offered a three-way split opinion. Members of the team offered different positions, varying from continuing therapy for up to a year or more, stopping therapy immediately, or continuing therapy on a less frequent basis until a few more anniversary dates had passed. Each team member provided rationale for his or her position based on Jane's comments during the session.

Session 9

At the beginning of the ninth session, 12 weeks later, Jane indicated she was feeling that she had mastered the worst of her grief but wanted to continue therapy on a less frequent basis until she had experienced the occasions leading up to the one-year anniversary of John's suicide.

Jane was troubled by a new relationship with a man she had been dating and by John's continued "presence" in her bed. Interventive questions asked to probe and perturb Jane's perceptions included: "What things do you do that keep John in bed with you?" "How will you know when it is time for John to leave your bed?" "If you were to believe that your experience of John in your bed were a form of self-control to help you from being intimate with someone else before you're ready, what would be different?"

Session 10

The tenth session took place 6 weeks later. In exploring the news since the last session, Jane reported that she had decided to spend Christmas at home with her family as she had traditionally done. In view of her previous strong, negative thoughts about spending Christmas at home, this was a major shift. The therapist asked questions that drew forth the differences and strengths that had enabled Jane to take such a big step: "What about yourself told you that you could do what had originally seemed to be impossible regarding Christmas?" "What would you need to notice about yourself regarding your handling of Christmas that would also tell you that you could handle New Year's Eve in your life?"

The potency of questions to invite new perspectives was dramatically demonstrated when the therapist asked Jane, "Looking back on the events of last New Year's Eve, what do you now tell yourself about John, about yourself, and about your relationship with John?" After careful thought, Jane responded that, John's priority was drinking, he had chosen not to seek help, he chose to end his life, and she could not have done anything to stop him. Jane's poignant statements reflecting a dramatic conceptual shift were immediately reinforced by commendations from the team. Congratulations and a handshake were offered to underline the importance of her new understanding. An end-of-session assignment for Jane requested that she think about the major change in her thinking that had occurred during the session and write the team a letter telling what she had learned.

Two weeks after the tenth session, a letter from Jane arrived at the Family Nursing Unit. It was addressed to John and read as follows:

> This is MY LIFE. I can't keep looking back nor over my shoulder, LIFE GOES ON. John, in the past 11 months, you have put me through absolute hell, made it unbearable at times. I guess I let you do this to me . . . John, you really owe me an apology, you are GUILTY and CHARGED WITH MENTAL CRUELTY. I am the victim in this case. *You* chose to leave, I had no control over your decision, but now, *I* am in control. It's my turn. I will be spending Christmas in my home with my family and friends and we will have a wonderful Christmas, mark my words. As for New Years, I still haven't made any definite plans as of yet, but I do know one thing for sure, as of just a day ago, I decided that I WILL NOT BE MOURNFUL. I am actually looking forward to 1990 as it will be a Brand New Beginning for ME, at long last.

Is there life after suicide? For Jane there is. Family Therapy opened space for Jane to grieve the death of her loved one and to begin a new chapter of her life.

SUMMARY

Family Therapy, as presented in this chapter, is based on a philosophical framework that views the family from a systemic view, looking for connections and reciprocal influences among systems of ideas, people, and events. The nurse's beliefs about problems, people, and change shape the nature of the interaction with the family. The role of the nurse is to intercede in ways that enable family members to discover their own solutions to their problems.

REFERENCES

Andersen T. 1987. The reflecting team: Dialogue and meta-dialogue in clinical work. *Family Process* 26:415–428.

Bateson, G. 1979. *Mind and nature.* New York: E.P. Dutton.

Bell, J.M., Watson L.W. and Wright, L.M. (eds.). 1990. *The cutting edge of family nursing.* Calgary, Alberta: Family Nursing Unit Publications.

Boscolo, L., Cecchin, G., Hoffman, L., and Penn, P. 1987. *Milan systemic family therapy: Conversations in theory and practice.* New York: Basic Books.

Fleuridas, C., Nelson, T., and Rosenthal, D. 1986. The evolution of circular questions: Training family therapists. *Journal of Marital and Family Therapy* 12(2):113–127.

Gurman, A., Kniskern, D.P., and Pinsof, W.M. 1986. Research on the process and outcome of marital and family therapy. In S. Garfield and A. Bergin (eds.), *Handbook of psychotherapy and behavior change* (3d ed.). New York: Wiley.

Haley, J. 1976. *Problem-solving therapy.* New York: Harper Colophon Books.

Hoffman, L. 1985. Beyond power and control: Toward a "second offer" family systems therapy. *Family Systems Therapy* 3(4):381–396.

Loos, F., and Bell, J.M. 1990. Circular questions: A family interviewing strategy. *Dimensions in Critical Care Nursing* 9(1):46–53.

Madanes, C. 1981. *Strategic family therapy.* San Francisco: Jossey-Bass.

Minuchin, S. 1974. *Families and family therapy.* Cambridge: Harvard University Press.

Piercy, F.P., and Sprenkle, D.H. 1990. Marriage and family therapy: A decade review. *Journal of Marriage and the Family* 52:1116–1126.

Selvini Palazzoli, M., Boscolo, L, Cecchin, G., and Prata, G. 1980 Hypothesizing-Circulatory-Neutrality: Three guidelines for the conductor of the session. *Family Process* 19, 3–12.

Selvini Palazzoli, M. Boscolo, L., Cecchin, G. and Prata, G. (1978). A ritualized prescription in family therapy: Odd days and even days. *Journal of Marriage & Family Counseling* 4(3):3–9.

Stanton D.M. 1988. The lobster quadrille: Issues and dilemmas for family therapy research. In L.C. Wynne (ed.), *The state of the art in family therapy research: Controversies and recommendations* (pp. 5–31). New York: Family Process Press.

Tomm K. 1988. Interventive interviewing: Part III. Intending to ask lineal, circular, strategic or reflexive questions. *Family Process* 27:1–15.

Tomm, K. 1980. Towards a cybernetic-systems approach to family therapy at the University of Calgary. In D.S. Freeman (ed.), *Perspectives on Family Therapy,* Vancouver, B.C.: Butterworth Co.

Tomm, K.M., and Wright, L.M. 1979. Family therapy training: perceptual, conceptual and executive skills. *Family Process* 18(3):227–250.

Watson, W.L. (Producer). 1989a. *Families and psychosocial problems* (videotape). Calgary: University of Calgary.

Watson, W.L. (Producer). 1989b. *Family systems interventions* (videotape). Calgary: University of Calgary.

Watson, W.L. (Producer). 1988a. *A family with chronic illness: A "tough" family copes well* (videotape). Calgary: University of Calgary.

Watson, W.L. (Producer). 1988b. *Aging families and Alzheimer's disease* (videotape). Calgary: University of Calgary.

Watson, W.L. (Producer). 1988c. *Fundamentals of family systems nursing* (videotape). Calgary: University of Calgary.

White, M. 1988. Saying hullo again: The incorporation of the lost relationship in the resolution of grief. *Dulwich Centre Newsletter.*

White, M. 1988–1989, Summer. The externalizing of the problem and the re-authoring of lives and relationships. *Dulwich Centre Newsletter,* 3–21.

White, M., and Epston, D. 1989. *Literate means to therapeutic ends.* Adelaide, South Australia: Dulwich Centre Publications.

Wright, L.M. 1989. When clients ask questions: Enriching the therapeutic conversation. *Family Therapy Networker* 13(6):15–16.

Wright, L.M., and Leahey, M. 1984. *Nurses and families: A guide to family assessment and intervention.* Philadelphia: F.A. Davis.

Wright, L.M., Watson, W.L., and Bell, J.M. 1990. The family nursing unit: a unique integration of research, education and clinical practice. In J.M. Bell, W.L. Watson, and L.M. Wright (eds.). *The cutting edge of family nursing.* Calgary, Alberta: Family Nursing Unit Publications.

31

ART THERAPY

ROBERT J. KUS
MARY ANN MILLER

> Vito was admitted to a chemical dependency center for cocaine abuse after getting into trouble with the law. From the day of admission, Vito has denied not only the seriousness of his problem but that he has any problem with drugs at all.

> Anne, the teenaged sister of cancer patient Helen, has been secretly upset at all the attention Helen has been receiving from their parents, friends, and relatives. Although intellectually she is able to accept Helen's receiving this attention, Anne is becoming resentful toward Helen, and this, in turn, is making her feel guilty.

> Carlos and Rita, as part of their family therapy experience, are asked to look at not only themselves individually, but to explore, together with their three children, what they are as a family unit.

In all three cases, Art Therapy was used to assist the clients complete their tasks. Vito, for example, became accepting of his chemical dependency after listing all of his losses and linking these to his cocaine use. This acceptance led him to be able to break down his denial and open his mind to treatment. Anne showed through her artwork how she was feeling insignificant due to Helen's illness. Helen's illness, portrayed as a dragon, was so huge that nobody was paying much attention to Anne. After she explained her art project in her sibling support group, the group members were able to offer her support and assurances that what she was experiencing was a natural reaction to a sibling's cancer. Finally, Carlos and Rita gleaned valuable insights into each other by engaging in the family coat-of-arms art project. Through creating an imaginary coat of arms for their family, they were able to identify common themes or threads running throughout their family life.

Art Therapy is an effective strategy that should be added to most nurses' repertoire of skills. Art Therapy has been used successfully with many populations to help persons heal and grow: dying persons (Misner 1979), families of dying persons (Junge 1985), adolescent substance abusers (Cox and Price 1990), adult chemically dependent persons (Allen 1985; Chen 1989; Johnson 1990; Miller 1987; Potocek and Wilder 1989), nursing staff (Misner 1979), chronic psychiatric outpatients (Green, Wehling, and Talsky 1987), children (Burns and Kaufman 1972; Kramer 1971), schizophrenics (Honig 1977; Young 1975), cancer patients (Johnson and Berendts 1986), and families of cancer patients (Johnson and Norby 1981).

TOWARD A DEFINITION OF ART THERAPY

Art Therapy is classified as one of the expressive or creative therapies. It is sometimes referred to as visual art therapy to distinguish it from the other expressive therapies, such as music therapy, dance/movement therapy, poetry therapy, and drama therapy. Sometimes bibliotherapy, horticulture therapy, and socio-drama and psychodrama are included in this list.

For our purposes Art Therapy will be defined as the creation of visual artwork for the purpose of healing or personal growth by individuals and the visual and verbal sharing of the resultant artwork in a group setting. This definiton excludes the use of artwork whose sole purpose is diagnostic, such as projective techniques used in psychological evaluation or coloring tools that childen use to show where they have pain. (For a thorough discussion of the various definitions, see Fleshman and Fryrear 1981, pp. 57–90.)

ART THERAPY AS A NURSING INTERVENTION

Most nurses do not have degrees in art therapy and therefore cannot be considered professional art therapists. Nevertheless, they can successfully do basic Art Therapy projects to help patients heal and grow as long as they keep certain things in mind.

First, nurses doing Art Therapy should adopt a "keep it simple" philosophy. Although many professional art therapists search art projects for hidden meanings that they believe they can find based on their education, nurses would do well to allow the clients to interpret their own artwork. The client is the primary therapist in personal growth and healing journeys, so their reality is what is most important. Nurses who want to explore the various schools of Art Therapy and how each approaches art interpretation are directed to such works as Rubin's *Approaches to Art Therapy: Theory and Technique* (1987).

Art Therapy by its very nature should be a joyful experience, which transcends the common, everyday life. It should be accomplished in a joyful atmosphere created not only by having an attractive place where art supplies are kept for clients but also by the nurse's presentation of self in relation to art therapy. Enthusiasm should shine through.

The focus should be on the healing or growth-producing nature of the artwork, not on its artistic value. Many clients initially are fearful of Art Therapy because they mistakenly believe that the goal is to produce a masterpiece or they mistakenly believe they "have no talent." Such fears should be laid to rest from the start. The purpose of doing Art Therapy is not to produce art masterpieces but to show one's life journey in a personally creative way.

Nurses need to discuss with clients the importance of sharing their finished artwork in a group setting both visually (showing the actual artwork) and verbally (explaining the artwork). Clients need to be reassured that there is no right or wrong thing to say because each individual's life journey is unique. The only "right" thing is to explain as best one can his or her project, and the only "wrong" thing to do is to not share with the group.

BENEFITS OF ART THERAPY

Benefits for Clients

For clients, Art Therapy has many benefits. First, it helps persons increase their self-understanding. It helps them see where they have been and may help to explore where they would like to go or would like to become.

Having a piece of art helps shy persons talk in a group setting. It is much easier to discuss something about which they know more than anyone else, and it is easier to talk when a prop, such as a piece of art, can be explained. Getting comfortable sharing self in group is a major task for many persons for whom Art Therapy has been used — chemically dependent persons who will be sharing self in groups such as Alcoholics Anonymous (AA), mentally ill persons who need to share self in psychotherapy groups, and couples who need to share themselves with other couples to gain better insight into their selves and relationships.

Art Therapy helps individuals explore relations with others. For example, when doing a family collage, clients often express surprise at how their behavior may be affecting other family members.

Art Therapy projects often help individuals recognize patterns of behaving, feeling, or thinking that they have not previously identified. By recognizing such patterns, clients are often able to break through the denial that has been serving as a roadblock to growth and recovery. The life stories of alcoholics, for example, often show that denial had to be overcome before a joy-centered life, a life of sobriety, could be lived (Alcoholics Anonymous 1976; Kus 1990a). A particularly powerful Art Therapy project, discussed in greater depth later in this chapter, is one dealing with loss. Often when chemically dependent clients see through their art project just how much they have lost and as they are able to link such losses to their addiction, they are able to cast off denial and begin the healing journey.

Art Therapy may help clients identify personal strengths as well as weaknesses. Many people who suffer, especially if they have a stigmatizing condition, may begin to see themselves, not just their condition, as worthless or negative (Kus 1990b). If this negative mind-set continues too long, such individuals may block out or not recognize any positive qualities in themselves. Nurses who use Art Therapy can assist such clients by having them do projects that focus on personal strengths. In the group setting, others can add their perceptions of the individual's strengths.

Art Therapy may help clients identify hopes and dreams for the future. Often clients who use Art Therapy have suffered greatly; their lives in the past and present may be sad. Projects focusing on dream making for the future may help rekindle the flame of hope for such clients. Identifying one's dreams and the ways to make such dreams come true is one of the most joyful uses of Art Therapy.

Clients can find an alternative mode of expressing themselves in Art Therapy. Those who have difficulty expressing feelings verbally are often able to share themselves on a feeling level for the first time. They may become more playful. How often do adults get to use crayons and colorful paper to express themselves? Rarely. Art Therapy allows the inner child to shine forth — the inner child who may have been buried under the avalanche of adult responsibilities and problems.

Many adults, after seeing how powerful Art Therapy can be in self-expression, often use it with their children to help them grow too.

Finally, Art Therapy may allow one to explore his or her blessings. Projects designed to assist clients look at the things for which they are grateful help clients put their life problems in a better perspective.

Benefits for Nurses and Other Helping Professionals

Art Therapy may assist clinicians in identifying and clarifying their clients' perceptions about their world. This is a critically important function of Art Therapy because people usually behave not on the basis of actuality, or what is happening in the universe, but rather on the basis of reality, or how they interpret what is happening in the universe (Kus, in press). Often clinicians come to see their clients in a very different light after hearing them describe their Art Therapy projects in a group setting.

Clinicians use Art Therapy to diagnose problems in their clients, especially when the insights gleaned in this way are combined with the insights gained from the other activities in which the client is taking part, activities such as individual therapy, group therapy, music therapy, or recreation therapy.

When clients share their Art Therapy projects in a group setting, the clinician can assess the client's ability to share in group settings and how others are responding to the client. Finally, this intervention can provide the clinician with the opportunity to give encouragement to the client's efforts at sharing in a group setting, thus increasing the likelihood that the client will continue to share self in groups in the future.

Benefits for Researchers

Art Therapy may help clinical researchers in two ways. First, it can help them identify common themes present in certain populations. For example, by examining the family collage artwork done by a group of battered persons, researchers could identify common threads that weave themselves in the lives of such persons. Moreover, Art Therapy projects generate an infinite number of research questions and challenge researchers to explore uncharted avenues.

LIMITATIONS OF ART THERAPY

Although the benefits of Art Therapy are legion, there are limitations also. Like any other treatment modality, it is not complete in itself. Rarely is it sufficient to treat an individual's problem. Nor is it designed to be the only thing necessary for individuals to grow. Rather, Art Therapy should be viewed as an important tool that may complement a host of others designed for healing and growth.

Art Therapy is often misunderstood by professionals and clients alike. Some confuse it with arts and crafts. Others misunderstand the purpose of it of helping persons heal and/or grow; they may mistakenly believe that the artwork itself is the end product as opposed to being merely a vehicle for growth and healing. These misunderstandings in both patients and staff can be dispelled with a minimal of education. Yet other clients (and staff, on occasion) may see Art Therapy as childish. They look solely at the concrete tasks of Art Therapy and neglect to see the therapeutic nature of the process. This, too, can be corrected with education. Most persons who participate in Art Therapy projects, especially when they share their projects verbally and visually in a group setting, come to see the therapeutic nature of Art Therapy and realize that their initial assessment of art therapy as childish was hastily made.

THE ART THERAPY CANDIDATE

Virtually all persons can benefit from Art Therapy because they have the potential to grow. To be more specific from a nursing perspective, though, we could say that certain nursing diagnoses are particularly amenable to being treated, in part, with Art Therapy:

Impaired Verbal Communication
Ineffectual Individual Coping
Ineffective Family Coping: Compromised

Ineffective Family Coping: Disabling
Family Coping: Potential for Growth
Diversional Activity Deficit
Altered Family Processes
Fear
Anticipatory Grieving
Dysfunctional Grieving
Powerlessness
Rape-Trauma Syndrome
Self Esteem Disturbance
Social Isolation
Spiritual Distress
Potential for Violence

SAMPLE ART THERAPY PROJECTS

Of the five Art Therapy projects described in this section, the first four have been part of the Art Therapy program at the University of Iowa Chemical Dependency Center, and the final one is a common project conducted in a large number of treatment centers around the world that deal with family therapy.

Nurses who wish to conduct Art Therapy projects need a number of common items at their disposal: plenty of magazines, especially magazines with pictures for patients to cut out for cut-and-paste projects; crayons; pencils (both colored and regular); scissors; glue; watercolor paints (if desired); multicolored construction paper or rolls of butcher paper; and plain paper bags of any size. There should be enough scissors, glue pots, crayon sets, and so forth so that clients do not have to become frustrated waiting to use supplies. When creating the necessary supply store, nurses may ask colleagues to contribute these items. They thus allow the other staff to feel useful and help to generate interest in Art Therapy.

Nurses doing Art Therapy should also provide space where completed projects, which have been shared in the group, may be displayed for staff and clients alike (provided that clients give their permission to have their works displayed). Clients often delight in showing off and explaining their projects to nursing and medical students, visitors, and other patients.

The Self-Image Project

The purposes of the self-image project are to assist clients in exploring how they are presenting themselves to others and how others perceive them; telling how they believe they "really" are; expressing their "real self" to others in an honest way; and learning, from peers that their self-image is not totally unique. The goals of this project are that clients will describe how they are presenting themselves to others or how they believe others are perceiving them; describe how they actually are "deep inside"; express feelings about themselves in an honest way; and listen to others tell about their self-images.

The typical supplies for this project are glue, scissors, magazines, crayons, drawing pencils, and a paper bag of any size.

Clients are told that on the outside of the bag they may draw or cut out images from magazines of how they think they come across to others—that is, how they present themselves to others and how others see them, either now or in the past. They may ask their peers how they see them. The inside of the bag is designed to place drawings, magazine pictures, and/or words that portray their "real selves" —their positive traits, weaknesses, secrets, wishes for the future and talents.

In the field of chemical dependency, clients often decorate the outside of their bags in a negative way. They decorate the bags with magazine pictures of whiskey bottles or beer cans, jail cells, handcuffed persons, passed-out winos, persons crying, and negative words such as *loser, drunk,* or *jailbird.* Another common theme, especially among men who have suffered much as a result of being in prison or jail, is toughness. They might decorate the outside of the bag with pictures of Rambo-like characters, strong animals such as lions, or prize fighters.

The insides of the bag are usually quite different. Instead of negative decorations, beautiful pictures and words appear. For example, it is common to see pictures of kittens, boys crying, and flowers on the inside of bags that have Rambo-like persons on the outside. The radical difference between one's "outside" self and "inside" self may be explained on the basis of the characterological conflicts that occur in chemical dependency. In other words, a good person does bad things as a result of the alcohol or other mind-altering drugs; one's behavior does not match his or her value system (Johnson 1980).

In the group sessions, clients often say that their real selves are much different from their outside selves. The nurse reminds clients that, in time, with sobriety, clients will more likely be perceived as gentle, kind, and good persons to match their interior or "real" self.

The Loss Project

The loss project was conducted with chemical dependency clients in 1989 and was designed by Lily Chen, a graduate student from China. This project was part of her clinical course requirements in the College of Nursing at the University of Iowa (Chen 1989). The purposes of the project were to assist clients in identifying the losses they had experienced in their lives and linking their losses (when appropriate) to their substance abuse. Although it was not listed as a purpose of this project, Chen found that this project had the effect of reducing some clients' denial of their addiction.

The goals listed were that clients would draw the losses they had experienced in life, show the completed artwork to the group, discuss the completed artwork in a group setting, and discuss how their chemical dependency was related or not related to their losses.

The supplies used were drawing paper, colored and regular pencils, crayons, glue, scissors, magazine pictures, and watercolor paints.

Clients were asked to show through artwork the various things they have lost in their lives: people, material objects, or abstract concepts such as health. They were told that these losses could be the result of their using mind-altering drugs or not. These losses would be shared in group setting.

This project turned out to be very powerful and, in many cases, very emotional. Many clients knew they had lost much, but had blocked out or minimized such losses. When they put all of them on paper, however, they were often amazed at the extent of their loss and the breadth of it: spouses, children, cars, money, freedom, mental health, physical health, spiritual values, jobs, and others. Tears were not uncommon when clients were discussing their losses, and the graduate nursing student used this opportunity to ensure the clients, most of them men, that crying is a wonderful thing to be able to do and is quite appropriate. Clients always gave each other positive strokes for sharing their loss projects, and when the clients shared particularly heart-wrenching stories in group, group members often gave the person sharing hugs.

Like other art projects, this one showed that clients often get to know each other on a much more intimate level from the sharing of Art Therapy projects. This increased intimacy helped them appreciate each others' life journeys and be more sensitive toward each other.

The Relationship Project

Relationships are an important part of life; they provide the spice of our lives and help produce our selves. It is useful at times, then, to take stock of our relationships. The relationship project helps clients explore their relationships and how their addiction is influencing, or has influenced, their relationships.

The purposes of the relationships project are to assist clients in identifying the most important relationships in their lives, classifying these relationships in terms of their positive or negative natures and showing how alcohol and other mind-altering drugs influenced these relationships. The goals are that the clients will identify the most important relationships in their lives; classify these relationships on the basis of whether they are mostly negative or mostly positive; determine how alcohol and other mind-altering drugs influenced these relationships; and share their artwork and insights in a group setting.

The clients are instructed to think of all the important relationships in their lives, past and/or present, and to decide whether each relationship is basically positive or negative. Then they show their most important relationships in an art project. One way to do this project is to start by choosing a color that most indicates their life. (Clients are assured that colors have different meanings to different people; a color that indicates anger to one person could indicate love to another.) They could give shapes to each of the important people in their lives (hearts, flowers, tombstones, ghosts, triangles, squares). They could trace these shapes on various colored paper, cut these out, and paste them on their background paper. For example, a client may indicate females as flowers and males as stars, and then indicate whether these were positive or negative relationships by making the negative men and women blue and the positive ones yellow. Another way of doing this project is to cut out pictures from magazines indicating important relationships and paste them on background paper.

Clients are asked to determine what role, if any, alcohol and other drugs played in these relationships and what effects they had. They were told that this project would be shared visually and verbally in group.

Like the loss project, this one often produces a great deal of emotion. For example, chemically dependent clients almost universally have a string of relationships destroyed or damaged due to their disease. The most common relationships that clients portray artistically and share verbally in group are lover and spousal relationships, parent-child relationships, friendships, and work relationships. Quite often they discuss how they have ruined the relationships because of their chemical dependency, while the other person in the relationship was blameless. Nurses may take this opportunity to explore with the clients how the past is past and to become stuck in one's past is an obstacle to growth. They may show how we can make up for past mistakes and reduce guilt feelings by sharing our past mistakes with others, making amends to persons we have harmed, and by asking for forgiveness, techniques used by followers of AA and other 12-step programs such as Overeaters Anonymous, Narcotics Anonymous (NA), Alanon, and Gamblers Anonymous.

The Spirituality Project

In the United States, virtually all chemical dependency centers have a 12-step base; that is, they follow the principles of AA and similar other groups. Because AA is a spiritual way of life, clients need to have some idea of what spirituality is and is not. Thus, the purposes of this project are to assist clients in identifying how they see spirituality and beginning to identify how their spirituality ideas can be incorporated into the 12-step framework. The goals of this project are that clients will express through art their conception of spirituality, which may include, but is not limited to, a higher power, ways of doing spirituality, and obstacles to achieving spirituality, and share their artwork in group visually and verbally.

Supplies most commonly used in doing this project are drawing paper, pencils and crayons, glue, scissors, magazines, watercolor paints, and pieces of nature, such as leaves, twigs, and pine cones.

Clients are first asked to create a project that reflects their personal spitituality. They are told that everyone has spirituality but not everyone has religion. (This idea is in harmony with the nursing belief that humans can be understood only in terms of mind, body, and spirit.) Some of the things they can think about before beginning their projects are their purpose in life, their basic values, the obstacles that get in the way of practicing their spirituality (their values and behaviors), the things that can help them increase their spirituality, and their conception of a higher power. They are also asked to consider how their illness has affected their spirituality, where their spirituality is now compared to what they would like it to be in the future, and how their religious ideas, if they have any, have changed over time.

Clients often find this project not only challenging but also very important. Some create artwork indicating a specific religious background, with crosses, pictures of Jesus, angels, clergy, rituals, and churches. A great number of projects show nature scenes because these individuals often see nature itself as their higher power. These clients often will create a project out of pine cones, leaves, twigs, rocks, and other natural materials. Often AA and NA are portrayed somewhere in the picture to show that they are an integral part of one's spirituality. Many persons divide their project into two parts: before treatment, characterized by negative images such as jails and words such as *bad, turmoil,* or *loser,* and after treatment, composed, in stark contrast, of positive images such as nature or good relationships and words such as *AA, winner,* and *serenity.*

The Family Coat-of-Arms Project

One of the most fascinating of all Art Therapy projects is the family coat-of-arms project, especially useful when whole families are involved. The purposes of this project are to help families identify basic themes in their family's history; identify how each member sees the family experience and how each individual's perception jibes with other family members' perceptions; cooperate with each other to produce a family coat of arms; become a more tightly-knit unit; identify negative family themes that can be prevented from continuing into the future; and identify positive themes of the family experience that can be nurtured and passed along to future generations. The goals of this project are that family members will identify the common themes in their family experience; cooperate with each other to create a family coat of arms; identify negative themes of the family experience that the family could eliminate if they wished; identify positive themes of the family experience that could be nurtured and handed down to future generations; and create a family coat of arms based on their family experience.

Supplies include colored paper, glue, scissors, crayons, colored pencils, and watercolor paints and brushes. Large rolls of butcher paper are useful because family members often work together on the floor and need room for creating, and recreating, their family coat of arms until they are satisfied.

Family members are instructed to explore their family experience and create a coat of arms that reflects their family experience. They may be shown examples of coats of arms from European cities or from fraternities and sororities. They are asked to explore their family experience in terms of the positive and negative thread or themes common to their family and to depict this experience graphically. Colors, symbols, and shapes are important in designing a coat of arms. This project is to be a work created by the whole family unit, not just one or two dominant members. Finally, they are told that they will be expected to discuss not only the finished product with the nurse (and other families if other families are involved) but also how creating this project affected the family unit as a whole and members individually.

Families always find this project enlightening. The sharing of the family's experience is never dull; in fact, the sharing can be counted on to be filled with laughter, perhaps a tear or two, and a sense of genuine pride. For many families, this is the first time in a long time they have seen themselves as a unit distinct from all other units.

CASE STUDY

Vito, a 29-year-old man, was admitted to a local chemical dependency center for treatment of his cocaine addiction at the direction of a judge.

Vito had been a high achiever throughout his childhood, and his goal orientation and achievements continued into adulthood. He had a keen sense of right and wrong, and he had always considered himself to be a good person — a perception shared by others. After finishing college at age 23, Vito passed his architect's exam and landed a good job at a prestigious architecture firm. In his job he was well liked by his co-workers and bosses, and he always did his best. He married a college sweetheart named Angie, and they had two sons, 6-year-old Tony and 3-year-old Dom.

At age 28, Vito began experimenting with cocaine and became hooked. Cocaine became the center of his life. He began neglecting his family and job, and his friends began avoiding him. After using cocaine for one year, the family's financial position was precarious. Vito was using all available cash for getting more cocaine. To get enough money for his ever-growing cravings, Vito began selling cocaine. This came to a halt when he was arrested in a drug bust.

Following his arrest, Vito was sued for divorce by his wife. After serving a 6-month shock sentence in prison, the judge recommended that Vito receive inpatient treatment for his cocaine addiction at a chemical dependency center.

When Vito came to the treatment center, his self-esteem was quite low. His outward presentation of self was that of a tough guy, but inwardly he was a scared young man. He denied that he had a cocaine problem: "I can take it or leave it." He blamed his arrest on the fact that he was caught. He blamed his impending divorce on Angie's lack of commitment to their marriage vows.

Upon entering treatment, Vito made it clear to the other patients that he fully intended to scam his way through the program. In individual and group therapy sessions, Vito shared minimally or superficially.

One experience, however, helped Vito begin to crack his wall of denial: a loss project done in Art Therapy. Vito listed the following things he had lost: his good name, freedom, legal status, job, friends, money, dreams, and spiritual compass. He also listed his probable losses as his wife, his children (whom he would probably lose in a custody battle), and his house (the court would probably give the house to his wife in a divorce battle). Vito's sharing of his art project in group was an emotional experience. Sobbing, he related all his losses, and he was able finally to admit that his cocaine abuse had led to all of these losses in some way. The other clients gave Vito a tremendous amount of positive strokes for his sharing.

From that day on, Vito began opening up in his treatment in his individual sessions, in groups, and in his AA and NA meetings. He advised newcomers to the program to make the most out of their treatment. Eventually, Vito and Angie sought marriage counseling and were able to save their marriage.

Today Vito is back working as an architect and gaining back his friends and self-respect. Although he and Angie are still in debt, they are paying off their bills little by little, and they have dreams for a bright future. Vito is living clean and sober one day at a time.

SUMMARY

Art Therapy is one of the creative therapies that can be used to assist clients heal and grow. Art Therapy, in particular, has been used successfully in helping clients gain special insights into various life issues such as spirituality, family relationships, self-esteem, mental health, and losses. This form of therapy, which is a blend of individual and group therapies, can be used by any client who wishes to explore psychosocial life issues in greater depth.

REFERENCES

Alcoholics Anonymous. 1976. *Alcoholics Anonymous* (3d ed.). New York: A.A. World Services.
Allen, P. 1985. Integrating art therapy into an alcoholism treatment program. *American Journal of Art Therapy* 24:10–12.
Burns, R.C., and Kaufman, S.H. 1972. *Actions, styles, and symbols in kinetic family drawings.* New York: Brunner Mazel Publications.
Chen, L. 1989. *Loss, the chemically dependent person, and art therapy.* Unpublished graduate paper, College of Nursing, University of Iowa, Iowa City.
Cox, K.L., and Price, K. 1990. Breaking through: Incident drawings with adolescent substance abusers. *Arts in Psychotherapy* 17:333–337.
Fleshman, B., and Fryrear, J.L. 1981. *Arts in psychotherapy.* Chicago: Nelson-Hall.
Green, B.L., Wehling, C., and Talsky, G.J. 1987, September. Group art therapy as an adjunct to treatment for chronic outpatients. *Hospital and Community Psychiatry* 38(9):988–991.
Honig, S. 1975. Art therapy used in treatment of schizophrenia. *Art Psychotherapy* 4:99–104.
Johnson, J.L., and Berendts, C.A. 1986, February. Arts and flowers: Drawing out the patients' bests: The WE CAN WEEKEND. *American Journal of Nursing,* 164–166.
Johnson, L. 1990. Creative therapies in the treatment of addictions: The art of transforming shame. *Arts in psychotherapy* 17:299–308.
Johnson J.L., and Norby, P.A. 1981. February. WE CAN WEEKEND: A program for cancer families. *Cancer Nursing* 4:23–28.
Johnson, V.E. 1980. *I'll quit tomorrow* (rev. ed.). San Francisco: Harper & Row.
Junge, X.M. 1985, March. "The book about daddy dying:" A preventative art therapy technique to help families deal with the death of a family member. *Art Therapy* 2:4–9.
Kramer, E. 1971. *Art as therapy with children.* New York: Schocken Books.
Kus, R.J. 1990a. *Gay men of Alcoholics Anonymous: First-hand accounts.* North Liberty, Iowa: WinterStar Press.
Kus, R.J. 1990b. Nurses and unpopular clients. In J.C. McCloskey and H.K. Grace (eds.), *Current issues in nursing* (3d ed., pp. 554–558). Philadelphia: W.B. Saunders.
Kus, R.J. and Carpenter, M.A. 1991, October. "Lance": A gay recovering alcoholic misdiagnosed as HIV-positive. *Archives of Psychiatric Nursing* 5(5):307–312.
Miller, M.A. 1987, June. *Art therapy, feelings, and the chemically dependent person.* Paper presented at the 33d International Institute on the Prevention and Treatment of Alcoholism, Lausanne, Switzerland.

Misner, S.J. 1979, August. Using art therapy techniques in staff and patient education. *Nursing Outlook,* 536–539.

Potocek, J., and Wilder, V.N. 1989. Art/movement psychotherapy in the treatment of the chemically dependent patient. *Arts in Psychotherapy* 16:99–103.

Rubin, J.A. (ed.). 1987. *Approaches to art therapy: Theory and technique.* New York: Brunner/Mazel.

Young, N.A. 1975. Art therapy with chronic schizophrenic patients of a low socioeconomic class in a short-term treatment facility. *Art Psychotherapy* 2:101–117.

SECTION IV

HEALTH PROMOTION

Overview: *Enhancing Client Health*

GLORIA M. BULECHEK
JOANNE C. McCLOSKEY

A growing desire for better health and more productive living has resulted in the wellness movement. There is increased awareness of physiological, psychological, sociological, and ecological factors and their impact on health. Clients desire to develop personal resources that maintain or enhance well-being. They seek protection from potential or actual health threats.

Organized nursing is calling for a restructuring of the health care system to achieve more balance between health promotion and prevention services and illness care. The role of the professional nurse in this evolving system is yet to be determined. One of three program areas of funding for the National Center for Nursing, National Institutes of Health, is health promotion–disease prevention. Research in this area is designed to decrease the vulnerability of individuals and families to illness or disability across the life span. Health promotion research addresses the general health of the population. Disease prevention research focuses on how to intercept the onset of a particular illness or disability. The aim is to develop the theory nurses need to guide practice in enhancing health.

Exercise is a frequently recommended health promotion intervention. Increasingly nurses are becoming involved in helping clients to initiate and monitor an Exercise Program such as that described in Chapter 32. Janet Davidson Allan, an adult health nurse practitioner, gives concrete guidance for assessing clients' suitability to undertake an Exercise Program. She describes the eight components of an exercise prescription, stresses the importance of helping the client to develop a positive attitude toward this life-style change before initiating any activity, and

403

acknowledges that long-term adherence to an Exercise Program is difficult to achieve; the time spent with motivation activities and in assisting the client with goal setting is crucial. Tables in the chapter give guidance for the progression of activity in a program of walking, jogging, or swimming. Strategies for maintaining the Exercise Program are presented, including an example of how a patient contract can help with maintenance. The chapter concludes with a case study of a 40-year-old man who desires to initiate a jogging program.

Patient Contracting is an intervention designed to assist clients in increasing desired behavior. The intervention, based on reinforcement theory, uses behavioral analysis to identify antecedent events that precede the behavior, introduce small steps that make up the behavior, and provide consequences that follow the behavior. Patients are taught to monitor themselves and thus learn the principles of behavioral analysis that can be applied in future behavior change. Susan Boehm has worked with this theory and intervention over a number of years and has summarized the research in Volume 7 of the *Annual Review of Nursing Research*. Here she provides a theory-based intervention with direction for clinical application, with a case study that illustrates its use. This intervention is placed in the Health Promotion section because of Boehm's emphasis on helping clients learn to analyze and shape their behavior.

Stress management is a health goal for many clients, and nurses can assist clients in learning this self-care activity. The hope is that stress management can be initiated as a preventive measure and become a life habit. Many clients need to learn to control stress overload in order to cope with symptoms or diseases. Acutely ill clients often experience stress overload because of the technology needed to sustain them. Stress management can sometimes assist clients in controlling long-term pain.

Two interventions for stress management are described in this section. The first, Relaxation Training, is defined in Chapter 34. The many relaxation techniques described in the literature are divided into two categories, external and internal, a useful classification because much of the literature on relaxation has been unclear about which technique is being utilized. Sharon Scandrett-Hibdon and Susan Uecker review both the general and nursing research related to Relaxation Training and present an assessment guide for screening clients and criteria for selecting appropriate clients. Associated nursing diagnoses are specified. The chapter describes a five-step nursing model for utilizing Relaxation Training, drawing from the techniques discussed. This eclectic model, utilizing both external and internal relaxation techniques, was developed by Scandrett-Hibdon and has been implemented by a group of psychiatric clinical nurse specialists at the University of Iowa. The intervention has been clearly defined and has been utilized with several hundred clients with a multitude of stress problems.

In Chapter 35, Susan Scandrett-Hibdon explores a second intervention, for coping with stress: Cognitive Reappraisal. Stress management has traditionally emphasized behavioral therapy — those techniques that treat a stress response. Cognitive Reappraisal, on the other hand, treats the stimulus that produces the stress response. Cognitive Reappraisal is a way of helping the client reorganize the way stressors are perceived. If the stressors can be perceived as less threatening, the amount of stress experienced should be decreased. A five-step model for implementing Cognitive Reappraisal is presented. Scandrett points out that a behavioral intervention, such as Relaxation Training, can be used in combination with the cognitive approach to achieve an immediate and long-range reduction in stress. This is illustrated effectively in her case study.

Efforts to assist clients to stop smoking have met with minimal success. Kathleen

A. O'Connell, a member of a research team studying health behavior at the University of Kansas, proposes that nurses are in key position to assist with this health promotion goal. She asserts that efforts to stop smoking must be self-directed and structures the intervention Smoking Cessation (Chapter 36) around six stages of self-change. The intervention is designed to help clients stop smoking rather than reduce it. The steps of the intervention are applied in a case study. O'Connell gives concrete help to nurses who are working with clients who desire or need to stop smoking.

The intervention of Weight Management, which Janet K. Crist describes, has evolved out of her personal experience in weight control and her experience with clients in her weight and wellness clinic. The theory explaining obesity has dramatically shifted recently. Crist begins Chapter 37 by overviewing the causal factors involved in obesity and uses this information in the design of the five-step intervention of Weight Management: focused assessment, eating plan prescription, energy utilization tactics, adherence strategies, and structured reinforcement and support. She provides the assessment tools and the daily menu planner she uses in her clinic and lists other resources useful in conducting the intervention. The case study's comments in the chapter illustrate the sensitivity that must be present to work with this client group. Nurses can provide the skilled communication needed to support clients who have had repeated failure and embarrassment. Because of this, private practice is an ideal setting to provide this intervention.

The chapter authors in this section have done an admirable job of developing six interventions to assist clients with health promotion. They have made explicit what is often only an implicit desire to deliver wellness care. A number of chapters in Section III, Life-Style Alteration, such as Patient Teaching and Mutual Goal Setting, are relevant to health promotion too.

32

EXERCISE PROGRAM

JANET DAVIDSON ALLAN

The need to change the sedentary habits of the adult American population is well recognized. Physical inactivity has been linked to premature cardiovascular disease, obesity, orthopedic problems, and emotional distress. Despite the tremendous public interest in exercise, nationwide participation in all types of physical activity increased only slightly (from 4% to 14%) between 1980 and 1990 (Dishman, Sallis, and Orenstein 1985). Less than 20% of U.S. adults get enough regular exercise to have a positive impact on their cardiovascular health (Rippe 1987). In addition, 40% of adults exercise intermittently, and 40% are sedentary (Stephens, Jacobs, and White 1985). Although great strides have been made in getting more Americans to be physically active, the percentage of exercising adults falls far short of the national fitness objectives for 1990 (Department of Health and Human Services 1980). Evidence for the role of regular exercise in the primary and secondary prevention of cardiovascular disease and numerous other prevalent health problems continues to accumulate (Pollock and Wilmore 1990; Rippe 1987). Most health promotion recommendations advocate modification of life-styles to include regular, moderate aerobic exercise and resistance training (American College of Sports Medicine 1990). Nurses, as part of their involvement in health promotion and risk reduction, need knowledge of exercise training in order to make appropriate assessments and develop Exercise Programs with clients.

WHAT IS EXERCISE?

Human physical performance capacity has three major determinents: capacity for energy output (aerobic and anerobic mechanisms), neuromuscular functions (strength, technique, and coordination), and psychosocial factors (motivation, social support) (Åstrand and Rodahl 1986; Muhlenkamp and Sayles 1986; Dishman, Sallis, and Orenstein 1985). Physical exercise is defined as action or activity involving physical and mental exertion. Sustaining such exertion physically involves muscular strength, muscular endurance, flexibility, and cardiopulmonary (aerobic) endurance (Åstrand and Rodhal 1986; Froelicher 1987). Muscle strength is the ability of a muscle group to produce a force against resistance (McArdle, Katch, and Katch 1986). Exercises involving muscle strength are often called isometric activities; common examples are weight lifting or carrying objects of all kinds. Flexibility refers to the range of movement of a joint(s) (Åstrand and Rodahl 1986). Exercises involving flexibility include arm swinging, neck rotation, and torso bending. These types of exercises are useful during warm-up periods prior to cardiac endurance activities. Muscle endurance is the ability of a muscle group to perform repeated action for an extended period of time (McArdle, Katch, and Katch 1986). Activities calling for muscle endurance include push-ups or jumping in place. Exercises that promote cardiopulmonary endurance or fitness are called aerobic exercises. These exercises are rhythmic, repetitive exercises that use large muscle groups and include jogging, biking, and race walking. In summary, cardiac endurance is the ability of the body to participate in vigorous exercise for an extended period of time (Froelicher 1987).

THE BENEFITS OF EXERCISE

The physical and psychological benefits of physical activity are well established (Pollock and Wilmore 1990; Siscovick, Laporte, and Newman 1985; Morgan 1985; Heyden and Fodor 1988). Physical activity is one of many health behaviors that has an impact on health status. The most extensively researched area has been the relationship between physical activity and coronary heart disease (CHD) (Morris et al. 1953; Fox, Naughton, and Gorman 1972; Brand et al. 1976; Paffenberger et al. 1970, 1977, 1986). Currently, there is strong, though not conclusive, evidence that regular physical activity can prevent or reduce the risk for CAD (Powell et al. 1987; Paffenberger et al. 1986; Kannel et al. 1986). Paffenberger and associates (1986), in a 16-year study of 16,936 male Harvard University alumni between the ages of 35 and 74 years, found that men who walked, climbed stairs, and played sports had fewer incidents of CHD than those who were less active. Supporting these results are the findings from the Framingham study of white men, which found that cardiovascular and coronary heart disease mortality decreased with increasing levels of physical activity at all ages, including the elderly (Kannel et al. 1986).

Other studies examine more broadly the association of health and activity. The Alameda County Study, known as the Alameda 7 (Belloc and Breslow 1972; Wiley and Comacho 1980), reported that seven health habits were related to both concurrent and subsequent health status. In this longitudinal study of 4000 adults aged 20 to 70 years, Belloc and Breslow initially identified seven health practices to be associated with a general index of health: no smoking, moderate drinking, 7 hours to 8 hours of sleep per night, regular meals, particularly breakfast, not eating between meals, moderate weight, and weekly physical activity. Physical activity, such as gardening or long walks, even at minimal levels was associated with positive health status. Wiley and Comacho, reporting on the same population 8 years later (1980), found that snacking and eating breakfast were less important than the other five habits and that individuals having more good habits tended to live longer. This classic study and other research (LaPorte et al, 1984; Paffenberger et al. 1986) emphasize the beneficial effect of lifetime physical activity habits. Schoenborn (1986) reported on the prevalence of the seven Alameda practices in the general population. She found that the practice of these habits varied with age, gender, education, and ethnicity; younger, less educated persons, men, and black women had the fewest healthy habits.

The elderly are particularly vulnerable to the effects of inactivity. Declining levels of physical activity have been implicated in bone loss in the elderly (Siscovick, LaPorte, and Newman, 1985). Only 7.5% of those over age 65 years meet the activity level defined in the 1990 national physical fitness and exercise objectives and fewer than 25% of noninstitutionalized adults aged 65 years and older participate in regular exercise (Caspersen, Christenson, and Pollard 1986). Accidents (particularly falls, which account for 60%) are the sixth leading cause of death among the elderly and can be attributed in part to a sedentary life-style that is not just the aging process (de Vries, 1979).

SPECIFIC BENEFITS OF AEROBIC EXERCISE

Regular, long-term aerobic exercise results in a number of physiological alterations that are beneficial to health. Physiological effects occur in three areas: hemodynamic (lower resting heart rate, lower blood pressure, increase in collateral cardiac circulation), biochemical (increase in fibrinolysis, decrease in catecholamines, increase in alpha lipoproteins), and morphologic (increase in muscle fiber size, increase in coronary vascularity) (Pollock and Wilmore 1990; Rippe 1987). Studies have suggested that elevated plasma levels of high-density lipoproteins (HDL) may be associated with a lower risk of CHD (Haskell 1986; Kannel 1983) and that vigorous exercise may result in elevated HDL levels (Haskell 1986). Hypertension increases the risk of CHD twofold. Decrease in blood pressure is one of the major positive hemodynamic effects of exercise (Rippe 1987). Moderate exercise seems to produce decreases in diastolic blood pressure in normal individuals (Pollock and Wilmore 1990; Raglin and Morgan 1987) and in hypertensive men (Seals and Hagberg 1984). Hagberg and Seals (1986), in a prospective study of 30 normotensive women, found that blood pressure was significantly lowered after training. Many of the hemodynamic changes seen with habitual aerobic exercise result from an increase in stroke volume and a lower heart rate.

Aerobic exercise has several other, less direct beneficial effects. For example, studies have suggested that exercise may reduce cigarette smoking, weight, and insulin levels (Hill 1985; Blair, Jacobs, and Powell 1985). Habitual exercise also reduces stress, improves psychological well-being, and reduces depression (Deobil 1989; Morgan 1985; Hayes and Ross 1986). Perri and Templer (1984), in a study of the effects of an exercise program on older adults, reported a significant increase in self-concept and perceived locus of control. In one nursing study, Goldberg and Fitzpatrick (1980) report increased morale among institutionalized elderly individuals after the initiation of a movement therapy program. These studies suggest that exercise training can be useful in the promotion of psychological as well as physical well-being.

CARDIAC FITNESS: QUANTIFICATION OF AEROBIC EXERCISE

The primary benefit of exercise training is related to improving cardiovascular efficiency and fitness. The amount of exercise necessary to accomplish cardiovascular fitness is related to the concept of maximum oxygen uptake (MVo_2)—the maximum amount of oxygen that can be utilized by the body. Maximum oxygen uptake measures the maximal amount of physical work that an individual can perform, using large muscles, in a given period of time. It is the most direct measure of exercise capacity. There is a maximal point for each individual. The amount of capacity required to provide beneficial effects on the cardiovascular system occurs at between 60% and 80% of the maximum aerobic capacity (Åstrand and Rodahl 1986). There is little added benefit to exercise beyond this 80% level. The major difference between sedentary and active individuals is the percentage of maximum cardiac used for a given amount of work.

Determination of the MVo_2, which is age related, is necessary in order to pre-

TABLE 32–1.   MAXIMUM HEART RATE AND TARGET ZONE, BY AGE

	MAXIMUM HEART RATE BEATS/MINUTE									
	208	200	194	188	182	176	171	165	159	153
85% level	177	170	165	160	155	150	145	140	135	130
70% level	146	140	136	132	128	124	119	115	111	107
Age	20	25	30	35	40	45	50	55	60	65

Sources: Zohman (1974); Hellerstein (1969).

scribe the appropriate amount of exercise. For each individual, there is an intensity (amount) of exercise that is enough to condition the muscles and the cardiovascular system. This is the concept of target zone. MVo_2 in clinical practice is not measured directly; however, there is a linear relationship between MVo_2 and heart rate. In normal individuals, the points of maximal oxygen uptake and maximal obtainable heart rate are positively correlated. Sixty percent to 80% MVo_2 correlates with 70% to 85% of the maximal obtainable heart rate.

The maximal obtainable heart rate can be determined from specific graded exercise tests, such as the treadmill, bicycle ergometer, step-test or, age-predicted heart rate charts (McArdle, Katch, and Katch 1986; Pollock and Wilmore 1990). Graded exercise testing provides information about the cardiovascular system that is unobtainable in a routine health assessment. In populations without coronary disease or major coronary risk factors, age-predicted heart rate charts (Table 32–1) can be used to determine maximum heart rate. Such charts can be used to calculate an individual's target zone and show the normal decline in maximal heart rate with age. Because of the variability of MVo_2 at any given age and the differences between men and women, these charts constitute rough approximations of target zone (Pollock and Wilmore 1990).

Table 32–1 shows the maximum attainable heart rate and the target zone for ages 20 years to 65 years. For example, an individual aged 45 years is predicted to be able to achieve a maximum heart rate of 176 at maximal exercise capacity. His or her target zone to be achieved during an exercise program would be a heart rate of 124 to 150. If an age-predicted chart is not available, the maximum heart rate can be calculated by subtracting the age in years from 220. For example, the predicted maximum heart rate for a 45-year-old would equal $220 - 45 = 175$. To find the target zone, find 85% and 70% of 175. DeVries (1974) suggests that elderly persons exercise in the 60% to 75% range by taking 60% of the maximal heart rate for an individual aged 60 years or 65 years.

ASSESSMENT

An Exercise Program must include a heart rate level so that the individual can monitor his or her own activity within an effective and safe zone. The decision whether to base the exercise prescription on the more accurate electrocardiographic exercise testing or an age-predicted chart should be made following a focused health assessment. Most adults, whether seeking help for an Exercise Program or for another concern, will have been leading sedentary lives and can be considered unconditioned. Most adults also have varying risk factors for cardiovascular disease or other functional impairments. Clear guidelines are needed to identify those clients who require extensive evaluation, including graded exercise testing or physician supervision, and those clients who might safely utilize the

TABLE 32-2.   HEALTH HISTORY FOR EXERCISE PRESCRIPTION

I.   Present Health Status (includes aspects of past health and family history)
    A.   Presence of Coronary Artery Disease (actual or suspected)
        1.   Do you have angina pectoris (or do you ever get a pressure or pain or tightness in your chest if excited, exercising, eating, or walking against a cold wind)?
        2.   Do you have or have you had palpitations or rapid heart beats or irregular heart beats?
        3.   Have you ever had a heart attack (myocardial infarction, coronary occlusion, or coronary thrombosis)?
        4.   Have you ever had rheumatic fever?
        5.   Have you had a cardiogram taken while exercising that was not normal?
        6.   Do you take or have you taken any of the following: nitroglycerin (small pill that you put under your tongue for chest pain), digitalis, or quinidine for your heart?
    B.   Risk Factors for Coronary Heart Disease
        1.   Do you have hypertension or high blood pressure? What is the treatment plan (diet, drugs, exercise, relaxation, herbal remedies)?
        2.   Do you have elevated cholesterol (high fat in the blood)? Are you on a special diet or taking medication?
        3.   Do you smoke now? How much? Did you ever smoke? When did you quit?
        4.   Has anyone in your family had a heart attack or heart trouble or high cholesterol before the age of 50?
        5.   Do you have diabetes mellitus or high blood sugar? What is the treatment plan (diet, oral agents, insulin)?
    C.   Other Potentially Limiting Conditions
        1.   Do you have any chronic illnesses?
        2.   Ask about: asthma, emphysema, hyperthyroidism, anemia, any arthritis, back, joint, visual, or auditory problems (current or past) that limit activity, renal disease, chronic infectious processes (chronic hepatitis), and obesity (greater than 30% of ideal weight).

II.   Past Health History
    Ask about any other major hospitalizations and surgeries; medications (prescribed and over the counter), major allergies, immunization status, and last skin test for tuberculosis.

III.   Personal Social History
    A.   Explore individual's health beliefs about health in general and exercise specifically. Include data on the following: general concern about health; priorities and positive health activities; past experience with health care system and providers; perceptions about susceptibility for heart disease and the potential severity of heart disease.
    B.   Explore reasons for wishing to start an exercise program and expectations. Include data on the following: past exercise experiences; knowledge about exercise; beliefs in the benefits of exercise; exercise interests: daily schedule (work and home); personal (financial) and community resources and client support systems (family and friends' concerns and knowledge about exercise).

age-related heart rate and for whom the nurse can help plan an Exercise Program. These guidelines will be useful whether the nurse has primary responsibility for a client's care or is working in collaboration with another health professional.

Assessment of the individual for an Exercise Program should include a focused health history and physical examination and selected laboratory parameters. The purposes of the assessment are to determine the presence of risk factors for or presence of CHD, to identify the existence of other health problems or functional difficulties that might modify or preclude exercise prescription, and to collect psychosocial and environmental data that would individualize the exercise plan. Table 32-2 outlines a health history to be used to evaluate an individual prior to exercise prescription. It incorporates a focused assessment for the presence of risk factors for coronary heart disease, actual CHD, and other health problems that might modify or preclude exercise. For the elderly, major hearing or vision losses are particularly important to evaluate. The psychosocial history provides important data about the individual's current health beliefs, life-style, and past experiences that will provide clues about motivation for exercising.

The physical examination should parallel the history by focusing primarily on the cardiac, respiratory, and musculoskeletal systems. Laboratory studies should include determination of lipid levels, urinalysis, complete blood count (for heavily menstruating women and the elderly), and any other studies indicated by the history and physical examination.

This assessment enables the nurse to identify individuals who can safely use the age-predicted heart rate and those who require further evaluation, perhaps even a physician-supervised Exercise Program. Fair, Allan-Rosenaur, and Thurston (1979) developed a useful client categorization scheme:

Category I: No Risk Factors or Disease. The nurse and client can utilize the age-predicted heart rate to plan an exercise program for the individual under 45 years old. Men over age 45 years should be referred for stress testing; if it is negative, exercise prescription can proceed utilizing the heart rate from the test (Pollock and Wilmore 1990). There is little evidence that asymptomatic women should be screened by exercise testing. Patients with a positive stress test should be referred to a physician for futher evaluation.

Category II: Risk Factors and/or Disease. Two questions should be answered: Does this client need stress testing? Can this client safely perform an exercise test?

For individuals under age 45 years old, the nurse should seek consultation to determine whether the risk factors or other health problems are slight enough to allow the use of age-predicted heart rate or severe enough to warrant exercise testing or physician consultation. A 30-year-old man who smokes and has moderate hypertension should be referred to a physician before being exercise tested. A 37-year-old woman with moderately elevated lipid levels who smokes five cigarettes per day and has chronic mild low back pain presents a common clinical situation for which the literature offers no clear guidelines. The health professional is left to apply clinical judgment and seek peer consultation in making decisions about these marginal situations.

All individuals over age 45 years old should undergo exercise stress testing. Consultation with a physician is advisable prior to referring any individual in Category II for testing (Froelicher 1987). Absolute contraindications to exercise testing or participation in a conditioning program include recent myocardial infarction, recent pulmonary embolism, congestive heart failure, heart block (second and third degree), aortic aneurysm, acute myocarditis, severe valvular disease (aortic stenosis), and uncontrolled arrhythmia (Froelicher 1987; Pollock and Wilmore 1990).

Within these broad parameters, there are clients with specific nursing diagnoses for whom the intervention of an Exercise Program is useful. The two most general diagnoses that can be applied to the vast majority of clients are Health Seeking Behaviors related to effective activity pattern and Altered Health Maintenance due to a sedentary life-style. More specifically, exercise is a useful intervention in clients with the following diagnoses (Carpenito 1989): Sleep Pattern Disturbance secondary to stress; Constipation secondary to decreased activity; Decreased Cardiac Output secondary to increased peripheral resistance or volume; Altered Nutrition secondary to more or potential for more than body requirements; and Impaired Physical Mobility Impairment secondary to pain, musculoskeletal neurological impairment, or anxiety and depression.

INTERVENTION ACTIVITIES

Translating an awareness of the need for physical activity into action or behavioral change is crucial to a successful exercise prescription. A successful exercise intervention includes the designing of an Exercise Program that has three major goals: increasing the likelihood that an individual will engage in an exercise program, teaching the individual how to achieve cardiovascular fitness safely, and assisting the individual to maintain the exercise program.

Increasing the Likelihood of Engaging in Exercise

Although there is a vast literature on health behavior, little is known about what motivates individuals to make changes in their life-styles. The behavioral and environmental determinants of exercise adoption and maintenance are still poorly understood. Dishman, Sallis, and Orenstein (1985) in an extensive review concluded that knowledge of and beliefs about health and activity, perceived needs and abilities, expectations, and environmental factors were the most relevant influences in adoption and maintenance of an exercise program. Persons who perceive their health as poor (Morgan, Shephard, and Finucane 1984) and believe that exercise has little value (Dishman 1982) are less likely to exercise. Environmental factors such as spousal support (Oldridge 1982) are important influences in initiating and maintaining an Exercise Program, whereas other environmental factors, such as time (Dishman 1982) and convenience of exercise site (Andrew et al. 1981), may outweigh personal intention (Dishman, Sallis, and Orenstein 1985).

Research that has focused on the determinants of health-protecting or health-promoting behavior provides some direction to the clinician in increasing the likelihood of an individual's participating in physical activity. The best-known health behavior models are the Health Belief Model (HBM) (Kasl and Cobb 1966; Becker et al. 1979) and Pender's (1987) Health Promotion Model. The Health Promotion Model, derived from social learning theory, provides a theoretical approach for predicting the likelihood of an individual's engaging in a health-promoting action such as exercise. The model argues that whether an individual will undertake a health action depends on specific personal perceptions as well as modifying factors and cues to action. The relevant cognitive-perceptual factors postulated to determine a health decision include individual perceptions concerning importance of health, self-efficacy, control of health, definition of health, health status, benefits, and barriers. For example, perceived self-efficacy in one's ability to exercise predicts exercise activity (Blair, Jacobs, and Powell 1985). Modifying factors that influence decision making include demographic, situational, behavioral, and interpersonal factors. Dishman, Sallis, and Orenstein (1985) identified past experiences with fitness programs as a major factor influencing involvement in exercise. The Health Promotion Model also stipulates that a cue to action or challenge must occur to trigger the appropriate behavior by making the individual consciously aware of his or her feelings about health. Cues can be internal, such as a desire to feel good, or external, such as messages from the mass media and interactions with family, friends, or health providers. Pender and Pender (1986) in a study of 377 adults found that exercising regularly was influenced by expectations of others. Although the Pender Health Promotion Model continues to be tested, the clinician can utilize the concepts from the model in assessing a client's readiness to engage in an exercise program. (See Table 32–2.)

In developing an exercise prescription with a client, the nurse must have knowledge of the factors that influence health behavior. The factors outlined in the Pender Model (1987) can be integrated into the health history and intervention plan. As research indicates, beliefs change as the individual has positive experiences with the health intervention (Dishman, Sallis, and Orenstein 1985). The nurse needs to reassess the client beliefs periodically during the monitoring phase of the intervention.

A challenge must occur to make an individual aware that a sedentary life-style constitutes a threat to health or well-being. The power of health assessment and health diagnosis in increasing individual awareness of the risks of a sedentary life-style should not be underestimated. There is notoriously little emphasis on health promotion in our medical care system. The nurse who focuses on health issues often receives a positive response. In that regard, the provision of health information, specifically about physical fitness, cannot be overemphasized. Harris and colleagues (1978) reported that while only 17% of patients received exercise information from a health professional, over 60% expected the provider to give such information.

Other techniques besides the actual health diagnosis and physical examination that the nurse can utilize to increase individual readiness for change involve decision-making theory and behavioral modification (Pender 1987; Farquhar 1978, Cobb-McMahon, Williams, and Davis 1984). Steps for self-directed change involve enhancing cognitive structure and motivation, teaching specific methods of achieving a particular change, and teaching specific methods of maintaining change over time.

Techniques for enhancing cognitive structure and motivation in relation to exercise include providing information about the benefits of exercise and the risks of a sedentary life-style and the ways of reducing such risks. Another useful technique is self-assessment (Cobb-McMahon, Williams, and Davis 1984). The individual should list his or her current beliefs about exercise, current activity patterns (weekdays, weekends, holidays), and barriers to making changes. The client can do this task orally or keep a written log and bring it to a subsequent visit. Farquhar (1978) also suggests a technique of self-monologues to identify belief barriers. These consist of paired positive and negative statements. An example of positive self-talk is, "Walking up three flights of stairs to the office will be good for me"; negative self-talk is, "I don't have time to exercise."

These steps are essential prior to developing an exercise plan with a client. Clients will be at different stages of readiness for proceeding to the second step, the actual exercise prescription. Often health professionals move directly from identification of the client as sedentary to exercise prescription and wonder why the client often does not adhere to the program or even return for future visits.

Achieving Fitness

The goal of the Exercise Program is to design with the client a training program that will safely achieve or maintain a conditioned cardiovascular system (Fair, Allan-Rosenaur, and Thurston 1979). The prescription has eight major aspects: type of activity, intensity, frequency, duration of the exercise, warm-up and cool-down exercises, education about conditions warranting cessation or modification of the program, method for monitoring intensity (Fair, Allan-Rosenaur, and Thurston 1979), and an individualized program, which also constitutes the third step of the nursing intervention. Table 32–3 summarizes the American College of Sports Medicine (1990) recommendations for exercise.

Type of Activity

A repetitive endurance type of exercise or one that uses large muscle groups is recommended—for example, rope skipping, cycling (rolling or stationary

TABLE 32–3.   RECOMMENDATIONS FOR EXERCISE PRESCRIPTION

Frequency	3 days to 5 days per week
Intensity	60% to 90% of maximal heart rate
Duration	20 minutes to 60 minutes of (continuous) aerobic exercise
Mode activity	Any activity that uses large muscles: walking-hiking, running-jogging, cycling-bicycling, dance, rope skipping, stair climbing, swimming
Resistance training	8 exercises to 10 exercises (1 set per exercise of 8 to 12 repetitions) that condition the major muscle groups at least 2 days per week

Source: American College of Sports Medicine (1990).

bicycle), swimming, brisk walking, jogging, running, stair climbing, skiing, and dancing. Physically disabled clients may utilize walking, modified stationary bicycles, or wheelchair propulsion (Lampman 1987; Shephard 1986). Walking and running are particularly suited to older clients because they avoid the isometric tension in upper body limbs created by cycling (de Vries 1979), a tension that increases blood pressure. Resistance and strength training enables all major muscle groups to be exercised—for example, weight lifting, push-ups, and sit-ups. Although weight training has been shown to be superior for strengthening, calisthenics are economic and provide reasonable training (Marcinik et al. 1985).

Frequency, Intensity, and Duration

Frequency refers to how many days per week the exercise should be performed. The majority of sports researchers recommend exercising 3 days to 5 days per week (Froelicher 1987; Pollock and Wilmore 1990). There should be an interval of no more than 1 day to 2 days between each exercise period. Persons at low levels of fitness and those in weight reduction programs should exercise at least 5 days per week (American College of Sports Medicine 1990).

Intensity is critical to improvement in cardiovascular fitness. It requires exercising at a heart rate within each individual's age-specified target zone—70% to 85% of maximal attainable heart rate (Table 32–1). Progression to a fitness level is crucial in exercise prescription and relies heavily on monitoring of heart rates during activity.

Duration refers to the specific length of time the individual should exercise and the amount of time required for conditioning. The majority of researchers conclude that each exercise session should be 20 minutes to 60 minutes in duration (Froelicher 1987; McArdle, Katch, and Katch 1986). Since duration is related to intensity, the greater the intensity, the shorter is the duration needed to achieve cardiovascular benefit: 20 minutes to 30 minutes of high-intensity (running) exercise and 40 minutes to 50 minutes of moderate exercise (walking). Since most persons are unconditioned, a less intense program of longer duration is realistic. Studies suggest that lower intensity is offset by increased duration and frequency (Wenger and Bell 1986; Pollock et al. 1977). It usually requires 20 weeks to 30 weeks of regular activity for adults to reach optimal training level.

Warm-up and Cool-down Phases

These two periods are an integral part of all exercise programs, although they do not provide a conditioning effect. The warm-up phase prepares the body for sustained activity by increasing blood flow and stretching postural muscles. It is a period of adaptation that prevents a sudden increase in workload on the heart, the circulatory system, and the muscles and joints. The warm-up sequence should be designed to increase the intensity of exercise gradually, include rhythmic exercises that stretch muscles, and put joints through their full range of motion (Safran, Seaber, and Garrett, 1989). For 5 minutes to 10 minutes, as the heart rate slowly reaches its target zone, this sequence should be followed:

1.   Initiate rhythmic movements starting with joint range of motion, such as performing a forward and backward crawl (circumduction, extension, and flexion of shoulder girdle); walk with hands clasped behind head, while twisting side to side (circulation, rotation of trunk); or do knee bends (Pollock and Wilmore 1990; Cantu 1980).

2.   Do stretching exercises, such as touching toes (hip, thigh, and back extensors), raising hands over head and bending from side to side (lateral trunk muscles), progressing to alternate knee hugs (back muscles), straight leg raises (knee and hip muscles), assuming sprinter's position with heel pointed (hamstrings), and walking rapidly in a circle (Wilmore and Costill 1988).

The cooling-down period is equally important after the period of endurance exercise to prevent syncope, which can result from a sudden decrease in the supply of blood to large muscle groups. For 5 minutes to 10 minutes, the individual should continue to use large muscle groups (for example, jogging but at a slower pace), slow down to a few minutes of walking, and employ range of motion, stretching, and static muscle contraction and relaxation activities (Pollock and Wilmore 1990).

Conditions Warranting Cessation of or Alteration in the Exercise Program

The nurse needs to provide clear instructions to clients to stop exercising and seek health advice if they experience any of the following conditions: pain in chest, arm, neck, or jaw; irregular heart rate; dizziness; persistent shortness of breath after exercise; nausea or vomiting during or after exercise; prolonged fatigue; uncoordinated gait or weakness; or muscle or joint swelling (Pollock and Wilmore 1990). Investigation of the cause of these symptoms must be made before a client resumes exercising. Every prescription should include a written list of these symptoms (Fair, Allan-Rosenaur, and Thurston 1979), which often occur because individuals do not progress slowly in their training program.

Clients need to consider discontinuation of their training program during episodes of minor illness. Deconditioning occurs very rapidly; studies report an initial loss beginning in 3 days and a 50% loss of the original improvement in 3 months (Froelicher 1987). The implication of these data is that the intensity of the exercise prescription needs to be decreased when the individual resumes an exercise program.

Monitoring Intensity and Individualizing the Program

Besides providing instruction about intensity, frequency, duration, and modifying circumstances, every client must be taught how to monitor the intensity of his or her exercise program. Intensity is based on exercising at a heart rate equal to 60% to 90% of the individual's maximal heart rate (target zone). The nurse must instruct the patient to monitor intensity by counting the pulse rate. Using a 10-second heart rate representative of his or her target zone, the client needs to count the pulse rate at the wrist or neck immediately upon stopping exercise. He or she must find the pulse quickly, count for 10 seconds, multiply times 6, and compare this number with the target zone range. If the pulse rate exceeds the target zone, the client needs to reduce the intensity of the exercise. If the pulse rate is lower than the target zone, the client needs to increase the intensity of the exercise. Intensity can be altered by manipulating two parameters: vigor and time.

Monitoring intensity also includes the concept of progressing to a fitness level. It is useful to think of an exercise program as consisting of two phases: a training phase to develop the individual to a desired level of fitness and a maintenance phase in which the individual tries to maintain optimal fitness. The client frequently moves too quickly into a fitness program during the training phase, exceeding his or her target rate, and often incurring injury and becoming discouraged.

In the training phase, the client with specific guidelines uses the 10-second pulse rate to develop an exercise pattern that includes a below-target zone 10-minute warm-up period, 20-minute to 60-minute aerobic exercise period within the target zone, and a 10-minute cool-down period in which the heart rate moves slowly out of the target zone. Initially, clients must monitor their pulse frequently so that they will not exceed their target zone. Providing specific written instructions to clients regarding progression is very useful. Fair, Allan-Rosenaur, and Thurston (1979) developed a written instruction sheet (see Figures 32 – 1 and 32 – 2). As illustrated in these figures, it is important for the nurse to provide detailed instructions concerning the 10-second heart rate, exercise schedule, warm-up and cool-down activities, and specific activities that lead to a sound progression into the conditioning exercise.

Most authors (Pollock and Wilmore 1990; Cooper 1972; de Vries 1979; Cantu 1980) recommend that all deconditioned individuals begin with a walking program. Such a program provides an opportunity not only to work out an exercise schedule but also to practice monitoring intensity. Tables 32 – 4 and 32 – 5 provide examples of a walking program for two different age groups. Walking is a particularly good exercise for the elderly; an individual who is not able to progress to jogging can receive major benefits from a walking program. For some individuals who are unable to be outside, a walking program can be carried out in a gym or recreation center. Younger individuals and some conditioned elderly persons may want to proceed to a jogging program once they are able to walk a mile in 13 minutes without exceeding their target zone. Table 32 – 6 illustrates a progressive jogging program.

Other conditioning exercises such as swimming, biking (indoor and outdoor), and rope jumping should be planned in a similar manner. Swimming is an excellent exercise for individuals of all ages. It has the advantage of being useful for clients who have musculoskeletal or neurological disabilities that make walking or jogging too difficult.

Research indicates that adults reach an optimal training level sometime after 20 weeks to 30 weeks of regular physical activity. At approximately 6 months, maximal aerobic power gains tend to plateau. The degree of improvement is related to the initial state of conditioning. Before delineating ways in which the nurse can help the client maintain a fitness program, clothing and the prevention of common injuries will be briefly discussed.

Preventing Common Injuries

Approximately 60% of all aches, pains, and injuries suffered by runners, joggers, and walkers are related to excessive speed work on hills, a lack of shock absorption,

Exercise Plan

Name: _____ John Smith _____ Age: _____ 30 _____

10 Second Exercise Heart Rate Prescription

Conditioning Exercise/Strength Training

a. Target Zone	136-155 bpm/25 beats/10 sec	Walking	Jogging
b. Stress ECG	NA	Swimming	Biking
		Other:	Local gym program 2X week

Frequency: Weeks 1-8: 4X Week (minimum): 3 Day Maximum Interval: Week 9 on: 3 X Week

Mon. 6:30-7:30 a.m.	Tues.	Wed. 6:30-7:30 a.m.	Thurs.	Fri. 6:30-7:30 a.m.	Sat.	Sun. 10-11 a.m.

EXERCISE ROUTINE: WALK/JOG

Warm-Up
5-10 min: forward/backward crawl; toe touching, side bending; straight leg raises and sprinter's position

Conditioning
Weeks 1-3: alternate jogging, walking 1 minute, then jogging and walking 2 minutes to cover one mile in 18 min. If exercise heart rate is exceeded, increase walking for 2 minutes, jogging 1 minute. Week 4 on: systematically increase pace to cover 1.5 miles in 22 minutes.

Cool-down
5-10 min: continue using large muscle groups, slower jogging 3 min; slow walking for 5 min. Then, 5 min period of alternating stretching and range of motion exercises.

STOP EXERCISE
Seek medical advice if any of these symptoms occur:
— Chest, arm, or joint pain
— Increased shortness of breath
— Irregular heart beat
— Lightheadedness, fainting
— Nausea and vomiting with exercise
— Unexplained weight changes
— Muscle or joint problems
— Prolonged fatigue
— Unexplained changes in exercise tolerance

Source: Adapted from Fair, J., Allan-Rosenaur, J., and Thurston, E. Exercise Management. *Nurse Practitioner*, 1979, May-June, pp. 13-18. Reprinted by permission.

FIGURE 32–1. Exercise Plan

and a lack of motion control (Johnson 1983). Low-impact activities should be emphasized for beginners and those susceptible to orthopedic injury, such as post-menopausal women, overweight persons, and the elderly (Dishman 1986). One survey (Powell et al 1986) reported that runners with the lowest percentage of injuries ran slowly, ran frequently, had low mileages, and ran on relatively soft surfaces such as grass, dirt, and asphalt. Shoes are the most important clothing investment for a runner, jogger, or walker for the prevention of injuries. Running shoes need to provide maximum cushioning to prevent overstretching of muscles and tendons and to provide strong support to control excess motion and guide the

Exercise Plan

Name: _Mabel Smithers_   Age: _60_

10 Second Exercise Heart Rate Prescription

		Conditioning Exercise/Strength Training

a. Target Zone*   _96-111 bpm/16 beats/10 sec_   Walking   Jogging

b. Stress ECG   _Negative_   Swimming   Biking

Other: _Calisthenics at YWCA 3X week_

Frequency: _Weeks 1-6: 4X Week (minimum): 2 Day Maximum Interval: Week 7 on 3X Week_

Mon.	Tues.	Wed.	Thurs.	Fri.	Sat.	Sun.
10 am-11 am		10 am-11 am		10 am-11 am		4 pm-5 pm

EXERCISE ROUTINE: WALKING

Warm-Up
5-10 min: range of motion (arms over head forward/backward crawl), stretching (touch toes knee bent, bend side to side), and walking in a circle.

Conditioning
Weeks 1-3: walk 1 mile/20 min. Weeks 4-6: walk 1.5 miles/24, 22, 21 min. Weeks 7-10: walk 2 miles in 32 min. If exercise heart rate not reached, increase pace of walking. If exercise heart rate exceeded, slow pace.

Cool-Down
5-10 min: continue to use large muscles - slower walking for 5 min. Then 5 min period of alternating muscle stretching exercise (raise hands over head).

STOP EXERCISE

Seek medical advice if any of these symptoms occur:
— Chest, arm, or joint pain
— Increased shortness of breath
— Irregular heart beat
— Lightheadedness, fainting
— Nausea and vomiting with exercise
— Unexplained weight changes
— Muscle or joint problems
— Prolonged fatigue
— Unexplained changes in exercise tolerance

*60-70% level of maximal heart rate
Source: Adapted from Fair, J., Allan-Rosenaur, J., and Thurston, E. Exercise Management. *Nurse Practitioner*, 1979, May-June, pp. 13-18. Reprinted by permission.

FIGURE 32–2. Exercise Plan

foot as it moves. (Readers desiring more information should seek other sources for specific details about running injuries, such as Blair 1985.)

Individualized Program: Maintaining the Exercise Program

Successful maintenance of a change in behavior or life-style is vital but notoriously difficult (Neale et al. 1990; Pender 1987). Attrition is a serious problem in most exercise programs, with over 50% of participants dropping out in the first 6

TABLE 32–4. PROGRESSIVE WALKING PROGRAM, AGED 50 YEARS
AND OVER

WEEK	FREQUENCY/WEEK	DISTANCE (MILES)	TIME/PLACE
1–2	4–5	1.0	18–20 min/slow
3	4–5	1.0	15–17 min/moderate
4	4–5	1.5	24 min/moderate
5	4–5	1.5	22½ min/moderate
6	4–5	1.5	21½ min/moderate
7	4–5	2.0	32 min/moderate
12	3	3.0	44 min/moderate-fast
16	3	4.0	55 min/moderate-fast

Sources: Blocker (1976); Cooper (1972); Pollock and Wilmore (1990).

months (Gillet 1988; Wankel 1985). Several reviews of research on adherence (Dishman, Sallis, and Orenstein 1985; Andrew et al. 1981; Martin and Dubbert 1984) suggest that self-motivation, personal feedback, and social support were key factors in maintenance of exercise programs. Gillet (1988), in a study of 38 overweight middle-aged women, reported 8 factors that influenced exercise adherence. These factors included commitment to a goal, group homogeneity, social networks, and pleasurable feelings associated with increased fitness. Although this aspect of exercise as a nursing intervention is discussed last, it is probably the most important. The process of individualizing or tailoring a prescription for the individual is the major strategy used not only for initiation of change but also for maintenance. This process of tailoring, which underpins the entire exercise intervention, is the cornerstone to successful initiation of and adherence to a particular plan, and it begins when the nurse first encounters the client. A variety of techniques can be utilized to individualize the intervention: focused nursing assessment, patient self-assessment, client self-monologues, and a specific weekly exercise program. Data related to daily patterns, preferences, past experience, health beliefs, personal resources, and social supports are utilized not only to increase client readiness but also to tailor the exercise plan.

Devising a plan with the client should involve an agreement about objectives or goals of care and mutual expectations. Goals of care are important because they provide clear direction for the nurse and client, guide the selection of specific intervention techniques, and provide a means for evaluation and recognition of change. One technique that is particularly helpful in developing a plan of action is the contract (Herje 1980; Steckel 1982; Kittleson and Hageman-Rigney 1988).

TABLE 32–5. PROGRESSIVE WALKING PROGRAM, AGED 30 YEARS
AND UNDER

WEEK	FREQUENCY/WEEK	DISTANCE (MILES)	TIME/PLACE
1–2	4–5	1.0	15.0
3	4–5	1.0	13.0
4	4–5	1.5	21½
5	4–5	1.5	21.0
6	4–5	1.5	20½
7	4–5	2.0	28.0
12	3–4	3.0	40.0

Sources: Blocker (1976); Cooper (1972); Pollock and Wilmore (1990).

TABLE 32–6. PROGRESSIVE WALKING PROGRAM, AGED 30 TO 50 YEARS

WEEK	FREQUENCY PER WEEK	DISTANCE	JOG	WALK	TIME (MIN)
1–3	4–5	1 mile	1 minute	1 min (130 yd)	18
			2 minutes	2 min (260 yd)	
			1 minute	1 minute	
			2 minutes	2 minutes	
			1 minute	2 minutes	
4–10	4–5	1.5 miles	Systematically increase week's 1–3 schedule of jog/walk		22
10–16	3	2 miles	Systematically increase week's 4–10 schedule of jog/walk		19

Sources: Blocker (1976); Cooper (1972).

Contracting as an intervention is specifically described in Chapter 33. An example of a contract for the intervention of exercise appears in Figure 32–3.

Contracting is an ideal strategy for providing clients with an individualized experience in behavioral change and concurrent means of developing positive health beliefs about that change. The use of other patient education techniques, the development of a positive therapeutic relationship, working with client's support networks, and regular follow-up visits may enhance the client's successful execution of the exercise plan (Dishman, Sallis, and Orenstein, 1985; Martin and Dubbert 1984).

CASE STUDY

CW is a 40-year-old married high school teacher who comes to the clinic concerned about being overweight and having a family history of heart disease. He feels that he is unhealthy and needs to change his life-style.

Goal: Establish regular walking program
Intermediate Behavior (Week 1):
1. Keep written diary of all activities for one week.
2. List pros and cons of exercise.
3. List resources in neighborhood and work.
4. List social support from work colleagues and family.

Contract:
I, Mr. Wiley, will bring diary of list of exercise activities, pros and cons, resources, and social supports from work and home to the next visit. The nurse will evaluate my current activities and help me plan a beginning walking program.

Signed: Ms. Franks, RN
Signed: Mr. Wiley
Date: 6/3/92
Reward: I will buy a new shirt.

FIGURE 32–3. Contract for Exercise

Mr. W, who is 6 feet tall, has weighed 200 pounds since age 30 years and has unsuccessfully attempted to lose weight numerous times using self-initiated fad diets. He eats two meals per day — lunch (at school) and dinner (at home) — and has a diet consisting of high cholesterol and high salt foods: bread or pasta products and few fruits and vegetables. He has never had blood cholesterol measured. Mr. W's father, who is living, had a myocardial infarction (MI) at age 45 years. Mr. W believes that he is at risk for an MI since he is fat and sedentary like his father. The rest of the family history is negative for diabetes, heart disease, hypertension, and hypercholesterolemia. Mr. W denies chest pain, high blood pressure, palpitations, or any history of rheumatic fever. He has never had an electrocardiogram (ECG). He has no history of rheumatic fever. He has no history of other chronic illness or current concerns. Mr. W. does not smoke, drinks 2 ounces of whiskey per day, and does not exercise regularly.

His history reveals no major surgeries or hospitalizations. Mr. W takes no prescribed medication, has no allergies, and was last skin-tested for tuberculosis and immunized in 1972.

Mr. W has been married for 15 years, has two children, aged 12 years and 10 years, and describes his relationship with his wife, who also teaches, as very good. Mrs. W in fact urged the client to have a checkup and get help with his concerns. Mr. W has taught science at the same school for 10 years and generally enjoys his job. He is financially secure. Until recently, Mr. W. felt that he was young, had no illnesses, and did not need to be concerned about his health. At a recent college reunion, he was shocked both by the early death of a few friends and by the youthfulness of others. As he stated, "I suddenly felt old, ugly, and worried that I'd have an MI like my dad and not be able to fully participate in life's activities." His past experiences with the health care system have been minimal but positive. With regard to exercise, Mr. W wishes to learn how to jog, because it will "improve my heart," but is afraid it will be too hard to maintain: "I'm lazy." He has not exercised since college and has never run. He would like to exercise at lunch but does not know how to go about this. He thinks that his family will be supportive of this plan.

Physical examination showed an overweight black male in no distress (blood pressure, 130/84; pulse, 84; respirations, 18), with the following findings:

Thorax Lungs: No lung abnormalities; equal expansion, and diaphragmatic excursion 3 cm bilaterally; resonant to percussion and clear to auscultation.
Cardiovascular: Normal sinus rhythm; $S_1 > S_2$; no murmurs or extra sounds; no bruits; Pulses 2+ and equal.
Musculoskeletal: No spinal deformities; full range of motion in all joints, good muscle mass.
Laboratory: ECG and urinalysis normal; cholesterol, 240 mg/dl.

Nursing Diagnoses for Mr. W are Altered Health Maintenance, secondary to sedentary life-style, Altered Nutrition: More Than Body Requirements, and Potential activity intolerance related to insufficient oxygenation.

The Exercise Program for Mr. W will begin with a progressive walking program (see Table 32–4) for 2 weeks to 4 weeks; when he is able to walk 1 mile comfortably in 13 minutes, he can begin the jogging program. Initially, to enhance cognitive structure and motivation and to obtain more specific data, a contract was established with Mr. W. In progressive visits, the nurse will move to assist Mr. W with specific aspects of initiating and maintaining an Exercise Program, teaching him how to monitor his pulse, helping him to develop a specific exercise plan, and selecting the appropriate time, climate, and clothing. Concurrently the nurse will work with Mr. W to develop a plan for improving his nutritional intake and weight loss.

SUMMARY

The need to change the sedentary habits of adult Americans is well recognized. With the increasing emphasis on exercise as an important health-promoting behavior, it is important that nurses have knowledge of exercise training in order to assess and develop management plans with the healthy exercising adult. This chapter provided a review of the fundamental elements of physical fitness and the beneficial effects of regular exercise; a model for assessing the adult client; and specific strategies for the development of a fitness program with the client. The mechanics of the exercise prescription are straightforward, but the tailoring of an individualized program that provides the guidance and support necessary for the initiation and maintenance of life-style change is more difficult.

Although there is a growing body of knowledge that nursing can utilize in developing Exercise Programs, more research needs to be done. We know very little about those factors that prompt individuals to make a decision to pursue a new course of action or to maintain this new behavior. Nurses have an important role as researchers and as skilled clinicians in taking leadership in the neglected area of promotion of health in the adult population.

REFERENCES

American College of Sports Medicine. 1990. The recommended quantity and quality of exercise for developing and maintaining cardiorespiratory and muscular fitness in healthy adults. *Medicine and Science in Sports and Exercise* 22(2):265–274.

Andrew G.M., et al. 1981. Reasons for dropout from exercise programs in post-coronary patients. *Medicine and Science in Sports and Exercise* 13(3):164–168.

Åstrand P.O., and Rodahl, K. 1986. *Textbook of work physiology* (3d ed.). New York: McGraw-Hill.

Becker, M., et al. 1979. Patient perceptions and compliance: Recent studies of the Health Belief Model. In R.B. Haynes, D.W. Taylor, and D. Sackett (eds.) *Compliance in health care* (pp. 78–109). Baltimore: Johns Hopkins University Press.

Belloc, N., and Breslow, L. 1972. Relationship of physical health status and health practices. *Preventive Medicine* 1:409–421.

Blair, S.N. 1985. Risk factors and running injuries. *Medicine and Science in Sports and Exercise* 17(2):xii.

Blair, S.N., Jacobs, D.R., and Powell, K.E. 1985. Relationships between exercise or physical activity and other health behaviors. *Public Health Reports* 100(2):140–152.

Blocker, W. 1976. Physical activities. *Postgraduate Medicine* 60:56–61.

Brand, R., et al. 1976. Job activity and heart attacks by logistic risk analysis. *Circulation* 54(Suppl. II):511.

Cantu, R.C. 1980. *Toward fitness: Guided exercise for those with health problems.* New York: Human Sciences Press.

Carpenito, L.J. *Nursing diagnosis: Application to clinical practice* (3d ed.). Philadelphia: J.B. Lippincott.

Caspersen, C.J. Christenson, G.M., and Polland, R.A. 1986. Status of the 1990 physical fitness and exercise objectives—evidence from NHIS 1985. *Public Health Reports* 101(6):587–592.

Cobb-McMahon, B.A., Williams, D.D., and Davis, J.H. 1984. Changing health behavior of community health clients. *Journal of Community Health Nursing* 1(1):27–31.

Cook, S.D., Brinker, M.R., and Poche, M. 1990. Running shoes: Their relationship to running injuries. *Sports Medicine* 10(1):1–8.

Cooper, K. 1972. *The new aerobics.* New York: Bantam.

Deobil, S. 1989. Physical fitness for retirees. *American Journal of Health Promotion* 4(2):85–90.

Department of Health and Human Services. 1980. *Promoting health/preventing disease: Objectives for the nation.* Washington, D.C.: U.S. Government Printing Office.

deVries, H. 1979. Tips on prescribing exercise regimens for your older patient. *Geriatrics* 4:75–81.

Dishman, R.K. 1982. Compliance/adherence in health-related exercise. *Health Psychology* 1:237–267.

Dishman, R.K. 1986. Exercise compliance: A new view for public health. *Physician and Sports Medicine* 14(5):127–145.

Dishman, R.K., Sallis, J.F. and Orenstein, D.R. 1985. The determinants of physical activity and exercise. *Public Health Reports* 100(2):158–171.

Fair, J., Allan-Rosenaur, J., and Thurston, E. 1979, May–June. Exercise management. *Nurse Practitioner,* 13–18.

Farquhar, J. 1978. *The American way of life need not be hazardous to your health.* New York: W. W. Norton.

Fox, S.M., Naughton, J.P., and Gorman, P.A. 1972. Physical activity and cardiovascular health. I. Potential for prevention of coronary heart disease and possible mechanisms. *Modern Concepts of Cardiovascular Disease* 41:17–20.

Froelicher, V.F. 1987. *Exercise and the heart: Clinical concepts* (2d ed.). Chicago: Year Book Medical Publishers.

Gillet, P.A. 1988. Self-reported factors influencing exercise adherence in overweight women. *Nursing Research* 37(1):25–29.

Goldberg, W., and Fitzpatrick, J. 1980. Movement therapy with the aged. *Nursing Research* 20:339–346.

Hagberg, J.M., and Seals, D.R. 1986. Exercise training and hypertension. *Acta Medica Scandinavica* (Suppl.):210–230.

Haskell, W.L. 1986. The influence of exercise training on plasma lipids and lipoproteins in health and disease. *Acta Medica Scandinavica* (Suppl.):25–37.

Harris, L., et al. 1978. *Health maintenance.* Mutual Pacific Life Insurance Co. N.Y.

Hayes, D., and Ross, C.E. 1986. Body and mind: The effect of exercise, overweight, and physical health on psychological well-being. *Journal of Health and Social Behavior* 27:387–400.

Hellerstein, H.K., et al. 1969. Walk, jog, run or play in shape. *Hospital Physician* 51:77–85.

Herje, P. 1980. Hows and whys of patient contracting. *Nurse Educator* January–February, 30–34.

Heyden, S., and Fodor, G. 1988. Does regular exercise prolong life expectancy? *Sports Medicine* 6:63–71.

Hill J.S. 1985. Effect of a program of aerobic exercise on the smoking behavior of a group of adult volunteers. *Canadian Journal of Public Health* 76:183–186.

Johnson, R. 1983. Common running injuries of leg and foot. *Minnesota Medicine,* 441–443.

Kannel, W.B. 1983. High-density lipoproteins: Epidemiologic profile and risks of coronary artery disease. *American Journal of Cardiology* 52:98–128.

Kannel, W.B., et al. 1986. Physical activity and physical demand on the job and the risk of cardiovascular disease and death: The Framingham study. *American Heart Journal* 112:820–825.

Kasl, S.V., and Cobb, S. 1966. Health behavior, illness behavior, and sick role behavior. Part I. *Archives of Environmental Health* 12:246–266.

Kittleson, M.J., and Hageman-Rigney, B. 1988. Wellness and behavior contracting. *Health Education* 19:8–11.

Lampman, R. 1987. Evaluating and prescribing exercise for elderly patients. *Geriatrics* 8(42):63–65, 75.

LaPorte, R.E., et al. 1984. The spectrum of physical activity, cardiovascular disease and health: An epidemiologic perspective. *American Journal of Epidemiology* 120:507–517.

McArdle, W.D., Katch, F.I., and Katch, V.L. 1986. *Exercise physiology, energy, nutrition and human performance* (2d ed.). Philadelphia: Lea and Febiger.

Marcinik, E.J., et al. 1985. Aerobic/calisthenic and aerobic/circuit weight training programs for navy men: A comparative study. *Medicine and Science in Sports and Exercise* 17:482–487.

Martin, J.E., and Dubbert, P.M. 1984. Behavioral management strategies for improving health and fitness. *Journal of Cardiac Rehabilitation* 4:200–208.

Morgan, P.P., Shephard, R.J., and Finucane, R. 1984. Health beliefs and exercise habits in an employee fitness programe. *Canadian Journal of Applied Sports Medicine* 9:87–93.

Morgan, W.P. 1985, February. Affective beneficence of vigorous physical activity. *Medicine and Science in Sports and Exercise* 17:94–100.

Morris, J., et al. 1953. Coronary heart disease and physical activity work. *Lancet* 2:1053–1057, 1111–1120.

Muhlenkamp, A.F., and Sayles, J.A. 1986. Self-esteem, social support, and positive health practices. *Nursing Research* 35:334–338.

Neale, A.V., et al. 1990. The use of behavioral contracting to incrase exercise activity. *American Journal of Health Promotion* 4(6):441–447.

Oldridge, N.B. 1982. Compliance and exercise in primary and secondary prevention of coronary heart disease: A review. *Preventive Medicine* 11:56–70.

Paffenberger, R.S., et al. 1970. Work activity of longshoremen as related to death from coronary heart disease and stroke. *New England Journal of Medicine* 282:1109–1114.

Paffenberger, R.S., et al. 1977. Work-energy level, personal characteristics, and fatal heart attack: A birth cohort affect. *American Journal of Epidemiology* 105:200–213.

Paffenberger, R.S., et al. 1986. Physical activity, all-cause mortality, and longevity of college alumni. *New England Journal of Medicine* 314:605–613.

Pender, N.J. 1987. *Health promotion in nursing practice* (2d ed.). Norwalk, Conn.: Appleton-Lange.

Pender, N.J., and Pender, A.R. 1986. Attitudes, subjective norms and intentions to engage in health behaviors. *Nursing Research* 35:15–18.

Perri, S., and Templar, D. 1984. The effects of an aerobic exercise program on psychological variables in older adults. *International Journal of Aging and Human Development* 5(20):167–170.

Pollock, M.L., et al. 1977. Effects of frequency and duration of training on attrition and incidence of injury. *Medicine and Science in Sports and Exercise* 9:31–38.

Pollock, M.L., and Wilmore, J.H. 1990. *Exercise in health and disease: Evaluation and prescription for prevention and rehabilitation* (2d ed.). Philadelphia: W.B. Saunders.

Powell, K.E., et al. 1986. An epidemiological perspective on the causes of running injuries. *Physican and Sportsmedicine* 14(6):100–114.

Powell, K.E., et al. 1987. Physical activity and the incidence of coronary heart disease. *Annual Review of Public Health* 8:253–287.

Raglin, J.S. and Morgan, W.P. 1987. Influence of exercise and quiet rest on state anxiety and blood pressure. *Medicine and Science in Sports and Exercise* 19(5):456–463.

Rippe, J.M. 1987. The health benefits of exercise (part 1 of 2). *Physican and Sports Medicine* 15(10):115–132.

Safran, M., Seaber, A., and Garrett, W. 1989. Warm-up and muscular injuries. *Sports Medicine* 8(4):239–249.

Schoenborn, C. 1986, November–December. Health habits of U.S. adults, 1985: The "Alameda 7" revisited. *Public Health Reports* 101(6):571–580.

Seals, D.R., and Hagberg, J.M. 1984. The effect of exercise training on human hypertension: A review. *Medicine and Science in Sports and Exercise* 16:207–215.

Shephard, R. 1986. Physical training for the elderly. *Clinics in Sports Medicine* 5:517–530.

Siscovick, D.S. Laporte, R.E., and Newman, J.M. 1985. The disease-specific benefits and risks of physical activity and exercise. *Public Health Reports* 100(2):180–188.

Steckel, S.B. 1982. *Patient contracting.* Norwalk, Conn.: Appleton-Century-Crofts.

Stephens, T., Jacobs, D., and White, C.A. 1985, March–April. Descriptive epidemiology of leisure-time physical activity. *Public Health Reports* 100(2):147–158.

Wankel, L.M. 1985. Personal and situational factors affecting exercise involvement: The importance of enjoyment. *Research Quarterly for Exercise and Sport* 56(3):275–282.

Wenger, H.A., and Bell G.J. 1986. The interactions of intensity, frequency, and duration of exercise training in altering cardio-respiratory fitness. *Sports Medicine* 3:346–356.

Wiley, J.A., and Comacho, T.C. Lifestyle and future health: Evidence from Alameda. *Preventive Medicine* 9:1–21.

Wilmore, J.H., and Costill, D.L. 1988. *Training for sport and activity: The physiological basis of the conditioning process* (3d ed.). Dubuque, Iowa: William C. Brown.

Zohman, L. 1974. *Beyond diet . . . exercise your way to fitness and heart health.* Mazola Corn Oil, CPC International.

PATIENT CONTRACTING

SUSAN BOEHM

Many individuals believe that patient contracts are an easy method of increasing patient adherence. It is all too frequently assumed that the nurse, building on patient education, can simply identify the necessary adherence behaviors and incorporate them into a contract. A contract written in this manner is essentially another set of directions for the patient to follow. Using this approach to identify behaviors for the contract may represent thoughtful nursing judgment, but it does not represent behaviors chosen by the patient. More important, such a contract has not seized the opportunity to teach the patient the behavioral principles underlying the use of the contract.

A patient contract that simply identifies behavioral goals for the patient will probably be no more successful in changing patient behavior than telling the patient what is expected of him or her. The success of Patient Contracting depends on the skills the patient learns during the process of developing a series of contracts. Patient contracts provide a unique opportunity for patients to learn to analyze their behavior in relationship to the environment and to choose behavioral strategies that will facilitate learning, changing, or maintaining a behavior. Hence, behavorial analysis provides the essential data for developing patient contracts.

THE CORE OF THE CONTRACT: BEHAVIORAL ANALYSIS

Behavioral analysis provides the foundation and core for the contract developed between the patient and the nurse. Behavioral analysis is the process by which the behavior is analyzed from three perspectives (Brigham 1982): antecedent events that precede the behavior, small steps that make up the behavior, and consequences that follow the behavior. The behavioral data used in the analysis are obtained by the patient through self-monitoring.

The behavioral analyses of these three perspectives provide direction for choosing behavioral strategies to support the patient's behavioral change. The behavioral strategies include rearranging antecedent events, practicing small steps of the behavior, and rearranging consequences (Barrett, Johnston, Pennypacker 1986). The strategies or techniques used to assist in the behavioral change are called behavioral strategies or behavioral techniques.

The behavioral analysis and strategies are not unfamiliar to most of us. These techniques have been integrated into programs for increasing exercise, managing time, developing study habits, controlling weight, and decreasing smoking (Nelson and Hayes 1986; Green 1984). Behavioral analysis and behavioral strategies have been the focus of many television talk shows and the subject of many books and have been widely reported in the popular press.

The behavioral analysis and strategies discussed in this chapter are based on research of psychological approaches to behavioral management exemplified by behavioral weight control programs. In the weight control model, individuals are taught to monitor behavior and to analyze the personal, social, and environmental variables that function as cues and reinforcers for their behaviors (Wilson and Brownell 1980; Farquhar 1978; Ferster, Nurnberger, and Levitt 1962; Stuart 1967).

Self-Monitoring and Behavioral Analysis

Behavioral analysis begins with the patient's self-monitoring the desired behavior. The goal of self-monitoring is to provide the patient and the nurse with a written record obtained by observing and counting the behavior. The behavior is observed and counted in order to identify and analyze the behaviors and their relationship to the environment.

Self-monitoring is a critical part of the behavioral change process since the patient's written observations and counting of the behavior provide essential baseline data. It is difficult to evaluate the effectiveness of the behavioral strategies in the absence of baseline measurements. Baseline data are important whether a behavior is being learned, decreased, eliminated, or maintained.

Thus, through self-monitoring, the patient collects data for analysis. Using the patient's self-monitored data, the nurse teaches and guides the patient to identify antecedent events that precede the behavior, small steps that make up the behavior, and consequences that follow the behavior. Based on these analyses, behavioral strategies are chosen that will assist in the behavioral change. Once these skills are learned, the patient will be able to use them for long-term maintenance, as well as for changing other behaviors.

Identifying Antecedent Events

An antecedent event precedes the behavior. When a behavior has been learned, having been followed by a reinforcing consequence, the antecedent event takes on the characteristics of a stimulus or cue that prompts the behavior. This stimulus may be strong enough to evoke the behavior even in the absence of a reinforcer. Sometimes the antecedent event becomes an extremely strong stimulus that actually controls the behavior. In this case, the behavior is described as being under stimulus control.

Thus, when the behavioral analysis indicates that the behavior the patient chooses to eliminate or decrease is strongly influenced by an antecedent event, the behavioral strategy is to rearrange, avoid, or eliminate the antecedent event. For example, it is not always apparent that thirst is often a cue for eating, especially between meals. Thirst can be identified as a cue for eating by observing and recording whenever one eats and how one felt before eating. In order to eliminate thirst as a cue to eat, the behavioral strategy is to provide easy access to fluids throughout the day.

In contrast, should the patient wish to increase a behavior, an antecedent event or cue can be arranged so as to prompt the behavior. For example, setting out one's jogging clothes and shoes in the morning may be an effective cue for jogging as soon as one gets home from work.

Identifying Small Steps in the Behavior

Counting the behavior is essential in order to measure progress. It also plays a critical role in identifying the multiple small steps that make up most of the complex behaviors patients need to learn or alter. When small steps are identified, the behavioral strategy is to practice a small step of the desired behavior for a designated period of time. When that small step has increased significantly and has been practiced regularly, the next small step can be added. Eventually the many small steps are chained together, resulting in the desired behavior. This behavioral strategy is particularly effective because patients are often overwhelmed by what is expected of them, which leads to lack of adherence.

Daily exercise, for example, is an extremely complex behavior that can be initiated in small steps. Some of the small steps include experimenting with several forms of exercise, exercising at a variety of times, and trying a variety of places to find the one most conducive to exercise. When the type of exercise is chosen, additional small steps include practicing the exercise for the shortest length of time and the fewest number of days per week. Each week the exercise is increased in small increments until the exercise routine adds up to the desired number and length of time.

Small steps can also be used to decrease or change a behavior. Small steps of a behavior can be practiced in a new pattern, thus changing the undesired behavior. For example, for a patient who wants to cut down on the number of calories eaten during a meal, a behavioral strategy is to put one's fork down between bites. This gives the body time to feel satisfied before too much food and calories are consumed. By altering small steps within the complex behavior of eating, behavior is changed and the consumption of calories reduced.

Identifying Consequences

Most behaviors are controlled or influenced by the consequences that immediately follow the behavior. If the consequences are important and pleasant, there is an increased likelihood of performing the behavior again. The only way to determine if a consequence has increased the behavior is to count the behavior and the presence of the consequence. If the behavior increases when the consequence has followed, the consequence is said to be reinforcing.

By analyzing the behavior, it is possible to identify consequences present in the environment that provide consistent reinforcement or support for numerous behaviors. Often the behavior that requires changing also requires that new consequences replace old ones. Behavioral analysis provides a means of identifying the reinforcing consequences and often provides clues for new consequences.

Frequently behavioral analysis indicates that the consequences need to be rearranged. Thus, the behavioral strategy is to provide adequate reinforcement for a new behavior or to eliminate old reinforcers for an undesired behavior. For example, each small step of initiating a daily exercise routine will be strengthened if followed by a reinforcing consequence. Reinforcing consequences could take many forms, including cognitive reinforcement as feelings of pride, social reinforcement as praise from a family member, or self-reinforcement as twenty-five cents toward a magazine. If the behavior is not increased or is not maintained, a new consequence needs to be tried.

In contrast, undesirable behaviors may require the elimination or substitution of consequences. For example, eating behavior is strongly reinforced by social consequences. If one is attempting to lose weight, it is often better to eat with others who are trying to lose weight than with those who do not need to lose weight. Those who are trying to lose weight are much more likely to praise efforts to eat smaller quantities and to praise choices of the correct foods.

Summary

Behavioral analysis of the data supplied by the patient's self-monitoring provides an opportunity to identify antecedents to the behavior, small steps of the behavior, and consequences of the behavior. By identifying these three perspectives of a given behavior, the appropriate behavioral strategy can be chosen.

The various steps in behavioral analysis and the practicing of the behavioral strategies become the focus for the patient contract. Specific behaviors chosen for the contract are behaviors that involve some aspect of the behavioral analysis and practice of the behavioral strategy.

CONTINGENCY CONTRACTING

The use of written contracts between therapist and client began in the early 1970s. The majority of articles and reports of research using contracts are found mainly in journals of psychology and social work. More recently it has been indexed under such key words as *behavioral strategies, behavioral interventions, contingency contracts, therapeutic contracts, treatment contracts, compliance/adherence,* and *behavioral health/medicine.*

The use of contracts in nursing has been reviewed in the *Annual Review of Nursing Research* (Boehm 1989). Research related to the effectiveness of patient contracts has been reported since the 1970s and has been used in a variety of settings and for a number of behaviors. These include maintenance of potassium levels for patients on dialysis, reduction of blood pressure in hypertension, reduction of blood sugar in diabetes, increase in patient knowledge, and increased use of contraceptives. Associated nursing diagnoses include Noncompliance, Knowledge Deficit, Ineffective Individual Coping, Altered Parenting, and Self-Care Deficit.

There are essentially two types of contracts: the contingency contract and the treatment or therapeutic contract. The treatment contract is structured in a more legalistic manner and is an attempt to formalize the treatment goals, a time limit, the treatment methods, personnel involved, and the degree of patient involvement. Like the contingency contract, the treatment contract is written and signed. Unlike the contingency contract, the treatment contract is focused on the therapeutic work to be accomplished between the patient and therapist (Rosen 1978). The treatment contract assumes that the therapist and client agree that the therapist will provide skills and time to the patient. In return, the patient will discuss the problem openly and honestly, will apply the therapist's advice, and will pay for the treatment (Rosen 1978).

In contrast, the contingency contract is based on the principle of positive reinforcement, which states that when a behavior is followed by a reinforcing consequence, there is an increased probability of that behavior's being performed again (Ayllon and Azrin 1968). Thus, providing a reinforcer for the performance of a specific behavior such as a written record of one's eating behavior will increase the probability that the patient will repeat the reinforced behavior. The contingency contract is a technique by which the desired behaviors are specified clearly and favorable consequences are identified in advance. Thus, appropriate reinforcers can be given when the behavior has been performed successfully.

In order to establish and maintain specificity of the behavior and the reinforcer, the contract is written. The patient makes the final choice of the behavior and the reinforcer. Whenever possible, the time frame for performance of the behavior is also identified. Both the patient and the nurse sign the contract.

This chapter will discuss the contingency contract and assumes that the behaviors chosen for it will have been identified during the continuing analysis of the patient's behavior conducted by the patient and nurse. The contingency contract is used to teach the patient how to analyze his or her own behavior and to reinforce the behaviors identified in the contract. The term *contract* will be used to refer to contingency contracts.

Choosing the Behavior for the Contract

The nursing process is a logical and effective basis in which to build the contract. It provides the nurse with the necessary clinical data which can be shared with the patient. The clinical data clarify for both the patient and nurse some of the priorities necessary to achieve wellness. A description of how to build the contract on the nursing process can be found in *Patient Contracting* (Steckel 1981). In contrast, developing the contract may seem false and contrived to the patient if the contract is introduced as something out of the ordinary and not as an integral part of the nurse's interaction with the patient.

It is also essential that the patient choose the target behavior to be monitored and analyzed. The self-monitoring and subsequent analysis are more likely to represent thoughtful ideas and plans initiated by the patient when the target behavior is the patient's choice.

The target behavior is the ultimate complex behavior that is to be learned. The target behavior is broken down into small steps, and as each step is practiced, it is reinforced, permitting it to be developed gradually and achieved by the patient. Over a series of contracts, the patient will have a variety of behaviors identified. They generally fall into categories that include self-monitoring, arranging, and rearranging antecedent events, practicing small steps of the target behavior, and arranging for reinforcing consequences.

In most cases, the first behavior identified for the contract will involve some type of self-monitoring that observes the target behavior. The patient may also include general notes designed to help identify antecedent events or consequences later in the process of the behavioral analysis. It is important, however, to start the self-monitoring in small steps. Because self-monitoring and the other behavioral strategies are new behaviors for the patient to learn, the principle of moving in small steps is a good rule to follow.

There are many forms of counting behavior and self-monitoring. The patient should be encouraged to choose the least intrusive method and the approach most likely to produce data. An example of a contract for self-monitoring might be:

I ___Beth___ will ___record between meal snacks 3 out of 7 days___

in return for ___an 8:00 AM appointment___

Signed ___Beth O'Hara___

Signed ___Sharon L. Worthington___

date ___1-2-91___ .

The results of the patient's self-monitoring become the focus of the next interaction with the nurse. The nurse and the patient go over the data together and consider ideas for breaking the behavior down into small steps. The self-monitored data may also permit a search for appropriate antecedents and reinforcers. The patient who has been encouraged to choose a behavior will have found the monitoring to be of particular interest and will have rich data, new insights, and suggestions for behaviors in future contracts.

The behavior for the second contract frequently involves more self-monitoring. Two to three contracts that focus on self-monitoring may be needed before one of the behavioral strategies is attempted. Such strategies will be related to arranging antecedent events, practicing a small step of the behavior, or arranging for reinforcing consequences. An example of such a contract might be:

I __Beth_____ will __substitute 2 apples for snacks_____

in return for __graph paper for recording my weight_____

Signed __Beth O'Hara_____

Signed __Sharon L. Worthington_____

date __1-25-91_____ .

A new contract is developed at each visit; however, that does not mean that a new behavior is chosen each time. Most of the time the patient will choose the same behavior over several contracts. New behaviors, even in small steps, require considerable time to practice, learn, and maintain.

The self-monitoring continues in some form even when the patient identifies other behaviors for the contract. The self-monitoring provides the data for analysis that will indicate whether the new antecedent events, the performance of small steps of the behavior, or new consequences are increasing the behavior. In other words, the ongoing behavioral analysis is dependent on these data.

In reality, the patient is given the reinforcer, identified in the contract, for producing the self-monitored records of the rearranged antecedents, the practice of small behavioral steps, and the provision of reinforcing consequences. A behavior can be reinforced only if it is observed, measured, and counted. Since the nurse is not in a position to observe the patient's practicing the behavioral strategies, the reinforcer cannot be a consequence for these behaviors. However, the reinforcer the nurse provided serves as the consequence for the self-monitored data used for the behavioral analysis. As a result, the patient is reinforced for participating in and learning the techniques of analyzing and changing behavior.

Choosing the Reinforcer for the Contract

The reinforcer identified for the contract provides the same function as the reinforcing consequences that support the patient's behavior identified during the behavioral analysis. However, it is a consequence that will be provided by the nurse in return for the self-monitored records the patient brings to the visit.

The form of reinforcement is a critical element and has several important characteristics. First and foremost, the patient must choose the reinforcement. Each reinforcer history is as personal as one's fingerprints, and what is reinforcing for one person will probably not be reinforcing for another. A reinforcer menu or list of potential reinforcers is an effective way of giving the patient an idea of available reinforcers. Sometimes these are written, but they can be simply named as suggestions.

The availability of reinforcers varies greatly by the settings and opportunities. However, each of us has a rich reservoir of potential reinforcers from which a patient can choose. For example, the nurse is in a unique position to make arrangements for more convenient appointments, parking arrangements, or a quiet place to work while waiting for an appointment. Reading to a patient, finding relatively new but used copies of magazines, locating a favorite newspaper, finding a partner for cards, lending a game, or arranging for a special food or dinner are but a few ideas for hospitalized patients. Volunteers in many settings are willing and helpful to provide time and items patients may request.

These more tangible reinforcers can also be earned. If a patient is practicing a repetitive behavior such as the small steps of a specific exercise, tokens or points can be given. These can be collected and exchanged for a larger reinforcer. Indeed, the counting or accumulation of tokens can be a powerful reinforcer since this serves as a form of counting behavior. Research data have demonstrated that people like to keep track of their own performance, and patients are no exception. Simple records kept with paper and pencil at the bedside or graph paper and colored felt-tip pens are eagerly kept. Children particularly like to paste stickers onto a calendar or a sheet of paper as a means of counting their behavior.

Nurses provide a considerable amount of social praise and reinforcement; however, they do not provide such praise in a systematic manner that is related to a very specific behavior and level of that performance. They have the potential to provide powerful forms of reinforcement through thoughtful and systematic attention and praise. It is critical, however, that such praise is clearly tied to the specific behavior the patient and nurse are attempting to increase. This needs to be thoughtfully planned and provided each time the behavior is performed and must be seen as separate and different from the usual praise and attention given daily to patients.

CASE STUDY

Margaret was 49 years old and married to an airplane pilot who was gone a good deal of the time. They had three teenaged sons and a small business that repaired golf clubs. Most of the responsibility for the children and the business was Margaret's.

During her annual physical, Margaret was diagnosed as having diabetes. Her physician had assured her that her blood sugar could be easily managed through diet and weight loss. Margaret was 50 pounds overweight, and her weight had been a lifetime battle for her. The diagnosis did not particularly worry her since there was a family history of diabetes.

The stress in her life contributed to Margaret's feelings of fatigue and a sense of being overwhelmed with responsibilities. Her physician and dietitian wanted her to measure her capillary glucose levels after she got up in the morning and before dinner in the evening. However, these were the two most harried times in her day, and she was never able to remember. Thus, she never brought her records of the glucose levels to clinic. "They were blank sheets of paper."

Nurse: Margaret, would you be willing to bring in your records next week, no matter if you tested your glucose only once?
Margaret: If you want to see a blank record, I guess I can do that.

Margaret and the nurse then wrote a contract: Margaret would bring her record of glucose levels to the clinic in return for a 15-minute appointment at 7:45 A.M. The appointment coincided with dropping one of her sons off at swim practice.

The following week Margaret's record indicated that she had tested her glucose three mornings out of seven and four evenings out of seven:

Nurse: Margaret, this is excellent! You measured your capillary glucose nearly half of the time. It is never easy to learn new habits at your age, much less with all the pressures and demands in your life. It must have taken some real effort to remember and then to measure your glucose. Do you have any ideas why it was easier for you on some days than on other days?

Margaret: My days are really crazy, and the mornings and mealtimes of the day are the worst. I have no idea why or how I did it on those particular days.

Nurse: From what you have told me, your days sound as if there is not time for yourself, much less time to think. If you are willing, though, I think we can gather some clues about your day that may help you plan for those days that are the worst. Want to give it a try?

Margaret: It has to be easy to do. I cannot fit one more thing into those times of the day. And if you want me to come back next week, it will have to be a 15-minute appointment at 7:45 A.M. as we did this morning.

Nurse: That is a deal. Let's make another contract. You will mark the graph indicating your glucose level as you did last week. But this time describe in four or five words what happened just before and just after you tested your glucose. On those days you don't have time to test it, try to recall what happened that prevented you from doing it. Then bring it back next week, and let's see what we find.

The following week as Margaret and the nurse reviewed the records, they noticed an increase in the monitoring. The record keeping itself seemed to be acting as a reinforcer. In addition, Margaret was more likely to measure her glucose on days that the children did not interrupt her and she had a few minutes of privacy in her bedroom.

Nurse: Margaret, do your notes give you any ideas as to circumstances you could rearrange so that you could more easily test your glucose?

Margaret: Who can control the kids or our schedules? I sure can't. Isn't there something easier I can try?

Nurse: For example? What do you have in mind?

Margaret: I could keep my record of the glucose but agree to test it just before I put on my makeup. I will not leave until my makeup is on so I could think of testing my glucose as a part of the makeup routine.

Nurse: That is a great idea. That is one of the best ways to learn a new behavior. Couple it with an old behavior or habit. You have really made progress. Over the last 2 weeks, you have significantly increased the number of times you have tested your glucose, and you have discovered some important clues about how you can increase it even more often. That is worth a bonus! Here is a token for the parking lot that you can use on your next visit.

Margaret: You have a deal. Next week, I want another parking token in return for measuring my glucose 6 out of 7 days.

Nurse: It is a deal!

Margaret continued to test her capillary blood glucose regularly. She did not measure her glucose six out of seven days the first week but in the following weeks she measured no less than six times a week. She became adept at readjusting the antecedents and reinforcing herself. She lost 50 pounds over the coming year, and her glucose was reduced significantly. It was eventually no longer necessary for her to check her glucose as often, but the skills she learned in doing so helped her to lose the weight and to maintain a lowered weight.

CONCLUSION

Besides providing a mechanism for assisting the patient to make behavioral changes, the successful use of contracts has several characteristics that translate into additional benefits. A series of written contracts provides a history of progress toward desired behaviors for both the patient and nurse. In order to be used successfully, the contract must be specific and explicit and stated in observable and measurable terms. If the behavior is not measurable and observable, it cannot be reinforced. A record provides evidence of progress and clarifies expectations of the patient. Consequently, the patient is clear as to what is expected. Specificity and clarity of expectations increase patient confidence and the likelihood of success in achieving desired behaviors.

As the nurse assists the patient in the behavioral analysis and in developing the contracts, it becomes clearer how the nurse's behavior can serve as a cue and a reinforcer for the patient's behavior. In other words, the nurse's behavior can function to stimulate patient responses and reinforce behaviors. By increasing awareness of how nurses' behavior influences the behavior of the patient, adjustments can be made so that nursing behavior stimulates and reinforces the behavior desired more effectively than would otherwise be possible.

REFERENCES

Ayllon, T., and Azrin, N. 1968. The token economy. New York: Appleton-Century-Crofts.

Barrett, B.H., Johnston, J.M., and Pennypacker, H.S. 1986. Behavior: Its units, dimensions, and measurement. In R.O. Nelson and S.C. Hayes (eds.), *Conceptual foundations of behavioral assessment* (pp. 156–200). New York: Guilford Press.

Boehm, S. 1989. Patient contracting. In J.J. Fitzpatrick, R.L. Taunton, and J.Q. Benoliel (eds.), *Annual review of nursing research* (pp. 143–154). New York: Springer.

Brigham, T. 1982. Self-management: A radical behavioral perspective. In P. Karoly and F.H. Kanfer (eds.), *Self-management and behavior change* (pp. 32–59). New York: Pergamon Press.

Carmody, T., Fey, S.G., Pierce, D.K., Connor, W.E., and Matarazzo, J.C. 1982. Behavioral treatment of hyperlipidemia: Techniques, results, and future directions. *Journal of Behavioral Medicine* 5 (1):91–116.

Farquhar, J.W. 1978. The community-based model of life style intervention trials. *American Journal of Epidemiology* (August) 108 (2):103–11.

Ferster, C.B., Nurnberger, J.I., and Levitt, E.P. 1962. The control of eating. *Journal of Mathetics* 1:87–109.

Green, L.W. 1984. Modifying and developing health behavior. *Annual Review of Public Health* 5:215–236.

Nelson, R.O., and Hayes, S.C. 1986. The nature of behavioral assessment. In R.O. Nelson and S.C. Hayes (eds.), *Conceptual foundations of behavioral assessment* (pp. 3–41). New York: Guilford Press.

Rosen, B. 1978. Written contracts: Their use in planning treatment programs for inpatients. *British Journal of Psychiatry* 133:410–415.

Steckel, S.B. 1981. *Patient contracting.* Norwalk, Conn.: Appleton-Century-Crofts.

Wilson, G.T., and Brownell, K.D. 1980. Behavior therapy for obesity: An evaluation of treatment outcome. *Advanced Behavior Research Therapy* 3:49–86.

34

RELAXATION TRAINING

SHARON SCANDRETT-HIBDON
SUSAN UECKER

Relaxation Training is composed of a group of varied and powerful techniques that are clinically accepted to counter the effects of stress. In this chapter, Relaxation Training techniques are reviewed and organized into a framework. A five-step program drawing from these techniques is presented as an effective nursing model for intervention.

First, the techniques are classified into two basic categories: externally oriented and internally oriented Relaxation Training procedures. Externally oriented relaxation techniques rely on a more outward focus. Procedures included in this category are progressive muscle relaxation, biofeedback, hypnosis, and healing touch. Internally oriented procedures have a more inner focus and include autogenic relaxation training, meditation, and self-hypnosis. The five-step program moves systematically from externally oriented relaxation techniques to internally oriented ones.

RELAXATION AS A RESPONSE TO STRESS

H. Benson, associate professor at Harvard Medical School and director of the Hypertension Section of Boston's Beth Israel Hospital, describing the relaxation response, claims:

> Each of us possesses a natural innate protective mechanism against "overstress," which allows us to turn off harmful bodily effects, to counter the effects of the fight or flight response. This response against "overstress" brings on bodily changes that decrease heart rate, lower metabolism, decrease the rate of breathing, and bring the body back into what is probably a healthier balance. (Benson and Klipper 1976, p. 26)

This response is proposed to be an integrated hypothalamic response resulting in decreased sympathetic nervous system activity and increased parasympathetic nervous system activity (Benson, Beary, and Carol 1974).

The relaxation response has the opposite effect of Selye's (1956) stress response. Early in the twentieth century, Cannon (1914) described the fight-or-flight response, or emergency reaction, which prepares the individual for fighting or running through increases in heart rate, blood pressure, breathing rate, metabolism, and levels of epinephrine, other hormones, and blood glucose; peripheral vascular constriction; dilation of the pupils; and decreased testosterone levels; Benson and Klipper 1976; Budzynski 1982; Cannon 1914; Mason 1980; Selye 1956). Studies demonstrate that regardless of the nature of stress (physical, chemical, or psychosocial), the final common pathways are stimulation of adrenocortical secretion with increase in serum glucocorticoids and sympathetic nervous system stimulation with a release of catecholamines (Khansari, Murgo, and Faith 1990). Benson and Klipper (1976) contend that when the fight-or-flight response is not used appropriately — for example, when minor stressors rather than catastrophic life events trigger this response — its repeated elicitation may lead to serious problems such as heart attack or stroke. For example, although you may become stressed and worried over events such as paying the rent, it is unlikely that you will die from not paying the rent. Your body, however, cannot distinguish the hypothetical threat that you create in your mind from an imminent real catastrophic event. In other words, the full stress response can be triggered by expectations, ideas, fears, memories, or emotions, as well as by life-threatening events.

Mason (1980) reports that some people get addicted to the rush of adrenaline (epinephrine) and need stress to keep the epinephrine flowing. He claims that such people will eat a lot of sugar quickly, which raises the blood glucose level, thus inducing a fight-or-flight physiological effect. This elevation causes the body to respond as if under threat; for example, "Eating a hot fudge sundae may elicit the same response as a roller coaster ride" (p. 3).

Many individuals tend to perpetuate or thrive on being tense or feeling this sense of rush. However, over time, the body responds by creating physical symptoms in an attempt to notify the individual that something is going wrong, and there is need to change the living conditions. For example, the heart may develop symptoms of tachycardia since it was not designed to be in stress 90° of the time. Symptoms or diseases often associated with stress include headaches, hypertension, tight or sore muscles, back pain, jaw tension, cold hands and feet, skin problems, allergies, asthma, arthritis, peptic ulcers, colitis, constipation, diarrhea, insomnia, fatigue, overeating, sexual dysfunction, fearfulness, forgetfulness, and cancer.

The immune response is affected by stress, particularly through neuroendocrine function and central nervous system interaction. Neurotransmitters and hormones with immunomodulatory properties suppressed by stress include glucocorticoids and catecholamines, which affect antibody production, natural killer cell activity, cytokine production, and lymphocyte proliferation to mitogen. Factors enhanced by stress include acetylcholine, met-enkephalin, dynorphin, thyroxine, prolactin, growth hormone, vasopressin, oxytocin, and melatonin which affect the number of lymphocytes and macrophages in bone marrow, T cell activation, phytohemagglutinin stimulation of T cell, plaque-forming cell, macrophage activation, interleukin 2 production and modulation, antibody synthesis and T cell proliferation. Other factors that may be suppressed or enhanced include sex hormones, beta-endorphin, corticotropin, vasoactivate intestinal peptide, and somatostatin (Khansari, Murgo, and Faith 1990).

The immune system weakens if stress is chronic, increasing susceptibility to illness (Budzynski 1982; Zegans 1982). Research findings show that altered moods, as in bereavement, suppress the ability of T lymphocytes to respond to mitogen stimulation or in major depressive disorders, which show depressed lymphocyte responses to mitogens, lymphocytopenia, and hypercortisolemia. Loneliness seems to result in suppression of natural killer cell activity, and immunologic abnormalities were seen in schizophrenics (Solomon 1981; Tecoma and Huey 1985). In contrast, survival time seems to be prolonged for some patients with cancer and acquired immune deficiency syndrome (AIDS) who have positive mental states (Derogatis, Abeloff, and Melisaratow 1979; Solomon, Temoshile, O'Leary, and Zick 1987).

In juxtaposition to the stress responses, relaxation elicits opposite physiological

TABLE 34–1.   COMPARISON OF PHYSIOLOGICAL STRESS AND
RELAXATION RESPONSES

PHYSIOLOGICAL EFFECT	STRESS	RELAXATION
Heart rate	Increased	Decreased
Breathing rate	Increased	Decreased
Metabolism	Increased	Decreased
Muscle tension	Increased	Decreased
Epinephrine	Increased	Decreased
Peripheral blood flow	Decreased	Increased
Blood pressure	Increased	Decreased

effects (Table 34–1). Other reported relaxation responses include an increase in alpha and theta brain waves, skin resistance, deep abdominal breathing, and decreased blood lactate levels. Pelletier (1976) suggests that healthy dealing with acute stressors includes four main states: baseline level, stress reaction (which corresponds to sympathetic nervous system stimulation), compensatory relaxation (which corresponds to parasympathetic stimulation), and return to baseline (Figure 34–1). In chronically stressed individuals—for example, the chronic worrier—the stress response stays elevated, with frequent intermittent stress excitation and absence of compensatory relaxation. This pattern of high excitation, Pelletier proposes, leads to disease or exhaustion, which is one way to break the pattern. In an extreme way, after chronic stress, illness produces a relaxation phase, "to let go of those excess levels of self-stressing neurophysiological activity and simply quiet themselves down" (Pelletier 1978, p. 5). When the relaxation response is elicited, the chain of deleterious physiological effects can be broken, preventing the development of symptoms. By altering the physiological stress response, relaxation allows the body to heal and rebalance itself.

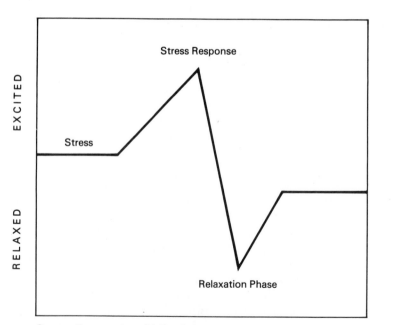

FIGURE 34–1. Healthy Response to Stress

Source: Conversation with Ken Pelletier. Medical Self-Care, 1976.
Reprinted with permission.

Psychological benefits of the relaxation response, which can be self-taught, are also reported: improved quality of life, better coping ability, peace of mind, insight into one's problems, lowered anxiety, and interruption of obsessive thought (Sims 1987). In general, a calming of thoughts and emotions also occurs.

Benson and Klipper (1976) contend that there are four essential elements in eliciting the relaxation response: "a quiet environment; a mental device such as a word or a phrase which should be repeated in a specific fashion over and over again; the adoption of a passive attitude . . . ; a comfortable position (p. 27). If various relaxation techniques are examined, usually all four elements are found to be present.

Externally Oriented Relaxation Techniques

Four types of externally oriented procedures—progressive muscular relaxation, biofeedback, hypnosis and healing touch—have an external component, for example, in progressive muscular relaxation there is externally visible active movement of gross muscle groups; with biofeedback, a biofeedback machine is used, and the external elements include the gauge, lights, or sound that indicates to the client the level of relaxation; in hypnosis and healing touch, there is the external dependence on another person to induce the state of relaxation.

Progressive Muscular Relaxation

Progressive muscular relaxation (PMR) is a systematic technique of tensing and releasing of gross muscle groups while attending to the differences in sensation of tension and relaxation (Berstein and Borkovec 1973). The goal is to increase the client's ability to identify even mild tension and to reduce it. This awareness is an important aspect of relaxation that needs to be developed in the client. Muscle tension may not be recognized consciously. In fact, most readers are unaware of the tension needed to maintain their posture to read this page. PMR is a process by which clients become more aware of and therefore become more in control of their tension levels. It can become a sensitivity program to increase the ability of the client to sense muscle tension and then more willfully let it go. Too often clients are not enough in touch with their bodies to sense tension until it is severe enough to create pain.

Progressive muscle relaxation began with the work of Jacobson in 1938 at Harvard University. He was looking for a technique that did not promote dependency on the part of the client. He also believed that suggestive measures as a rule have failed to induce more than "transitory emotional improvement" (Jacobson 1970). Jacobson discovered that by systematically tensing and releasing the various muscle groups and by learning to discriminate between the resulting sensations of tension and relaxation, a person can almost completely eliminate muscle contraction and experience a feeling of deep relaxation. In this procedure, a cognition or awareness of the difference between tension and relaxation is developed, and the cerebral effect is to attend to relaxation, which signals the muscle to relax.

PMR is based on the underlying assumption that anxiety and relaxation are mutually exclusive; anxiety cannot exist if the muscles are truly relaxed. Jacobson defined anxiety from his later work in having people imagine triggering a telegraphic key with their finger and then getting measurable electrical activity without actual motor activity. He viewed anxiety as the result of the person's seeing or imagining the anxious situation consciously or subconsciously, which then sets the muscles of the person's body into a particular pattern of tension (Jacobson 1970).

Jacobson's original program (1934) required too much time for practical application. Each of 15 muscle groups was worked on for 1 hour to 9 hours daily, for a total of 56 sessions. Wolpe modified Jacobson's program so that the basic training program could be completed in six 20-minute sessions, with two 15-minute periods of daily home practice (Bernstein and Borkovec 1973). Wolpe's technique generally dealt with phobias or fear response, but he helped to originate the modifications that make the technique so widely applicable today. Bernstein and Borkovec were major contributors in refining and shortening the technique (1973). Since then, numerous authors have adapted Jacobson's progressive muscle relaxation technique. Progressive muscle relaxation is a relatively simple technique that can be taught by a trained nurse in a short amount of time.

Biofeedback

Biofeedback, a recent development, evolved from animal experimentation (Miller 1969) in which researchers discovered that "involuntary" responses mediated by the autonomic nervous system could be conditioned. Following World War II, technological advances devised instrumentation that could detect, record, and amplify the body's internally generated electrical impulses and provide a corresponding signal that the subject could interpret. Discovered by individuals in separate laboratories (Budzynski and Stoyva 1969; Green, Walters, Green, and Murphy 1969), biofeedback in relaxation was recognized as helpful in learning deep muscle relaxation (Tarler-Benlolo 1978). Biofeedback research and clinical applications have mushroomed, and the Biofeedback Research Society was formed in 1969 (Gaardner and Montgomery 1977). Certification in biofeedback practice is offered through the Biofeedback Certification Institute of America.

In biofeedback, an artificial closing of the external feedback loop occurs; for example, looking in a mirror provides information for the viewer. Information about biological functions of which an individual ordinarily is unaware is presented to the person so that it can be used to alter the biological function (e.g., reduce muscle tension or lower blood pressure). Voluntary control over automatically regulated body functions allows the person to learn about and to alter the body's response in a more healthful way. In addition to the principle of feedback, Ashby's information theory (1963), which says that a variable cannot be controlled unless information about that variable is available to the controller, applies here. The information is delivered to the person in a neutral way, thus differentiating biofeedback from operant conditioning, in which feedback information is either reinforcing or aversive (Gaardner and Montgomery 1977). The person can utilize the information received in any of several ways.

The feedback process is as simple or as complex as the feedback designer desires. Most feedback systems include physiological monitors, amplification of the physiological stimuli, a processor that selects pertinent physiological information, a feedback generator that alters information into meaningful units, and a feedback display (Breeden and Kondo 1975). The feedback information can be continuous (analog) or discontinuous (digital). Physiological parameters utilized most often include electromyography (EMG), temperature, sound, electroencephalography (EEG), psychogalvanometer, and cardiovascular monitoring. In Relaxation Training, the physiological parameters utilized most often are muscle tension, heart rate, blood pressure, and hand temperature. Feedback information reported to be utilized most frequently in clinical settings involves continuous or discontinuous tones reflecting muscle tension, heart rate, blood pressure, or skin temperature.

An example of use of EMG biofeedback for Relaxation Training involved having the client sit in a comfortable position with limbs supported. Silver–silver chloride electrodes are placed over the client's frontalis muscle, which has been cleaned, removing loose epidermis and oil from the skin. EMG levels are monitored prior to turning on the feedback machine so that a microvolt scale can be selected that allows fluctuation of muscle tension levels. The client is asked to listen to a continuous tone feedback in which the pitch reflects the tension in the muscle. The goal is for the client to lower the pitch of the sound, utilizing any relaxation technique he or she chooses. The client is asked to focus on how the body feels when the pitch is low. Home practice is encouraged and may involve utilizing a portable biofeedback machine or simulating the body sensations felt during the lowest-pitched sounds of the training sessions. One of the difficulties with this approach is that transfer of learning from the machine must be carefully planned and reinforced. Dependence on the biofeedback machinery has been noted and a return to previous tension patterns observed within a 6-month period.

Hypnosis

Hypnosis can be very useful in nursing. Techniques are not discussed in detail here because the use of hypnosis requires supervised practice by qualified professionals. We all have experienced naturally occurring hypnotic states — for example "spacing out" in a boring class or during a Sunday sermon (Grinder and Bandler 1981). Also, most of us have some erroneous notions of what hypnosis is, according to our experiences with a stage hypnotist, television show, movie, or book, which have made hypnosis seem like magic or mind control.

According to LeCron (1971), it is difficult to define hypnosis but easy to describe it. This difficulty perhaps contributes to the distortions and confusion. In a hypnotic state, subjects are aware of their environment, but the focus is internal. Clients are more suggestible than at other times but still behave within the limits of their own moral codes. Persons who are hypnotized are actually quite protective of themselves but may be surprised at their resourcefulness in coming up with creative solutions to their problems or in seeing different perceptions of situations (LeCron 1971). It is useful to think of hypnosis as an advanced stage of relaxation, since relaxation techniques are a usual part of the induction process.

Common phenomena in hypnosis are hyperamnesia, an ability to remember past details forgotten in the conscious mind; age regression, the ability to reexperience a previous event; increased suggestibility; hypnotic anesthesia, the ability to block pain; and time distortion, the sensation that time is contracted or lengthened (LeCron 1971).

Although there are indications that hypnosis has been used throughout history, credit for the discovery is given to Franz Anton Mesmer in 1734. Mesmer, a Viennese physician, is reported to have learned this technique from a Catholic priest. Mesmer's theories were attacked by his colleagues, and he died in obscurity in Austria (Daley and Greenspun 1979; LeCron 1971). Interest in hypnosis has waxed and waned over the years.

Following World War I, use of hypnosis increased, as it did again after World War II, especially in the treatment of battle neurosis. More recently, the influence of Erickson's hypnotic technique, based on story telling and use of metaphor, has been felt as his followers carry on his work (Zeig 1982). In addition, the work done by Grinder and Bandler (1981), who studied and analyzed Erickson's unique style, is having a widespread impact on the practice of hypnosis.

Hypnosis is a powerful procedure for qualified nurses to use — for example, when clients are in such painful or anxious states that they cannot attend to learning PMR or autogenic techniques. Chronic anxiety also can be addressed using hypnotic suggestions, especially in dealing with habits, enhancing patients cooperation, and altering physiological processes. The promotion of comfort and relieving stress are prime considerations for using hypnosis.

Therapeutic Touch

Therapeutic Touch, a nursing intervention, described in Chapter 15, promotes relaxation in a manner well suited to nursing care in acute-care settings. Its use is particularly helpful when the recipient is unable to attend to relaxation instructions. Derived from laying on of hands by Kunz and taught by Krieger (1979), Therapeutic Touch involves the nurse's becoming centered and passively listening with the hands as the hands scan the body of the client in an effort to determine the client's condition. Then energy is smoothed and modulated to wherever the client needs. Research on Therapeutic Touch has demonstrated significant reductions in anxiety, physiological indicators of stress in premature infants, and tension headache pain (Heidt 1981; Quinn 1982; Keller and Bzdek 1986; Fedoruk 1984).

A variation of Therapeutic Touch that involves light fingertip stroking of major energy lines or meridians in the body is called the Scutter technique. It uses long, sweeping motions along the meridians and scooping energy from selected joints (elbows, knees, hands, and feet). This technique promotes deep relaxation and is particularly useful to assist the client in experiencing relaxation in one part of the body while the remainder remains more tense. Clients needing to be touched respond readily to this procedure. Children are especially responsive to Scutter relaxation, particularly at bedtime.

A third technique, developed by Janet Mentgen (1991), produces a deep relaxation. This procedure, called magnetic unruffling, involved 20 to 30 long, slow sweeps of the hands across the whole body field moving from head to toes. An unlayering of energy occurs, with the recipient's slipping into deeper states of relaxation. This procedure dramatically releases blockages and balances the physical body.

Each of these techniques relies heavily on the facilitator since the recipient is passive during the activity. All of these relaxation procedures work well on hospitalized clients who are experiencing distress, pain, restlessness, and agitation. In addition, healing touch works well with outpatients, who can often learn some of the procedures to use on family or themselves.

Internally Oriented Relaxation Techniques

The three internally oriented relaxation techniques—autogenic training, meditation, and self-hypnosis—rely on an inward focus. With these methods, the path to the relaxed state is more passive than with the methods of the externally oriented techniques. Once the internally oriented methods have been learned, clients can use the techniques without the nurse's help. This fact is appealing to nurses in their goal of maintaining control by the client or returning it to the client. This type of intervention is also consistent with the nursing theory of self-care (Orem 1980).

Autogenic Training

Autogenic training, derived from the self-suggestive techniques, was developed by the German psychiatrist and neurologist Schultz in the 1930s. Schultz had been influenced by Vogt, a brain physiologist, who noted that some of his hypnotic subjects could overcome effects of stress such as tension, fatigue, and headaches (Green and Green 1977).

Schultz was attracted to this technique because he was looking for a way to achieve a similar state to hypnosis without the need for the hypnotist. He was intrigued by the idea that the technique did not promote a lack of responsibility by the client and overdependence on the therapist or hypnotist. Schultz found that subjects who experienced the hypnotic state reported two major physical responses: heaviness sensation correlates with relaxation of the muscles, and the warmth is a psychophysiological perception of the vasodilation of the peripheral vessels (Schultz and Luthe 1969).

Autogenic training, then, consists of suggestions to oneself about the relaxing feelings of heaviness and warmth. It is viewed as a self-regulatory mechanism, a way to balance mental and physical functions. Autogenic training is built on the concept of "self-induced passivity or passive concentration" (Schultz and Luthe 1969, p. 14). This idea is similar to that of passive volition, which is often referred to in the literature on relaxation. Passive volition is allowing the sensations to take over rather than an active striving for the relaxation state. This passive opening up of the body to experience these physical sensations is desired; an active pursuit of the desired state is not likely to meet with success.

Schultz and Luthe developed two basic series of exercises. The first series included six components: heaviness (neuromuscular system), warmth (vascular system), heart rhythm (steady, strong), respiration (effortless), warmth (in the abdominal area), and coolness (of the forehead). The second series consists of certain meditative procedures that are not generally used except by advanced followers of Schultz's methods.

Schultz's and Luthe's joint work was built on and modified by Kleinsorge and Klumbies (1964), who looked at specific symptoms and developed specific phrases to use. For example, with headaches, they suggested such phrases as, "My head feels free and light and my forehead pleasantly cool," or "I feel fresh air circulating around my head." The idea of warmth in the face and head is not usually suggested, especially with headaches, because of the resulting vasodilation and the possibility of increased pain.

Investigators inadvertently discovered the usefulness of autogenic training in controlling migraine headaches. During a laboratory session on autogenic warmth, a subject relieved her own migraine when she was able to warm her hands. It is thought that the vascular system tends to rebalance in response to the hand-warming exercise, pulling blood into peripheral circulation; that is, as the hand warms, the head cools and pain is decreased (Green and Green 1977).

Meditation

In Eastern countries meditation has a religious as well as cultural connotation. In Western countries, use of meditation practices has not been common but is increasing. Meditation is being recommended as a relaxation technique, especially in the wellness or holistic health literature. Mason (1980) notes that meditation focuses the individual's attention and alters the level of awareness. During meditation, the person's attention is specifically directed to an image or thought, and the person is entirely involved in the technique.

LeShan (1974) states that meditation may be structured or unstructured. In one type of unstructured meditation, the individual chooses an idea and simply thinks about it, trying to experience the idea fully. This type of meditation requires discipline; the person is to remain focused on the idea rather than allow the mind to go off on distracting thoughts. This is called reflective meditation, in which deeper meanings of an idea are revealed (Meditation group for the new age, 1978). LeShan (1974) suggests that an individual use his or her own response to a technique to determine which meditation is best.

One type of structured meditation is to focus on specific objects, such as a seashell or candle. This type of meditation, called concentration, trains the individual to focus the mind at will and to attend to the present moment (Meditation group for the new age, 1978). Another form makes use of a mantra, a word or phrase repeatedly chanted. An example of mantra meditation is transcendental meditation (TM). Benson and Klipper (1976) chose to study TM subjects after they reviewed the various forms of meditation, finding TM to be basically a yoga technique done in a simple, consistent way. In TM, a trained instructor gives the individual a specific mantra, which is to be kept secret. The meditator repeats this mantra, which helps to prevent distracting thoughts, while sitting in a comfortable position. TM practitioners are usually instructed to meditate 20 minutes twice daily, before breakfast and before dinner.

Another type of meditation is call receptive; this practice opens the individual's receptivity to intuition, insight, aspects of personality, guidance, inspiration, and knowledge. The person silences himself or herself utilizing a mantra, breath, or visualization and then sits in quiet expectancy. Information may be received through seeing, hearing, feeling, inner knowing, or an urge to act (Meditation group for the new age, 1978).

Benson and Klipper (1976) studied TM subjects, noting that they produced a hypometabolic or restful state, in contrast to the physiological. Changes of the fight-or-flight (hypermetabolic) state: a quiet environment, use of a mental device, a passive attitude, and a comfortable position.

In their book, *The Relaxation Response* (1976), Benson and Klipper propose the following meditative technique:

1. Sit quietly in a comfortable position.
2. Close your eyes.
3. Deeply relax all of your muscles, beginning at your feet and progressing up to your face. Keep them relaxed.
4. Breathe through your nose. Become aware of your breathing. As you breathe out, say the word "one" silently to yourself. Breathe easily and naturally.
5. Continue for 10 to 20 minutes. You may open your eyes to check the time, but do not use an alarm. When you finish, sit quietly for several minutes, at first with eyes closed and later with your eyes opened. Do not stand up for a few minutes.
6. Do not worry about whether you are successful in achieving a deep state of relaxation. Maintain a passive attitude and permit relaxation to occur at its own pace. When distracting thoughts occur, try to ignore them by not dwelling upon them and return to repeating "one." With practice the response should come with little effort. Practice the technique once or twice daily, but not within two hours after any meal, since the digestive processes seem to interfere with the elicitation of the relaxation response. (Benson and Klipper, 1976, p. 163)

Self-Hypnosis

Self-hypnosis is the internal half of external hypnosis; it is the result of returning the control and responsibility back to the client after the acuteness of the situation has ceased and the person is ready to learn the technique.

In self-hypnosis individuals induce themselves into a hypnotic state, for example, by reading an induction script into a tape recorder and playing it back when the person wishes to do self-hypnosis or by thinking or saying aloud the hypnotic induction. Generally this technique requires disciplined practice for a person to become comfortable using it. The individual maintains self-control and, to end the hypnotic state, simply says something like, "I am ready to return to my normal state, and on the count of 4, I will open my eyes and feel alert."

Self-hypnosis is similar to autogenic training, but it is usually learned after the person has learned hypnosis. In addition, self-hypnosis, like hypnosis, allows for time in the altered state for the person to solve a problem or get a new perspective on a situation rather than just experience relaxation.

LITERATURE REVIEW

A tremendous number of studies on relaxation have been done in nursing and other areas since the early 1980s, with emphasis specification of effects and uses of relaxation. Three review articles of studies indicated that both biofeedback and autogenic or progressive muscular relaxation, alone or in combination, are effective in treating people with tension and migraine headaches with no evidence that biofeedback is superior to autogenic or PMR (Beaty and Haynes 1979; Tarler-Benlolo 1978; Turner and Chapman 1982). Snyder (1988), in a review of 24 nursing studies, found positive outcome measures in four areas: comfort, improved physiological status, improved psychological status, and combined conditions. Use of at least four training sessions was found to have significant results, and mastery in relaxing muscle groups was found to be important. Common findings of the review articles indicate that home practice is important in maintaining reduction of tension headaches, although effective comfort was evidenced even without home practice. Migraine headaches have responded well to finger-warming biofeedback, a procedure in which the subjects warm fingers using autogenic training and a feedback system to let subjects know of the temperature change. TM was most helpful in elderly residents who were taught one of three procedures (TM, mindfulness training, and relaxation) and examined for improved functioning. Mindfulness produced the next most improved conditions (Alexander, Chandler, Langer, Newman, and Davies 1989).

A meta-analysis by nurses tested the effects of relaxation training on clinical symptoms (Hyman, Feldman, Harris, Levin, and Malloy 1989). Forty-eight non-mechanical-assisted relaxation techniques used to control a variety of clinical symptoms were examined. Findings revealed that treatments of any type, except Benson's relaxation technique, brought improvement in problems such as hypertension, headaches, and insomnia. A series of studies found relaxation to be helpful to clients in reducing sensation and distress of cholecystectomy clients, overall sickness absenteeism, anxiety of adults and children, state and trait anxiety, urinary cortisol levels and wound erythema postsurgically, and diastolic as well as systolic blood pressure (Bailey 1984; Kolkmeier 1982; Lamontagne, Mason, and Hepworth 1985; Levin, Malloy, and Hyaan 1987; Munra, Creamer, Haggerty, and Cooper 1988; Pender 1984, 1985; Holden-Lund 1988; Scandrett, Bean, Breeden, and Powell 1986). Tamez, Moore, and Brown (1978) explored the effect of PMR training on the frequency of use of medications to reduce tension. They also compared the effect of live versus taped relaxation instructions. No significant differences were found in the three groups (control, live instructions, taped instructions), but there were indications that live instructions were more effective than taped instructions. Others have noted the superiority of live instruction

(Berstein and Borkovec 1973; Paul and Trimble 1970). Relaxation with guided imagery was reported useful in reducing state anxiety for a short time (King 1988). Teaching clients combined relaxation techniques is reported to be effective (Bowles, Smith, and Parker, 1979; Garrison and Scott 1979).

Pender (1985) reported that locus of control shifted to a more internal one with the progressive relaxation training in hypertensive patients. This finding differed in a study using a five-step relaxation procedure on three populations (psychiatric, cardiac and cancer), where no significant changes were reported on locus of control (Scandrett-Hibdon, Lomenick, Sachse, and Hart 1983).

Concern over limitations and side effects was reported (Lazarus and Mayne 1990). Some of these concerns were that in tense subjects taught progressive relaxation, paradoxical increases in anxiety can occur while similar subjects who focused on pleasant images showed significant improvement. Matching type of relaxation technique with client was strongly indicated.

Meditation may be effective in reducing the cognitive aspects of anxiety (Lehrer, Schoicket, Carrington, and Woolfolk 1980). Lehrer, Hochron, McCann, Swartzman, and Rebar (1986) noted that studies with asthma subjects failed to distinguish between asthmatics with symptoms mediated by diminished sympathetic activity and those with increased parasympathetic activity. Relaxation decreases sympathetic activity; thus, only large-airway obstruction may be helped. Those with small-airway obstruction may find relaxation countertherapeutic because these airways tend to dilate with sympathetic autonomic nervous stimulation. Other variables in asthma need to be taken into account.

In gastrointestinal problems, autogenic training, which involves passive concentration on warmth in the abdominal area, may cause problems with the hypermotility of peristalsis, increase in blood flow in gastric mucosa, and augmentation of acidity in gastric juices. Even with progressive muscular relaxation, parasympathetic rebound can occur, with decreases in sympathetic tone leading to nausea and vomiting due to increased vagal tone (Lazarus and Mayne 1990). Headaches seem to be responding better to cognitive interventions as an adjunct (Holroyd, Androsik, and Westbrock 1977; Murphy, Lehrer, and Jurish 1990). Relaxation-induced anxiety may occur, with fear of loss of control being reported. Side effects were also seen in that relaxation may be fatiguing for weak patients, such as those with cancer (Sims 1987). Some clients may have difficulty acquiring skill, some cardiac irregularities may have increased irregularity, dyspnea may not respond to focus on breathing, and psychotics may decompensate (Donovan 1980). Withdrawal from life, symptoms of insomnia, and hallucinations can occur when relaxation is used more than twice a day (Sims 1987). In acutely ill cardiac patients, PMR was seen to initiate the Valsalva response with the breath held for 15 seconds (Herman 1987).

An interesting study with disturbed psychiatric patients (major depression and schizophrenic) was completed using passive and progressive muscle relaxation to determine differences in side effects (Richard, McCoy, and Collier 1989). No significant differences in side effects was found, with the incidence of these being infrequent and consisting mostly of unwanted thoughts, falling asleep, feeling anxious, and having muscle cramps.

Hypnosis has been reported to be effective in reducing or eliminating pain, but many of the articles are in case study form, so comparisons are difficult. Turner and Chapman, in their review article on hypnosis, note that although hypnosis has been used longer than any other psychological intervention in pain, the research is sparse: "Until controlled research demonstrates otherwise, we are forced to take a posture of skepticism toward the clinical lore that hypnosis is a powerful method of chronic pain alleviation" (Turner and Chapman 1982, p. 30). Other researchers have found hypnosis to be useful in psychosomatic disorders such as asthma, hyperventilation, insomnia, and stress management (Wilkson 1981; Daley and Greenspun 1979). Benson and colleagues (1978) studied the effectiveness of self-hypnosis and a meditation relaxation technique on anxiety and found both procedures to be equally effective.

In general, much more specific information is being cultivated about the indications and side effects of Relaxation Training. Methodologies of studies have improved, although there remain in nursing no programs of research on relaxation. Findings indicate that the type of relaxation procedure needs to be specified for the client, live as opposed to taped instructions are better, multiple training sessions work best, and home practice remains important in maintaining positive results. Research is needed to determine techniques best suited for particular symptoms. Study of preferred sequences in clients is another area of needed study; for example, does the client begin with sensation, followed by imagery, and then cognition, or is there another order better suited for a client (Lazarus and Mayne 1990)? Training is designed to maximize effective learning by using the client's preferred sequencing. The influence of personality traits of the trainer as well as the clients need study as well.

ASSESSMENT TOOLS

Before employing these techniques, the nurse must make a careful assessment of the client. Symptoms need to be carefully identified, perhaps by using an anxiety scale or anxiety symptom checklist. Baseline data on blood pressure, pulse, and respirations are recommended, as well as posttraining measures of the same vital signs to validate the physiological changes associated with relaxation. In addition, it is vital to use an organized assessment guide. Essential components of an interview guide include the following:

1. Client's identification of the most bothersome symptoms.
2. Onset and duration of symptoms.
3. Full description of symptoms.
4. Family history of similar complaints.
5. What the client has previously tried that helped and what did not help.
6. What causes the client to seek relief now.
7. Current and past medications—including over-the-counter drugs.
8. Any physical illnesses.
9. Physical limitations (e.g., low back pain, neck pain).
10. Previous experience with any relaxation training.
11. Pattern of alcohol use or use of any other mind-altering drugs.
12. Dietary pattern, including use of caffeine, sugar, and alcohol.
13. Sleep pattern.
14. Exercise pattern.
15. Overview of daily routine, including environmental and psychological stressors.
16. Any psychiatric history, including means to screen for major depressive disorders.
17. Motivation to learn and willingness to practice at home.

Item 16 is particularly important because people who also are severely depressed may be referred for Relaxation Training to relieve their anxiety. If the depression is not treated, Relaxation Training will not be successful in relieving anxiety.

If the focus of the training is stress management, an assessment such as the Travis Wellness Inventory (Travis 1977), the Holmes-Rahe Social Readjustment Rating Scale (Holmes and Rahe 1967), or Breeden's symptom checklist (Scandrett, Bean, Breeder, and Powell 1986) may be useful. These tests may be repeated at the end of the training sessions to assist in evaluation.

All six of the Relaxation Training techniques presented in this chapter are skill based and must be learned by nurses in an experiential format. Training with specific feedback on technique delivery, voice tone, timing, and word choice are essential. This training is being offered in nursing continuing education programs, as well as in college of nursing curricula. Other potential trainers are professionals from fields such as psychology.

The nurse's own beliefs and personal use of these techniques are essential in conveying to the client the effectiveness of the technique. Relaxation is not magic; learning it requires work. The reward of this intervention can be the effective modification of symptoms and the regaining of body control.

ASSOCIATED NURSING DIAGNOSES AND APPROPRIATE CLIENT GROUPS

In determining the appropriate client group, it is useful to keep in mind the three basic criteria of being able to use Relaxation Training: The client needs to be able to attend to body sensations, follow instructions, and follow through with home practice. One technique might be more effective over another with a particular client. The advantage of the Scandrett five-step program is that it allows the nurse and the client to examine several techniques and to progress from gross motor movement to thought-induced relaxation.

Utilizing the previously outlined assessment guides, the nurse would likely arrive at one or more nursing diagnoses. The ones that seem most likely are the following:

Anxiety
Sleep Disturbance
Activity Intolerance
Powerlessness
Ineffective Breathing Pattern
Pain
Ineffectual Individual Coping
Impaired Physical Mobility
Fear

Relaxation Training is useful in all of these diagnoses.

Because of the feature of muscular passivity, autogenic training has been most useful in clients who have pain, burns, traction, and bleeding tendencies. Active tensing and releasing of gross muscle groups, as in PMR, may be painful or impossible for these clients. All of the techniques can be used to combat the feelings of loss of control, powerlessness, and fear that can overwhelm clients at times. For example, autogenic relaxation used with a 54-year-old man with testicular cancer who was feeling overwhelmed by the impact of numerous changes in his life created by his disease helped him to regain control of his response to his disease progression. He modified his work environment to accommodate his relaxation practice sessions at work by having his secretary hold calls and setting aside a specific time to practice daily. He was able to carry on his work and as a result felt better about himself.

This example also illustrates how autogenic training is helpful in intervening in a pain-fear-anxiety cycle. The client can use the autogenic training to extend the period of pain relief and thereby decrease the amount of analgesics required. A client who had suffered from frequent headaches was helped by a combination of PMR and autogenic relaxation. Autogenic training was used to reduce the pain after the headache developed. PMR was used during the day to release tension that built up in the client's muscles as a result of particular positions she had to maintain in her work.

Meditation has been reported to be particularly useful in stress management and in optimizing good health. Many regular meditators report an increased sense of well-being, increased energy levels, decreased anxiety, and an overall positive attitude (Benson and Klipper 1976; LeShan 1974). Many people using meditation as part of their daily routine report that it helps to lessen the effects of the fight-or-flight response on the various body organs. One client who prior to her admission to the hospital had practiced TM for a number of years was concerned that the hospital routine would not allow her to continue this practice. In this situation, the client was not taught any new relaxation technique; instead her existing one was reinforced by determining with her the schedule and educating the staff about the technique to ensure their cooperation.

Hypnosis seems more appropriate in situations in which there are acute time limitations, such as pain. Pain can impair the client's ability to concentrate on Relaxation Training. For example, hypnosis helped a young man to cope with his back and neck pain caused by injuries in an automobile accident. The hypnosis provided relief initially; throughout his hospitalization, he was taught other techniques as his ability to concentrate improved.

POSSIBLE CLIENT RESPONSES

There are some possible drawbacks to use of Relaxation Training techniques. One is a fear of loss of control. Clients need to be reassured that they are still in control and can choose to stop the procedure at any time by opening their eyes. Actually, clients are less in control if they are unable to elicit the relaxation response. Some clients fall asleep before the procedure is completed; they may need to be instructed to get more sleep. In addition, a finger clue system may have to be set up in the training session to indicate whether a person is still alert. To use the finger cue, the nurse makes a statement like the following one during the training session: "As you continue to hear my voice, raise the index finger on your left hand to indicate you can still hear me" (Bernstein and Borkovec 1973).

Another possible effect is becoming labile. Emotions are discharged when the body is more relaxed. The client may need to be reassured that this is normal and be allowed an opportunity to deal with these feelings, with the nurse or another appropriate person.

Orthostatic hypotension may occur. The client needs to be instructed to get up slowly and to flex and tighten muscles slightly before standing. Sometimes there are other unfamiliar body sensations, which may be unsettling to the client—for example, feeling very light, warm, heavy, or floating. It is important to let the client know that these feelings are normal and are signs that the person is relaxing. It is useful to remind clients that they are always in control.

Guilt may arise. Too often if a psychological activity is used, assumptions are made that the symptoms are all in the client's head. It is important to accept the clients as they are, without judging their symptoms. Inducing feelings of guilt in clients by implying they are causing their symptoms is unfair; instead, gently show them ways in which they can choose not to contribute to these symptoms and how to use relaxation methods to relieve symptoms and enhance their health.

FIVE-STEP RELAXATION PROCEDURE

A sequential learning procedure evolved from the senior author's years of studying relaxation procedures, especially comparing EMG biofeedback and PMR (Breeden and Kondo 1975; Scandrett et al. 1986). Application of autogenic and meditative procedures ensued in clinical practice, and it was noted that many clients did best when relaxation techniques began with muscle tension procedures. The progressive muscle procedures were especially helpful in instructing the clients to tune into their own body sensations. As the senior author began increasing the complexity of tasks, two autogenic procedures were added, which involved mental suggestion and autogenic switch-over. The sequence of autogenic instruction was expanded and modified to follow the same body routine, so there was consistency in training procedures. These three short, calming procedures were taught to elicit a quick relaxation response in any setting. The five-stage procedure is as follows:

1. Progressive muscle relaxation.
2. Shortened muscle relaxation.
3. Autogenic heaviness.
4. Autogenic warmth.
5. Calming techniques.

Step 1: Progressive Muscle Relaxation

Step 1 consists of tensing and releasing 12 major muscle groups, modified from Bernstein and Borkovec (1973). Jacobson introduced this progressive relaxation procedure in 1938 in a book entitled *Progressive Relaxation*. Jacobson believed that a decrease in muscle tension would lead to a decrease of autonomic (especially sympathetic) nervous system activity. The outline of muscle systems utilized in the training program is presented in Appendix 34A.

The therapist's goal is to have the client focus on the sensation in the muscles. Therefore, the training might begin with the direction, "Focus all of your attention on the muscles of your right hand." The therapist stimulates the onset of the tension cycle by saying, "Make a tight fist now, noting how the muscles feel when they are tensed." This assists the client to pay attention to body sensations. This tension is maintained for 7 seconds to 10 seconds (with only 5 seconds for the feet).

At a predetermined cue, such as saying quickly, "Relax now," the muscle group is released. The client is encouraged to continue focusing on the muscle group as it relaxes — for example, "Notice how the muscles feel as they relax." The therapist provides a relaxation pattern, such as, "Allow the muscles to relax," for about 20 seconds to 30 seconds.

At this point, the state of relaxation can be assessed by having the therapist ask if the muscles are relaxed: "If the muscles in your right hand feel completely relaxed, signal by lifting the little finger of your left hand." After the initial check, the therapist can compare the muscle groups to determine the state of relaxation, for example: "If the muscles in your face are as deeply relaxed as those in your arm, lift the left little finger." Checking periodically with the client is extremely important, for having any muscles tensed can be distracting for the client. If tension remains in a muscle group, the same muscle group is tensed again for 7 seconds and then relaxed.

The next sequence of tensing occurs after the muscle relaxation check, or after the 20 seconds to 30 seconds of relaxation patter, depending on where one is in the training. The training occurs through all 12 muscle groups. The muscles of the feet should not be tensed longer than 5 seconds to avoid cramping. It is best not to mention to the client that cramping might occur but rather to shorten the time and lessen the intensity of the tensing. In cramping, deficiencies of calcium or potassium may be occurring, therefore the nurse may recommend that the clients increase their consumption of calcium by adding a glass of milk. In some cases additional potassium is also needed. After all muscle groups appear relaxed, the client takes four deep breaths, releasing any remaining internal tension. Smooth muscle relaxes in approximately 20 minutes. This tensing-relaxing procedure takes about 15 minutes to 20 minutes, and the client then sits relaxed for 10 minutes to 20 minutes.

Clients gain several consistent results from this procedure. They report more awareness of their body, and they learn that they can control the tension response. Many clients are quite impressed with the dramatic differences between the two feeling states of tension and relaxation. This procedure is useful for individuals who have a short attention span or who are agitated. Individuals with neck and shoulder tension often report a dramatic response to this procedure.

The nurse should carefully screen clients who have neck or back orthopedic injuries because hyperextension of the upper spine adds discomfort and complicates this condition. Clients with increased intracranial pressure, capillary fragility, bleeding tendencies, severe acute cardiac difficulties with labile hypertension, or any other condition in which tensing muscles might produce greater physiological injury need to be screened and taught more passive procedures. Some clients report muscle soreness after beginning the procedure. Many clients have been tense for many years, and it takes time to work out the various tensions in some parts of the body.

Step 2: Shortened Muscle Relaxation

The aim of this step is to show the client that the relaxation response can be elicited more quickly by combining groups of muscles. It is taught after the client has mastered the first 12 muscle group procedures. Sometimes clients mass the muscles on their own. The focus remains on how the muscles feel when tensed or relaxed, and the tensing-relaxation procedure usually takes about 5 minutes to 10 minutes, after which the client relaxes for another 10 minutes to 20 minutes.

The muscles are grouped in the following manner, utilizing the same tensing descriptions as in step 1:

1. Both hands, upper and lower arms (Check for relaxation)
2. Face
3. Neck and upper back (check for relaxation)
4. Abdomen and buttocks
5. Both legs (Check for complete relaxation)

Deep breaths are taken at the end of the procedure to release inner tension. Clients are encouraged to keep the legs on the floor, chair, or bed instead of lifting both simultaneously, especially if they have low back pain. If it suits the client better, one can be lifted at a time.

Checks are made for tension, and any spots that still seem troublesome are again tensed and released several times. Certain muscle groups may remain tense over several weeks. Persistent tension in certain muscle groups may need additional exercises prior to these procedures. Some clients have tremendous tension in their necks. They are encouraged to do gentle yoga neck stretches prior to beginning the relaxation procedure if they have no structural defects in the neck or spine.

Clients sometimes report that the relaxation is not as complete when the shortened procedure is used. They can be encouraged to practice daily, suspending judgment about the procedures until 1 week has passed. Usually satisfaction is reported after daily home practice. Slight setbacks in depth of relaxation response may occur as each new procedure is learned; however, increased proficiency usually occurs with consistent home practice.

Step 3: Autogenic Heaviness

When the client produces deep relaxing of the various muscle groups, physical tensing is dropped from the training procedures. At this point in the training, mental suggestion is emphasized, allowing the client to learn how the mind can facilitate a relaxed body. The purpose is to obtain a psychophysiological shift to an autogenic state, fostering recuperative processes in the body through stimulating self-normalizing brain mechanisms.

This step requires an individual to concentrate on relaxation, with various body parts eliciting a feeling of heaviness. Heaviness cues the muscular system specifically. The procedure consists of reading a statement and then pausing for enough time for the statement to be internally repeated (Appendix 34B). The client is instructed to repeat the statement and to elicit the feeling within the body part being directed. Reading with the script should take 15 minutes to 20 minutes.

Heaviness is the first sensation emphasized because it seems to be a predominant feeling that accompanies deep relaxation. Most clients report this subjective feeling, although a few say they feel lightness or floating sensations instead of heaviness. For an obese client, a feeling of lightness may be more pleasing to them, and *lightness* can be substituted for *heaviness*. Usually clients report a deepened state of relaxation with this first autogenic procedure. Sometimes other mental imagery may be used—For example, to feel heaviness, "Imagine that your arm is a sand bag; allow it to fall limp and loose."

Home practice instructions include having clients review the script and then making the suggestive statements to themselves. With clients who are highly distractible or have difficulty concentrating, it is sometimes helpful to audiotape this session and have them practice once daily for 3 days with the tape. During the remainder of the week, the client can try the procedure without the tape.

Step 4: Autogenic Warmth

Autogenic warmth cues relaxation in the vascular system. The feeling of warmth is elicited after the person releases tension from the muscles and senses a feeling of heaviness. The script for this step is given in Appendix 34C. Some persons tend to have difficulty in eliciting warmth. Additional imagery is often helpful in such cases, such as, "Feel the sun shining upon your skin, "Feel the skin warming," or "Recall how your hands feel in warm dishwater." A client who continues to have difficulty can be asked to feel the warmth of his or her palm as it rests on the arm of the chair and then to feel that warmth spread over and throughout the arm. Utilizing common, simple images seems to be more helpful than building more elaborate ones. This procedure takes the same amount of time as the third step and replaces it.

A shortened list is provided for the client to review the key points for home practice. The key points include tension release, relaxation, heaviness, and warmth. Most clients are able to learn the procedure easily.

Step 5: Calming Techniques

When clients have mastered the previous steps, they are ready to learn the short procedures of eliciting the relaxation response. Three major procedures are taught (Appendix 34D), allowing clients to select one that is most attractive and helpful to them. The first procedure combines yoga breathing with mental suggestions, the second procedure counts and relaxes the body parts, and the third uses repetition of a word that symbolizes relaxation to the client.

We have seen staff nurses attempt to train clients to relax by using quick procedures, such as tensing the whole body and then releasing it. From our experience, learning to relax is a reconditioning process that is most effectively trained by continued practice. When a person is trained in relaxation, deep relaxation response occurs quickly. Starting with the quick calming techniques, however, bypasses the reconditioning of training and often fails to elicit as deep a relaxation response. In an emergency situation, 7 to 15 abdominal breaths can provide temporary relief.

Appropriate Candidates

The five-step procedure has been utilized for over 16 years with a wide variety of inpatients and outpatients of a large university hospital. Successful training with positive patient self-reports has occurred in patients with orthopedic, neurological, blood dyscrasia, bone marrow transplant, psychiatric, obstetric, surgical, cardiac, pediatric, oncologic, and medical problems. The key symptoms utilized to select candidates from these patient populations are difficulties with tension and anxiety. Complete elimination of tension headaches, pain, and general tension has been noted repeatedly in individual cases.

We found it best to exclude persons with chronic pain, acute psychoses, spastic torticollis (stiff neck), alcohol, and drug problems and those taking psychotropic medications. However, if the trainer feels there is sufficient motivation by the clients to learn or to gain from the training, these clients need not be refused. We have successfully utilized tapes rather than live training with clients with paranoid personalities. From clinical observation, it appears that a more externally controlled person (one who believes that others control his or her fate) seems to respond better with the muscle tensing procedures; the more internally controlled person (one who is in charge of his or her own destiny) does best with autogenic or meditative procedures.

GUIDELINES FOR PRACTICE

Certain guidelines or recurring themes help ensure the success of the Relaxation Training. One is the need for home practice once or twice a day. Compliance with home practice becomes a key factor in motivation to learn. Another is to allow the client to progress to the next step only after the previous one is mastered. When possible, it is preferable to let clients practice at one level for a week. In inpatient settings, clients have been trained in all five steps in a 10-day period, with 2 days of practice between each session.

Occasionally a client masters only one stage, for example, PMR, and has great difficulty with the next step. Acknowledging that a client has learned a procedure well appears to be helpful and allows the client to progress or maintain skills at his or her own rate. Some clients are doubtful or become discouraged easily and need reassurance. Explaining that symptom development took years so altering the symptoms also requires time is helpful. Reinforcement of daily home practice often assists in reducing this doubt.

Providing relaxation consultation in a variety of hospital settings often means modifying the basic training procedures to fit the client's needs. The selection of relaxation techniques must take into account the client's biological state, for example, offering only the autogenic and calming procedures to clients with high blood pressure, acute burns, increased intracranial pressure, or bleeding difficulties. In intensive care, a client with C-2 vertebral fracture on an automatic respirator was taught to use autogenic calming and warmth, visualizing her breath flowing easily and effortlessly. This procedure helped her feel that she had some control in her life, and she left the rehabilitation hospital without respiratory assistance.

Some clients express fears or discomfort in being asked to relax. Some are fearful of losing control when they become relaxed. The latter clients can open their eyes, demonstrating that they remain in control. We also suggest to the clients that if they cannot relax, they lack control over their range of responses.

Other persons occasionally report dizziness or orthostatic hypotension upon arising after the session. These persons should tense their muscles by stretching and rising slowly. In fact, it is a good practice to have all clients stretch their muscles prior to walking.

Although audiotapes are often used, we believe in the value of having a client experience personal, individualized training and being able to observe the relaxed state of the trainer. Audiotapes are given to the client to take home only when difficulty with a particular procedure is encountered, and then the "in vivo" session is recorded. Budzynski (1982) claims that use of audiotapes works best with the Western-oriented individual. Good response has occurred with our approach, which discourages dependence on audiotapes. Usually use of the tape is suggested for only half of the week, with self-instruction encouraged for the remainder of the time.

Some clients have difficulty controlling extraneous thoughts. Utilizing mental images, such as placing worries in a box in the mind or letting the thoughts drift by, as in the autogenic warmth script, or paying no attention to them can reduce these. If after several weeks a client continues to experience trouble with intrusive thoughts, training the client to "stop" thoughts may be indicated. Thought stopping is a behavioral procedure in which the client practices interrupting thought processes and replacing them with the desired state or thought. Intrusions may occur from disrupting external noises or family members. Encouraging the client to negotiate with the family for uninterrupted times and unplugging the telephone are very helpful.

Another response the client may have is recalling emotionally painful situations, old conflicts, or emotional discharges. It is best not to bring this possibility to the client's attention beforehand, but if it occurs, the client needs to be reassured that it is a normal response. The psyche will take advantage of the relaxed muscles and emotions by bringing to awareness unresolved conflicts for the person to release.

Providing a nondistracting and nondisrupting environment is critical for success in training clients in relaxation. Sitting in a comfortable reclining chair with a footstool is the best position, although lying down also promotes relaxation (sometimes too much, so that the overtired client sleeps). Dim, nondirect lighting, quiet, and comfortable temperatures are important factors.

Training a person to relax takes a certain amount of self-discipline by the instructor. The best effect is produced if the pitch of the voice is lowered (unless the voice is already low), the pace of words is slowed, and speaking is rhythmical. The voice should not be so soft that the client must strain to hear. Even more helpful (yet sometimes difficult in dimly lit rooms) is to pace the words with the client's breathing. Going through the procedure with the client is helpful, using the body response as guide. The nurse can tape the instructions and not her own relaxation response to the directions. She should be quite careful to observe the client closely, utilizing the body's responses to pace the training. Difficulty with drowsiness, inattention, and drifting off can occur in the trainer when experiencing the procedure simultaneously with the client.

One of our biggest concerns with Relaxation Training is the misuse of the procedures, when the client is trained in one procedure in only a single session with instructions for home. This single-session approach violates good learning principles because periodic training increases chances for successful behavioral alteration. Often the trainers themselves discredit relaxation as an intervention when the client does not show symptom change. Yet it is the trainer who has not offered optimal behavioral training. When we train in relaxation procedures, we are altering chronic habits, which takes a period of time. Also, some trainers present relaxation as the final answer to the problem instead of acknowledging it as a part of a more holistic approach.

The five-step Relaxation Training procedure needs to be studied for effectiveness with a variety of clients. It has been utilized with differing clients in a major university hospital. Four research projects have tested this procedure with three populations: individuals with cardiac, oncologic, and psychiatric problems (Scandrett-Hibdon, Lomenick, Sachse, and Hart 1983). Positive significant changes were found for blood pressure, respiratory, pulse, Breeden Anxiety Scale, state, and trait anxiety symptoms. Internal and external locus of control did not change significantly. Relaxation certainly is not a panacea for living stress free, but it can provide an alternative to being anxious. It also allows the client the opportunity to prevent more permanent structural problems in the body.

CASE STUDIES

Case Study 1

A young woman who as a result of a severe automobile accident suffered two crushed ankles and a broken arm in addition to facial lacerations experienced much physical discomfort and anxiety as the healing process ensued. I was called to teach her relaxation techniques. She readily learned the five steps and found that her pain and discomfort were reduced as she elicited the relaxation response. In addition, she felt calmer and more in control of her situation. She utilized the Relaxation Training even after leaving the hospital to assist in dealing with anxieties related to her healing process.

Case Study 2

A psychiatric outpatient experienced much free-floating anxiety that interfered with his ability to concentrate on his studies in his doctoral program. In addition, he tended to find it difficult to care for his son while his wife worked and became anxious and felt overwhelmed or irritable. Relaxation Training was difficult for him, but he practiced diligently and was able, with encouragement, to relax fairly well. He used the relaxation to calm himself whenever he became anxious, and he found that with regular practice, he had less anxiety and in general felt more in control.

CONCLUDING REMARKS AND RECOMMENDATIONS

Maintaining the highest quality of client care in a cost-effective manner is one of the biggest challenges facing nurses. The cost of Relaxation Training is minimal, and the results are great. With the shorter hospital stay, anxiety often plays a larger part in slowing a client's recovery; Relaxation Training can greatly enhance the progress.

Nursing can make a major contribution if nurses themselves begin to practice and to train others in the use of relaxation techniques. A tremendous change would occur in the climate of hospitals, clinics, and health service agencies, and it would be noticed by other members of health teams as well as by clients. Perhaps some real healing and refuge could take place in healing centers. Bustle, stress, and burdens on the part of nurses certainly do not uplift our clients or promote healing.

It is imperative that nursing clinicians as well as nursing researchers write and publish results of their work. There is greater wealth of knowledge than is apparent in the literature. Nurses practicing in a variety of settings need to report their use of and results with Relaxation Training. Because of the wide application of the Relaxation Training techniques and our own positive results in some similar situations, we see many opportunities for nurses to use relaxation techniques. For example, oncology nurses could use Relaxation Training to help clients cope with the stress and anxiety accompanying changes caused by pain, radiation, chemotherapy, and the disease itself. Psychiatric nurses could use it in intervening with sleep disturbance and anxiety in their clients. Obstetrical nurses can use relaxation techniques in childbirth classes. Surgical nurses can explore the influence of relaxation on their clients' postoperative recovery. Cardiovascular nurses may use these techniques in cardiac rehabilitation. Some of these settings already use relaxation in their program, yet more needs to be done.

In the future, nurse clinicians and nurse academicians need to work together to study the effects of Relaxation Training. Many research questions remain: What techniques are appropriate for which person? How long do the effects last? Is the technique effective to cope with symptoms only if home practice is continued even when symptoms are not present? Would regular and early use of Relaxation Training prevent stress-related disease? Nurses are the appropriate people to ask and answer these questions.

REFERENCES

Alexander, C.N., Chandler, H.M., Langer, E.J., Newman, R.J., and Davies, J.L. 1989. Transcendental meditation, mindfulness and longevity: An experimental study with the elderly. *Journal of Personality and Social Psychology* 57(6):950–964.

Ashby, W.R. 1963. *An introduction to cybernetics.* New York: John Wiley & Sons.

Bailey, R.D. 1984. Autogenic regulation training and sickness absence amongst student nurses in general training. *Journal of Advanced Nursing,* 581–587.

Beaty, E.R., and Haynes, S.N. 1979. Behavioral interventions with muscle-contraction headache: A review. *Psychosomatic Medicine* 41(2):165–180.

Benson, H., Beary, J., and Carol, M. 1974. The relaxation response. *Psychiatry* 37:37–46.

Benson, H., and Klipper, M.Z. 1976. *The relaxation response.* New York: Avon Books.

Benson, H., Frankel, F.H., Apfel, R., Daniels, M.D., Schneiwind, H.E., Nemiah, J.C., Sifneos, P.E., Crassweller, K.D., Greenwood, M.M., Kotch, J.B., Arns, P.A., and Rasner, B. 1978. Treatment of anxiety: A comparison of the usefulness of self-hypnosis and a meditational relaxation technique. *Psychotherapeutic Psychosomatics* 30:229–242.

Bernstein, D.A., and Borkovec, T.D. 1973. *Progressive relaxation: A manual for the helping professions.* Champaign, Ill.: Research Press.

Bowles, C., Smith, J., and Parker, K. 1979. EMG biofeedback and progressive relaxation training: A comparative study of two groups of normal subjects. *Western Journal of Nursing Research* 1(3):179–189.

Breeden, S.A., and Kondo, C.Y. 1975. Using biofeedback to reduce tension. *American Journal of Nursing* 75(11): 2010–2012.

Budzynski, T.H. 1982, Spring. Presentations at the Memphis Medical Association Meeting, Memphis Tennessee.

Budzynski, T.H., and Stoyva, J.M. 1969. An instrument for producing deep muscle relaxation by means of analog information biofeedback. *Journal of Applied Behavior Analysis* 2:231–237.

Cannon, W.B. 1914. The emergency function of the adrenal medulla in pain and major emotions. *American Journal of Physiology* 33:356–372.

Conversation with Ken Pelletier. 1978. *Medical Self-Care* 5:3–9.

Daley, T.J., and Greenspun, E.L. 1979. Stress management through hypnosis. *Topics in Clinical Nursing* 1:1.

Derogalis, L.R., Abeloff, M.D., and Melisaratow, N. 1979. Psychological coping mechanisms and survival time in metastatic breast cancer. *Journal of the American Medical Association* 242(14):1504–1508.

Donovan, M. 1980. Relaxation with guided imagery: A useful technique. *Cancer Nursing.*

Eppley, K.R., Abrams, A.I., and Spear, J. 1989. Differential effects of relaxation techniques in trait anxiety: A meta-analysis. *Journal of Clinical Psychology* 45(6):957–974.

Fedoruk, R.B. 1984. *Transfer of the relaxation response, therapeutic touch B as a method for reduction of stress in premature neonates.* Unpublished doctoral dissertation, University of Maryland.

Gaardner, K.R., and Montgomery, P.S. 1977. *Clinical biofeedback: A procedural manual.* Baltimore: Williams & Wilkins.

Garrison, J., and Scott, P.A. 1979. A group self-care approach to stress management. *Journal of Psychiatric Nursing* 6:9–14.

Green, E., and Green, A. 1977. *Beyond biofeedback.* New York: Dell Publishing.

Green, E.E., Walters, E.D., Green, A.M., and Murphy, G. 1969. Feedback technique for deep relaxation. *Psychophysiology* 6:371–377.

Grinder, J., and Bandler, R. 1981. *Trance-formation.* Moab, Utah: Real People Press.

Heidt, P. 1981. An investigation of the effect of therapeutic touch on anxiety of hospitalized patients. *Nursing Research* 30:32–37.

Herman, J.A. 1987. The effect of progressive relaxation on Valsalva response in healthy adults. *Research in Nursing and Health* 10:171–176.

Holden-Lund, C. 1988. Effects of relaxation with guided imagery on surgical stress and wound healing. *Research in Nursing and Health* 11:235–244.

Holmes, T.H., and Rahe, R.H. 1967. The social readjustment rating scale. *Journal of Psychosomatic Research* 11:213–218.

Holroyd, K.A., Androsik, F., and Westbrock, T. 1977. Cognitive control of headaches. *Cognitive Therapy and Research* 1:121–133.

Hyman, R.B., Feldman, H.R., Harris, R.B., Levin, R.F., and Malloy, G.B. 1989. The effects of relaxation training on clinical symptoms: A meta analysis. *Nursing Research* 38(4):216–220.

Jacobson, E. 1934. *You must relax.* New York: McGraw-Hill.

Jacobson, E. 1938. *Progressive relaxation.* Chicago: University of Chicago Press.

Jacobson, E. 1970. *Modern treatment of tense patients.* Springfield, Ill.: Charles C. Thomas.

Keller, E., and Bzdek, D.A. 1986. Effects of therapeutic touch on tension headache pain. *Nursing Research* 35(2):101–105.

Khansari, D.N., Mrugo, A.J., and Faith, R.E. 1990. Effects of stress on the immune system. *Immunology Today* 11(5):170–175.

King, J.V. 1988. A holistic technique to lower anxiety: Relaxation with guided imagery. *Journal of Holistic Nursing* 6(1):16–20.

Kleinsorge, H., and Klumbies, G. 1964. *Technique of relaxation.* Bristol, England: John Wright.

Kolkmeier, L.G. 1982. Biofeedback–relaxation therapy for hypertension. *Topics in Clinical Nursing* 3(4):69–73.

Kolkmeier, L.G., 1989. Clinical application of relaxation, imagery, and music in contemporary nursing. *Journal of Advanced Medical-Surgical Nursing* 1(4):73–80.

Krieger, D. 1973. The relationship of touch with the intent to help or to heal to subjects in-vivo hemoglobin values: A study in personalized interaction. In *Proceedings of the Ninth Association Regional Conference,* Kansas City: American Nurses' Association.

Krieger, D. 1979. *The therapeutic touch.* Englewood Cliffs, NJ: Prentice-Hall.

Lamontagne, L.L., Mason, K.R., and Hepworth, J.T. 1985. Effects of relaxation in anxious children: Implications for coping with stress. *Nursing Research* 34:289–292.

Lazarus, A.A., and Mayne, T.J. 1990. Relaxation: Some limitations, side effects and proposed solutions. *Psychotherapy* 27(2):261–266.

LeCron, L. 1971. *The complete guide to hypnosis.* New York: Harper & Row.

Lehrer, P.M., Hockron, S.M., McCann, B., Swartzman, R., and Rebar, P. 1986. Relaxation decreases large airway but not small airway asthma. *Journal of Psychosomatic Research* 30:13–25.

Lehrer, P.M., Schoicket, S., Carrington, P., and Woolfolk, R.L. 1980. Psychophysiological and cognitive responses to stressful stimuli in subjects practicing progressive relaxation and clinical standardized meditation. *Behavior Research and Therapy* 18:298–303.

LeShan, L. 1974. *How to meditate.* New York: Bantam Books.

Levin, R.F., Malloy, G.B., and Hyaan, R.B. 1987. Nursing management of post operative pain: Use of relaxation techniques with female cholecystectomy patients. *Journal of Advanced Nursing* 12:463–472.

Mason, L.J. 1980. *Guide to stress reduction.* Culver City, Calif.: Peace Press.

Meditation group for the new age. 1978. Kent, England: Courier Company.

Meehan, M. 1985. *The effect of therapeutic touch on the experience of acute pain in post operative patients.* Unpublished doctoral dissertation, New York University.

Miller, N.E. 1969. Learning of visceral and glandular responses. *Science* 163:434–445.

Munra, B.H., Creamer, A.M., Haggerty, M.R., and Cooper, F.S. 1988. Effect of relaxation therapy on post-myocardial infarction patients' rehabilitation. *Nursing Research* 37(4):231–236.

Murphy, A.I., Lehrer, P.M., and Jurish, S. 1990. Cognitive coping skills training and relaxation training as treatment for tension headaches. *Behavior Therapy* 21:89–98.

Orem, D.E. 1990. *Nursing concepts of practice.* New York: McGraw-Hill.

Parkes, B. 1985. *Therapeutic touch as an intervention to reduce anxiety in elderly hospitalized patients.* Unpublished doctoral dissertation, University of Texas, Austin.

Paul, G., and Trimble, R. 1970. Recorded versus live relaxation training and hypnotic suggestion. *Behavioral Therapy* 3:285–302.

Pelletier, K. 1976. *Mind as healer, mind as slayer.* New York: New York.

Pender, N.J. 1984. Physiologic responses of clients with essential hypertension to progressive muscle relaxation training. *Research in Nursing and Health,* 197–203.

Pender, N.J. 1985. Effects of progressive muscle relaxation training in anxiety and health locus of control among hypertensive adults. *Research in Nursing and Health* 8:67–72.

Quinn, J.F. 1982. An investigation of the effect of therapeutic touch done without physical contact on state anxiety in hospitalized cardiovascular patients. *Dissertation Abstracts International.* 43(6):1797–1798.

Randolph, D. 1984. Therapeutic and physical touch: Physiological responses to stressful stimuli. *Nursing Research* 33:33–36.

Richard, H.C., McCoy, A.D., and Collier, J.B. 1989. Relaxation training side effects reported by seriously disturbed inpatients. *Journal of Clinical Psychology,* 446–450.

Scandrett, S.L., Bean, J., Breeden, S., and Powell, S.R. 1986. A comparative study of biofeedback and progressive relaxation in anxious patients. *Issues in Mental Health Nursing* 8:233–249.

Scandrett-Hibdon, S.L., Lomenick, E., Sachse, D., and Hart, C. 1983. [Using the five step relaxation process on three populations.] Unpublished study.

Schultz, J.H., and Luthe, W. 1969. *Autogenic therapy.* (Vol. 1) Autogenic methods. New York: Grune & Stratton.

Selye, H. 1956. *The stress of life.* New York: McGraw Hill.

Sims, S.E.R. 1987. Relaxation training as a technique for helping patients cope with the experience of cancer: A selective review of the literature. *Journal of Advanced Nursing* 12:583–591.

Snyder, M. 1988. Relaxation. *Annual Review of Nursing Research* 6:111–128.

Solomon, G.F. 1981. *Psychoneuroimmunology.* New York: Academic Press.

Solomon, G.F., Temoshik, L., O'Leary, A, and Zick, J. 1987. An intensive psychoimmunologic study of long-surviving persons with AIDS. Annals New York Academy of Sciences 496:647–655.

Tamez, E.G., Moore, M.J., and Brown, P.L. 1978. Relaxation training as a nursing intervention versus pro re nata medication. *Nursing Research* 27(3):160–165.

Tarler-Benlolo, L. 1978. The role of relaxation in biofeedback training: A critical review of the literature. *Psychological Bulletin* 85(4):727–755.

Tecoma, E.S., and Huey, L.Y. 1988. Psychic distress and the immune response. *Life Sciences* 36:1799–1812.

Travis, J. 1977. *Wellness workbook for health professionals.* Mill Valley, Calif.: John Travis Wellness Resource Center.

Turner, J., and Chapman, C.R. 1982. Psychological interventions for chronic pain: A critical review. II. Operant conditioning, hypnosis and cognitive-behavioral therapy. *Pain* 12:23–46.

Wilkson, J.B. 1981. Hypnotherapy in the psychosomatic approach to illness: A review. *Journal of Royal Society of Medicine,* 525–530.

Zeig, J. 1982. *Eriksonian approaches to hypnosis and psychotherapy.* New York: Brunner/Mazel.

Zegans, L.S. 1982. Stress and development of somatic disorders. In Goldberger L., and Brezwitz, S. (eds.), *Handbook of stress: Theoretical and clinical aspects.* New York: Free Press.

APPENDIX 34A: INSTRUCTIONS TO CLIENTS FOR PROGRESSIVE MUSCLE RELAXATION

HAND: Tighten the dominant hand into a fist. Tighten the nondominant hand into a fist. (Check for relaxed state.)

UPPER AND LOWER ARM: Bend elbow of the dominant arm and point it to the ceiling, tensing both upper and lower arm. (Repeat with the nondominant arm. Check for relaxation.)

FOREHEAD: Raise eyebrows toward top of head.

EYES AND NOSE: Squint your eyes and wrinkle your nose.

MOUTH: Purse your lips into a little round "O" and push out in an accentuated "Kiss." (Check for relaxation.)

NECK: Hyperextend your head, grit your teeth, and make wide smile.

UPPER BODY: Try to touch your shoulder blades; arch your back.

ABDOMEN: Suck in your abdomen.

BUTTOCKS: Tighten your buttocks. (Check for relaxation.)

THIGH: Raise your dominant leg about 6 inches from the floor; tighten your upper leg. Repeat with the nondominant leg.

CALF: Pull your dominant foot toward your head. Pull your nondominant foot toward your head.

FOOT: Point your dominant foot away and curl your toes. Point your nondominant foot away and curl your toes. (Check for relaxation.)

If tense, raise little finger of right or left hand.

APPENDIX 34B: INSTRUCTIONS TO CLIENTS FOR AUTOGENIC HEAVINESS

Please place yourself in a comfortable position; close your eyes. Repeat to yourself the following statements, and allow your body to experience the suggested feelings.

I am completely at rest, at rest, and my whole body is relaxed.

My thoughts are directed only at this rest; everything else is immaterial— insignificant—nothing can disturb me.

Rest and relaxation.

Each muscle is relaxed and limp.

Nothing can disturb me.

I am completely at rest.

My right arm is limp and relaxed.

My right arm feels heavy.

My right arm feels relaxed and heavy.

A leaden heaviness spreads throughout my whole right arm, through the upper arm, through the lower arm, through the hands, and into the fingertips.

My right arm feels pleasantly relaxed and heavy.

My left arm is limp and relaxed.

My left arm feels heavy.

My left arm feels relaxed and heavy.

A leaden heaviness spreads throughout my whole left arm, through the upper arm, through the lower arm, through the hands, and into the fingertips.

My left arm is pleasantly relaxed and heavy.

The muscles in my head and face are limp and relaxed.

The muscles in my head feel heavy.

My head seems to sink into the couch.

My head is relaxed and heavy.

The muscles in my face grow limp and relaxed.

The muscles soften, and a youthful quality comes over my face.

The muscles of my head and face are pleasantly relaxed.

The muscles of my neck and shoulders grow limp and relaxed.

These muscles feel heavy.

The muscles feel relaxed and heavy.

A leaden heaviness spreads throughout the muscles of the neck and shoulders, from the base of the skull, down the neck, out into the shoulders and upper back.

These muscles are pleasantly relaxed and heavy.

The muscles of my chest and middle back grow limp and relaxed.

These muscles feel heavy.

The muscles of my chest and middle back feel relaxed and heavy, and a very pleasant heaviness spreads throughout all the muscles of my chest and around back to all the muscles of my back.

The muscles of my chest and of my middle back are pleasantly relaxed and heavy.

The muscles of my buttocks and of my genitals are limp and relaxed.

These muscles feel heavy.

The muscles of my buttocks and my genitals feel relaxed and heavy.

A leaden heaviness spreads throughout all these muscles, relieving the tension.

The muscles in my buttocks and in my genitals are relaxed and heavy.

My right leg is limp and relaxed.

My right leg feels heavy.

My right leg feels relaxed and heavy.

A leaden heaviness spreads throughout my whole right leg, through the upper leg, through the lower leg, through my foot, and into my toes.

My right leg is pleasantly relaxed and heavy.

My left leg is limp and relaxed.

My left leg feels heavy.

My left leg feels relaxed and heavy.

A leaden heaviness spreads throughout my whole left leg, through my upper leg, through my foot, and into my toes.

My right leg is pleasantly relaxed and heavy.

My left leg is limp and relaxed.

My left leg feels heavy.

My left leg feels relaxed and heavy.

A leaden heaviness spreads throughout my whole left leg, through my upper leg, through my lower leg, and into my foot and toes.

I am completely at rest.

A feeling of rest and well-being is coming over me.

Rest envelopes me like an ample cloak.

Rest protects me.

I surrender completely to the rest and relaxation—I am completely at rest.

This inner rest is of great benefit and helps me relax.

This process deepens with each exercise.

This inner rest will accompany me everywhere.
I will gain confidence and strength from it.
I will feel refreshed as if after a deep and peaceful sleep.
I will feel alert and renewed — ready to handle my tasks.
Breathe deeply.
Be aware of where your body is now, stretch, and open your eyes.

Modified from: Kleinsorge, H., and Klumbies, G. Technique of relaxation. Bristol, England, John Wright, 1964. Used with permission.

APPENDIX 34C: INSTRUCTION TO CLIENTS FOR AUTOGENIC WARMTH

As before, place any concerns or worries in a little box in your mind so that you may now center yourself to help yourself relax. Take four deep breaths, sensing the deepness of your breath as you release any tension.

As before, repeat the following phrases to yourself, beginning with your dominant arm and hand. I focus on the tightness in my arm and hand, and I release it. I see the tension moving out from the body and feel again that slowing sense of relaxation. With the sense of heaviness, I feel my arm and hand become more and more limp. I allow a very gentle, comforting warmth to begin to slow down, starting at my shoulder and gently moving across my upper arm, down into my lower arm, and into my hand and fingertips. I move now to the other arm and hand, and again I release the tightness. I feel relaxation and heaviness flowing in. I allow the very limpness to become more and more accentuated. I again feel that gentle sense of warmth, beginning at my shoulder and moving down my arm, into my hand and into my fingertips. Now both of my arms are limp and relaxed and somewhat warmer than the rest of my body.

Moving now to my head and face, I release any tension, release any lingering worries away from my head and face. I know that my mind can do anything I choose to do. I feel the deep sense of relaxation flowing to the muscles of my head and face. I know that the heaviness of my head is too heavy to move or shift, unless I really want to. I allow the muscles of my face to become very smooth and very soft, taking on a youthful, creaseless quality. I do not warm my head, since I did not pull blood to that area, but instead I allow myself to feel a very gentle coolness, as if a breeze, a summer breeze, was caressing my face, bringing refreshment.

Next, I move down to the area of my neck and shoulders, again releasing the tension. With extra tightness in my shoulders and neck, I imagine that they are like knotted ropes, and I begin now to untie the knots, so that the fibers may lie lazily side by side. I feel the heaviness coming into these areas, and beginning at the base of my skull, I note the warmth slowly coming around and down the neck, bathing this area with deeper relaxation and increased blood flow.

I move now to the area of the shoulders, my upper chest, and upper back, let go of my tension, and allow the relaxation to begin flooding this area. I feel the heaviness becoming more apparent, and I feel the comforting warmth flowing down my neck to my upper chest and across my upper back and shoulders. It is very comforting and warming.

I note that as I relax these areas, I feel less burdened. I now let go the tightness from my middle chest and abdomen, and my middle back and lower back, and I feel the relaxation flooding on down, bringing with it comforting heaviness. I allow the warmth to continue on down, bathing these areas with increased relaxation and rest. I now allow myself to release tightness in my buttocks and genitals, and again allow the relaxation to flow into these areas, bringing with it the sense of heaviness and comforting warmth. I'm aware now that the upper portion of my body feels relaxed, heavy, and very deliciously warm, except for my head and face, which feel refreshed.

I now release tightness and discomfort from my legs, and from all the joints in my legs, and my feet, and toes. I feel relaxation moving on down with a very comforting heaviness and limpness. I feel the warmth following, flowing on down into my legs and feet. I again take several deep breaths, feeling the fresh air flowing into my lungs, and releasing any remaining inner tension. I notice an increasing calmness coming over the center of my abdomen. This feeling grows, as if my stomach were the center of calmness within me. I feel its warmth. I feel how soothing it is. (At this point, the client is instructed to rest for 10 to 20 minutes).

APPENDIX 34D: THREE ALTERNATIVES FOR CALMING TECHNIQUES: INSTRUCTIONS TO CLIENTS

Breath Control

Heaviness

1. Allow yourself to be comfortably supported by the chair (or couch or floor) with your arm on the armrests.
2. Close your eyes, and begin to relax.
3. Take a deep breath, then another, overfilling your lungs.
4. As you slowly exhale, experience a band of heaviness move down through the body, from your head to your feet. It may take two to three breaths to complete this.

Warmth

1. Keep your eyes closed. Again take a deep breath, then another, overfilling your lungs. Hold the breath.
2. As you slowly exhale, experience a band of warmth move down through your body from your head to your feet, taking a couple of breaths, if necessary, to complete the feeling.

Count Back

Relax each body part as you count from 1 to 10.

Head	1
Face	2
Neck	3
Upper back	4
Arms	5
Lower back	6
Stomach	7

Buttocks	8
Legs	9
Release inner tension	10

Take two to three deep, cleansing breaths.

Cue Word

Simply repeat one word, such as *relax* or *calm*, several times to yourself as you recall the feeling of being relaxed.

35

COGNITIVE REAPPRAISAL

SHARON SCANDRETT-HIBDON

Minds are powerful. What we frame the world to look like through our perceptions strongly colors our actions. In essence, we create our world through our own thoughts. If we see it as threatening, then we relate to everything with caution and fear; if we see it as peaceful and loving, our actions correspond. Not only do perceptions color our world, but others respond to our behavior, amplifying the "vibrations" we initiate.

An individual's emotional and behavioral response to a situation is determined by how the event is interpreted and what meaning is assigned to the situation. Interpretations and meanings are influenced by individual values, schemas, and learned response patterns to stressors. Usually a person experiences psychological distress when perceiving a situation as threatening. When people are psychologically distressed, their perceptions and interpretations of events become highly selective, egocentric, and rigid. Their normal cognitions are impaired by decreasing their ability to turn off idiosyncratic thinking, to concentrate, to reason, or to recall. In addition corrective functions are lessened (Beck and Weishaar 1989).

The world contains actual problems; divorce, crime, and unemployment are all realities that threaten everyone. But everyone must learn how to take care of themselves just as primitive peoples learned to protect themselves from the threats from their environment. People often react to small events as if they were immense. Being late for an appointment or a meeting may be met with the same intensity of emotion as lack of money to buy food; criticism from a colleague may be dealt with in the same depth as a major disaster, such as a fire or an accident. People also create forces in the environment that amplify stresses, because part of each person thrives on the fear. The predominance of disaster and doom in the reports of mass media is a good example of this phenomenon. Advertising portrays the opposite extreme—the beautiful image of which most people often fall short.

Nurses tend to deal mainly with the physical effects of these undiscriminating cognitions; however, the physical effects are only the symptoms of the problem. Nurses can and should do more to deal with clients' thoughts, feelings, and beliefs. Nurses need to go beyond treating symptoms and offer clients an opportunity to alter cognitions that contribute to the stress response in the body. As nurses see clients who experience stress, they can ask if the client desires to do anything about the situation causing the symptoms. If so, the nurse can offer the client assistance in several ways: by exploring and evaluating the causes of the stress by teaching how to relax in response to the stress, and by changing the perception of the situation.

The intervention whereby a nurse helps the client deal with stress by changing the perception of the situation is termed Cognitive Reappraisal. Reappraisal is an evaluative process in which stressful stimuli are examined for their impact and meaning and are placed in perspective of the whole. Thought patterns are consciously altered by reinforcing responses that are most holistically adaptive. Pragmatic strategies for facilitating alternative ways of coping are explored and rehearsed. Other names for this approach are *cognitive restructuring* and *cognitive therapy.*

Cognitive therapy stresses the primacy of cognition, entering the change process from thoughts and images. Information processing is directed toward modifying biased selection of information and distorted interpretations. Examination of symptoms, experiences, and conscious beliefs is explored, and basic beliefs are examined for accuracy and healthy coping. New beliefs are constructed, with the therapist's supporting the client in testing how these ideas function (Beck and Weishaar 1989).

LITERATURE REVIEW

Cognitive theory dates back to Greek philosophers such as Epictetus, who wrote, "Men are distressed not by things, but by the views which they take of them" (Epictetus 1948, p. 19). The individual's view of self and his or her personal world is central to how he or she behaves. Beck (1963, 1964, 1967) found a negative bias in the cognitions of depressed patients rather than Freud's long-held idea that anger is against the self. The scientific community has refocused its attention on cognitive theory since the mid-1970s. Rotter (1954), Kelly (1955), and Beck (1963) are early cognitive learning cultivators who developed theories, conducted research, and taught these notions. They are considered the founding fathers of the cognitive revolution in psychotherapy. Ellis (1962) confronted the client's belief systems as unrealistic and gained lay popularity with his rational-emotive therapy. Some other "thought management" writers who emphasized thinking were Bain (1928), Carnegie (1948), Coue (1922), Dubois (1909), Maltz (1960), and Peale (1960). Bandura (1969) ushered in the shift in behavior therapy to a cognitive and information processing model of behavioral change. Other behaviorists supported the cognitive approach, including Goldfried (1967) and Meichenbaum (1972). Beck (1967) developed a cognitive model of depression. The importance of cognitive theories of emotion was developed by Arnold (1960) and Lazarus (1984).

Most writers on cognitive theory believe that maladaptive feelings are caused by maladaptive thoughts. Some basic assumptions of cognitive theory include the following:

1.   Adaptive and maladaptive behavior and affective patterns are developed through cognitive patterns.
2.   Moods and feelings are influenced by current thoughts.
3.   Cognitions include inner dialogue, perceptions, and fantasies, which represent meanings the client attaches to experiences.
4.   Pessimistic thoughts that cause anxiety are frequently unrealistic, illogical, and distorted.
5.   Many clients have underlying assumptions or cognitive schema that predispose them to anxiety or depression (Childress and Burns 1981).

The cognitive approach to emotion emphasizes the appraisal of the situation as a kind of mediator between the environmental stimulus and the emotional response (Murray 1964). The appraisal of a situation depends on information available to the person, contextual as well as immediately relevant, and how the person processes and deals with that information. The emotional response, positive or negative, is viewed as part of adaptation to a situation.

If, for example, a person who is turned down for a desired job claims, "This shows how undesirable I am; I'll never amount to anything," the resulting emotions most likely will be feelings of worthlessness, hopelessness, and guilt. Others might perceive the rejection differently—as an opportunity to learn why they were not selected for the job—and use that information to seek a position that is better suited for them. This person may feel disappointed but not overwhelmed or have a compromised self-esteem because of the episode.

Burns (1980) identified some cognitions that are self-defeating for: cognitive distortions, including all-or-nothing thinking (black or white); overgeneralization (seeing one negative event as evidence for defeat in other areas); dwelling on a single negative detail, excluding other things; disqualifying positive experiences; jumping to conclusions (such as predicting negative outcomes); catastrophizing or minimizing, assuming one's negative emotions are a valid reflection of the world; using "should" statements; labeling oneself negatively; and personalizing (claiming things are caused by oneself). Another cognitive distortion is subjective reasoning in which feelings are equated with facts. Arbitrary inferences draw a specific conclusion without supporting evidence. Systematic bias in information processing can also occur in which the bias is applied to external information or to internal messages—for example, a depressed person has a negative view of self, the hypomanic individual sees the self as better than others, and the panicking individual catastrophizes bodily and mental experiences (Beck 1989).

Cognitive appraisals may be influenced by information from multiple sources, with resulting bodily reactions and emotions. Bodily reactions can be seen as preparatory for upcoming behavioral demands. The person must appraise the bodily arousal itself for consistency with other information being processed. In addition, the person evaluates his or her own ability to cope with the threat. The anxious client typically has a distorted worldview in terms of imminent danger from future events, predicting dire consequences and treating them as fact. This client is often blind to these negative predictions, which can become self-fulfilling prophecies. In one study, 90% of the anxious patients reported negative visual images before and during the anxious episode (Beck, Laude, and Bohnert 1974). Another example is a person who sees himself or herself as unlovable and may not interact with other people, even briefly. Avoiding others creates a sense of loneliness, undesirability, and lack of love. Physical sensations of emptiness, agitation, and general discomfort may result. Reinforcement of the irrational belief that one is unloveable is supported.

Cognitive Reappraisal is a "structured short-term treatment for depression and anxiety, based on helping the client to identify and change distorted thought patterns that trigger and perpetuate one's distress" (Childress and Burns 1981, p. 1024). Clients are taught to recognize cognitive distortions and to observe their bodily reactions. Awareness is the first step in gaining control over one's behaviors. Alteration of a person's reaction to a seemingly threatening stimulus can occur by providing a benign interpretation of the event. If people view a stressor as manageable with their coping abilities, their defensive behavior is no longer necessary. Mastering one problem area increases a person's confidence in being able to cope with other problems, including those that are more threatening (Murray and Jacobson 1978).

Behavioral techniques are used to assist clients to reinforce changes in their beliefs about the feared stimuli and to reduce anxiety response habits. It is important to develop coping skills. Those encouraged are relaxation training, meditation, self-distraction, assertion, and behavioral rehearsal. In essence, this approach encourages behavioral self-control—an act that the individual regulates.

One phenomenon that may be operating in positive self-control is self-reward, which researchers have found to be effective. This self-reward can be simply self-praise (Mahoney and Arnkoff 1978). A sizable amount of research shows that self-talk—messages one tells oneself—can dramatically influence an individual's performance of widely varying tasks (Meichenbaum 1974, 1977). Meichenbaum combined cognitive modification and skill training in a coping skills paradigm that is useful in treating anxiety, anger, and stress. Cognitive therapy is efficacious in the treatment of unipolar depression (Beck and Rush 1978; Ernst 1987). Studies from seven independent centers compared the efficacy of cognitive therapy to antidepressant medications and found that cognitive therapy alone was superior to drugs alone or equal to antidepressants. Additionally, cognitive therapy was seen to have greater long-term effects than drug therapy alone (Beck 1989).

In his cognitive approach, Ellis focused on core irrational ideas (Ellis and Harper 1975); Meichenbaum was more interested in idiosyncratic thoughts. Beck (1970a + b, 1976) emphasized self-discovery by the client more than direct confrontations by the therapist, which Ellis emphasized. The use of cognitive therapy has been studied with other pathological conditions, such as anxiety disorders, panic, drug abuse, anorexia, bulimia, geriatric depression, dysphoric disorder, psychosomatic illnesses, and pain (Beck 1989; Blinchik and Grzesiak 1979; Kolata 1981; Biran and Wilson 1981). Studies of behavioral techniques demonstrate that cognitive and behavioral changes occur together (Williams and Rappaport 1983; Gournay 1986). Bandura (1977) focused on changing performance, one of the most effective ways to change cognitions. Beck, Rush, Shaw, and Emery (1979) demonstrated that desired cognitive changes did not necessarily follow changes in the behavior of depressed clients. The therapist must know the client's expectations, interpretations, and reactions to events. Psychiatric nurses have long used both cognitive (e.g., assertiveness training) and behavioral (e.g., relaxation training) interventions, yet few studies report the effectiveness of cognitive approach. Use of a cognitive intervention was reported in Alzheimer's disease (Geiger 1988). Cognitive appraisal of stress among family caregivers has been examined, as have assessments of cognitions in coping (Oberst, Thomas, Gass, and Ward 1989; Nyamathi, Dracup, and Jacoby 1988; Nyamathi 1989; Pagana 1988).

REAPPRAISAL TOOLS

Nurses can use five tools to assist clients in reappraising their thoughts and perceptions.

Stress Identification

The first part of this intervention consists of an evaluation process: an assessment of the client's stresses, fears, hurts, and problems. The nurse asks questions to elicit the meaning, function, usefulness, and consequences of the patient's beliefs. Stress identification tools, such as Holmes and Rahe's Life Change Scale (1967) or Wolpe and Lang's Fear Survey (1969), can assist the client in identifying problematic areas. "While all stressors represent change of some sort, many of them involve the loss of something valued" (Brallier 1982, p. 6). When clients list the specific stressors, they can more fully examine their world and the forces impinging upon them. Sometimes individuals cannot define what is upsetting them, perhaps because they are unable or unwilling to examine the disturbing force. Often the vagueness of a stressor is distressing in itself. Frequently examination of all the things the client is attempting to deal with brings clarity and focus to the client's thoughts. This clarity by itself may reduce tension. In addition, the clients may relax their self-expectations when the stressors are seen in perspective. Some clients may find themselves even more overwhelmed and feel unable to move beyond the emotion.

Stress Evaluation

The nurse can assist the client in examining specific stressors by listening and by clarifying areas that seem vague. Information can be obtained about the following areas: incidence of stressors, frequency of occurrence, meaning of the stressor to the client, relation to belief system, pervasiveness of the threat or amount of actual risk to the client's well-being, and the placement of stimuli in relation to other things in life. Brallier (1982) claimed that generally individuals give in to the cumulative effects of stress, whereas some may utilize defense mechanisms or healthy adaptations to a long-term stressor. Often some stressors will be diffused in the process of evaluation as the client sees the amount of focus or energy already expended on a stressor. Clients tend to put the stressors into perspective and may decrease the amount of energy wasted on unimportant stressors.

Hierarchy of Cognitions and Stressors

Cognitions are organized in a hierarchy, with each differing from the next in accessibility and stability. The most accessible and least stable are voluntary thoughts, which are temporary. Next are automatic thoughts, which are triggered by circumstances and accompanied by emotions. Usually these thoughts are internally consistent with individual logic and are given credibility without challenge. A client can be taught to recognize and monitor these thoughts. Automatic thoughts come from underlying assumptions, so they shape one's perceptions, determine goals, and provide interpretations and meanings of events. Automatic thoughts are more stable and often out of awareness. The deepest cognitions are the core beliefs that define the person's worldview or schemas. Change that occurs at this level renders the client less vulnerable to future distress (Beck 1989). Understanding the levels of cognitions assists the nurse and the client to determine what needs to be changed.

Stressors are assigned priorities by the client, from the most upsetting to the least upsetting. The client may be able to let go of minimally disturbing stressors or less stable cognitions at this time, focusing more fully on the most important stressors or cognitions.

Assessment of Coping

Clients then focus on the ways they react to particular important stressors. They can discern the facilitative skills that allow healthy adaptation in relation to a specific stressor and recognize their own resources and strengths more consciously. Brallier (1982) suggests that the client's perceptions of his or her ability to control a stressor is an important factor. Individuals who have a strong sense of internal control can prevent distressing experiences, and those with only a moderate sense of control manage a stressor more adaptively. In addition, clients can examine the weaknesses in their coping styles. These coping styles may include

TABLE 35-1.   DESCRIPTION OF BEHAVIOR ALTERATION APPROACHES

Decatastrophizing: Decreasing avoidance behavior by considering alternatives
Decentering: Moving away from thinking that the self is the focus of everyone's attention
Extinction: Learning through consequences of a response in which no aversion or strong reinforcers occur
Persuasion or direct guidance: Encouraging the client to utilize more adaptive behavior methods
Reattribution: Considering alternative causes of events, reality testing
Redefining: Making problems more concrete or specific
Vicarious learning: Observing successful handling of a stressful situation by others
Imagery or covert modeling: Utilizing mental images to experience or rehearse behaviors prior to actual attempts
Desensitization: Using relaxation to cope with actual and imaginary anxiety-arousing situations
Problem solving: Resolving situational difficulties utilizing a specific process

avoidance of stressors, accommodation to stressors, or adjusting mentally and emotionally to stressors (Brallier 1982). The nurse can assist the client to learn more facilitative coping strategies or can refer the client to another resource for this information and training. This step assists the client in moving from being a passive victim to an active participant in handling life.

Another component of this step is allowing the client to see the aspects of the stressor that can be altered through individual action and those that are beyond change. Once the person has acknowledged what can and cannot be changed, the process of acceptance of unchangeable events can begin. If one cannot change a stimuli, the only alternative is changing one's response. Clients may also have to work on their typical response pattern. Sometimes clients learn that they like to scare themselves and thrive on fear. The rush of adrenalin can be addicting. Others may see themselves as crisis prone, living as victims most of the time, and may create crises when life becomes too quiet.

Behavioral Management Techniques

Cognitive therapy fosters change in clients' beliefs. Through the appraisal process, clients decide whether to reject, modify, or maintain personal beliefs, being well aware of their emotional and behavioral consequences. The changes are based in reality and can assist to alter biased views. Behavioral change is promoted by cognitive changes. Cognitive changes can occur in voluntary thoughts, continuous or automatic thoughts, or assumptions (Beck 1989).

Alteration of socially and symbolically threatening cognitions or situations sometimes requires specific techniques that assist the client in letting go of these stressors; among these techniques are decatastrophizing, extinction procedures, persuasion, reattribution, reality testing, redefining the problem, decentering, task assignment, activity scheduling, vicarious experiences, behavioral rehearsal, imagery, and problem solving. Some are described more fully in Table 35-1. Referral to counselors or other psychotherapists may be necessary with some of these techniques. As the stressors are decreased, changes in the client's life adaption style are required. Long-term personality factors, such as a tendency to appraise every setback as a catastrophe, may have to be dealt with to produce significant emotional changes. Individuals with psychosomatic disorders tend to deny that emotional factors are connected with their physical symptoms. In some cases, the nurse can only plant seeds about contributory factors to a particular psychosomatic condition; actual change may occur much later in the client's life through another helper or psychotherapist.

SELF-CONTROL TECHNIQUES

The nurse can assist the client to modify either the stressor or the response. The stressor can be defused by clarification and examination from a broader perspective or by assisting the client to focus on more adaptive thoughts or desired behaviors, such as the use of affirmations or positive thoughts. Another technique is to recondition the stressor through systematic desensitization (Wolpe and Lazarus 1967). In this reconditioning process, the stressor is paired with the relaxation response, thus counteracting the anxiety response. Through relaxation, the client gains control over the physical response to a stressor. Another tool that can assist in gaining control of responses is to keep a journal in which the client writes self-negating statements and explores their opposites (Burns 1980). Use of imagery — that is, visualizing oneself as successfully handling stressors — can be of assistance, as can the use of role playing. The nurse can teach the client these techniques.

NURSING DIAGNOSES AND CASE STUDY

The following nursing diagnoses are pertinent to Cognitive Reappraisal:

Fear
Powerlessness
Ineffective Individual Coping
Altered Thought Processes
Altered Health Maintenance

Clients who suffer from stress and anxiety may benefit from Cognitive Reappraisal. Those who have incorporated stress into their lives so much that they have developed psychosomatic illness or experience chronic anxiety are prime candidates. Often the symptoms these clients experience are treated but with no attempt made to eliminate the cause or contributory factors. Reappraisal can lessen their fear by shifting perspective and allowing them to regain maximum control of their response to the fearful stimuli. A sense of powerlessness can be reduced if these clients clarify a stressor and their response to it. Identifying areas in which to seek assistance, to grow, or to make decisions assists clients in recognizing where they have control over a stressor.

Health maintenance alteration is also addressed by this intervention. Any individual attempting to facilitate health by changing a life-style is susceptible to stressors that may be perceived as blocks to living harmoniously with oneself. The life changes necessary for health maintenance are often seen as stressful in themselves. Activities that can alter these perceptions can ensure greater success in producing the desired life-style change. Methods of reappraisal allow the individuals to change their cognitive frame or glasses, permitting them to see the world differently.

CASE STUDY

A 34-year-old, moderately overweight male dentist on faculty at a University was referred to me for relaxation training and stress management. He was interested in reducing his hypertension, which developed a year previously when he found that his work was becoming highly stressful. Although he was in supportive counseling with a psychiatrist and planned major life changes to alleviate the situation, he continued to be anxious. Although his blood pressure had been reduced by medications (Inderal, Proglycem, and Minipress) and a weight-reduction diet, it still fluctuated to high levels whenever some upsetting incident occurred at work. To help the client gain control of both the stressors and his response, Relaxation Training and Cognitive Reappraisal were used.

A five-step Relaxation Training program was instituted (see Chapter 34). Initially the dentist was impatient for his blood pressure to become lower. In general, his blood pressure fluctuated less with stress as he continued to practice the relaxation at least five times a week. For example, on February 10, his blood pressure was 190/120 following a very stressful event at work, whereas by mid-March, his blood pressure 130/90 after a very stressful clinic morning. By the end of March, he reported feeling much more relaxed a greater percentage of the time, and he could quiet himself within 3 minutes to 5 minutes when previously it had taken him 20 minutes to 30 minutes. In April his hypertensive medications were reduced, and in May he could maintain his blood pressure at 130/90 in upsetting events.

Concurrently with Relaxation Therapy, Cognitive Reappraisal was used. The client identified all stressors plaguing him at the time and prioritized the list for work and for home from the most stressful to least stressful:

Work
1. Interactions with department chairman and dean.
2. An individual at work.
3. Some dealing with a passive-aggressive hygienist.

Home
1. All interactions with parents, especially father.
2. Arguments with wife (infrequent).
3. Selling of house and moving.
4. Children vying for attention, especially at mealtimes.
5. Misplacing things.

After review of each item, in-depth work was done on two main areas: interactions with his father and interactions with his department chairman. Imagery was enlisted to assist the relaxation response to counter upsetting stimuli. In addition, keeping his focus on the here and now was encouraged, since fear is often anticipatory. A third area was addressed: his impatience with the slowness of the sale of his house. His typical response to this problem was reviewed in depth. His pattern was first to worry and feel helpless and angry about failing to influence his realtor effectively. Using Cognitive Reappraisal, he cited all of the good points about his house and argued with himself that it should sell easily. After this process of reviewing his feelings and examining all he had done about the house, he was able to relax and let go of the worry. By the end of March, he reported that while many upsetting stimuli still existed, his response to them had changed. His list of stressors became shorter. It still included stressful interactions with his parents, which he decided he did not want to change, his children still seeking attention at meals, and avoidance of his department chairman. Signs of his anxiety were reflected mainly in the shallowness of his breathing, which we worked on with Relaxation Training, encouraging him to breathe deeply of life in each moment. In general, he reported feeling better and calmer. The relaxation assisted him to gain control over his physical response and to see that he could control anxiety, at least at the physical level. However, if we dealt only with that level, he would most likely still feel hurt by the emotionally painful stressors. Cognitive Reappraisal has reduced the emotional pain.

RECOMMENDATIONS FOR RESEARCH

Research is needed on using cognitive approaches in nursing practice. What types of clients respond best to Cognitive Reappraisal? What cognitive techniques are most helpful with illogical versus valid thoughts? Are symptoms reduced by changed thinking? What coping styles are most helpful in reducing signs of stress? For what types of clients do combined approaches of cognitive and behavioral approaches work best? Does a person gain more internal control using these procedures? Methods of diffusing stress or releasing fear and stress also need to be validated, and efficacy for nursing practice in various settings needs to be studied.

REFERENCES

Arnold, M. 1960. *Emotion and personality* (vol. 1). New York: Columbia University Press.

Bain, J.A. 1928. *Thought control in everyday life.* New York: Funk and Wagnalls.

Bandura, A. 1969. *Principles of behavior modification.* New York: Holt, Rinehart and Winston.

Bandura, A. 1977. Self efficacy: Toward a unifying theory of behavioral change. *Psychological Review* 84:191–215.

Bandura, A. 1977. *Social learning theory.* Englewood Cliffs, N.J.: Prentice-Hall.

Beck, A.T. 1963. Thinking and depression. I. Idiosyncratic content and cognitive distortions. *Archives of General Psychiatry* 9:324–333.

Beck, A.T. 1964. Thinking and depression II. Theory and therapy. *Archives of General Psychiatry* 10:561–571.

Beck, A.T. 1967. *Depression: Clinical, experimental and theoretical aspects.* New York: Haeber.

Beck, A.T. 1970a. Cognitive therapy. Nature and relation to behavior therapy. *Behavior Therapy* 1:184–200.

Beck, A.T. 1970b. Role of fantasies in psychotherapy and psychopathology. *Journal of Nervous and Mental Disease* 150:3–17.

Beck, A.T. 1976. *Cognitive therapy and the emotional disorders.* New York: International Universities Press.

Beck, A.T., Laude, R., and Bohnert, M. 1974. Ideational components of anxiety neurosis. *Archives of General Psychiatry* 31:319–325.

Beck, A.T., and Rush, A.J. 1978. Cognitive approaches to depression and suicide. In G. Serban (ed.), *Cognitive defects in the development of mental illness* (pp. 235–257). New York: Brunner/Mazel.

Beck, A.T., Rush, A.J., Shaw, B.F., and Emery, G. 1979. *Cognitive therapy of depression.* New York: Guilford Press.

Beck, A.T., and Weishaar, M.E. 1989. Cognitive therapy. In R.J. Corsini and D. Wedding (eds.), *Current psychotherapies.* Itasca, Ill.: F.E. Peacock Publishers.

Biran, M., and Wilson, G.T. 1981. Treatment of phobic disorders using cognitive and exposure methods: A self-efficacy analysis. *Journal of Consulting Clinical Psychology* 49(6):886–899.

Blackburn, I.M., Bishop, S., Glen, A.I.M., Whalley, L.J., and Christie, J.E. 1981. The efficacy of cognitive therapy in depression: A treatment trial using cognitive therapy and pharmacology, each alone and in combination. *British Journal of Psychiatry* 139:181–189.

Blinchik, E.R., and Grzesiak, R.C. 1979, December. Reinterpretative cognitive strategies in chronic pain management. *Archives of Physical Medical Rehabilitation* 60:609–612.

Brallier, L. 1982. *Transition and transformation: Successfully managing stress.* Los Altos, Calif.: National Nursing Review.

Burns, D.D. 1980. *Feeling good: The new mood therapy.* New York: William Morrow.

Carnegie, D. 1948. *How to stop worrying and start living.* New York: Simon and Schuster, 1948.

Cautela, J.R. 1971. Covert conditioning. In A. Jacobs and L.B. Socks (eds.), *The psychology of private events: Perspectives on covert response systems.* New York: Academic Press.

Childress, A.R., and Burns, D.D. 1981. The basics of cognitive therapy. *Psychosomatics* 22(12):1017–1020, 1023–1024, 1027.

Coue, E. 1922. *The practice of autosuggestion.* New York: Doubleday.

Dubois, P.C. 1909. *The psychic treatment of nervous disorders.* New York: Funk and Wagnalls.

Ellis, A. 1962. *Reason and emotion in psychotherapy.* New York: Stuart.

Ellis, A., and Harper, R.A. 1975. *A new guide to rational living.* Englewood Cliffs, N.J.: Prentice-Hall.

Epictetus. 1949. *The enchiridon.* New York: Bobbs-Merrill.

Ernst, D. 1987. A review of systematic studies of the cognitive model of depression. Unpublished manuscript, Center for Cognitive Therapy, Philadelphia.

Geiger, B.F. 1988. Cognitive interventions in Alzheimer's disease. *Journal of Rehabilitation* 54(3):21–24.

Gelb, L.A., and Ullman, M. 1967. Instant psychotherapy offered at an outpatient psychiatric clinic. *Frontiers of Hospital Psychiatry* 4:14.

Goldfried, M.R. 1967. Systematic desensitization as training self-control. *Journal of Consulting and Clinical Psychology* 11:213–218.

Gournay, K. 1986. *Cognitive change during the behavioral treatment of agoraphobia.* Paper presented at the meeting of the Congress of European Association for Behavior Therapy, Lucerne, Switzerland.

Holmes, T.H., and Rahe, R.H. 1967. The social readjustment rating scale. *Journal of Psychosomatic Research* 11:213–218.

Kelly, G.A. 1955. *The psychology of personal constructs.* New York: Norton.

Kolata, G.B. 1981. Clinical trial of psychotherapies is under way. *Science* 212(4493):432–433.

Kovacs, M. 1980. The efficacy of cognitive and behavior therapies for depression. *American Journal of Psychiatry* 137(12):1495–1501.

Lazarus, A.A. 1971. *Behavior therapy and beyond.* New York: McGraw-Hill.

Lazarus, R. 1984. On the primacy of cognition. *American Psychologist* 39:124–129.

Mahoney, M.J., and Arnkoff, D.B. 1978. Cognitive and self-control therapies. In S.L. Garfield and A.E. Bergins (eds.), *Handbook of psychotherapy and behavior change.* (pp. 689–722). New York: John Wiley and Sons.

Maltz, M. 1960. *Psycho-cybernetics.* Englewood Cliffs, N.J.: Prentice-Hall.

Meichenbaum, D. 1972. Cognitive modification of test anxious college students. *Journal of Consulting and Clinical Psychology* 1(39):370–380.

Meichenbaum, D. 1974. *Cognitive behavior modification.* Morristown, N.J.: General Learning Press.

Murray, E.J. 1964. Sociotropic-learning approach to psychotherapy. In P. Worchel and D. Byrne (eds.), *Personality change.* New York: John Wiley and Sons.

Murray, E.J., and Jacobson, L.I. 1978. Cognition and learning in traditional and behavioral therapy. In S.L. Garfield and A.E. Bergins (eds.), *Handbook of psychotherapy and behavior change* (pp. 661–687). New York: John Wiley and Sons.

Nyamathi, A. 1989. Comprehensive health seeking and coping paradigm. *Journal of Advanced Nursing* 14(4):281–290.

Nyamathi, A., Dracup, K., and Jacoby, A. 1988. Development of a spousal coping instrument. *Progress in Cardiovascular Nursing* 3(1):1–6.

Oberst, M.T., Thomas, S.E., Gass, K.A., and Ward, S.E. 1989. Caregiving demands and appraisal of stress among family caregivers. *Cancer Nursing* 12(4):209–215.

Pagana, K.D. 1988. Stresses and threats reported by baccalaureate students in relation to an initial clinical experience. *Journal of Nursing Education* 27(9):418–424.

Peale, N.V. 1960. *The power of positive thinking.* Englewood Cliffs, N.J.: Prentice-Hall.

Platt, J., and Spicack, G. 1927. Problem-solving thinking of psychiatric patients. *Journal of Consulting and Clinical Psychology* 39:148–151.

Rotter, J.B. 1954. *Social learning and clinical psychology.* Englewood Cliffs, N.J.: Prentice-Hall.

Strupp, H.H. 1980. A multidimensional analysis of techniques in brief psychotherapy. *Psychosomatics* 21(7):595–601.

Williams, S.L., and Rappaport, A. 1983. Cognitive treatment in the natural environment for agoraphobics. *Behavior Therapy* 14:299–313.

Wolpe, J. 1958. *Psychotherapy by reciprocal inhibition.* Stanford, Calif.: Stanford University Press.

Wolpe, J., and Lang, P.J. 1969. *Fear survey schedule.* San Diego, Calif.: Educational and Industrial Testing Services.

Wolpe, J., and Lazarus, A.A. 1967. *Behavior therapy techniques.* New York: Pergamon Press.

36

SMOKING CESSATION

KATHLEEN A. O'CONNELL

Thousands of studies have demonstrated that smoking is hazardous to the health of smokers and those around them. Despite the scientific consensus and the increased public awareness, about 25% of the U.S. population continues to smoke. Rates among low-income groups are considerably higher.

Although there is consensus on the dangers of smoking, there is less agreement on how to get people to stop smoking. Research has consistently shown that programs frequently succeed in the short term but that 80% to 85% of those in the programs relapse within 12 months of their attempt (Schwartz 1987). While such findings are discouraging, over 33 million people in the United States have succeeded in quitting smoking since 1964. Research indicates that numerous attempts at cessation are often necessary; in other words, people can quit, but they have to keep trying.

Nursing interventions for smoking cessation is promising for several reasons. First, nurses are frequently in contact with groups most in need of help: those suffering from smoking-related diseases, pregnant women, and those in lower-income groups. Moreover, nurses in primary care and community health settings often follow clients for much longer periods of time than traditional cessation approaches. This familiarity may make it possible to identify appropriate techniques and to help clients through several cessation attempts.

The intervention described here is designed to help individual clients stop, rather than reduce, smoking. Abstinence is the generally accepted goal of smoking control programs because smoking reduction has not been shown to reduce disease risk.

RELATED LITERATURE

Few published studies of nursing interventions for smoking are available (O'Connell 1990). However, antismoking program studies abound in the literature. Schwartz (1987) has reviewed some 416 studies conducted between 1959 and 1985. Success rates appear low across all programs; 33% abstinent at 12 months is the best that can be expected, with much lower rates generally prevailing. Studies of programs similar to the one described here are frequently termed minimal interventions. These studies were undertaken in outpatient facilities and involve

Case studies and examples were drawn from research project NR 10675 entitled Reversal Theory and the Motivations for Health Behavior funded by the National Center for Nursing Research, Mary Cook, Ph.D., Principal Investigator.

physician's advice during a regularly scheduled office visit to quit smoking. This may also include take-home reading materials for the clients and follow-up inquiry by the physician at subsequent appointments. Controlled studies indicate that such minimal programs, consisting of only advice by a physician, yield about a 6% success rate at 1-year follow-up. When the advice is supplemented by tips on how to quit and by follow-up support, success rates were 22.5% (Schwartz 1987). A study of a minimal program that involved both nurses and physicians in outpatient settings demonstrated a 6-month success rate of 15% when clients received advice from both physician and nurse and a 25% rate when they received advice and a self-quit manual (Janz, Becker, Kirscht, Eraker, Billi, and Woolliscroft 1987). Although these programs have low success rates, when they are applied to large numbers of clients, they yield significant gains across the population. In addition, clients who fail can learn valuable information that may help them succeed subsequently.

Other programs with outpatients may include the use of Nicorette gum, which provides nicotine replacement during the initial abstinence period. Research has indicated that nicotine gum alone (without any behavioral components to the program) yields a median success rate of 11% but that nicotine gum along with a behavioral program can raise abstinence rates to 29% one year after cessation (Schwartz 1987).

INTERVENTION TOOLS

Assessments of smoking history and of quitting history are useful to guide Smoking Cessation. The following questions can be asked during an interview or by questionnaire:

1. How many cigarettes do you currently smoke per day?
2. How long have you been smoking regularly?
3. What brand and type of cigarette do you smoke? filters? menthol? nicotine level? tar level?
4. Do you use tobacco other than cigarettes (cigars, pipes, smokeless tobacco)?
5. How many times have you tried to quit smoking?
6. If you have tried to quit, what was the longest time you went without a cigarette?
7. How long ago was your most recent attempt to quit?
8. How many smokers do you live with? work with?
9. How many of your friends are smokers?
10. How soon after awakening do you smoke your first cigarette of the day?
11. Have you ever tried Nicorette (nicotine) gum?

Intercurrent and postprogram assessments are also necessary in order to determine if the clients (and the program) have been successful. Such assessments should use interviews or questionnaires to determine self-reported cessation. The questions should include the following:

1. Have you smoked any tobacco at all, even a puff, since you quit smoking?
2. If so, when was the first time you smoked?
3. How many cigarettes did you smoke at that time?
4. When was the next time you smoked?
5. How many cigarettes a day are you smoking now?

In addition to self-reported cessation, it is necessary to obtain an objective measure. Numerous studies have shown that smokers trying to quit tend to underreport their smoking behavior. Objective indicators of cessation include expired-air carbon monoxide and salivary or serum cotinine (a metabolite of nicotine). Expired-air carbon monoxide can be determined with a portable instrument, which costs $1200 to $1500. Nonsmoker values are usually less than 8 parts to 10 parts per million. Being outdoors in traffic, faulty car exhaust systems, and faulty furnace systems can raise carbon monoxide levels and may be responsible for some false-positives. Salivary and serum cotinine levels are more expensive but also more specific indicators of smoking behavior. These assays are not easily performed, however, and usually require professional laboratory services. If the client is using Nicorette gum, cotinine levels will not be a useful indicator of smoking cessation.

ASSOCIATED NURSING DIAGNOSES

Smoking Cessation can be an appropriate intervention for several nursing diagnoses (North American Nursing Diagnosis Association [NANDA] 1990). Because of the risks of smoking, all smokers can be considered to have a diagnosis of Altered Health Maintenance. In addition, smokers with Activity Intolerance and Ineffective Airway Clearance are likely to benefit from Smoking Cessation. Those who have independently decided that they need to quit smoking—Health Seeking Behaviors: Smoking Cessation—would also benefit.

Introducing Smoking Cessation may put the patient at risk for some other nursing diagnoses: Constipation, Diarrhea, Sleep Pattern Disturbance, Anxiety, and Altered Nutrition: Potential for More Than Body Requirements. These diagnoses are related to the withdrawal symptoms and to the finding that most recent ex-smokers gain weight as they stop smoking. Although the average weight gain of 6 pounds is of no clinical significance, some clients gain 20 pounds or more. Most health care providers agree that the advantages of stopping smoking far outweigh the health disadvantage of weight gain; however, the psychological impact of the weight gain may predispose some clients to relapse.

THE INTERVENTION

Like many other health promotion activities, Smoking Cessation must be a self-directed process. The nurse can encourage and inform, but the client ultimately decides whether to undertake Smoking Cessation. Prochaska and DiClemente (1983) have identified five stages of self-change: precontemplation (unmotivated to quit smoking), contemplation (considering quitting), action (the act of quitting), maintenance, and relapse. Individuals may go through the entire cycle numerous times before they are able to remain in the maintenance stage. The program described here is designed to be carried out by nurses who are practicing in clinics or community health settings where they have the opportunity to interact with clients directly. Different activities are described for each of the stages. The practitioner may elect to institute only the first stage with the entire caseload of smoking clients. The nurse may undertake a more active role in the other stages as well. In either case, the practitioner should be encouraging and optimistic and yet remain aware of the numerous difficulties faced by clients who attempt to give up smoking.

Prepare the Practice Setting

The first step to prepare the practice setting is to contact national and local resource organizations to find out how they can help. For instance, the American Cancer Society (ACS) has sponsored a program, Tobacco-Free Young America, which enlists the aid of health care providers, including nurses. ACS provides a kit containing suggestions for methods that practitioners can use with their clients, and it has produced numerous written materials, booklets, and audiovisuals. The American Lung Association (ALA) and the federal Office of Smoking and Health have a variety of materials, and these and other organizations are constantly updating their selections. Much of the material is directed at special groups (pregnant women, Hispanics, teen-agers) and must be selected carefully for those that are especially helpful to a specific client group. Community resources for quitting smoking might include smoking cessation clinics, hot lines, or referral services.

The next step is to set up a system to record the smoking status of all clients. The records must contain a section to record the specific techniques tried and the outcomes of these and to record the client's smoking history information.

The nurse next initiates plans to identify smokers in her caseload by asking each client directly about his or her smoking history. Clients who have ever smoked should complete a smoking history questionnaire. Charts of those who have been abstinent for more than 2 years are flagged with "Successful Ex-smoker" stickers. "Recent Ex-smoker" stickers are used for those who have abstained for less than 2 years, and "Smoker" stickers for those who are currently smoking, at any level. Recent ex-smokers should be given continued attention and encouragement. Records on successful ex-smokers and nonsmokers should be updated periodically in case their status changes.

Help the Client in the Precontemplation and Contemplation Stages

Current smokers must be given clear advice to quit smoking. Reviewing the clients' smoking history, quitting history, and the current smoking behavior is a good way to begin the interchange. Relating smoking to the client's current health problems or concerns is often effective in personalizing the message. In addition, the nurse needs to continue to demonstrate interest and concern about the client's smoking status at subsequent patient visits. It is common to hear smokers say that a health care provider told them to quit once (perhaps when they had a respiratory infection) but that the provider had not brought up the subject since. The health care provider might have concluded that advising the client to quit was useless, while the client simultaneously thought that the health care provider was not serious because it was mentioned only once. Continued interest provides a message to the client that smoking remains a concern.

Clients in the precontemplation phase are those who do not appear interested in quitting at this time. They might be given a pamphlet about the benefits of quitting but should not be berated for smoking. Most smokers are aware of the general health effects of smoking; many feel guilty or out of control where smoking is concerned, and others may behave defiantly in response to a nurse's concerns. Exploring clients' experiences with smoking and with trying to quit may help to illuminate specific concerns or problems. The client needs to know that help is available when he or she is ready to quit smoking.

Help the Client Get Ready for Action

When the client is considering giving up cigarettes, the nurse can help him or her choose the best method among group programs, individual therapy, and self-quit programs.

The ACS and the ALA and many hospitals and health care agencies sponsor group programs. Group programs offer social support and structure to clients. Nurses interested in running group programs can take advantage of special training sessions offered by these organizations. However, group programs may be inappropriate for some clients. Clients with adequate resources may prefer individual therapy with a hypnotist, counselor, or behavioral therapist. Other clients prefer a self-quit method. Self-help materials are available from several sources. If the client wishes to embark on an individual self-help program, the nurse can facilitate the program by doing some or all of the following, depending on the client's needs and the nurse's availability:

1. Suggest or provide the written self-help materials.
2. Offer to review the self-help materials with the client to identify specific aspects of the program with which the client may need help.
3. Offer to help the client select a specific quit day and to sign a contract stating that he or she will stop smoking on that day. The contract could include the nurse's promise to call the client on quit day (or the day before).
4. Help the client identify sources of social support, plan specific coping strategies for a variety of situations, and make a list of rewards. Follow-up appointments at regular intervals to discuss progress and problems may be indicated. The exact nature of the nurse's involvement should depend on the needs of the client and on the setting where services are provided.

Manage Nicotine Replacement

Nicotine replacement therapy is thought to be the most helpful to people who are highly dependent on nicotine. Markers of high dependence include smoking more than a pack (20 cigarettes) per day and consistently smoking within 30 minutes of awakening. If the client's previous attempts at quitting caused numerous withdrawal symptoms, such as extreme irritability, anxiety, difficulty concentrating, insomnia, drowsiness, or dizziness, or if the client was unable to abstain from cigarettes for more than 24 hours, nicotine replacement should be considered.

Several types of nicotine replacement therapy have been under investigation. These include a patch, an inhalant, and nicotine gum. Since nicotine gum was the first to be introduced commercially, more is known about its use than other forms of nicotine replacement. Nicotine is destroyed in the gastrointestinal tract. Therefore, the nicotine in the gum must be absorbed through the mucous membranes of the mouth. Chewing the gum vigorously and rapidly will cause most of the nicotine to be swallowed. Therefore, the gum should be chewed slowly and intermittently over a period of 30 minutes. Some authors suggest that the gum should be chewed until the taste or tingling in the mouth is evident; then the gum should be held in the mouth, until the taste disappears (about 1 minute) when the gentle chewing cycle should be repeated.

In order to be effective in allaying withdrawal symptoms and smoking urges, at least 12 to 15 pieces of the gum (2 mg dose) should be chewed every day. Gum use should not exceed 30 pieces a day and should be tapered off 3 months to 6 months after cessation.

Side effects of gum use include nausea, sore mouth or jaw, heartburn, sore throat, mouth irritation, and palpitations. Persons with dental problems who have trouble with regular gum may have difficulty with Nicorette gum. Another side effect of nicotine gum is that the addiction to cigarettes may be replaced with the addiction to nicotine gum. Although most scientists agree that gum use is less hazardous to one's health than cigarette smoking, remaining addicted to nicotine still has untoward consequences. Moreover, nicotine gum is more expensive and harder to obtain (it requires a prescription) than cigarettes. The gum is contraindicated in clients who are unable to chew, have severe angina, have recently had a myocardial infarction, or have life-threatening arrhythmias. Like virtually all other medications, nicotine gum use is contraindicated for pregnant and lactating women.

Most users of nicotine gum report that it helps with their withdrawal symptoms but does not eliminate craving for cigarettes. Nicotine gum has a much slower course of action and does not provide the bolus effect (sharp rise in nicotine levels) that is delivered by inhaled nicotine. Thus, it is clear that even with the help of a pharmacological agent such as nicotine gum, eliminating the smoking habit is no easy task.

Support the Client in the Maintenance Phase

The experience of smoking cessation changes as abstinence proceeds. Paul, one of the subjects in our recent study of smoking cessation, described the experience at several different points in the cessation process: "The first 3 weeks were kind of a steady level of discomfort that you could ignore, with sharp peaks of an alarm, your brain telling you to get that nicotine back into your system." During the fourth week, Paul reported, "The alarms have been going off a lot more frequently, but they are different. In the beginning, the urges were like a crushing weight that took minutes to go away. Now [in the fourth week], it's just quick little jabs in the chest." Eight weeks after cessation, Paul reported having "2 or 3 million desires to smoke"—mostly when seeing someone smoking. "Now," he said, "they are like cap gun explosions as you go through a day and they don't seem to be as severe as they were." At 6 months after cessation, Paul reported that his urges were not as strong as they used to be. "They're still somewhat frequent," he reported, "but certainly easier to ignore."

Reviewing the client's most tempting situations and assessing the frequency and strength of urges to smoke is an excellent method of determining the types of problems the client is having with the cessation attempt. It is important to congratulate the client for coping successfully and to help the client identify circumstances that remain problematic or that might pose problems in the future, such as an upcoming deadline or a big party. The nurse should continue to follow the client for at least 2 years, congratulating and encouraging at each visit. Many ex-smokers complain that they never get enough credit for quitting. While they are still struggling, their nonsmoking friends forget that they might still need encouragement. Follow-up should also include methods to verify abstinence with carbon monoxide readings or other objective measures.

Support the Client During the Relapse Phase

The relapse phase typically begins with a lapse, defined as a single smoking occasion after which abstinence is resumed. Thereafter, the individual engages in a period of struggle during which occasional smoking alternates with complete abstinence. Gradually the smoking becomes more frequent until regular smoking is resumed. Most lapses occur during the first 2 weeks after cessation. Two examples from a recent study we have conducted (Cook 1990) illustrate the subjects' experiences early in the cessation process.

Home alone 2 days after she quit smoking, Eileen was cleaning the family room when she found a cigarette, left by her husband, still a smoker. Apparently it had fallen out of his pocket or pack and was lying on the sofa. Eileen recalled the incident:

> When I saw it, then the hunger for a cigarette just got overwhelming at that point. I felt like there was no way I couldn't smoke it. I should have picked it up and run to the bathroom and thrown it into the toilet but I couldn't let myself do that, it was just a real addiction, a real need to smoke that cigarette. I don't think I would have smoked a cigarette if it hadn't just been there. It was just there. It was like being on a diet, walking into a room and a chocolate chip cookie is lying there, I mean you know, you just can't resist. At the time, I didn't do anything I had been taught to do [to resist smoking]. As far as deep breathing or take time out, move from the situation, all that. It was just a total reaction of *I've got to smoke this cigarette.*

Working late one evening 13 days after quitting smoking, Paul encountered a pack of cigarettes on a nearby desk apparently left by a janitor. Paul reported,

> It was like being surprised . . . the only way I can describe it is if you discovered that there was a Ferrari in your garage and you had no idea how it got there. The hottest car in your imagination is sitting there. And you just jump. You can't believe it. What's going on? Where did this come from? There is even a Bic lighter sitting on top of them. Everything I need to fire one up is right here, right now. Then it was like physically kind of welling up into the chest. It was just like . . . it almost made you want to stand on your tiptoes cause it's almost lifting you off the ground.

Despite his overwhelming desire, Paul resisted the urge to smoke: "You've got to come back down and to do that I just screamed and said a cuss word. I think it was the 'F' word. I didn't care who heard me. And I had a feeling that I want it but I dare not do that. It's a bit like knowing that if you touch them, something bad is going to happen to you. You want them so bad, but it's like putting your hand in a bear trap." When asked what prevented him from smoking, Paul replied, "I screamed and I cussed. . . . and I tried not to look at them. I told myself, 'Just keep walking, just keep walking down the hall. Keep your feet in front of each other and get out of here.'"

These examples illustrate the importance, and the difficulty, of eliminating cigarettes from the environment, especially early in the cessation process. A cigarette is a strong stimulus to smoke, particularly if no one else is around to observe the behavior. These examples also illustrate the role of strategies in preventing lapses. Shiffman (1982) has found that strategy use is the major factor in resisting the temptation to smoke. Eileen admitted that she used no strategies, while Paul spoke of the strategies that he used, including cussing, screaming, and getting away from the stimulus. Thus, helping the client to identify strategies that he or she could use in a tempting situation is an important component to successful Smoking Cessation.

Although the early phases of cessation are especially problematic for some, the later phases present problems as well. Several studies have shown that temptations to resume smoking often occur in negative-affect situations (Cummings, Gordon, and Marlatt 1980; O'Connell and Martin 1987; Shiffman 1982). However, recent research using concepts from the theory of psychological reversals shows that lapses in abstinence are more likely to occur when the ex-smoker was in paratelic states (playful, sensation oriented, and preferring high arousal levels) than in telic states (serious minded, goal oriented, preferring low arousal) (O'Connell, Cook, Gerkovich, Potocky, and Swan 1990). A single lapse after cessation is highly predictive of relapse. Several studies (Brandon, Tiffany, and Baker 1986; O'Connell and Martin 1987) indicate that 90% of those who smoke a single cigarette within the first 3 months of cessation will return to regular smoking within the year. The reasons are unclear. Marlatt and his colleagues posited the Abstinence Violation Effect, which occurs when an individual attributes a lapse to personal and uncontrollable weakness. This attribution leads the individual to resume smoking. On the other hand, a single lapse might reinitiate withdrawal symptoms, which the individual may not be accustomed to dealing with. Or the lapse might convince the ex-smoker that he or she can have a cigarette now and then.

A client's report that he or she has lapsed (smoked but resumed abstinence) or is smoking occasionally is a warning sign of impending relapse but also a sign that the subject is still exercising considerable control over smoking. The initial lapse situation can be explored with the client to determine what factors contributed to the lapse, including times the subject is currently smoking. The client can be advised to institute (or reinstitute) rigorous stimulus control procedures, including disposing of all cigarettes and avoiding places where others are smoking or where cigarettes are available. The client should be informed that the lapses and occasional smoking tend to increase withdrawal symptoms and might make it harder to resist smoking. Different strategies include initiating or stepping up nicotine replacement and helping the client find different ways of remembering to use strategies. Clients who have lapsed need support in understanding that the lapse is not a sign that the client is meant to return to smoking and help in reviewing the reasons for quitting and the benefits. Other techniques that might treat some of the nursing diagnoses caused by stopping smoking might be instituted. Any smoking during a cessation attempt is cause for concern, and the nurse should explain this to the client while being careful not to overreact to admissions of smoking since such reactions may influence the client's tendency to tell the truth in the future.

For the client who returns to regular smoking, the nurse should be supportive, conveying that she knows how difficult it is to stop smoking, reviewing with the client what he or she may have learned about himself or herself or about smoking, encouraging the client to try again, and reminding the client that most people who succeed at quitting must try numerous times before they succeed.

CASE STUDY

Doris was a 43-year-old professional who was going through a divorce at the start of Smoking Cessation. Although she expected to be tempted to smoke when she was dealing with her estranged husband, these incidents were not associated with highly tempting situations. During the first 6 weeks of cessation, her only significant temptation occurred when she was bowling with friends who were smoking. Eleven weeks after quitting, Doris was at a bar for her birthday celebration. She described herself as euphoric, relaxed, and flirtatious. When she asked a member of the band with whom she was chatting for a cigarette, her girlfriend objected strenuously. "I think that I was trying to prove that I can have one and still stay smokeless," Doris said, "that I'm not addicted, or anything, I'm in control of the situation, and whatever it comes to I know that just one little cigarette is not going to put me back on that trodden path." She resumed abstinence after smoking a single cigarette.

About 2 months later (5 months after cessation), Doris began to have problems with her daughter. These problems had been of concern to her for several weeks, but they were especially on her mind one evening when she was discussing the situation with friends. One of the friends was smoking, and

Doris asked him for a cigarette. A few days later she was given some sample cigarettes at a convention she was attending, and thereafter she resumed smoking on a regular basis.

Doris's experience illustrates some of the perplexing aspects of stopping smoking. The stress of dealing with her husband, which occurred frequently during this period and which she expected, did not appear to induce an urge to smoke. However, Doris relapsed in a stressful situation that included a type of stress (problems with her daughter) that she was not prepared to deal with. Although she had resisted temptation in situations where others were smoking and in stressful situations, the combination of a new stressor, smoking cues, and easy availability proved too much to control. It is unclear if her prior lapse at the bar influenced her subsequent relapse. Although Doris resumed abstinence after the lapse in the bar, during which she "proved" that she had control over her smoking habit, the feeling of control may have also given her a false sense of security. Control was demonstrated only for situations in which she was in a specific positive mood. Control in a negative mood is a different psychological experience. This example demonstrates that resisting smoking requires a variety of coping skills, because the skills that work in one situation may be ineffective or inappropriate in another.

CONCLUSION

Smoking Cessation can be carried out at different levels of intensity. The lowest level of intensity involves consistent tracking of the smoking status of clients, encouraging them to quit smoking, referring those who are ready to quit to smoking cessation programs, and following up on their progress. Higher-intensity interventions involve the nurse's involvement in the actual cessation process. The practitioner needs to have appropriate expectations about the success rates of such programs, which are likely to be discouragingly low, and to remain motivated to continue the program despite setbacks. Keeping abreast of new techniques might be helpful, along with self-congratulations for successes. Maintaining a Smoking Cessation intervention is quite similar to maintaining smoking cessation. A significant behavioral change will be demanded, overcoming disappointments and setbacks will be necessary, but the rewards will be significant and compelling.

REFERENCES

Brandon, T.H., Tiffany, S.T., and Baker, T.B. 1986. The process of smoking relapse. In F.M. Tims and C.G. Leukefeld (eds.), *Relapse and recovery in drug abuse* (pp. 104–117). Rockville Md.: U.S. Public Health Service. (NIDA Research Monograph No. 72)

Cook, M.R. 1990. *Reversal theory and the motivations for health behavior* (Final Report: Grant NR 10675). Kansas City, Mo.

Cummings, C., Gordon, J.R., and Marlatt, G.A. 1980. Relapse: Strategies of prevention and prediction. In W.R. Miller (ed.), *The addictive behaviors: Treatment of alcoholism, drug abuse, smoking, and obesity* (pp. 291–321). New York: Pergamon Press.

Janz, N.K., Becker, M.H., Kirscht, J.P., Eraker, S.A., Billi, J.E., and Woolliscroft, J.O. 1987. Evaluation of a minimal-contact smoking cessation intervention in an outpatient setting. *American Journal of Public Health* 77:805–809.

Marlatt, G.A., and Gordon, J.R. 1980. Determinants of relapse: Implications of the maintenance of behavior change. In P.O. Davidson and S.M. Davidson (eds.), *Behavioral medicine: Changing health lifestyles* (pp. 410–452). New York: Brunner/Mazel.

North American Nursing Diagnosis Association. 1990. *Taxonomy I Revised — 1990 with Official Nursing Diagnoses.* St. Louis, Mo.: NANDA.

O'Connell, K.A. 1990. Smoking cessation: Research on relapse crises. In J.J. Fitzpatrick, R.L. Taunton, and J.Q. Benoliel (eds.), *Annual Review of Nursing Research* (vol. 8, pp. 83–100). New York: Springer.

O'Connell, K.A., Cook, M.R., Gerkovich, M.M., Potocky, M., and Swan, G.E. 1990. Reversal theory and smoking: A state-based approach to ex-smokers' highly tempting situations. *Journal of Consulting and Clinical Psychology* 58:489–494.

O'Connell, K.A., and Martin, E.J. 1987. Highly tempting situations associated with abstinence, temporary lapse, and relapse among participants in smoking cessation programs. *Journal of Consulting and Clinical Psychology* 55:367–371.

Prochaska, J.O., and DiClemente, C.C. 1983. Stages and processes of self-change of smoking: Toward an integrative model of change. *Journal of Consulting and Clinical Psychology* 51:390–395.

Schwartz, J.L. 1987. *Review and evaluation of smoking cessation methods: The United States and Canada 1978–1985.* Bethesda, Md.: U.S. Department of Health and Human Services. (NIH Publication No. 87-2940)

Shiffman, S. 1982. Relapse following smoking cessation: A situational analysis. *Journal of Consulting and Clinical Psychology* 50:71–86.

37

WEIGHT MANAGEMENT

JANET K. CRIST

Weight Management is necessary because of the age-old "disease" obesity. In the past, many health care professionals viewed obesity as a simple result of overeating, which could be treated by adherence to a low-calorie diet. Finding the willpower to control gluttony was the obese person's challenge. Others saw the disease as occurring because of psychological problems that caused overeating. Most health care professionals regarded obesity as a problem requiring minimal attention on their part; therefore, the patient's problem was neglected. "Only in recent years has obesity been defined and recognized as a puzzling disorder or group of disorders with major health implications" (Van Itallie 1988, p. xviii). One-quarter of American adults—27% of women and 24% of men—are overweight.

The disease of obesity is associated with high blood pressure, elevated blood cholesterol, diabetes, heart disease, stroke, some cancers, gallbladder disease, and osteoarthritis of the weight-bearing joints (Mason 1990). Evidence is mounting that obesity in adults is associated with certain health risks. Persons with a history of moderate obesity and a generalized distribution of fat may be quite healthy, but there is considerable evidence that central or upper body (truncal) obesity is associated with heart disease, stroke, diabetes, and hypertension. Additionally, orthopedic-related disorders, psychological problems, and much social agony can accompany obesity. Some studies have linked obesity with uterine cancer. Breast, prostate, and colon cancers have been linked not necessarily to obesity but to high fat content in diets. Because smoking was not eliminated as a variable, some of the results from these studies may be questionable. Nevertheless, there is strong evidence that fat in the diet contributes to health problems; thus, there are many factors affecting an individual's weight and that person's attempt to modify weight. Help is needed for the obese person as well as health care professionals to understand the complexities of these problems. Although many of these difficulties seem insurmountable, there is general agreement among researchers that people with weight problems must strive to lose the unwanted pounds through altered lifestyles and more healthful eating habits.

Managing this difficult problem requires attention to the scientific information. Recent research has focused on the physiological causes and the influence of social and environmental aspects. The nurse requires a thorough understanding of nutrition, exercise, and the complex set of problems that cause people to become overweight and unable to lose the weight.

I gratefully acknowledge Jane M. DeNio, RN, BSN for her writing assistance.

OVERVIEW OF OBESITY

Psychological Aspects

For many years obesity was considered to be the result of the inability to cope with psychological problems. The inability to cope manifested itself through eating to feel better or eating to become fat, thereby avoiding certain relationships. Those long-standing theories contributed to prevalent perceptions that the fat person lacks willpower, is lazy, and does not care how he or she looks or feels. Fat people who asked for help were usually referred to a psychiatrist or psychologist, enrolled in a group session, and counseled to learn to deal with their problems. This approach was intended to decrease the person's reliance on food and to make the person feel better. The psychological approach met with some success but did not get to the crux of the problem.

Physiological Aspects

Researchers in the biological sciences have focused on how physiological disorders might affect weight. Greenwood and Vasselli's (1981) studies with animals contributed to the understanding that psychological problems may not be the only reason for overeating. A person may overeat because of certain metabolic changes that occur in the body several months prior to the onset of that behavior. Among the possible physiological causes of obesity are genetics, number and size of fat cells, the regulatory system in the body, the fat storing enzyme (lipoprotein lipase), and taste for fat.

Studies (Stunkard, Foch, and Hrube 1986; Stunkard, Thurkild, Sorenson, Hanis, Teasdale, Chakraborty, Schull, and Schulsinger 1986) involving identical twins and adopted children documented the genetic influence of obesity in humans. Because of their identical genes, identical twins were more likely to have similar weight than were fraternal twins. Adopted children were more likely to have weights similar to their biological parents than to their adoptive parents with whom they had no genes in common.

Studies with Zucker rats, which inherit their obesity as a recessive trait, graphically demonstrated the early onset of obesity and helped explain a theory that involves number of fat cells versus size of fat cells. Hirsch and Knittle (1970) reported on differences in the number of fat cells versus the differences in fat cell size as a factor in obesity in humans. People who became obese as adults had much larger fat cells than normal-weight people. Child-onset obese people were found to have larger numbers of fat cells; their fat cells may have been normal but usually were larger than normal. Their findings led them to conclude that people with the least likely success in losing weight were those with the greatest number of fat cells, predisposing them to obesity in adulthood.

Studies on obesity have demonstrated that the weights of animals and humans remain steady over periods of time. These findings have led to a set-point theory (Keesey 1986; Keesey and Corbett 1984), which states that the human body, under stable environmental and physiological conditions, tends to regulate its weight within fairly narrow limits. It is theoretically possible to change the set point by lowering caloric intake or increasing physical activity. For the set point to be changed permanently, however, the new caloric intake and activity level must remain constant. If either is modified, the body returns to its original set point. This theory is used to explain why it is difficult for obese persons who have lost weight to maintain that lower weight. These people "diet" over a period of time and then revert to their former eating patterns. This return to higher calorie counts puts them back to their original set point. It is unknown where the set-point mechanism resides—within the brain or adipose tissue.

Others (Yost and Eckel, 1988) have explored the possibility that the regulatory mechanism for obesity exists in the adipose cell itself, specifically within the lipoprotein lipase (LPL) enzyme which the adipose cell manufactures. The LPL enzyme is used to pull the fat from food. When a person of normal weight consumes fat, the body lowers the LPL level and attempts to use the fat for energy before storing it in the fat cells. When a formerly obese woman is given fat in her diet, the level of LPL increases dramatically above her already high level; she pulls the fat out of the food and stores it rather than allowing it to be used for energy.

Drewnowski, Brunzell, Sande, Iverius, and Greenwood (1985) explored people's tastes for fatty food. They found that overweight people prefer the taste of fat to that of sugar, in contrast to lean people, who prefer the taste of sugar. Their studies also showed that overweight people consumed no more calories than their thinner counterparts, but because of their desire for the taste of fat, they consumed more of their calories in that form.

Others (Brownell, Greenwood, Stellar, and Schraeger 1986; Gray, Fisler, and Bray 1988) who have studied obesity have dealt with the body's adaptive response to energy expenditure. Changes in metabolic rates and enzyme production are examples of the adaptive changes of the body to deal with thermogenesis, the body's production of heat and use of fuels. Some or all of these adaptive mechanisms appear to be involved when a person attempts to lose weight. We no longer need to use energy to hunt for food, and, in most cases, the quality of our food has increased, so we do not need large quantities of it to meet caloric requirements. Many people, however, continue to eat large quantities and then experience the problem of excess calories and little or no activity. LPL is produced for fat storage, but seldom is that fat storage needed for energy. People usually have plenty of food; therefore, the fat is stored, sometimes permanently. Periods of famine can be simulated by cutting calories to lose weight. This self-imposed famine may increase the production of LPL, causing more fat to be stored instead of using it for energy. Instead of having an energy deficit during the times that calories are reduced, the body adapts by lowering its metabolic rate. This adaptive mechanism, once necessary to survival, now causes some people to have problems getting their weight down and keeping it down. Liebel and Hirsch (1984) suggest that once obese people lose weight, the resulting slowdown in their metabolic rate will make it more difficult to maintain their lower weight. The mechanism to maintain the body's volume of water and sodium is also stimulated when attempting to cut calories to lose weight; as fat is lost, water is retained. This and other adaptive mechanisms, which are physiologically induced, contribute to the psychological frustrations associated with losing weight.

Social and Environmental Aspects

While much has been done and is continuing to be done to study the physiological aspects of obesity, research is being conducted on the external influences to obesity. Approximately 34 million adults in the United States are obese, and the incidence of obesity in children is increasing. Studies have shown that obese children are prone to be obese adults; the obesity problem is only going to increase.

Wadden, a prominent researcher in obesity, stated in an interview with Liebman (1987) that the percentage of obese persons in the United States has steadily increased during the twentieth century. He believes it is not the gene pool that has changed; rather, the environment which tends to support obesity. At the same time that money is being spent to research and treat obesity, the country's food industry is spending more to advertise and encourage people to eat fattening foods. The fast food industry, known for its high-fat, -sugar, and -sodium foods, has grown by leaps and bounds to meet the needs of our rushed society. Conversely, the level of physical activity has decreased due to increased use of cars and public transportation, sedentary jobs, and decreased leisure time for sports.

NURSING DIAGNOSES AND APPROPRIATE CLIENT GROUP

Weight management is an appropriate intervention for several nursing diagnoses:

Altered Nutrition: More Than Body Requirements
Knowledge Deficit (Nutrition)
Knowledge Deficit (Exercise)
Impaired Physical Mobility
Activity Intolerance
Altered Health Maintenance
Powerlessness
Self Esteem Disturbance
Ineffective Individual Coping
Social Isolation

The most appropriate client groups for Weight Management are adults with no major health problems requiring diet therapy. If a patient has a medical condition necessitating diet therapy, the assistance of a dietitian may be required. Many clients have difficulty complying with the list of foods to be eaten and not eaten to manage their health condition. But with the nurse's knowledge, understanding, and guidance, many clients are able to follow the dietitian's prescription through their daily living patterns. Adults with ineffective coping mechanisms, feelings of anxiety and powerlessness, disturbances in self-concept, and social isolation may require additional psychological counseling in addition to Weight Management. Here, again, the nurse's knowledge, understanding, and guidance may help facilitate the work being done toward the psychological problems.

Research continues to identify the need for childhood weight management programs because the overweight child is more likely to mature into an overweight adult. Traditionally, children have been included in weight management programs, but their growth factor has not been factored into the equation of energy requirements versus caloric requirements; thus, the potential exists for risking future growth and health problems. These potential risks may require the direct attention of dietitians and physicians.

WEIGHT MANAGEMENT PROGRAM

Treatment for obesity is based on understanding the many problems faced by the obese. Mandell stated (1986 p. 21), "For me (and other physicians holding similar views that obesity is mainly a result of overeating), obesity is a wonderful thing. Once we have decided we don't know what's wrong with an obese patient and don't know how to treat his or her symptoms, we can take the offensive and blame the patient." This honest statement demonstrates the need for health professionals to become knowledgeable about what causes obesity, as well as the feelings of the obese—of failure, guilt, frustration, and loneliness—that they have faced probably most of their life.

Knowledge of the research into obesity is basic to understanding the complexities of the problem. Instructional strategies based on these findings are more likely to motivate the client to make the behavioral changes necessary to succeed. Knowledge of the body's nutritional needs, the components of a good balanced diet, where exercise fits into this formula, as well as strong communication skills and counseling techniques are necessary to help the client succeed in losing weight and, in turn, lowering the health risks associated with obesity. Weight Management is accomplished by a five-step program.

Focused Assessment

Grommet (1988) describes a widely accepted approach to data gathering and states that a multi-disciplinary approach to Weight Management is necessary. An entry questionnaire and a physical examination can cover the areas of nutrition and food behaviors, energy expenditure assessment, psychosocial assessment, and medical assessment. The nutrition and food assessment arises from a self-reported food record. The record includes not only the kind of food eaten but also the amounts consumed, how it was prepared, and the caloric value. The context or situation in which the food was eaten, the duration of the eating, location and physical position while eating, mood while eating, presence of others, or associated activities while eating need to be recorded. If the assessment is only on the caloric intake and not on energy expenditure, the client may not link the importance of activity and obesity. An assessment of the energy balance will encourage the obese not to focus on intake alone. Grommet's energy expenditure assessment plan also includes multiple physiological measures of daily activities and their resulting energy costs.

The psychosocial assessment consists of an interview or questionnaire that considers why a person wants to lose weight, how many times he or she has tried, length of maintenance, if food is used to stifle negative emotions (anger, anxiety, boredom, depression, rejection, and loneliness), how other family members feel about obesity, and how this weight loss treatment will be different from others. Grommet suggests using other standardized psychosocial instruments toward cognitive and affective assessment to ascertain other underlying psychological aspects. Grommet's medical assessment includes a medical history and physical examination, as well as selected blood chemistry tests and urinalysis. The history covers a weight history, drug therapies, and estimate of body composition with skin fold testing.

Grommet's approach to assessment is thorough; however, I have found that the obese resent all the extended questionnaires, probing, and expense in order to "just lose weight." This may explain why people continue to use commercial weight businesses. In many of those businesses, they go in, pay a fee, and are instructed how to follow the program, using the business's own foods in many cases. There is little to no emphasis on health or exercise. In order for Weight Management to be lasting, a life-style change is required. Therefore, I use modifications to Grommet's model in my clinic.

The assessment data I use are listed in Table 37–1. The data are obtained from a self-report questionnaire (Figure 37–1), which includes a 1-day sample menu. The questions are carefully stated to lessen the possibility of offending the client. Following the completion of the questionnaire, I clarify the written information and

TABLE 37-1. ASSESSMENT QUESTIONS

Demographic information
Name
Age
Occupation
Marital status and who you live with
Setting (city versus rural)

Family history
Age and weight of parents and siblings
Occupation of parents
Health history of parents, grandparents
Cultural background

Health of patient
Height and current weight
Where do you carry your weight?
Any diseases or health conditions?
Allergies
Medications currently taking
Cholesterol level
Did physician recommend weight loss? Why?

Patient's diet history
Weight as a child
Have you tried weight reduction?
What methods?
Success of these methods?
How long did you maintain this weight?
What would you like to weigh?
When did you last weigh that amount?

Food or eating history
What is a typical day's eating pattern?
What are problem times of the day for eating?
What are the problem foods?
How much water do you drink per day?
What situations cause you the most problems with eating?
What influences your eating habits the most?
How did you learn to plan your meals?
What influences you the most when grocery shopping?
How do you decide what you will eat each day?

Exercise history
Exercise regularly?
How many times per week?
What kind?
How long and what intensity?
What keeps you from doing an exercise?

Motivational history
Why do you want to lose weight?
Why did you decide to get assistance to lose weight?
Did any one help you to make that decision?
Does anyone know you are asking for assistance?

obtain any additional information through an initial interview. The interview demonstrates a personal interest that a written questionnaire cannot provide.

Clients seem to resent being told they have to have a physical examination before they start a weight management and exercise program. Their usual reply is "Why? He told me I needed to lose weight when I last saw him. Do I have to pay for another exam?" An examination is probably not essential unless the client has significant health problems or has not seen a physician for several years. Interview questions pertaining to activity level at work, occupation, activities at home, leisure-time activity, and regular exercise pattern usually reveal if their caloric intake exceeds their energy expenditure. Additionally, excessive figuring of formulas makes the client feel like an object rather than a human with likes, dislikes, and feelings.

The psychosocial assessment is probably one of the most important aspects in assisting the obese person to be successful in losing weight. I do not believe that the psychology of the person is the reason he or she gained weight in the first place, but it can be one of the most important aspects in losing weight. Many clients are trying to lose weight again. They have been made to feel like failures not only by family members and friends but by many health professionals, all because very few people fully understand the complexities of the problem. Obese clients need to be told that their problem is probably not their fault; genetics, adaptive mechanisms caused by previous weight problems, and socioenvironmental influences all contributed to their problem. They also need to be told that no one can offer anything to correct

WEIGHT & WELLNESS

M A N A G E M E N T   320 East Benton • Iowa City, Iowa 52240 • (319)338-9775

CLIENT HEALTH QUESTIONNAIRE

NAME _____   HOME PHONE _____

ADDRESS _____   BUSINESS PHONE _____

CITY _____ STATE _____ ZIP _____

AGE _____ HEIGHT _____ OCCUPATION _____

Please check any diseases or conditions you have had:

___ Alcohol related problems	___ Epilepsy
___ Anemia	___ Fractures (within past 6 mos.)
___ Anorexia	___ Gall bladder problems
___ Arthritis	___ Gastric reduction
___ Asthma	___ Gout
___ Bronchitis	___ Heart attack
___ Bulimia	___ High blood pressure
___ Cancer	___ Hypoglycemia (low blood sugar)
___ Chest pains	___ Kidney disorders
___ Chronic cough	___ Nervous disorders
___ Chron's disease	___ Osteoporosis
___ Circulatory disorders	___ Pancreatitis
___ Colitis	___ Pneumonia
___ Colostomy	___ Rheumatoid arthritis
___ Coumadin therapy	___ Shortness of breath
___ Diabetis	___ Stroke
___ Diverticulitis	___ Thyroid disorders
___ Depression	___ Ulcers
___ Emphysema	

Please list any other conditions not included above _____

WOMEN ONLY:
Are you now pregnant?   Yes ____ No ____
Are you currently breast feeding?   Yes ____ No ____

GENERAL INFORMATION:
Have you been hospitalized within the last two years?   Yes ____ No ____
If so, when and for what reason? _____

List any medications and dosages of such you are currently taking
(Also include any non-prescription drugs.) _____

List any allergies (Food, drug or seasonal) _____

Are you subject to headaches, dizziness or fainting spells?   Yes ____ No ____

Do you take any vitamin supplement?   Yes ____ No ____

Have you had your cholesterol level measured recently?   Yes ____ No ____
How long ago? _____ What were the results? _____

Are you currently under a physician's care?   Yes ____ No ____
If so, please describe: _____

Has your physician recommended that you lose weight?   Yes ____ No ____
If yes, did he/she recommend a particular weight?   Yes ____ No ____ Amount _____

Name of your personal physician _____ City _____

May we notify your physician that you are participating in our weight
reduction program?   Yes ____ No ____

Have you ever consulted a psychologist, counselor or pyschiatrist?
Yes ____ No ____ If so, please state reason. _____

What previous methods of weight reduction have you attempted? _____

What results did you obtain? _____ How long did you maintain your
loss? _____

Are other members of your immediate family overweight?   Yes ____ No ____
If yes, who? _____ by approximately how many pounds? _____

What would you like to weigh? _____ When did you last weigh that amount? _____
Do you exercise regularly?   Yes ____ No ____ What type of exercise do you do? _____
_____ How many times per week? _____

Write a typical day's eating pattern below.
TIME	MEAL	FOODS AND DRINKS CONSUMED
___	Breakfast	_____
___	Break	_____
___	Lunch	_____
___	Break	_____
___	Dinner	_____
___	Evening snacks	_____

Please indicate any problem times or problem foods _____

How much water do you drink daily? _____
How much coffee or tea do you drink daily? _____
How much pop do you drink daily? _____

How did you learn about our clinic? _____

I understand that the information provided above will be kept confidential
unless a medical problem is discovered. Should such a problem be
identified, necessary portions of the information I have provided may be
shared with my physician. I have answered all questions as truthfully and
completely as possible. My signature in no way obligates me to participate
in the programs of WEIGHT & WELLNESS MANAGEMENT.

FOR COUNSELOR'S USE ONLY

Current weight _____

Client's signature _____

Counselor's signature _____

Date _____

FIGURE 37–1.   Client Health Questionnaire

those measures but they can get help in learning how to make good choices in eating, how to increase physical activity without "killing" themselves, and how to handle the social and environmental aspects.

The Eating Plan Prescription

The next step is implementing a plan of action for the individual. The caloric plan can be determined by counting the usual calories eaten and subtracting 500 calories from their count. Another method is increasing the energy expenditure so there is an energy deficit of approximately 500 calories per day. Using these methods, the client will lose approximately 1 pound per week. These are the ideal methods to figure caloric plans, but seldom can a person give an actual calorie count for each day. They usually say that their food intake varies each day depending on whether they take their lunch to work, eat out at noon or in the evening, where they eat, and with whom. I have found it best to put most females with a medium build and height on a 1200 calorie program based on the U.S. Department of Agriculture minimum requirements for an adult. For the men, a 1500 calorie program is recommended, with the additional calories consisting of servings in the fruit, vegetable, and starch categories. Both programs are based on an exchange program, with the client making the choices in each food group. These levels of calorie intake allow the person to begin the Weight Management program with some success. If they are averaging more than a 2-pound loss per week, their calorie count is increased. If they are losing less than an average of 1 pound per week, they are encouraged to increase their energy expenditure each day.

Energy Utilization Tactics

A person who is starting an exercise program should be evaluated by a physician, but if that is required before starting, many individuals will not follow through. To begin this part of the program, I explore with them where they work, the activity level required for the job, and where they live in relationship to their place of employment. I avoid the use of the term *exercise* initially. Many people can begin to increase their activity by taking stairs instead of an elevator. For example, if they work on the sixth floor, they will be instructed to begin by walking the first flight and then pick up the elevator on the second floor. When they have mastered that level of activity, they can take two flights up, and so forth. Others will be encouraged to walk to work instead of driving or riding the bus. If they have been riding the bus, the same progression can be used as taking the stairs. When they feel better about this activity, the term *exercise* may be added, such as a walk. Instruct the person to take at least a 30-minute walk daily. This exercise may need to be a stroll at first, with the client resting if necessary. The speed of exercise will increase over time, which will necessitate a longer distance to be covered. The client needs to be instructed to continue exercising for at least 30 minutes per day.

Much of the literature states that exercise is needed only three times per week, but I have found that clients usually do not find the time to exercise unless it is planned into each day. It should become an every-day habit, just like brushing teeth. Along with the encouragement to exercise, teachings about health precautions are necessary. At a minimum, clients should be instructed that feelings of lightheadedness, chest pain, or muscle or joint pain require that exercise must stop until the pain is properly evaluated by a physician.

The term *exercise* to most obese people is a "dirty" word. They say, "How can I exercise when I don't even have enough energy to do my daily work?" I have found that increasing activity gradually works, but I also insist on seeing some improvement on a weekly basis. Many clients need suggestions on how to incorporate exercise into their lives, such as through family leisure activity. Ideas for this kind of activity include a walk in the park, a walk to the library, or a game of softball with the children and neighbors.

Adherence Strategies

Laguartra and Danish (1988) identify five variables to explain why a client does not adhere to prescribed treatments: characteristics of the client, characteristics of the illness, characteristics of the clinical setting, quality of interaction between the expert and the client, and characteristic of prescribed regimen. These variables can play a significant part for an individual to follow a regimen for Weight Management and for incorporating this regimen into his or her life-style so the changes can be permanent. Additionally, any one of these characteristics can be the impetus or excuse for a client to discontinue the program. To help people who have had lifelong problems with obesity and weight control, the last three variables need to be emphasized through counseling and education.

The characteristics of the clinical setting are important. The clinic should be convenient and easily within driving or walking distance. It should have a conference room that affords privacy and is pleasantly appointed for comfort and mood elevation. The client should not have to wait for long periods of time before being seen; they are usually fitting their counseling sessions into an already busy schedule. The scheduling should allow flexibility so that a client feels free to bring up problems without feeling rushed.

The quality of interaction between the nurse and client is of primary importance. Rogers (1959) states there must be an atmosphere of empathy, genuineness, and unconditional positive regard as conditions of helping. Because these clients have been judged negatively by society, there has to be warmth, friendliness, and an ability to understand the feelings of the client so that he or she feels satisfied with the interaction and will adhere to the teachings and recommendations. I do not necessarily feel that the nurse has to have experienced the problems of obesity, but it helps to be able to say, "I know, I have been there," when the client asks, "How do you know how I feel? Have you ever been fat?" It is extremely important that no judgmental statements are made during the counseling. These clients are sensitive to body language. They have been the recipients of jokes, snickers, and name calling for probably much of their lives or have imagined them because they feel so negative about themselves. Obese people are extremely sensitive about how they look. Regardless of what other people think, they have not "let themselves go." They are a victim of a disease that is not necessarily of their own doing.

If clients are to follow a Weight Management program for a lifetime, the characteristics of the prescribed treatment must be adjusted to fit their life-style as much as possible and not be complex. For example, if a client and her husband have a favorite place to eat every Friday evening after work, she will need to be taught how to order from the menu without having to find out the calorie count of every food item ordered. She should be taught the appearance of serving sizes so it is not necessary to weigh and measure each item (for example, "A protein serving should be the size of the palm of the hand"). She needs to be guided to the most appropriate selections. Instead of a hamburger and french fries, a grilled chicken breast sandwich and a side salad are better choices. If she does not like those selections, she may need to make a decision as to how often to eat out. These should be her decisions, not the counselor's.

Because family dynamics enter into the decisions to be made, many changes in the client's life-style may not be altered too much if the client is to be able to follow them for a lifetime. Adjusting the treatment plan to meet the individual's needs may require inserting a strenuous exercise program rather than decreasing the calorie intake significantly. Another option is to decrease calories fairly significantly when accompanied by an exercise program consisting of a walk or a bike ride with the family three to five times per week. Since the purpose is to obtain a permanent change in weight management, the decision regarding treatment plans should be left up to the client and family.

Structured Reinforcement and Support

Brownell (1984) felt that the best way to give reinforcement and support to overweight clients is through group sessions. Group interactions give the necessary support to the individuals so they will continue. From my experience, however, group sessions put the person in a competitive situation. As the etiology of obesity is varied, so the weight loss will also be varied. Although individual weight losses are not mentioned, group sessions cause people to compare their progress. A group member whose weight loss is not as rapid as the next person's may become discouraged and feel like a failure.

I have found individual counseling to be the most effective choice in my clinic. Many clients have stated, "Good! I don't have to sit in a group meeting again." Individual sessions allow the program to be adjusted to that particular client and to handle his or her problems as they arise. Having the client keep a daily eating and exercise diary allows me to teach and adjust the program as needed. The diary is not time-consuming for the client and is a good method for monitoring eating. Additionally it is an effective teaching tool. Although teaching topics such as good fats versus bad fats, cholesterol versus fat, and how to read labels might be easier in a group, the individual counseling allows those subjects to be introduced when the client is ready. Individual counseling also permits sessions as often as the client and nurse feel are necessary. Some clients require daily sessions because they feel sure they will fail again; others may need to be seen only weekly or twice a week.

Most recommendations in weight loss plans say that the client should not be weighed more than once per week. That may be true in theory, but I have found it is reinforcing to have at least two weights weekly. It is important to most clients to have the tangible reward the scale shows to keep them progressing in their program. If they have been eating and exercising properly for a week, they need to see the weight loss to prove they have done well. Additionally, monitoring twice a week assists in keeping the client on the program by not allowing the person to eat out of control for a couple of days and then fast for 2 days to lose weight. That kind of behavior does not indicate good changes in eating habits.

INTERVENTION TOOLS

Information on the nutritional needs of the body can be found in literature from the U.S. Department of Agriculture and Human Services, the National Dairy Council, the National Council of Nutrition, and university extension bulletins, as well as other agencies. Much of this literature is available from local public health departments. A poster of the four food groups, available from many of these agencies, is necessary to provide instruction on nutrition.

The client needs to keep a daily food and exercise planner/diary; an example is shown in Figure 37–2. This planner is used to monitor the client's eating. The planner can be used to plan meals before eating and/or to record what has been eaten on a daily basis. Clients need to list what food group the specific item belongs in so that they eventually learn to make good choices in their diet. Many clients need assistance in planning meals; the use of cookbooks with nutritional analyses listed for each recipe can be helpful. To assist in the reading of food labels, actual labels should be used for instructional purposes.

Other tools used for teaching exercise and other health matters are university newsletters and books, which can be loaned to the clients to reinforce what is taught by the nurse. Books written for the layperson that are widely available include *Jane Brody's Nutrition Book; Jane Brody's Good Food Book; Reader's Digest Eat Better, Live Better; Reader's Digest: The Complete Manual of Fitness and Well-Being; The Aerobic Program for Total Well-Being; Fit or Fat;* and *Fit or Fat for Women.* The nurse's responsibilities when suggesting books is to be sure the information is accurate and not just the current popular information.

	Monday	Tuesday	Wednesday	Thursday	Friday	Saturday	Sunday	Weekly Allotments
BRKFST								Beef Eggs Cheese **Weekly Weight Record**
LUNCH								Last Weight _____ Monday _____ Tuesday _____ Wednesday _____ Thursday _____ Friday _____ Saturday _____
DINNER								
SNKS								TOTAL LOSS _____ FOR WEEK Questions & Notes
	Water Coffee/tea Diet drinks Extras	Water Coffee/tea Diet drinks Extras	Water Coffee/tea Diet drinks Extras	Water Coffee/tea Diet drinks Extras	Water Coffee/tea Diet drinks Extras	Water Coffee/tea Diet drinks Extras	Water Coffee/tea Diet drinks Extras	
	Proteins Vegetables Fruits Breads Milk Fat Salad dressing	Proteins Vegetables Fruits Breads Milk Fat Salad dressing	Proteins Vegetables Fruits Breads Milk Fat Salad dressing	Proteins Vegetables Fruits Breads Milk Fat Salad dressing	Proteins Vegetables Fruits Breads Milk Fat Salad dressing	Proteins Vegetables Fruits Breads Milk Fat Salad dressing	Proteins Vegetables Fruits Breads Milk Fat Salad dressing	*WEIGHT & WELLNESS* M A N A G E M E N T 320 East Benton • Iowa City, Iowa 52240 (319) 338-9775
	Exercise: Kind Time	Exercise: Kind Time	Exercise: Kind Time	Exercise: Kind Time	Exercise: Kind Time	Exercise: Kind Time	Exercise: Kind Time	

FIGURE 37–2. Daily Menu Planner

CASE STUDY

Betty, a 43-year-old single woman who lived alone, worked as a data programmer in the community. She was referred to the clinic by a social worker because she was grossly overweight. She was seeing the social worker at the mental health center because of feeling so isolated. She did not have the confidence to ask others out for an evening of fun, and nobody ever asked her to join them. She spent most of her time at work or in her apartment. When she sat in my office, she would not look me in the eye and made repeated references that she was so ashamed of herself because of her weight.

She grew up on a farm and was the youngest of 12 siblings. Her father died at age 72; she did not remember the cause. She remembered him as healthy and quite thin. Her mother was overweight by approximately 50 to 75 pounds. Betty remembered her as always in that size range and that she always seemed tired and never had any fun. Her mother died in a car accident at age 62 years. Betty stated that six of her siblings are also overweight by 20 pounds to 50 pounds.

Betty weighed 298 pounds at the clinic and was 5 feet, 10 inches tall, with a large body frame. Her weight was not localized to any certain place on her body. She stated she had always been fat. Her blood pressure was 169/92. She did not know her cholesterol count but assumed it was normal since her doctor had not said anything about it. She had seen a physician approximately 3 months ago and had received instructions to lose weight because of her blood pressure. He had not suggested how to do it or where to get help. A person at work had suggested the mental health clinic might be a place to start. Betty stated she "dieted" all her life, but never seemed to succeed: "I always seemed to fail at that." She did not have any planned exercise, and her activity at work was sedentary. She drove to work and anywhere else she needed to go. "I could not walk. My feet and legs hurt too much, and besides I jiggle. My clothes always seem too small. I'm afraid people will make fun of me. I don't want people to see me."

Betty said it did not seem as if she ate very much, but "I suppose I do because look how FAT I am." She did not eat breakfast "because I'm not hungry then." Many times she did not eat lunch because she did not have time at work; "besides, if I eat then, I seem to be starved the rest of the day." She started eating when she got home, "and then I eat until I go to bed. Many times I wake up at night really hungry. I eat so I can get back to sleep." Her evening meal consisted of food picked up at a fast-food drive-up or a large, delivered pizza.

Betty came for help because of the mental health referral (a requirement to continue that counseling) but stated, "I really have to make some changes. I can't live like this anymore, but where do I start?" We started with the nursing diagnoses: Altered Nutrition: More Than Body Requirements, Powerlessness, Self Esteem Disturbance, Ineffective Individual Coping, Knowledge Deficit (Nutrition), Activity Intolerance (because of self-concept) and Knowledge Deficit (Exercise), Social Isolation, and Altered Health Maintenance.

Betty completed the health questionnaire, and additional information was obtained during our face-to-face interview. I usually orient females to a 1200 calorie weight management program, but in Betty's case, I started her on a 1500 calorie program. I felt she would be too hungry with only 1200 calories of food, and hunger might cause temptation to eat foods not on the program. As she progressed, we determined she could eat between 1500 and 1800 calories a day and still lose weight. But by starting her at the lower end of her range, she lost weight and felt comfortable with the eating plan. She liked to have milk at each meal, so we included that in her plan, along with an additional serving of yogurt or cheese. Over time, Betty was allowed to increase the amount of fruits, vegetables, and starches as she felt she needed them. Because she had been eating fast foods and pizzas in the past, I worked with her to plan grocery lists and 2 weeks of sample menus. As she became more comfortable with the program, I began to share recipes with her to add variety to her diet. I taught her how to figure combination dishes, such as casseroles, tacos, and chili, into her daily diet. Later instruction included how to judge whether a recipe she found in the newspaper was a good choice for her diet or how to modify it to make it acceptable. I instructed her to use the menu planner/diary to record everything she ate. I explained that it was not my approach to reprimand her if she ate something that was not on the program. Using her diary, we discussed alternative choices based on the nutritional values of what she had eaten and the circumstances that caused her to make certain food selections. Later in the program, we talked about eating in restaurants and in other people's homes.

The biggest problem I had was trying to convince Betty that exercise was just as important to the overall program as what she was eating. She kept saying she would start exercising after she lost some weight. I explored her work setting with her to identify exercise availability. The first suggestion was for her to park in the farthest space of the parking lot so she would have to walk into the building. She was hesitant because she had an assigned space fairly close to the building. She was afraid that changing spaces could cause problems for the other personnel with assigned spots. She worked on the first floor, so climbed no stairs, and she had a sedentary job. She could not walk or ride the bus to work because her plant was outside the city limits, with no bus service. Further, there were no sidewalks to use for walking during breaks. Because of her weight, the ideal exercise would have been water exercise to ease the stress on her lower joints, but she would not consider it. She did not have a swimming suit and would not buy one because she would not be "caught dead in a swimming suit."

Because of her resistance to any of these options, I modified my approach. I was able to convince her to buy a good pair of walking shoes, stressing the more expensive brands versus those from a discount store, because she needed the support and cushioning the better brands provide. I suggested she go to a store that specialized in clothing for larger women and buy an exercise outfit sized to fit her. When she had the proper equipment, I encouraged her to start exercising by strolling around the block where she lived two to three times per day. Her first goal was to be able to stroll for 30 minutes at one time. Then we worked toward obtaining an aerobic effect. The speed of her walking was increased with the use of walking tapes. Because she did not know how to take her pulse, I instructed her to regulate her speed according to her breathing; she was not to be so breathless that she could not carry on a conversation with another person. Her clue to knowing she was exercising rather than simply walking was that she should be perspiring, at least around her hairline.

The fact that I see all my patients through individual sessions was ideal for Betty. I do not believe she would have continued her program if she had to be in a group session. In the beginning, I encouraged Betty to see me six times a week. I wanted her to know that there was always someone she could talk to about her problem. In our initial encounters, Betty never asked any questions, and she was very slow answering mine. She would not look at me when she talked, and she cried easily. Eventually, as she understood that I have had a weight problem, she became more open, initiating the conversation and looking at me as she talked. One day she announced that she and her counselor at the mental health clinic felt she no longer needed that counseling. She talked about social outings with people at work and how she could not remember when she had so much energy.

At the beginning of her program I asked Betty's permission to contact her physician and her mental health counselor. I talked to her physician about her blood pressure and cholesterol count. He felt both would come down if she lost weight. The counselor stated that if I could help her feel positive about herself and her actions with regard to her weight, her other problems would fall into place. I worked with Betty for 13 months as she lost 108 pounds. Following her weight loss, her blood pressure was 120/80–130/84, and her cholesterol count was 184. I continue to see Betty approximately once per month, and she remains at her desired goal weight.

SUMMARY

My suggestions for Weight Management do not completely adhere to the literature recommendations; I have modified the protocol based on my experience as a nurse and formerly obese person. There is a pressing need for more research in this area, particularly from the nursing point of view. I am frequently asked as clients move to other locations in the country, "Is there a nurse like you where I'm going to live?" I strongly suggest that nurses take an interest in this community-based type of client care.

REFERENCES

Bailey, C. 1977. *Fit or fat?* Boston: Houghton Mifflin.

Bailey, C., and Bishop, L. 1989. *Fit or fat for women.* Boston: Houghton Mifflin.

Brody, J.E. 1985. *Jane Brody's good food book: Living the high carbohydrate way.* New York: Bantam Books.

Brody, J.E. 1987. *Jane Brody's nutrition book: A lifetime guide to good eating for better health and weight control.* New York: Bantam Books.

Brownell, K.D. 1984. The psychology and physiology of obesity. Implications for screening and treatment. *Journal of the American Dietetic Association* 84(4):406–414.

Brownell, K.D., Greenwood, M.R.C., Stellar, E., and Schraeger, E. 1986. The effects of repeated dieting on metabolism and food efficiency. *Physiological Behavior* 38:459–464.

Cooper, K.H. 1982. *The aerobics program for total well-being: Exercise, diet, emotional balance.* New York: Bantam Books.

Drewnowski, A., Brunzell, J.D., and Sande, K., Iverius, B., and Greenwood, M.R.C. 1985. Sweet tooth reconsidered: Taste responsiveness in human obesity. *Physiology and Behavior* 35:617–622.

Gardner, E.J. (ed.). 1982. *Reader's Digest eat better, live better: A commonsense guide to nutrition and good health.* Pleasantville, N.Y.: Reader's Digest Association.

Gray, D.S., Fisler, J.S., and Bray, G.A. 1988. Effects of repeated weight loss and regain on body composition in obese rats. *American Journal of Clinical Nutrition* 47:393–399.

Greenwood, M.R.C., and Vasselli, J.R. 1981. In R.F. Beers and E.G. Bassett (eds.), The effects of nitrogen and caloric restriction on adipose tissue, lean body mass and food intake of genetically obese rats: The LPL hypotheses. *Nutritional factors: Modulating effects of metabolic processes.* New York: Raven Press.

Grommet, J.K. 1988. Assessment of the obese person. In R.T. Frankle and M.U. Yang (eds.), *Obesity and weight control* (pp. 111–132). Rockville, Md.: Aspen.

Hirsch, J., and Knittle, J.L. 1970. Cellularity of obese and nonobese human adipose tissue. *Federation Proceedings 29,* 1516.

Horn, B. (ed.) 1988. *Reader's Digest: The complete manual of fitness and well-being: A lifetime guide to self-improvement.* Pleasantville, N.Y.: Reader's Digest.

Keesey, R.E. 1986. A set-point theory of obesity. In K.D. Brownell and J.P. Foreyt (eds.), *Handbook of eating disorders* (pp. 63–87). New York: Basic Books.

Keesey, R.E., and Corbett, S. 1984. Metabolic defense of the body set-point. In A.J. Stunkard and E. Stellar (eds.), *Eating and its disorders* (pp. 87–96). New York: Raven Press.

Laguartra, I., and Danish, S.J. 1988. A primer for nutritional counseling. In R.T. Frankle and M.U. Yang (eds.), *Obesity and Weight Control* (pp. 205–224). Rockville, Md.: Aspen.

Liebel R.L., and Hirsch, J. 1984. Diminished energy requirements in reduced-obese patients. *Metabolism* 33(2):164–169.

Liebman, B.F. 1987. Fated to be Fat? *Nutrition Action Health Letter* 14:(1)4–6.

Mandell, T. 1986. Obesity—a boon to us physicians. *Post Graduate Medicine* 80(7):21, 25.

Mason, J.O. (ed.). 1990. Conference edition: Summary. In *Healthy people 2000. National health promotion and disease prevention objectives.* Washington, D.C.: U.S. Department of Health and Human Services, Public Health Service.

National Institutes of Health Consensus Development Conference Statement, H., Jules (Chairman). 1985. Health implications of obesity. *Annals of Internal Medicine* 103(1):147–151.

Rogers, C.R. 1959. A theory of therapy, personality, and interpersonal relationships, as developed in the client-centered framework. In S. Koch (ed.), *Psychology: A study of science* (pp. 184–256). New York: McGraw-Hill.

Stunkard, A.J., Foch, T.T., and Hrubec, Z. 1986. A twin study of human obesity. *Journal of the American Medical Association* 256(1):51–54.

Stunkard, A.J., Thorkild, I.A., Sorenson, T.I.A., Hanis, C., Teasdale, T., Chakraborty, R., Schull, W., and Schulsinger, F. 1986. An adoption study of human obesity. *New England Journal of Medicine* 314(4):193–198.

Van Itallie, T.B. 1988. Foreword to R.T. Frankle and M. Yang (eds.), *Obesity and weight control.* (pp. xvii–xviii). Rockville, Md.: Aspen.

Wadden, T.A., and Stunkard, A.J. 1985. Social and psychological consequences of obesity. *Annuals of Internal Medicine* 103:1062–1067.

Yost, T.J. and Eckel, R.H. 1988. Fat calories may be preferentially stored in reduced-obese women: A permissive pathway for resumption of the obese state. *Journal of Clinical Endocrinology and Metabolism* 67(2):259–264.

SECTION V

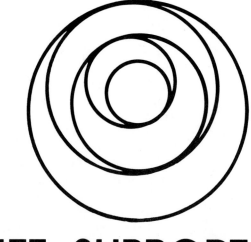

LIFE SUPPORT

Overview: Commitment to Healing and Caring

GLORIA M. BULECHEK
JOANNE C. McCLOSKEY

Critical care nurses make up the largest group of nurse specialists. The autonomous nature of their practice, however, is not generally understood. Practice as a critical care nurse requires an in-depth understanding of normal body function, compensatory mechanisms for alterations in function, and the use of technology and drugs to treat dysfunction. In addition, it is the nurse who makes the situation human for the patient and family. As knowledge and technology have increased, many specialized arenas of critical care practice have developed, among them, dialysis, neuroscience, and coronary care. Too often it is assumed that nurses in these units are technicians practicing strictly by protocol. The seven interventions explored in this section refute this assumption. The interventions are presented at a more abstract level than is typical of critical care literature. The collection illustrates the complex nature of clinical judgment required by critical care nurses and the comprehensive responsibility they assume.

The Surveillance chapter provides a classic description of autonomous nursing action in critical care settings. Surveillance includes both cognitive and behavioral nursing activities to collect information, synthesize that information, and take appropriate action. A nurse using Surveillance, the subject of Chapter 38, must know when to look, what to look for, and why to look. Frequently expert technical skills are required to manage the technology used in indirect measurement. Systematic documentation is required so patterns in data can be identified. Expert clinical judgment is required in order to decide whether to continue monitoring, whether to adjust medications or equipment, whether to institute a new protocol, or whether to collaborate with other health professionals. Cynthia M. Dougherty points out a number of nursing diagnoses for which this intervention could be used and a variety of settings where nurses could use the intervention.

Marita G. Titler and Gerry A. Jones define Airway Management in Chapter 39 as the initiation and maintenance of airway patency. It is accomplished in several ways, from correct positioning to use of various artificial airway devices. The authors organize these many activities into an intervention with four components: monitoring, positioning, insertion and management of the airway, and secretion removal. They draw from a vast literature in nursing and medicine to formulate recommendations for nursing practice. A considerable amount of nursing research has been conducted on the techniques described, and much more remains to be studied. Titler and Jones recommend the intervention for three respiratory nursing diagnoses and point out potential risks from instituting the intervention.

Mechanical ventilation is a common life support measure in critical care units. Nurses are responsible for managing the care of these patients in collaboration with a variety of health team workers. The nurse needs a broad perspective for dealing with all components of the intervention of Ventilatory Support as described by Jane S. Knipper and Michele A. Alpen in Chapter 40: initiation of mechanical ventilation, management of the equipment, monitoring patient response and management of complications, and weaning from mechanical ventilation. The authors provide tables that are helpful in understanding the technology used in artificial ventilation and refer readers seeking practice protocols in authoritative references. Two case studies are provided—one dealing with routine use of the intervention and a second dealing with a more complex situation.

The next chapter, describing Hemodynamic Regulation, begins with an overview of the interrelationship of the heart, vascular structures, and intravascular volume. Nursing diagnoses are related to this physiological triad. Marla Prizant-Weston and Kathleen Castiglia structure the three-part intervention around three goals for treatment. The nurse needs to select the appropriate part of the intervention based on the nursing diagnosis and treatment goal. Most of the nursing actions described are implemented autonomously by the nurse; a few require collaboration with a physician. Research supporting various actions is integrated with the description of the intervention.

Large numbers of individuals, often young productive adults, are afflicted with brain injury from events such as trauma, stroke or tumor. Nurses are largely responsible for preventing or minimizing secondary brain injury, a syndrome resulting from high intracranial pressure or volume. Pamela H. Mitchell and Laurie L. Ackerman have developed an intervention they call Secondary Brain Injury Reduction (Chapter 42) that is designed to protect the patient's brain from further neurologic insult resulting from compression or ischemic damage. It is composed of three parts: ongoing monitoring of the patient's status, promotion of cerebral perfusion, and controlling stimuli in the patient's environment. A sound knowledge of physiology is needed to implement this intervention. The nurse is required to synthesize data, recognize emerging patterns, and take action immediately because the patient's condition can change very quickly. Many of the parameters being monitored interact, so the nurse must manage respiratory and cardiac function as well as neurological status. The American Association of Neuroscience nurses has developed a core curriculum to assist nurses to learn this area of specialization. A sizable body of research is beginning to direct nursing practice.

In Chapter 43, Meg Gulanick and Carol Ruback overview the various types of shock and outline the nursing diagnoses associated with this life-threatening event. They describe Shock Management as an intervention with four components:

providing surveillance, maintaining tissue perfusion, maintaining vital organ function, and providing emotional support. Numerous nursing activities are required to carry out the components of the intervention. The authors describe these activities and overview them in a protocol for Shock Management. The case study illustrates that nursing judgment and action to implement the intervention are the key factors in patient survival.

Over 80,000 persons in the United States with end-stage renal disease are being treated with dialysis. Nurses have been integral to the management of care for these patients since the technology became available in the 1960s. In Chapter 44, Margery O. Fearing and Laura K. Hart have conceptualized the nursing intervention of Dialysis Therapy as preparing patients for treatments, managing the technology, monitoring the treatment and possible complications, and collaborating with the patient, family, and health team members in developing a plan of care. The priority clinical conditions that Dialysis Therapy can correct are fluid, electrolyte, and acid-base imbalances. The NANDA terminology is currently incomplete in describing these physiologic diagnoses. There are also many psychosocial problems related to this life-sustaining treatment, and Fearing and Hart identify these associated nursing diagnoses. The bulk of the chapter overviews the protocols for hemodialysis and peritoneal dialysis. This introduction to the technology will be valuable to nondialysis nurses to understand this field of nursing and also to be familiar with the type of care a patient receives while in a dialysis unit. A core curriculum to help nurses learn the detailed protocols has been prepared by the American Nephrology Nurses' Association. Many patients are on home dialysis. Nurses are doing the family education needed to prepare the patient and caretakers to manage this technology outside the dialysis center. The chapter concludes with two case studies that provide typical profiles of patients receiving center and home hemodialysis treatment.

Critical care nurses work with each patient as a unique individual while coordinating the multitude of technological devices and the variety of specialized caregivers. The relationship with the physician has become collaborative. Research has shown that the amount and quality of communication between nurses and physicians in critical care units is predictive of patient welfare. The chapters in this section demonstrate that nursing is an essential element in determining positive patient outcomes in critical care units.

38

SURVEILLANCE

CYNTHIA M. DOUGHERTY

We are at a time in nursing science and nursing practice where the link between nursing diagnostic categories and nursing interventions is possible and necessary to determine. The nursing intervention Surveillance is important in many areas of nursing practice, and particularly in the critical care setting. This intervention is also widely used in community health care, psychiatric, and long-term-care settings.

The work is ongoing to define the autonomous interventions that nurses implement, especially those that focus on the management of physiological processes and complex medical technology. Surveillance is one intervention that nurses can implement independently and be held accountable for in their daily nursing practice in the care of critically ill individuals.

DEFINITION AND DESCRIPTION

Surveillance is defined as the application of behavioral and cognitive processes in the systematic collection of information used to make judgments and predictions about a person's health status. *Webster's New World Dictionary, College Edition* defines surveillance as "to watch over, a close watch, a vigil, to look over and examine closely, or to view or study as a whole." Surveillance is similar to observation, defined by Webster as "an act or the power of seeing or fixing the mind upon something; gathering information by noting facts or occurrences." Surveillance thus encompasses observation in that the gathering of information through watching, feeling, or touching is part of this intervention. Both observation and surveillance are oriented toward collecting as much information as necessary to achieve a particular purpose. Surveillance extends beyond observation in two ways: it utilizes more and different types of methods to gather the data and includes an evaluation or judgment. The evaluation is essential to establishing a nursing diagnosis and predicting patient outcomes. Surveillance is the same as monitoring but not the same as assessment. Nursing assessment implies the gathering of information in order to formulate a diagnosis at one point in time. A global assessment of health status is made at the time of initial contact with the health care institution, such as at hospital admission or an annual physical examination. After the initial assessment is complete, a decision is made about surveillance of future signs or symptoms in order to identify a problem, observe the progress of a current problem, or deem that no problem exists.

Thus, Surveillance is both a behavioral and a cognitive process. Information is gathered to determine how to deal with future developments and to make estimates about a certain situation that deserves close scrutiny (Dulles 1963). The behavioral component of Surveillance involves the collection of information from both primary and secondary sources. Direct data collection includes inspection, palpation, percussion, and auscultation (Yacone 1987; Timerding 1989). Secondary sources of information may involve the use of several types of highly technical equipment. Recently nursing research has focused on the most reliable methods to obtain valid data from hemodynamic monitoring equipment (Quaal 1988). Nurses are concerned with what types of activities and techniques alter cardiopulmonary monitoring results and how these results are used to change treatment. New monitoring parameters and devices used in the care of the critically ill are always becoming available. SVO_2 monitoring and transcutaneous oxygen sensing have become widely used in monitoring and evaluation of patients with cardiac disorders (Timberding 1989; White, Winslow, Clark, and Tyler 1990).

The cognitive component of Surveillance includes studying, interpreting, analyzing, evaluating, and intercepting data to indicate a range of possibilities and to isolate those factors influencing a situation (Dulles 1963). This process involves knowing where to look for information, remembering how frequently certain observations are required, and when to expect a change in response to treatment (Reyes 1987; Carrieri, Stotts, Levinson, Murdaugh, and Holzemer 1982). A basic understanding of normal and abnormal findings is essential (Thompson 1989; Chan 1989). Perception and the ability to relate sensory stimuli to some relevant knowledge or previous experience are two important elements of Surveillance. From direct study and from a theoretical orientation, we accumulate factual knowledge that gives relevance to what we see. Nurses are responsible for interpreting signs and symptoms with a high degree of accuracy and reporting abnormalities to those responsible for changing treatment (Yacone 1987; Papenhausen 1981). It is vital to know what to look for, because the most obvious sign may not be the most important one to monitor.

RELATED LITERATURE

The concept of surveillance has been abstracted from literature primarily in the field of intelligence related to espionage. In this field, surveillance suggests that a judgment has been made by some governmental unit that the behavior being monitored is outside the range of legitimate political activities. In the case of the person being watched, the class of events under surveillance is categorized as potentially threatening and the individual functions appropriately in terms of avoiding or minimizing possible negative consequences. Intelligence, a synonym of *surveillance*, involves the process of information gathering followed by evaluation, judgment, or prediction, and then reporting the findings to an organization or group participating in the policymaking process (Blum 1972).

In Eastern Europe, the Soviet Union, and Nazi Germany, surveillance has been used as a control to maintain the governmental structure. Political surveillance has been used to describe a set of techniques employed in the collection of political information about a subject. These activities have been used to produce a set of political assumptions (Askin 1973). Blum (1972) has defined surveillance as "watching, recording, and compiling information about another person's activities and movements, for whatever purposes such information can be used by the person for whom it is gathered" (p. 98). Surveillance has an open-ended meaning, with control of information clearly left to the one who has undertaken the surveillance activity.

The process of surveillance has involved an ongoing development of information about events, persons, groups, and even attitudes of large segments of the public (Blum 1972). Surveillance must have planning and structure. Objectives are outlined, priorities established, and obstacles examined. Information that is gathered is of little value unless it reaches the hands of the decision makers. In priority cases, someone has to decide what constitutes important information. Special watch is kept to scan incoming data for anything of critical nature, clues are sorted, and ideas are exchanged as to the development of an impending crisis. Because there is not time to submit every item for detailed analysis, raw intelligence can be dangerous without an understanding of the circumstances from which it was gathered. Therefore, information must be interpreted within a context (Dulles 1963).

Because the concept of surveillance has emerged in the field of intelligence, implications of deviance and secrecy have been associated with it. When viewed in the light of police operations, criminal investigations, and political or intelligence activities, surveillance stigmatizes or labels those behaviors under close watch as deviant. When applied to a hospital situation, where patients have voluntarily placed themselves in the care of professionals for the purpose of remedying a health problem, the act of Surveillance is legitimate and appropriate. In this instance the information that is gathered forms the basis for monitoring a diagnosis and instituting prompt intervention. Therefore, in the hospital setting, Surveillance is both legitimate and necessary for the patient in a life-threatening situation. The purpose for collecting information is to resolve a health problem.

Critical care units were established for the purpose of monitoring carefully specific signs or symptoms in order to intervene quickly in life-threatening situations (Timerding 1989). The development of highly technical equipment and complex devices for monitoring has expanded over the last decade. Mechanical assist devices are sometimes used to keep the heart beating while an organ donor is sought or to sustain life until cardiogenic shock subsides. This rapid growth of technology related to critical care has resulted in increased complexity and cost in the care of those who are seriously ill.

Surveillance of the critically ill patient is important because the information gathered is used to benefit the patient, including preventing death. Patients in critical care settings receive more frequent and detailed surveillance activities than patients with less acute health problems. In complex organ dysfunction or life-threatening conditions, many aspects of the patient's symptoms and response to treatment are carefully monitored in order to intervene quickly when necessary (Miller, Garrett, McMahon, and Ringel 1989).

For the acutely ill patient, systematic observing and recording will increase the nurse's ability to predict physiological instability. Because complications can occur rapidly, a baseline from which to recognize changes in the patient's condition is needed. In these situations, systematic assessment of vital signs and symptoms can save lives (Chan 1989). Without Surveillance in the critical care situation, important information is likely to be overlooked, and problems of life-threatening proportion may be either missed altogether or misidentified. The essence of successful Surveillance involves the piecing together of minute amounts of information that, evaluated separately, may appear unrelated and insignificant.

Behavioral Component

The behavioral component of Surveillance comprises those activities undertaken by the nurse in order to collect information. In the intelligence field, information may be obtained from primary and secondary sources, such as governmental records and people (neighbors, business associates, acquaintances, family, and relatives). People watching and listening are basic behavioral activities of surveillance. Information may also be gathered by means of digging through letters, notes, bills, memoranda, newspapers, security indexes, books, codes, and journals or by checking garbage contents or traffic routes (Blum 1972; Askin 1973). Surveillance may be carried out by physically following another person's actions for a specific time period or by collecting data through the use of electronic devices such as wiretaps, tape recorders, videotapes, cameras, or closed circuit television (Dulles 1965).

In the critical care situation, the behavioral component of Surveillance includes direct observation of the patient to survey mental and physical status. Methods include checking pupils; observing behavior, color of skin, and mucous membranes; noting external jugular veins for distension; taking vital signs, auscultating heart and lung sounds; palpating pedal pulses; observing edema and temperature of extremities; and recording reactions to medications (Gardner 1989; Papenhausen 1981). It also includes indirect observation with the use of invasive electronic equipment, such as cardiac output computers, ventilators, fluoroscopic equipment, intravenous pumps, and pressure lines (Sedlock 1981; Thompson 1989; Watson 1987).

Cognitive Component

The cognitive aspect of Surveillance involves the collection and evaluation of data to draw conclusions and make predictions. In order to do this, the act of gathering information must be a reliable process (Abbey 1990). All observations should be tailored to suit the individual circumstance. Recognition of inappropriate signs becomes easier when the exact nature of what is being looked for is known. Thus, a theoretical knowledge base underlying the information collection is an essential part of the cognitive component of Surveillance because one must know what to look for and when to look. Establishing baseline data for future comparison is part of this cognitive process. This baseline assessment serves as the basis for decisions on what parameters will be surveyed over time.

Relatively minor changes in the critically ill patient are often very important and if detected quickly enough may make it possible to avoid further complications, including death (Chan 1989). In order to do this, the ordering of priorities in critical care needs to be systematic and routinized. Treatments need to be set into motion without delay, and data must be extracted as rapidly as possible, speedily analyzed, and acted upon.

The cognitive component of Surveillance requires the nurse to possess certain attributes or skills. Among these are the theoretical knowledge base and clinical skills to implement the behavioral components of Surveillance (Itano 1989). The attributes required of the nurse using Surveillance in the critical care area are similar to those of an effective intelligence officer: the ability to be perceptive about people, to work well with others in difficult situations, to discern between essentials and nonessentials, to be ingenious, intelligent, and inquisitive, to pay close attention to detail, to express concerns clearly and directly, to make rapid decisions, and to be nonjudgmental (Dulles 1963). The nurse must have mastered certain technical skills necessary for operating equipment safely and performing physical assessment accurately.

RECOMMENDATIONS FOR PRACTICE AND RESEARCH

Very little research has been reported in which Surveillance has been tested as an appropriate intervention for specific nursing diagnoses. Most descriptions of Surveillance as a nursing intervention are embedded within the nursing assessment section of physical assessment textbooks and they label it as a monitoring activity. Recently, the American Association of Critical Care Nurses (AACN) published a manual of outcome standards for nursing care of the critically ill that included Surveillance as a nursing intervention for every nursing diagnosis listed in the publication (AACN 1990).

Three related studies (Dougherty 1985; Hubalik 1981; Wessel 1981) have demonstrated that Surveillance activities are legitimate and important in critical care situations involving patients with severe cardiovascular disorders. Nurses used both medical and nursing diagnoses to determine the parameters of interest for their Surveillance activities. These studies described the practice of medicine and nursing in Surveillance during treatment of patients with decreased cardiac output as collaborative. All studies reported dependent, collaborative, and independent interventions for this patient group. Many of the independent and collaborative interventions were Surveillance activities. For example, taking vital signs, evaluating laboratory values, monitoring electrocardiogram changes, and regulating fluid intake were independent (Wessel 1981).

In critical care situations, nurses actively and independently monitor numerous patient responses to illness and treatment (Roberts 1987). Some of the parameters of interest are identified through physician orders, and others are determined independently by the nurse. The responsibility for collecting all the information at an appropriate time is the responsibility of the nurse.

The major research activity implied by this intervention is to test the two indexes of the intervention tool (time and parameters of interest) with different patient groups, who have different nursing diagnoses and show differences in acuity of condition. Short-term goals and outcomes of Surveillance could also be derived from and tested for various patient groups, with the results of these research efforts used to verify the appropriateness of Surveillance as a nursing intervention for different nursing diagnoses. Research findings could be used to refine nursing diagnoses and derive new interventions for testing. Systematic collection of data should help improve standards of care, as well as help with the cognitive component of this intervention. That is, more reliable and valid data should lead to better evaluation, prediction, and practice in maintaining the health status of individuals in life-threatening situations.

INTERVENTION TOOLS

Two elements are essential to any Surveillance tool: time, measured in seconds, minutes, or hours, and parameters of interest, such as vital signs or blood gases. Several examples of tools exist in the form of flow sheets used in critical care areas. Standard monitoring procedures for cardiac patients are sometimes established by clinical protocols in each hospital. These protocols provide clues as to the appropriate parameters of interest to monitor for various types of cardiac problems. Standards of practice for critical care nursing might also be used to determine parameters of interest.

The medical and nursing diagnoses help to determine the frequency of data collection, as well as the types of information needed in the Surveillance effort. In general, the more critical or life-threatening the situation is, the more frequently the parameters of interest should be monitored and evaluated.

Successful Surveillance used to prevent complications and promote physiological stability in the critical illness situation depends on the nurse's ability to diagnose the problem requiring the intervention of Surveillance and the ability to choose the appropriate parameters of interest to use for information gathering.

ASSOCIATED NURSING DIAGNOSES AND CLIENT GROUPS

The target population for Surveillance is any person in a life-threatening condition, those who are not able to care for themselves independently, and those who may exhibit self-destructive behaviors. Types of patient groups for whom Surveillance is appropriate include those in critical care situations, ranging from the emergency room to the psychiatric unit, those who are members of at-risk groups in the community, and those who because of physical or mental impairments are not able to care for themselves safely.

The following primary diagnoses often require this intervention:

Impaired Adjustment
Ineffective Airway Clearance
Potential Altered Body Temperature
Ineffective Breathing Pattern
Decreased Cardiac Output
Diarrhea
Fluid Volume Deficit
Impaired Gas Exchange
Potential for Suffocation
Impaired Swallowing
Altered Thought Processes
Potential for Violence.

The degree to which the potential or actual problem is life threatening or poses a problem of safety will determine whether Surveillance, alone or in combination with other interventions is indicated. To focus this discussion, the illustrations of Surveillance in this chapter will apply specifically to a patient with congestive cardiomyopathy who has the nursing diagnosis of Decreased Cardiac Output.

SUGGESTED PROTOCOLS FOR SURVEILLANCE

After the individual has been admitted to the hospital or other health care institution, a quick determination of the life-threatening problems are diagnosed, and appropriate interventions are instituted. After the general history and physical assessment has been completed, the body systems that are most problematic are targeted, and Surveillance parameters are determined. The exact parameters of interest that will be subsequently monitored are sometimes determined by the types of monitoring devices that are placed on the patient by the physician. For example, a person with chest pain and subsequent cardiac arrest will most likely be monitored with invasive cardiac output equipment. Thus, cardiac output will be one of the priority parameters of interest when initiating Surveillance for this person. The only other decision to be made about the parameter of interest is the frequency of monitoring. This decision depends on the stability of the cardiovascular system, the baseline cardiac output, and the response to treatment. If invasive monitoring equipment is not used, cardiac output is not one of the parameters of interest for this person. Other parameters of interest for this person would be determined when admitted to a particular nursing unit.

Once baseline determinations for the parameters of interest are made, the frequency of subsequent monitoring is determined. The time of the parameters may change as further information is collected or a pattern in the data becomes apparent. New parameters may be selected for monitoring and/or the time interval changed to increase or decrease the frequency of monitoring. When greater stability is achieved, the frequency of the monitoring interval can be safely decreased. The decision to change a parameter of interest or the frequency of monitoring is most often made by the nurse.

CASE STUDY

Bill is a 27-year-old construction worker who developed congestive cardiomyopathy following a viral infection. He contracted a subsequent respiratory infection, which exacerbated his congestive heart failure, placing him in a life-threatening condition. In order to save his life, he was hospitalized in the coronary care unit and intra-aortic balloon pumping (IABP) was instituted in order to resolve cardiogenic shock. The primary nursing diagnosis for Bill was Decreased Cardiac Output, defined as a decrease in volume of blood ejected from the heart due to factors influencing stroke volume or heart rate. The antecedent condition leading to Bill's decreased cardiac output was a decreased ventricular contractility resulting from the cardiomyopathy.

This episode of decreased cardiac output was not the first for Bill, but this time it was complicated by continued enlargement and dilation of the heart. Compensatory mechanisms that normally aid in increasing cardiac output when a decrease in stroke volume has occurred were ineffective in maintaining a steady state because Bill's cardiac reserve had been depleted. Because his cardiac output could not be maintained on the medical regimen, Bill was being considered for a heart transplant as the only remaining medical treatment that could improve his condition.

After Bill returned from the cardiac catheterization laboratory, where right and left catheterization was completed and an intra-aortic balloon pump was inserted, he was reattached to all monitoring capabilities in the coronary care unit. Equipment used for monitoring included left femoral Swan-Ganz catheter, left femoral arterial line, right femoral IABP, two right femoral intravenous lines, urinary catheter, cardiac monitor, ventilator, nasogastric tube, and left subclavian intravenous lines. At the time the primary nurse first came in contact with Bill, he was experiencing a further decrease in his cardiac output, indicating that cardiogenic shock and death were imminent if prompt action was not instituted.

A number of factors led to the selection of the nursing intervention of Surveillance for Bill. Desired outcomes included early detection of an impending cardiopulmonary disaster, early detection of complications, successful resolution of the decreased cardiac output, detection of minor changes in hemodynamic state, establishment of priorities of care so important areas would not be overlooked, development of a plan to deal with future developments in care, and resolution of the instability in cardiac function long enough for Bill to receive a cardiac transplant. These goals have been found to be of primary importance for critically ill cardiac patients (Chan 1989; Gardner 1989; Timerding 1989; Yacone 1987).

The nurse began the intervention of Surveillance immediately after the patient history and physical examination were completed. The physician outlined to the nurse the specific parameters of interest that medicine considered most

Time Sequence

Parameters	1600	1700	1800	1900	2000	2100	2200	2300	2400
Temperature (°C)	37.2		37.9		38.5		38.5		38.8
Apical Pulse	125	124	125	129	126	131	130	133	135
Respirations	12	12	12	12	12	12	12	12	12
Blood Pressure	104/33	105/41	104/33	115/21	104/22	86/36	80/33	81/32	84/32
Pulmonary Artery Systolic/Diastolic/Mean	42/35/39	37/28/30	35/24/30	48/30/42	48/33/37	36/20/29	32/18/26	32/20/28	35/18/24
Pulmonary Artery Wedge	30	28	30	34	32	25	19	20	24
Cardiac Output	5.25		2.86		2.74		3.78		3.07
Urine Output/cc	7	17	55	13	12	18	15	38	22
Rhythm	RSR	RSR	RSR	RSR	RSR	RSR	RSR	RSR	RSR
Ventilator TV/FIO$_2$/Rate	800/40/12	800/40/12	800/40/12	800/40/12	800/40/12	800/40/12	800/40/12	800/40/12	800/40/12
Dopamine 1600 mg/500 cc	10	20	20	20	20	28	32	32	32
Dobutamine 1000 mg/500 cc	--	--	10	10	--	--	--	--	--
Nipride 200 mg/500 cc	--	--	--	14	10	18	18	18	14
IABP	1:2	1:2	1:2	1:2	1:2	1:2	1:2	1:2	1:2
Heparin units/hr	1000	1000	1000	--	1000	--	600	600	600
Lungs	clear R rales L	same	bi-basilar rales	same	congestion	bi-basilar rales	same	rales & ronchi	same
Heart	S$_1$ = S$_2$ 4/6 Systolic murmur	same	4/6 Systolic murmur	same	S$_1$ = S$_2$ S$_4$	same	4/6 Systolic murmur	same	same
Pedal pulses R/L	none	+ / +	+ / +	none	none	none	− / +	− / +	doppler + / +
Skin temperature/color	cool/pale	same	dry/pale	same	cold/pale	same	same	same	same
Movement	paralysis	same	same	same	restless	paralysis	same	same	same
Pupils	PERL 2/2	same	same	same	same	same	same	same	same
JVD	4-5 flat	same	same	6 flat	same	same	same	same	same
Secretions	--	oral	oral & nasal	--	ET suction oral	--	oral bloody	--	--
Abdomen	flat 0 sounds	same	same	same	same	same	same	same	same
Dressings	dry	dry	changed	dry	changed	dry	changed	dry	dry
Edema R ankle/L ankle	+ 3/ + 2	+ 3/ + 2	+ 3/ + 2	+ 3/ + 2	+ 3/ + 2	+ 3/ + 2	+ 3/ + 2	+ 3/ + 2	+ 3/ + 2
Nose & Mouth Care	/	/	bloody/	bloody/	bloody/	/	/	/	/
Medications	MS 10 mg	Valium 5 mg	Maalox 30 cc	Lasix 80 mg	Heparin 10,000 Dilantin 300 mg	Pavulon 10 mg MS 10 mg	--	--	--

IABP = Intra-aortic balloon pump
JVD = Jugular venous distension
MS = Morphine sulfate

FIGURE 38–1. Basic Parameters of Interest Monitored during Surveillance of Bill

Parameters	Time Sequence				
	0300	0850	1320	1725	2235
Na		136			
K		4.9			
CL		92			
BUN		62			
Cr		2.6			
PT	32		30	28	28
PTT	> 150	118	57	53	77
LDH	> 2000	4290			
AST	> 3080	> 3080			
CPK	2450	3420			
CPK-MM	100	100			
CPK-MB	0	0			
Hg/Hct	$\frac{13.1}{40}$	$\frac{11.6}{34.9}$			
WBC	21.9	18.7			

FIGURE 38–2. Additional Parameters of Interest Monitored during Surveillance of Bill (24-Hour Period)

salient for Bill. These are listed as the first 15 parameters on the Surveillance flow sheet, beginning with temperature and ending with heparin (Fig. 38–1). All other observation parameters included on the flow sheet were determined to be important by the nurse (Figures 38–1 through 38–3). The time frame selected for the intervention was also determined by the nurse during this critical period. (Because of the vast amount of data collected during the ensuing 4-day period, the information presented here is limited to a brief period to illustrate the implementation of the intervention.)

Implementation of this intervention is summarized on the flow sheet presented in Figure 38–1. The behavioral aspect of Surveillance included inspecting, palpating, percussing, and auscultating Bill's body, equipment, and environment. This encompassed vital signs, pulmonary artery pressure, cardiac output, urine output, oxygen status, medication titration, heart and lung sounds, peripheral circulation, skin color and temperature, secretions, hygienic care, intravenous titration, and laboratory values. The parameters that the nurse identified as most important to observe were in agreement with those identified in the literature for acutely ill cardiac patients. The physician was primarily interested in data concerning Bill's hemodynamic and medication status, parameters that were also of priority to the nurse. Although the physicians were notified when significant changes occurred in Bill, they were not generally aware of the frequency of observations made, the titration of

Parameters	Time Sequence					
	0030	0430	0850	1225	1630	2030
PH	7.40	7.38	7.46	7.44	7.48	7.50
PCO_2	40	40.7	42	40	40	34
PO_2	77	72.4	88	86	77	94
HCO_3	24	23	29	26	28	25
O_2 delivery	40% ventilator					
Chest film	ET tube and Swan-Ganz in good placement cardiac silhouette enlarged-pulmonary vascular congestion					
EKG 12-Lead	sinus tachycardia rate 120 pr .20 notching of R waves, ischemia V_1-V_6, poor R wave progression					

FIGURE 38–3. Additional Parameters of Interest Monitored during Surveillance of Bill (24-Hour Period)

medication according to observations, the administration of prn medications, or the results of all laboratory data.

The cognitive component of Surveillance for Bill included looking, seeing, estimating, knowing, understanding, interpreting, analyzing, and evaluating all of the parameters identified. These cognitive aspects may not always be readily apparent to someone observing the nurse who is doing Surveillance, particularly if the nurse is merely standing at the patient's bedside and thinking. But because the frequency of recording and reporting is common to nurses in critical care, this cognitive component is often reflected in the nurse's notes that imply that judgments are made. This cognitive component is also observable when the nurse notes abnormality and either reports it to the physician, expecting collaboration and decision making, or acts independently by titrating medications, changing the position of the patient, increasing the rate of intravenous fluids, giving emergency drugs, implementing protocols, collecting subsequent laboratory samples, or making a conscious effort to continue to survey a particular parameter.

The Surveillance flow sheet for Bill shows that the nurse was busy manipulating cardiac monitoring equipment and adjusting intravenous fluids, medications, and various other equipment. It is also demonstrated that changes in Bill's blood pressure, cardiac output, and pulmonary artery pressure were associated with changes in medication administration (1800 and 2100); changes in laboratory values were associated with changes in medication

(1900 and 2200); changes in arterial blood gases prompted positioning and suctioning (1600, 1800, 2000); and neurological status changes were associated with medication administration (1700 and 2100). In noting these associations, the cognitive aspect of Surveillance becomes observable, and the actions that followed careful and consistent watching become apparent.

In this case study, Surveillance was implemented as a nursing intervention for the purpose of preventing cardiopulmonary disaster. Surveillance was operationally defined as physically observing the parameters of temperature, pulse, respiration, blood pressure, pulmonary artery pressure, urine output, cardiac rhythm, ventilator settings, medications, IABP, lung and heart sounds, peripheral pulses, skin temperature and color, movement, pupil size and reaction, dressings, jugular venous distension, edema, secretions, abdomen, and mucous membranes; surveying serum electrolytes, coagulation times, enzymes, blood counts, arterial blood gases, chest films, and electrocardiograms; interpreting the findings as normal or abnormal; and reporting significant findings regarding Bill's life status in order to act early and plan subsequent care.

The final step of the process involves an evaluation of the success of the intervention in reducing Bill's problem of decreased cardiac output and in the rapid detection of changes in stability. It would be unrealistic to think that Bill's cardiomyopathy could be resolved by Surveillance; however, rapid detection and evaluation of changes in the cardiovascular system prompted immediate action. From the time that the nursing intervention was instituted, Bill remained alive and reasonably stable for 4 days. By close monitoring and early action, it was hoped that the cardiogenic shock would be stabilized so that Bill could be transferred for a heart transplant. Surveillance over hemodynamics, urine, laboratory values, and medications prevented major cardiopulmonary complications until approximately 1 hour before his death. Surveillance prompted prioritizing needs, quick intervention, detection of minor changes, and most likely extended the life span of Bill beyond what would have been expected. This intervention allowed time for family members to begin the grief process in coping with this crisis.

Although decreased cardiac output was not ultimately relieved by this intervention, Bill's condition was maintained and stabilized at a level that was compatible with life for a critical time period. For this nursing diagnosis of Decreased Cardiac Output, Surveillance provided the best overall results that could be expected. The general goal of increasing cardiac output was not met because an overwhelming infection kept Bill from receiving a heart transplant in time to save his life. Nevertheless, at points along the way, major decreases in cardiac output were prevented. Surveillance was an important nursing intervention for this critically ill patient.

SUMMARY

The nursing intervention of Surveillance is described as an independent intervention important for individuals facing life-threatening conditions, those who are unable to independently care for themselves, and those exhibiting self-destructive behaviors. The application of both cognitive and behavioral processes are used to make judgments about a person's health status. Perception and the ability to relate sensory stimuli to some relevant knowledge or previous experience are two important elements of Surveillance. Nurses are responsible for interpreting signs and symptoms as accurately as possible and reporting abnormalities. It is vital to know what to look for, because the most obvious sign may not be the most important one to monitor.

REFERENCES

American Association of Critical Care Nurses. 1990. *Outcome standards for nursing care of the critically ill.* Laguna Niguel, Calif.: AACN.

Abbey, J.C. 1990. Development of instruments to measure physiologic variables in clinical studies. *Critical Care Nursing Quarterly* 12(4):21–29.

Askin, F. 1973. Surveillance: The social perspective. In Columbia Human Rights Law Review (ed.), *Surveillance, dataveillance, and personal freedoms.* Fair Lawn, N.J.: R. E. Burdick.

Blum, R.H. 1972. *Surveillance and espionage in a free society.* New York: Praeger.

Carrieri, V., Stotts, N., Levinson, J., Murdaugh, C., and Holzemer, W.L. 1982. The use of cardiopulmonary assessment skills in the clinical setting. *Western Journal of Nursing Research* 4(1):5–17.

Carroll-Johnson, R.M. 1989. *Classification of nursing diagnosis: Proceedings of the Eighth National Conference.* Philadelphia: J.B. Lippincott.

Chan, E.S. 1989. Nursing assessment following cardiac resuscitation. *Nursing* (England) 3(36):30–31.

Contrades, S. 1987. Altered cardiac output: An assessment tool. *Dimensions in Critical Care Nursing* 6(5):274–282.

Dougherty, C.M. 1985. Decreased cardiac output. *Nursing Clinics of North America* 20(4):787–799.

Dulles, A. 1963. *The craft of intelligence.* New York: Harper & Row.

Gardner, P.E. 1989. Cardiac output: Theory, technique, troubleshooting. *Critical Care Nursing Clinics of North America* 1(3):577–587.

Hubalik, K.T. 1981. *Nursing diagnosis associated with heart failure in critical care nursing.* Unpublished master's thesis, University of Illinois, Chicago.

Itano, J.K. 1989. A comparison of the clinical judgment process in experienced registered nurses and student nurses. *Journal of Nursing Education* 28(3):120–126.

Miller, P., Garrett, M.J., McMahon, M., and Ringel, K. 1989. Strategies to promote valid and reliable nursing interventions in research. *Western Journal of Nursing Research* 11(3):373–378.

Mirvis, D.M., Berson, A.S., Goldberger, A.L., Green, L.S., Heger, J.J., Hinohara, T., Insel, J., Krucoff, M.W., Moncrief, A., Selvester, R.H., and Wagner, G.S. 1989. Instrumentation and practice standards for electrocardiographic monitoring in special care units. *Circulation* 79(2):464–471.

Papenhausen, J.L. 1981. Data based criteria for cardiovascular nursing intervention. *Critical Care Quarterly* 4:1–7.

Quaal, S.J. 1988. Hemodynamic monitoring: A review of the literature. *Applied Nursing Research* 1(2):58–67.

Reyes, A.V. 1987. Monitoring and treating life-threatening ventricular dysrhythmias. *Nursing Clinics of North America* 22(1):61–76.

Roberts, S.L. 1987. The role of collaborative nursing diagnosis in critical care. *Critical Care Nurse* 7(4):81–86.

Sedlock, S. 1981. Cardiac output: Physiologic variables and therapeutic interventions. *Critical Care Nurse* 1:14–22.

Thompson, C. 1989. The nursing assessment of the patient with cardiac pain on the coronary care unit. *Intensive Care Nursing* 5(4):147–154.

Timerding, B.L. 1989. Cardiopulmonary monitoring and sudden cardiac death. *Topics in Emergency Medicine* 11(2):12–22.

Watson, J.E. 1987. Fluid and electrolyte disorders in cardiovascular patients. *Nursing Clinics of North America* 22(4):797–803.

Wessel, S.L. 1981. *Nursing functions related to the nursing diagnosis decreased cardiac output.* Unpublished master's thesis, University of Illinois, Chicago.

White, K.M., Winslow, E.H., Clark, A.P., and Tyler, D.O. 1990. The physiologic basis for continuous mixed venous oxygen saturation monitoring. *Heart and Lung* 19(5):548–551.

Yacone, L.A. 1987. Cardiac assessment. *RN* 50(5):42–48.

39

AIRWAY MANAGEMENT

MARITA G. TITLER
GERRY A. JONES

Airway patency is necessary for life. Nursing activities to achieve airway patency can be traced to the early 1900s when nurses tried several methods to maintain a tight seal between the patient's neck and Drinker respirator. During the 1940s, nurses began to suction tracheostomies using a variety of techniques (Adler 1979). Today nurses continue to use various practices to maintain airway patency, with controversies surrounding these techniques.

Airway patency is achieved through the intervention of Airway Management, a necessary prerequisite to ventilatory support. Airway Management is accomplished in several ways, ranging from correct positioning of the patient to use of various artificial airway devices. This chapter focuses on Airway Management in adults.

AIRWAY MANAGEMENT AND NURSING DIAGNOSES

Although Airway Management is used for many patients with a variety of diagnoses, it is most applicable for those with Ineffective Airway Clearance, Impaired Gas Exchange, and Ineffective Breathing Pattern. These three diagnoses have been the focus of several scholarly publications and investigations in which Airway Management activities are described (Hanley and Tyler 1987; Hoffman 1987; Kim and Larson 1987; Lareau and Larson 1987; Openbrier and Covey 1987; Shekleton and Nield 1987; York 1985).

Instituting this intervention has some potential risks that may lead to nursing diagnoses of Potential for Infection, Potential for Injury, Potential for Aspiration, Impaired Tissue Integrity, Altered Nutrition: Less Than Body Requirements, Potential for Altered Oral Mucous Membrane, Impaired Swallowing, Body Image Disturbance, and Impaired Verbal Communication (Carroll-Johnson 1989).

OVERVIEW OF RESEARCH AND RELATED LITERATURE

Medical research about Airway Management has focused on complications associated with the insertion and use of artificial airways, types of suction catheters, magnitude of negative pressure use for suctioning, and complications associated with various types of airway cuffs and materials (Bernhard, Yost, Joynes, Cothalis, and Turndorf 1985; Bradstater and Muallem 1969; El-Naggar, Sadagopa, Levin, Kantor, and Collins 1976; Hunsinger, Lisnerski, Maurizi, and Philips 1980; Kastanos, Miro, Perez, Mir, and Agusti-Vidal 1983; Klainer, Turndorf, Wu, Maewal, and Allender 1975; Kuzenski 1978; Landa, Kwoka, Chapman, Brito, and Sackner 1980; Magovern, Shively, and Fecht 1972; Marsh, Gillespie, and Baumgartner 1989; Mathis and Wendley 1974; Pardowsky and Guthrie 1983; Plum and Dunning 1956; Polacek and Guthrie 1981; Rashkin and Davis 1986; Rosen and Hillard 1962; Routh, Hanning, and Ledingham 1979; Sackner, Hirsch, and Epstein 1975; Sackner, Landa, Greeneltch, and Robinson 1973; Stauffer, Olson, and Petty 1981; Via-Reque and Rattenburg 1981).

Much of the nursing research concerning Airway Management is on endotracheal suctioning (ETS) (Ackerman 1985; Barnes and Kirchhoff 1986; Riegel and Forshee 1985; Rudy, Baun, Stone, and Turner 1986; Stone 1989; Stone and Turner 1988). Major independent variables investigated include methods of preoxygenation (hyperoxygenation and hyperinflation), suction duration, intratracheal instillation of saline, and use of open versus closed suction techniques. Major dependent variables investigated are hypoxemia, oxygen desaturation, changes in hemodynamic pressures, and increases in intracranial pressures (Adlkofer and Powaser 1978; Baker, Baker, and Koen 1983; Baun 1984; Belknap, Kirilloff, and Zullo 1980; Belling, Kelley, and Simon 1978; Bodai 1982; Bodai, Walton, Briggs, and Goldstein 1987; Bostick and Wendelgass 1987; Buggy, Hanson, Flynn, and Baun 1980; Carlon, Fox, and Ackerman 1987; Campbell, Byram, Chulay, Hepburn, Tribett, Johnson, Rosenthal, Stridor, Chase, Dellasanta, and Annanian 1990; Chulay and Graeber 1988; Conforti 1982; Craig, Benson, and Pierson 1984; Hanley, Rudd, and Butler 1978; Hardie and Kirchhoff 1989; Harken 1975; Hess and Easter 1986; Lucke 1982; Naigow and Powaser 1977; Pierce and Piazza 1987; Preusser, Stone, Gonyon, Winningham, Groch, and Karl 1988; Rindfleisch and Tyler 1983; Rogge, Bunde, and Baun 1989; Rudy, Baun, Stone, and Turner 1986; Skelley, Deeren, and Powaser 1980; Stone and Turner 1988; Stone, Vorst, Lanham, and Zahn 1989; Taggart, Dorinsky, and Sheahan 1988). A pioneering study by Nelson (1989) provides an initial organization and naming of nursing activities used in Airway Management. Based on Nelson's study, Airway Management is defined as the initiation and maintenance of airway patency.

AIRWAY MANAGEMENT TOOLS

Several devices are used for Airway Management. Naso/oropharyngeal airways enhance nasotracheal suctioning and prevent obstruction of the posterior pharynx by the tongue. Although nasopharyngeal airways are more tolerable than oral airways in semicomatose or awake patients, their use is contraindicated in patients with maxillofacial trauma and sinus infections. Naso/oropharyngeal airways are changed every 24 hours to prevent the buildup of secretions and to decrease risk of iatrogenic infections. Malpositioning of these airways results in increased dyspnea, snoring respirations, or inspiratory crowing (Brooks-Brunn 1986; Elpern and Bone 1990; McHugh 1985; Persons 1987).

Esophageal obturator airways (EOA) are most frequently used in the field or emergency room. When properly placed in the esophagus, the EOA blocks air flow into the stomach and allows ventilation through apertures at the pharyngeal level. This device is a temporary measure, used only until an artificial airway is no longer needed or until an endotracheal (ET) tube can be inserted. Prior to removal of the EOA, regurgitation should be anticipated and prevented by patient positioning or insertion of a nasogastric tube (McHugh 1985; Persons 1987).

An ET tube is the most commonly used artificial device for providing short-term

Airway Management. ET tubes come in various sizes and designs. Most are made of polyvinyl chloride, silicone, nylon, or some combination of these materials. Factors that must be considered when selecting an ET tube are the size of the patient, cannulation route (oral or nasal), and reason for insertion. Tubes with large-volume, low-pressure cuffs that create a seal with less than 20 mm Hg pressure are preferred (Bernhard et al. 1985; Brooks-Brunn 1986; McHugh 1985).

No data are available to guide size selection of ET tubes. Sizes are individualized, with smaller tubes producing less laryngeal damage and less nasal trauma than larger tubes but increasing resistance to gas flow. In contrast, larger tubes facilitate suctioning and bronchoscopy, permit use of lower cuff pressures, and are less likely to become obstructed by secretions (Plummer and Gracey 1989).

Special endobronchial (EB) tubes are available for differential lung ventilation. They allow for the delivery of high pressures to the "diseased" lung while maintaining adequate ventilation and perfusion to the normal lung. Each lumen is connected to a separate ventilator, and two low-pressure cuffs are located at different positions on the tube (Traver and Flodquist-Priestley 1986).

Tracheostomy tubes are used to prevent or reverse upper airway obstruction, facilitate secretion removal, and cannulate the airway for long-term mechanical ventilation (Heffner 1990; King 1988; Lane 1990). These tubes also come in various sizes and designs. Metal tubes have been used for many years and are still made of sterling silver or silverplate. Their use is currently limited because of their inflexibility, patient discomfort, and high risk of associated pressure necrosis. In addition, metal stimulates mucus production and tissue irritation. Patients who have a permanent tracheostomy following laryngectomy may use a metal tracheostomy (Lane 1990).

Single-lumen, double-lumen, and fenestrated tracheostomies are among the types most commonly used. Single-lumen tubes have one tube with a built-in cuff and an obturator, which is used during tube insertion. The double-lumen tube is like the single-lumen tube with the addition of an inner cannula that can be removed for cleaning of built-up secretions. The need for an inner cannula is a current source of debate, as the use of materials and enhanced humidification techniques decrease secretion adherence to the inside of the tube. Single-lumen tubes provide a larger inside diameter for air flow than double-lumen tubes (Lane 1990; McHugh 1985). Fenestrated tracheostomy tubes are a special type of double-cannula tube that permit patients to speak when the inner cannula is removed (McHugh 1985). A common rule in selecting the size of a tracheostomy tube is that it should be about two-thirds the size of the trachea (McHugh 1985).

ET and tracheostomy tubes with low pressure–high volume (soft) cuffs minimize tracheal wall trauma (Bernhard et al. 1985; Heffner 1990; Kastanos et al. 1983; Klainer et al. 1975; Magovern, Shively, and Fecht 1972; Mathis and Wendley 1974; Nordin 1977; Routh, Hanning, and Ledingham 1979; Sackner, Hirsch, and Epstein 1975; Stauffer and Silvestri 1982). Proper use of such cuffs prevents leakage of inhaled air, prevents significant aspiration, and minimizes pressure on the surrounding trachea. The cuff is normally inflated during mechanical ventilation in patients unable to defend their airway and in most cases during and after feeding (Hoffman and Maszkiewicz 1987; Lane 1990). Soft cuffs are being refined, resulting in third-generation cuffs with thinner walls and smaller diameters. These changes reduce the contact area with the trachea and eliminate the folds and invaginations that contribute to aspiration (Goodnough 1988; Lane 1990).

Self-inflating silicone (foam) cuffs are found on some tracheostomies. Following insertion, the port to the cuff is left open, the cuff inflates automatically, and a constant pressure of 20 mm Hg is maintained. There is some evidence that the ability to maintain a constant pressure declines as cannulation time increases (Hoffman and Maszkiewicz 1987; Lane 1990; McHugh 1985).

Devices used for endotracheal suctioning include sterile gloves, a suction catheter, manual resuscitation bag (MRB), ventilator, oxygen source, and negative pressure source. These devices are discussed as part of the Airway Management intervention.

THE INTERVENTION

Airway Management is a four-part intervention composed of monitoring, positioning, insertion and management of artificial airways, and secretion removal. These four components encompass specific activities nurses do to carry out this intervention. Pharmacological interventions used to assist with airway management are beyond the scope of this chapter (see Brooks-Brunn 1986 for further information).

Monitoring

Monitoring for early signs of airway obstruction is among the best forms of Airway Management. Airway obstruction should be suspected with (1) inability to speak; (2) lack of chest movement; (3) absence of breath sounds and air movement; (4) abnormal or coarse breath sounds (e.g., crowing, wheezing, stridor); (5) prolonged expiration, (6) pharyngeal gurgle, (7) supraclavicular and intercostal retractions; (8) increased restlessness, (9) anxiety, (10) air hunger, and (11) increased system pressures and decreased tidal volume in the mechanically ventilated patient (Amborn 1976; Brooks-Brunn 1986; Capps and Schade 1988; Knipper 1986; Persons 1987; Smith 1983).

Noting the patient's ability to clear secretions is an essential part of Airway Management. This includes monitoring the patient's ability to take a deep breath and to generate high expiratory air flows and velocities (Cosenza and Norton 1986; Traver 1985). Slow vital capacity and maximal inspiratory force (MIF) are useful to determine deep-breathing ability. Normal vital capacity is dependent on the patient's age, size, and sex, with 15 mL/kg recommended for maintaining spontaneous ventilation. MIF, the amount of negative pressure the patient can generate, is usually -60 cm H_2O in a healthy adult, but a MIF of at least -20 cm H_2O is needed to maintain effective spontaneous ventilation (Traver 1985). Forced expiratory volume in 1 second (FEV_1) and the ratio of FEV_1 to forced vital capacity (FVC) helps determine the patient's ability to generate high air flow and velocities needed for effective coughing. Markedly reduced FEV_1 and FEV_1/FVC (normally more than 70%) means that the patient will have difficulty generating and conducting air flow (Traver 1985).

Monitoring the need for suctioning is an important part of Airway Management. Suctioning should not be done routinely in the absence of positive indicators because of adverse consequences of microatelectasis, tissue damage, hemoptysis, bronchospasm, hypoxia, cardiac arrhythmias, and even death (Knipper 1986; Riegel and Forshee 1985). Auscultation of adventitious sounds (crackles and ronchi) over the large airways is associated with significant amounts of secretions and is a reliable indicator for tracheal suctioning (Amborn 1976; Bulechek, Knipper, Titler, and Alpen 1991; Knipper 1986; Smith 1983). Coughing and increased inspiratory pressure on mechanical ventilators also indicate presence of airway secretions (Hoffman and Maszkiewicz 1987; McHugh 1985).

Pulse oximetry, capnometry, and arterial blood gas findings can be useful airway monitoring indicators. However, these physiological indexes of oxygenation are influenced by ventilation and oxygen transport, as well as airway patency (Cecil, Thorpe, Fibuch, and Tuohy 1988; McCauley and Von Rueden 1988; Szaflarski and Cohen 1989; Yelderman and New 1983).

Positioning

Relaxation of the oropharyngeal muscles allows the tongue to block the airway, a common cause of airway obstruction (Brooks-Brunn 1986; Cordora, Hurn, Mason, Scanlon-Schlip, Veise-Berry 1988). According to the American Heart Association, the head tilt, assisted by the chin lift, is the most important step in opening the airway in the adult. If cervical spinal injury is suspected, the jaw thrust technique is recommended instead of the head tilt – chin lift technique. If positioning is unsuccessful in opening the airway, or if the patient is unable to maintain a patent airway following this acute action, artificial means of maintaining airway patency must be considered.

Artificial Airway Insertion and Management

Cannulation of the trachea can result in various injuries, including airway trauma, pulmonary infection, laryngeal edema, tracheal stenosis, dilatation, necrosis, tracheomalacia, tracheoesophageal fistula, and tracheoinnominate artery fistula (Bishop 1989; Heffner 1990; Heffner, Miller, and Sahn, 1986a, 1986b; Lane 1990; Mackenzie 1983; Marsh, Gillespie, and Baumgartner 1989; Shekleton and Nield 1987). A variety of nursing activities are used to manage patients with artificial airways in an effort to minimize these complications. These include facilitating insertion of ET and tracheostomy tubes, stabilizing the tubes, administering hydration, managing cuff pressures, and administering tracheostomy care.

Inserting Artificial Airways

Nurses routinely insert oral and nasopharyngeal airways. Oral airways are inserted into the mouth laterally and then rotated downward to pull the tongue forward. Nasopharyngeal airways are inserted into the nostril and should fit comfortably, extending from the external nares to the base of the tongue. Care should be taken to prevent injuring the mucosa with insertion. EOAs are routinely inserted by nurses and other health care personnel who have passed Advanced Cardiac Life Support Training. Instructions for procedures for insertion of EOAs are readily available (McHugh 1985; Persons 1987).

Insertion of ET tubes is limited to those who are trained and credentialed (Plummer and Gracey 1989). Indications for ET intubation include airway management of patients who develop obstruction despite presence of a naso/oropharyngeal airway, removal of airway secretions, prevention against aspiration, and provision of mechanical ventilatory support (Brooks-Brunn 1986; Lane 1990; Plummer and Gracey 1989).

ET tubes can be placed via the oral or nasotracheal route. The oral route provides quick and certain airway control in emergent situations. Nasotracheal intubation provides airway access in patients with oral trauma and is purported to be more comfortable than the oral route. However, a study of postoperative cardiac surgery patients demonstrated no difference in the degree of discomfort or amount of sedation required in the orotracheal and nasotracheal groups (Fletcher,

Olsson, Helbo-Hansen, Nihlson, and Hedestrom 1984). Although the nasotracheal route is believed to cause less laryngotracheal injury, this is not supported by research (El-Naggar et al. 1976; Rashkin and Davis 1986; Stauffer, Olson, and Petty, 1981; Via-Reque and Rattenburg 1981). Nasotracheal cannulation is associated with a high incidence of purulent sinusitis and sepsis, which adversely affects patient outcomes (Deutschman, Wilton, Sinow, Dibbell, Kontantinides, and Cerra 1986; Kronberg and Goodwin 1985; O'Reilly et al. 1984). Unless contraindicated by the patient's condition (e.g., oral trauma), the oral route is favored by most experts (Heffner 1990).

The length of time that an ET tube can be left in place prior to performing a tracheostomy has been the point of lively conversation among researchers and clinicians for several years (Heffner 1990; King 1988; Marsh, Gillespie, and Baumgartner 1989; Stauffer, Olson, and Petty 1981). Experts attending a consensus conference initiated by the National Association of Medical Directors of Respiratory Care recommend that an ET tube be used when the anticipated length of time for an artificial airway is 10 days or less. If the anticipated need for an artificial airway is greater than 21 days, a tracheostomy is preferred. When the length of time for artificial airway management is unclear, ongoing monitoring is required to determine whether conversion to a tracheostomy is indicated (Plummer and Gracey 1989). Despite these recommendations, researchers continue to question the value of a tracheostomy when an artificial airway is required for periods as long as 3 weeks (Marsh, Gillespie, and Baumgartner 1989; Stauffer, Olson, and Petty 1981). Thus, there does not seem to be an absolute time limit for converting an ET tube to a tracheostomy (Heffner 1990; Marsh, Gillespie, and Baumgartner 1989).

Techniques of endotracheal tube insertion are reviewed elsewhere (Brooks-Brunn 1986; McHugh 1985; Persons 1987; Stauffer, Olson, and Petty 1981). Nurses assist with insertion of an ET tube by preparing the necessary equipment (laryngoscope, endotracheal tube, stylet, oxygen source, 10 mL syringe), ensuring optimal positioning of the patient, informing the patient about the procedure, administering appropriate medications as ordered, and monitoring for complications during insertion (e.g., cardiac arrhythmias, esophageal intubation). Auscultation of the chest and postintubation radiographs are necessary to ensure correct placement of the tube. The tip of the endotracheal tube should be 2 cm to 4 cm above the carina (Persons 1987).

Unsuccessful intubation efforts in the nonapneic, awake, or semiawake patient most frequently result from insufficient administration of topical anesthesia, general sedation, and/or muscle paralyzing agents. Patients with increased intracranial pressure, increased anxiety, extreme sensitivity to airway stimulation, or agitation benefit from receiving general sedation with or without muscle paralysis. Drugs commonly used for intubation include short-acting barbiturates (thiopental), narcotic analgesics (fentanyl), benzodiazepines (midazolam), and muscle relaxants (succinylcholine). Ensuring that adequate ventilation can be maintained by face mask is extremely important prior to administering paralyzing agents (Heffner 1990).

Following insertion, validation of placement, and stabilization of the tube, the nurse marks the ET tube at the centimeter markings corresponding to the position of the lips or nares. The practitioner can then tell at a glance whether the tube has slipped farther into the trachea or has become dislodged (Brook-Brunn 1986; Hoffman and Maszkiewicz 1987; Stauffer and Silvestri 1982).

Insertion of a tracheostomy tube is most valuable when done as an elective surgical procedure. Emergent tracheostomy has a fivefold increased rate of complications and should be avoided in preference of cricothyroidotomy if immediate surgical airway access is required (Heffner 1990). Many patients are converted from an ET tube to a tracheostomy to improve airway suctioning, patient comfort, and mobility; facilitate more rapid reintubation following spontaneous decannulation; and clear the mouth for speech and eating (Heffner 1990). Because tracheostomies are preferentially inserted as an elective surgical procedure in the operating room, nursing responsibilities focus on assisting with performance of emergent tracheostomies and monitoring for complications following completion of the procedure (Persons 1987).

Stabilizing Artificial Airways

Movement of ET and tracheostomy tubes causes abrasions to tracheal mucosa and contributes to laryngeal injury (Bishop 1989; Brooks-Brunn 1986; Mackenzie 1983). Although various methods and techniques are advocated to secure artificial airway devices, little research has been done to test the efficacy of these methods (Dunleap 1987; Hoffman and Maszkiewicz 1987; Hravnak 1984; Mackenzie 1983; McHugh 1985). Naso/oropharyngeal airways are taped in place to prevent them from becoming dislodged and obstructing the posterior pharynx (Elpern and Bone 1990; Persons 1987). ET tubes can be secured with commercially available ET tube holders, twill ties, or adhesive tape (Dunleap 1987; Hoffman and Maszkiewicz 1987; McHugh 1985; Persons 1987). Tapes and ties are changed daily, and oral ET tubes are moved to the other side of the mouth to prevent tissue necrosis. It is important to minimize motion between the tube and patient, administer meticulous mouth care, and monitor the integrity of oral mucous membranes during this process. Tube holders are loosened at least daily and skin care is administered. Breath sounds are noted after the tape or twills are changed.

Tracheostomy tubes are stabilized with twill tape. According to one author, this is a most unappreciated aspect of caring for patients with tracheostomies (Dunleap 1987). It is recommended that tapes be changed every 24 hours and/or following performance of routine tracheostomy care, old tapes be left in place while new tapes are inserted, tapes be tied at the side of the neck with a piece of gauze or foam placed between the patient's skin and the tie, and the tapes be tied snuggly enough to prevent slippage of the tracheostomy but loose enough to prevent neck irritation and erosion (can fit one to two fingers between the ties and the patient's skin) (Brooks-Brunn 1986; Dunleap 1987; McHugh 1985). Specific procedures for changing ties are published elsewhere (Dunleap 1987; McHugh 1985).

Leverage and traction on ET and tracheostomy tubes should be minimized by suspending the ventilator tubing from overhead supports, using flexible catheter mounts and swivels, and supporting tubes during turning, suctioning, and ventilator disconnection and reconnection (Heffner, Miller, and Sahn 1986b; McHugh 1985; Mackenzie 1983; Stauffer and Silvestri 1982). A unique procedure for securing the ventilator tubing of tracheostomized patients has been described (Hravnak 1984). Prolonged coughing, breathing out of phase with the ventilator, agitation, and decerebrate or decorticate posturing cause trauma to the tracheal mucosa and should be avoided by rectifying the cause, providing sedation, and, if necessary, administering muscle relaxants for mechanically ventilated patients (Heffner, Miller, and Sahn 1986b; Mackenzie 1983). Precautions should be taken to avoid self-extubation and spontaneous dislocation of airways. Use of arm restraints and appropriate sedation are two such activities (Stauffer and Silvestri, 1982).

Hydration

Bypassing upper air passages with an artificial airway causes mucosal drying, interferes with the mucociliary transport system, diminishes the cough reflex, and creates dry, thick secretions that are difficult to remove (Lane 1990; Shekleton and Nield 1987; Wanner 1977, 1986). Warming and humidifying inspired air is necessary to minimize these complications. However, no consensus exists as to the most efficacious way to provide humidification for patients with artificial airway devices (Shekleton 1987). Although cold humidifiers can be employed, they supply only about 50% of the humidification of warm humidifiers (Lane 1990). The cascade type of bubble humidifier heats and humidifies 100% of the inspired gas and is the type most frequently found in ventilator circuits.

Adequate systemic hydration is among the most reliable way to reduce the risk of inspissation of mucus production (Cosenza and Norton 1986; Shekleton and Nield 1987). Rehydration of dehydrated patients has been demonstrated to increase mucociliary clearance rates (Chopra, Talpin, Simmons 1977; Hirsh, Tokayer, and Robinson 1975). Therefore, oral and intravenous fluids are administered to maintain an adequate systemic fluid balance.

Nebulizers create a vapor mist and are used when inspired air/gas is delivered via a T piece or tracheostomy mask (Shekleton and Nield 1987). Controversy exists regarding the efficacy of mist therapy and ultrasonic nebulizers (USN). Major problems with mist therapy include chilling of the patient, and infection, particularly with Aerobacter and Pseudomonas organisms (Cosenza and Norton 1986; Shekleton and Nield 1987). USN have several drawbacks. In a sample of 10 persons with asthma or bronchitis and 10 controls, all subjects experienced an increase in airway resistance following use of USN (Cosenza and Norton, 1986). This type of device can also deliver too much fluid; if this fluid is plain water, mucosal edema can develop.

Managing Cuff Pressures

Because tracheal mucosa capillary perfusion pressure is about 20 mm Hg to 30 mm Hg, cuff pressures should be maintained below 15 mm Hg to 20 mm Hg (Bernhard et al. 1985; Goodnough 1988; Heffner 1990; Lane 1990; Snowberger 1986). Two methods are used for placing the correct amount of air into the cuff (Brooks-Brunn 1986; Lane 1990; Snowberger 1986). The minimal occlusive volume (MOV) technique is achieved by injecting air slowly during the inspiratory phase of ventilation until the patient receives the prescribed tidal volume on the ventilator or until an air leak cannot be auscultated over the trachea. The minimal leak technique is like the MOV technique but .1 mL to .5 mL of air is withdrawn following insertion of the minimal occlusive volume to allow a small leak. A small leak should be auscultated over the trachea during the inspiratory and expiratory phase of ventilation (Brooks-Brunn 1986; Hoffman and Maszkiewicz 1987).

Cuff pressures are monitored every 4 hours to 8 hours during expiration using a three-way stopcock that is simultaneously connected to the cuff, a calibrated syringe, and a mercury manometer or commercially available pressure manometer. Cuff pressure are also checked after general anesthesia to minimize the effect of nitrous oxide diffusion into the cuff. Procedures for inflating and measuring cuff pressures are described in detail by several experts (Goodnough 1985, 1988; Lane 1990; McHugh 1985; Persons 1987; Snowberger 1986).

Tracheostomy Care

Meticulous tracheostomy care is necessary to minimize accompanying complications, such as infection, skin breakdown, and airway obstruction. Little research exists on the best method of tracheostomy care. Generally, care includes keeping the area around the stoma clean, dry, and open to air; preventing traction on the tubing; and cleaning the inner cannula as often as necessary to prevent buildup of secretions. Sterile technique is recommended to decrease the risk of infection. Tracheostomy ties are changed following cleansing of the stoma site and inner cannula. A tracheostomy dressing is not used unless there is an excessive amount of exudate because wet dressings promote infections and tissue breakdown (Brooks-Brunn 1986; McHugh 1985; Persons 1987). Procedures for tracheostomy care are readily available in the literature (McHugh 1985; Persons 1987).

Secretion Removal

Removal of secretions, an important component of Airway Management, is accomplished by endotracheal and nasotracheal suctioning and chest physical therapy (chest percussion, postural drainage, chest vibration, and cough promotion).

Endotracheal Suctioning (ETS)

Various methods of ETS have been investigated in an attempt to prevent or reverse side effects, particularly suction-induced (SIH) hypoxemia and hemodynamic compromise. These methods include preoxygenation, hyperinflation, hyperoxygenation, hyperventilation, manual inflation, and oxygen insufflation. Using these terms interchangeably and without conceptual clarity has led to confusion and variation in research findings. These terms, as defined by Barnes and Kirchhoff (1986), are listed in Table 39–1 to provide a common ground for discussion of ETS activities.

Universal precautions are recommended as part of the suction protocol, particularly with high-risk patients. According to Centers for Disease Control guidelines, universal precautions apply to blood and other body fluids containing visible blood (Update: Universal precautions, 1988). Because suctioning may result in blood-tinged secretions and it is difficult to predict when this will happen, wearing gloves and goggles for protection is advisable.

Sterile suction equipment is used in the hospital for each suction procedure. The ratio of the catheter diameter to internal diameter of the tube should be less than .5 to prevent excessive negative pressure and atelectasis (Baier, Begin, and Sackner 1976; Rosen and Hillard 1962). The magnitude of negative pressure applied to the catheter affects the amount of hypoxemia, secretion recovery, endotracheal mucosal damage, and negative airway pressure (Kuzenski 1978; Pardowsky and Guthrie 1983; Plum and Dunning 1956; Polacek and Guthrie 1981; Sackner, Landa, Greeneltch and Robinson 1973). A negative pressure setting of 100 mm Hg to 120 mm Hg is recommended. Greater pressure is no more effective in removing secretions and greatly increases tracheobronchial trauma (Hunsinger et al. 1980). High negative airway pressure may result in removal of intrapulmonary gas and airway collapse (Bradstater and Muallem 1969; Rosen and Hillard 1962).

Use of suction devices that permit the patient to remain on the ventilator during suctioning (oxygen insufflation devices, OID; closed tracheal suction system, CTSS) are controversial but thought to be beneficial for patients on greater than

TABLE 39 – 1.   TERMS AND TECHNIQUES USED TO REDUCE SUCTIONING-INDUCED HYPOXEMIA

TERM	DEFINITION	TECHNIQUE
Manual inflation	Lung inflation by means of a resuscitation bag; does not imply an increase in percentage of oxygen and/or pressure	Bagging
Preoxygenation	Administration of oxygen before suctioning; does not imply an increase in percentage of oxygen and/or pressure	Bagging Change in ventilation rate Mechanical sigh
Insufflation	Delivery of oxygen through the double lumen of a suction catheter or the sidearm of an endotracheal tube adapter; allows oxygen to be administered simultaneously with suctioning	
Hyperoxygenation	Administration of oxygen at an FIO_2 greater than the patient is receiving or is usually required; may be performed before, during, and/or after suctioning	Bagging with supplemental O_2 Increasing the ventilator FIO_2
Hyperinflation	Lung inflation by means of a resuscitation bag or ventilator can be at a volume equivalent to the ventilator setting or as much as one and one-half times the preset ventilator value; does not imply a change in oxygen concentration	Bagging Sighing
Hyperventilation	An increase in rate of ventilation; does not imply an increase in volume or oxygen concentration	Bagging Increasing the ventilator rate

Source: Barnes and Kirchhoff (1986).

10 cm H_2O of positive end-expiratory pressure (Carlon, Fox, and Ackerman 1987; Langrehr, Washburn, and Guthrie 1981). A review of research findings reveals that PaO_2/SaO_2 decline was either equivalent or greater in studies that used hyperoxygenation (100%) combined with manual resuscitation bag hyperinflation (Baker, Baker, and Koen 1983) or hyperinflation at the preset tidal volume with subsequent removal from the ventilator for suctioning (Brown, Stansbury, Merrill, Linden, and Light 1983; Naigow and Powaser 1977) as compared to studies employing an adapter that permits the patient to remain on the ventilator with no additional hyperinflation or hyperoxygenation (Bodai 1982). However, there are potential risks with the use of these devices. Excessive negative airway pressure created by the CTSS can cause a decrease in functional residual capacity and a tendency toward alveolar collapse (Craig, Benson, and Pierson 1984), especially in the assist control mode of ventilation (Taggart, Dorinsky, and Sheahan 1988). Additional issues associated with use of the CTSS are the cost-effectiveness of the system, infection control, and amount of secretion recovery (Bodai et al. 1987; Noll, Hix, and Scott 1990; Ritz, Scott, Coyle and Pierson 1986). Further studies are needed using larger sample sizes and better control of extraneous variables to determine the efficacy and side effects of OID and CTSS.

The appropriate method for hyperinflation and hyperoxygenation before, during, and following passage of the suction catheter remains controversial. Most clinicians use either the MRB or the ventilator to deliver additional oxygen and volume. Belknap, Kiriloff, and Zullo (1980), and Buggy and associates (1980) found greater increases in PaO₂ using the MRB. However, other studies (Baker, Baker, and Koen 1983; Conforti 1982; Lucke 1982) demonstrate that ventilator "sigh" and uninterrupted oxygenation during passage of the suction catheter provides a greater increase in PaO₂. Hemodynamic changes associated with hyperinflation followed by ETS include decreases and increases in mean arterial pressure (Campbell et al. 1990; Goodnough 1985; Stone, Preusser, Groch, and Karl 1988) and increases and decreases in cardiac output (Preusser et al. 1988; Walsh et al. 1989). Although recent research indicates that hyperinflation with an MRB and ventilator prevents SIH, use of the MRB increases mean airway pressure and mean arterial pressure significantly more than use of the ventilator in postoperative open heart surgery patients (Campbell et al. 1990; Chulay 1988; Preusser et al. 1988; Stone et al. 1989). This is dangerous for people with new grafts and those with increased intracranial pressure (Rudy, Baun, Stone, and Turner, 1986), particularly when these findings are combined with those indicating a 27% mean increase in oxygen consumption during ETS (Walsh et al. 1989).

Although further research is required to determine the optimal methods for hyperoxygenation and hyperinflation for ETS, current data suggest that the patient be hyperoxygenated with the ventilator FiO₂ setting at 1.0 (100%) and hyperinflated using the ventilator set at one and a half times the present tidal volume. The nurse should note that it can take up to 3 minutes for the oxygen delivery to reach 100% following an increase in ventilator FiO₂ to 1.0 (Hess and Easter 1986). This washout time is variable and depends on the rate, flow, and tidal volume settings on the ventilator, as well as the length and diameter of the ventilator tubing (Stone and Turner 1988). If the nurse decides to use a MRB, the patient may receive less than 100% oxygen (Barnes and Watson 1982, 1983). It is recommended that the oxygen flow rate to the reservoir be set to flush, a reservoir of between 1000 cc and 2600 cc be used, and sufficient time be allowed to refill the MRB from the reservoir (Preusser 1985; Stone 1989).

Ten seconds to 15 seconds is the recommended duration for each suction pass (Lane 1990). An observational study of clinical practice revealed a 7-second mean suction duration with the majority of fall in PaO₂ occurring during the first 5 seconds. Suction durations of 10 seconds and 15 seconds did not significantly increase the fall in PaO₂ (Rindfleisch and Tyler 1983).

Number of consecutive suction passes seems to have an insignificant effect on tidal volume and hypoxemia, with the greatest fall occurring after the first suction pass (Hipenbecker and Guthrie 1981). However, if the MRB is being used for hyperinflation, increases in mean arterial pressure seem to be cumulative and thus increase from one hyperinflation-suction sequence to the next (Stone et al. 1989). Although further research is indicated, it seems that the number of suction passes is insignificant if the ventilator is used for hyperinflation.

Intratracheal instillation of 2 cc to 5 cc of normal saline is often used in conjunction with suctioning to facilitate removal of secretions. Normal saline instillation is not efficacious for thinning, mobilizing, or removing dried secretions (Ackerman 1985; Bostick and Wendelgass 1987; Hanley, Rudd, and Butler 1978). At best, it stimulates a cough that further irritates the mucosa and contributes to bronchospasm but may bring a small amount of dried secretions to the bronchi for retrieval with a suction catheter (Ackerman 1985; Elpern and Bone 1990).

Most studies on ETS have used convenience samples, acutely ill but stable patients, and post–open heart surgery patients with minimal pulmonary complications. Studies report improved oxygenation of most patients with use of a certain suction procedure but also list outliers whose oxygenation was decreased using the same technique (Bodai, Walton, Briggs, and Goldstein 1987; Chulay 1988). Individual patient variables reported as contributing to SIH are greater than 75 pack-year smoking history, elderly (over age 70 years), presence of arrythmias prior to ETS, PaO_2 less than 70 mm Hg, a wide alveolar to arterial (A-a) gradient, acid-base imbalances, and cardiovascular instability (Chulay 1988; Chulay and Graber 1988; Fell and Cheney 1971; Jones 1989; Lane 1990). Responses to ETS vary based on types of patients studied; therefore, the nurse must monitor and evaluate each patient's oxygen (SaO_2, SvO_2) and hemodynamic status (MAP, cardiac rhythm) immediately before, during, and after suctioning. If adverse consequences occur during suctioning, the suction procedure is terminated, and supplemental oxygen is administered. Suctioning techniques should be varied, based on the clinical response of the patient. The amount and type of secretions retrieved are noted.

Nasotracheal Suctioning (NTS)

NTS is indicated in patients with coarse breath sounds over large airways who are unable to cough effectively to remove secretions yet do not have an ET or tracheostomy in place. Many of the same principles of ETS apply to NTS. Hyperoxygenation and hyperinflation are necessary before, during, and following each suction pass. These maneuvers can be accomplished with a MRB or by instructing the patient to take deep breaths through an oxygen delivery system (e.g., nasal cannula, face mask). Slow advancement of the catheter avoids damage to nasal mucosa and turbinate bones. It is important to elicit the cooperation of the conscious patient prior to insertion of the catheter. Instructing the patient to take slow, deep breaths reduces the gag reflex and feelings of suffocation and helps retract the epiglottis, thereby facilitating catheter passage through the vocal cords into the trachea (Elpern and Bone, 1990).

Chest Physiotherapy

Chest physiotherapy (CPT) is directed at improving mucus and sputum clearance from the airways. It includes postural drainage, chest percussion, chest vibration, and cough enhancement (Kirilloff, Owens, Rogers, and Mazzocco 1985; Lane 1990; Shekelton and Nield 1987). Chest physiotherapy is a well-entrenched standard in pulmonary nursing care and has been used with a variety of acute and chronically ill populations. However, a recent research review by Kirilloff and colleagues (1985) reveals that CPT is not always efficacious. It appears to be beneficial for acutely ill patients who have large volumes of secretions and patients with lobar atelectasis. It is not efficacious in people with exacerbations of chronic bronchitis, patients with pneumonia who have limited amounts of secretions, and status asthmatics. CPT used in acutely ill patients is associated with bronchoconstriction and hypoxemia. It is contraindicated in patients with seizures, resectable carcinoma, recent hemoptysis, severe hypertension, unstable hemodynamics, and increased intracranial pressure (Lane 1990). CPT should not be performed within 1 hour after eating because of the increased risk of regurgitation and aspiration.

Postural drainage is administered by positioning the patient with the lung segment to be drained in the uppermost position. This facilitates movement of secretions toward major bronchi for clearance (Brannin 1974; Brooks-Brunn 1986; Norton and Conforti 1985; Techlin 1979).

Percussion is done with cupped hands held rigid so that a hollow sound is produced when an area of the chest wall is clapped. The purpose is to loosen and dislodge secretions from the airways. The amount of force used is relative to the person's body physique.

Chest vibration is the delivery of vibratory movements to the chest wall as the patient exhales. It can be delivered with the nurse's flat hand or with a machine (Brooks-Brunn 1986; Lane 1990). Mechanical vibratory devices have not been sufficiently evaluated to reach a conclusion about their efficacy (Kirilloff et al. 1985). Although percussion and vibration are used widely, empirical evidence demonstrates little efficacy in their use (Kirilloff et al. 1985).

Cough enhancement (improving cough effectiveness) is one of the most important strategies of Airway Management. Although the physiology of cough is beyond the scope of this chapter, several important points necessary to promote effective coughing are reviewed here (Cosenza and Norton 1986; Traver 1985).

An effective cough requires a deep breath that expands airways so that air can flow distal to any secretions, closure of the glottis, contraction of the muscles of expiration with a subsequent increase in intrathoracic pressure, and sudden opening of the glottis. Coughing is best facilitated in the sitting position with the head slightly flexed, shoulders relaxed, and knees flexed (Traver 1985).

The first activity in promoting an effective cough is encouraging the patient to take a deep breath. Firm placement of the nurse's hands on the lateral basal area of the chest wall is used to encourage deep breathing. The nurse should be careful to avoid restricting chest movement with the hands; rather, the hands are placed to encourage the individual to push them out as far as they can with each inspiration. Several deep breaths are taken before the actual cough maneuver, and the individual is given positive feedback with each deep breath. Incentive spirometers can be used to encourage deep breathing.

Several cough techniques are used to stimulate the normal cough reflex. The patient is taught not to suppress this reflex when it occurs. To elicit a cascade (normal) cough, the nurse instructs the patient to take a deep breath, followed by a succession of three to four coughs until almost all of the air is out of the lungs. This maneuver is repeated several times. Cascade coughing moves secretions from the periphery of the lungs to the central airways (Cosenza and Norton 1986; Janson-Bjerklie 1983; Oldenburg, Dolovich, Montgomery, and Newhouse 1979).

The hugh cough (forced expiration technique) is a simple modification of the cascade cough. The patient inhales deeply, bends forward slightly, and then performs a series of three to four huffs against an open glottis. The goal of this technique is to clear bronchial secretions with less airway compression than occurs with a cascade cough. Investigators have found a significant amount of secretion expectoration using this maneuver (Pryor, Webber, Hodson, and Batten 1979; Sutton, Parker, Webber, Newman, Garland, Lopez-Vidriero, Pavia, and Clark 1983).

The end-expiratory cough is a modification used for patients with bronchiectasis (Traver 1985). The patient does several deep inspirations followed by a prolonged slow exhalation. On the third or fourth breath, the patient exhales to a lung volume below normal resting lung volumes and then coughs without inhaling. This empties mucus from bronchiectic dilations of the airways (Traver, 1985).

Augmented cough is used in patients who are unable to generate sufficient expiratory muscle force. For patients with chest wall pain, a large towel is folded in thirds lengthwise and positioned on the chest to cover the painful area, with the ends of the towel crossing in front. The patient holds the right towel edge with the left hand and the left towel edge with the right hand, thus crossing the arms across the chest. As the patient coughs, the towel is pulled tight and subsequently loosened with each inspiration. Patients who are fatigued or have muscular weakness can be assisted by use of the lateral chest wall rib spring applied during the expiratory phase of the cough maneuver. The nurse's hands are placed on the chest wall and abruptly compressed against the chest wall as the patient coughs. For patients who do not have the ability to contract the abdominal muscles adequately, the nurse places her flat hand on the upper abdomen just below the xiphoid with the other hand placed on the patient's shoulders. As the patient coughs, the abdomen is abruptly compressed and the patient is flexed forward (Traver, 1985).

After coughing, the patient performs a voluntary maximal inhalation of 3 seconds to 10 seconds to aid in reinflating collapsed alveoli. Maximal inhalation following coughing helps avoid complications of pooled mucus, decreased oxygenation, and increased risk of infection. The use of incentive spirometer for these inspiratory efforts has proved to be twice as effective as any other method (Bartlett, Gazzaniga, and Geraghty 1973).

CASE STUDY

Alex Knight is a 59-year-old male with a 10-year history of chronic obstructive lung disease. He has a 65 pack-year smoking history but quit smoking 5 years ago. This is his third hospital admission within 6 months for respiratory distress. Three days prior to this admission, Alex noted increasing fatigue, shortness of breath, and increased sputum production. He is admitted to his local community hospital after his grandson called the paramedics when finding him slumped over the washbasin, conscious but extremely tachypneic. Upon arrival in the emergency room, a number 8 oral endotracheal tube is placed, and he is admitted to the intensive care unit with respiratory distress. He is placed on a mechanical ventilator, and an arterial line is inserted. His arterial blood gases are pH 7.30, PaO_2 65 torr, $PaCO_2$ 50 torr, HCO_3 30. He is connected to a pulse oximeter for ongoing monitoring of SaO_2. He has coarse breath sounds scattered throughout his chest, and endotracheal suctioning results in large amounts of thick, yellow, tenacious sputum.

Nursing diagnoses include Ineffective Airway Clearance related to fatigue, chronic air flow limitations, and presence of an artificial airway; Ineffective Breathing Pattern related to respiratory muscle fatigue and air flow limitations; and Impaired Gas Exchange related to chronic air flow limitation and retention of secretions. Projected outcomes are to maintain a clear airway, return arterial blood gases to baseline values, and wean from mechanical ventilation.

Airway Management is carried out by ongoing monitoring of SaO_2 values, auscultating for the presence of coarse breath sounds over major airways, and noting increases in inspiratory pressures. These findings indicate a need for ETS. The nurse initially uses an open suction technique with hyperoxygenation and hyperinflation using the MRB. This is poorly tolerated, as evidenced by short runs of ventricular tachycardia, increasing blood pressure from 140/87 to 182/104, and decrease in SaO_2 from 95% to 87%. The nurse then applies a CTSS, which allows Alex to remain ventilated during suctioning. Hyperinflation and hyperoxygenation are achieved by setting the ventilator to an FiO_2 of 1.0 for 3 minutes prior to suctioning and delivering three breaths with the ventilator set at one and a half times the present tidal volume. The suction pressure is set at 120 mm Hg. ETS results in a return to normal breath sounds and inspiratory pressure. Suction-induced hypoxemia and hemodynamic compromise are limited by using the CTSS, accompanied by hyperoxygenating and hyperinflating with the ventilator.

Humidification and heating of inspired oxygen are achieved via the water cascade on the ventilator. Alex's intravenous intake is increased to 3000 cc in the first 24 hours to correct the underlying dehydration that is contributing to thick, tenacious secretions.

Every morning prior to daily chest X-rays, the tape is removed from the ET tube, the tube is moved to the other side of the mouth, oral care is administered, oral mucosa are evaluated, and the tape is reapplied. Cuff pressures are noted every 8 hours and maintained at 18 mm Hg based on the minimal occlusive volume technique. By the third day, the amount of secretions declines. Weaning trials are begun on the fifth day, and Alex is weaned from the ventilator in 4 days. He is successfully extubated after 24 hours on a T piece. Nursing activities following extubation focus on cough enhancement and proper hydration through administration of intravenous and oral fluids.

SUMMARY

Airway Management is a critical life support nursing intervention, which encompasses monitoring, positioning, insertion and management of artificial airways, and secretion removal. It is applicable in many areas of nursing practice, particularly in emergency and critical care. The challenge for the future is to continue testing the efficacy and side effects of the various activities used in Airway Management.

REFERENCES

Ackerman, M. 1985. The use of normal saline instillations in artificial airways: Is it necessary or useful? *Heart and Lung* 14:505–506.

Adler, D.C. 1979. Pulmonary nursing, 1900–1979, and future projections. *Heart and Lung* 8:882–890.

Adlkofer, R.M., and Powaser, M.M. 1978. The effect of endotracheal suctioning on arterial blood gases in patients after cardiac surgery. *Heart and Lung* 7:1011–1014.

Amborn, S.A. 1976. Clinical signs associated with the amount of tracheobronchial secretions. *Nursing Research* 25:121–126.

Baier, G., Begin, R., and Sackner, M. 1976. Effect of airway diameter, suction catheter, and the bronchofiberscope on airflow in endotracheal and tracheostomy tubes. *Heart and Lung* 5:235–238.

Baker, P., Baker, J., and Koen, P. 1983. Endotracheal suctioning techniques in hypoxemic patients. *Respiratory Care* 28:1563–1568.

Barnes, C., and Kirchhoff, K. 1986. Minimizing hypoxemia due to endotracheal suctioning: A review of the literature. *Heart and Lung* 15:164–176.

Barnes, R., and Watson, M. 1982. Oxygen delivery performance of four adult resuscitation bags. *Respiratory Care* 27:139–146.

Barnes, T, and Watson, M. 1983. Oxygen delivery performance of old and new designs of the Laerdal, Vitalograph, and AMBU adult manual resuscitators. *Respiratory Care* 28:1121–1128.

Bartlett, R., Gazzaniga, A., and Geraghty, T. 1973. Respiratory maneuvers to prevent postoperative pulmonary complications. *JAMA* 224:1017–1020.

Baun, M. 1984. Physiological determinants of clinically successful methods of endotracheal suction. *Western Journal Nursing Research* 6:213–225.

Belknap, J., Kirilloff, L., and Zullo, T. 1980. The effect of preoxygenation technique on arterial blood gases in the mechanically ventilated patient. *American Review of Respiratory Diseases* 121:210–213.

Belling, D., Kelley, R., and Simon, R. 1978. Use of the swivel adaptor during suctioning to prevent hypoxemia in the mechanically ventilated patient. *Heart and Lung* 7:320–322.

Bernhard, W.N., Yost, L., Joynes, D., Cothalis, S., and Turndorf, H. 1985. Intracuff pressures in endotracheal and tracheostomy tubes. *Chest* 87:720–725.

Bishop, M.J. 1989. Mechanisms of laryngotracheal injury following prolonged tracheal intubation. *Chest* 96:185–186.

Bodai, B.T., Walton, C.B., Briggs, S., and Goldstein, M. 1987. A clinical evaluation of an oxygen insufflation/suction catheter. *Heart and Lung* 16:39–46.

Bodai, I. 1982. A means of suctioning without cardiopulmonary depression. *Heart and Lung* 11:172–176.

Bostick, J., and Wendelglass, S. 1987. Normal saline instillation as part of the suctioning procedure: Effects on PaO_2 and amount of secretions. *Heart and Lung* 16:532–537.

Bradstater, B., and Muallem, M. 1969. Atelectasis following tracheal suction in infants. *Anesthesiology* 31:468–473.

Brannin, P. 1974. Oxygen therapy and measures of bronchial hygiene. *Nursing Clinics of North America* 9:111–121.

Brooks-Brunn, J. 1986. Respiration. In L. Abels (ed.), *Critical care nursing: A physiologic approach* (pp. 168–253). St. Louis: Mosby Co.

Brown, S., Stansbury, D., Merrill, E., Linden, G., and Light, R. (1983). Prevention of suction-related arterial oxygen desaturation. *Chest* 4:621–627.

Buggy, E., Hanson, V., Flynn, K., and Baun, M. 1980. Effects of two oxygenation methods during suctioning at zero, 10, and 20 cm. of positive end-expiratory pressure (PEPP). *American Review of Respiratory Diseases,* 121:211–215.

Bulechek, G., Knipper, J., Titler, M., and Alpen, M. 1991. [Adventitious lung sounds as an indicator for endotracheal suctioning]. Unpublished data.

Campbell, G., Byram, D., Chulay, M., Hepburn, D., Tribett, D., Johnson, S., Rosenthal, C., Strider, V., Chase, D., Dellasanta, L., and Annanian, L. 1990. Physiological changes associated with endotracheal suctioning (ETS). *Heart and Lung* 19:303.

Capps, J.S., and Schade, K. 1988. Work of breathing: Clinical monitoring and considerations in the critical care setting. *Critical Care Nursing Quarterly* 11(3):1–11.

Carlon, G.C., Fox, S.J., and Ackerman, N.J. 1987. Evaluation of a closed-tracheal suction system. *Critical Care Medicine* 15:522–525.

Carroll-Johnson, R.M. (ed.) 1989. *Classification of nursing diagnoses: Proceedings of the Eighth Conference.* Philadelphia: J.B. Lippincott.

Cecil, W.T., Thorpe, K.J., Fibuch, E.E., and Tuohy, G.F. 1988. A clinical evaluation of the accuracy of the Nellcor N-100 and Ohmeda 3700 pulse oximeters. *Journal of Clinical Monitoring* 4(1):31–36.

Chopra, S., Talpin, G., and Simmons, D. 1977. Effects of hydration and physical therapy on tracheal transport velocity. *American Review of Respiratory Diseases* 115:1009–1014.

Chulay, M. 1988. Arterial blood gas changes with a hyperinflation and hyperoxygenation suctioning intervention in critically ill patients. *Heart and Lung* 17:654–661.

Chulay, M., and Graeber, G.M. 1988. Efficacy of hyperinflation and hyperoxygenation suctioning intervention. *Heart and Lung* 17:15–22.

Conforti, C. 1982. The effect of two preoxygenation techniques in minimizing hypoxemia during endotracheal suctioning. In *Proceedings of the Ninth National Teaching Institute* (p. 309). Newport Beach, Calif. American Association of Critical-Care Nurses.

Cordora, V., Hurn, P., Mason, P., Scanlon-Schlip, A., and Veise-Berry, S. 1988. *Trauma nursing: From resuscitation to rehabilitation.* Philadelphia: W.B. Saunders.

Cosenza, J., and Norton, L. 1986. Secretion clearance: State of the art from a nursing perspective. *Critical Care Nurse* 6(4):23–27.

Craig, K., Benson, M., and Pierson, D. 1984. Prevention of arterial oxygen desaturation during closed-airway endotracheal suction: Effect of ventilator mode. *Respiratory Care* 29:1013–1017.

Deutschman, C.S., Wilton, P., Sinow, J., Dibbell, D., Kontantinides, F.N., Cerra, and F.B. 1986. Parasinal sinusitis associated with nasotracheal intubation: A frequently unrecognized and treatable source of sepsis. *Critical Care Medicine* 14:111–118.

Dunleap, E. 1987, August. Safe and easy ways to secure breathing tubes. RN, 26–27.

El-Naggar, M., Sadagopa, S., Levin, H., Kantor, H., and Collins, V.J. 1976. Factors influencing choice between tracheostomy and prolonged translaryngeal intubation in acute respiratory failure: A prospective study. *Anesthesia Analog* 55:195–201.

Elpern, E., and Bone, R. 1990. The technique of nasotracheal suctioning. *Journal of Critical Illness* 5:993–999.

Fell, T., and Cheney, F.W. 1971. Prevention of hypoxia during endotracheal suction. *Annals of Surgery* 174:24–28.

Fletcher, R., Olsson, K., Helbo-Hansen, S., Nihlson, C., and Hedestrom, P. 1984. Oral or nasal intubation after cardiac surgery? A comparison of effects on heart rate, blood pressure, and sedation requirements. *Anaesthesia* 39:376–378.

Goodnough, S. 1985. The effects of oxygen and hyperinflation on arterial oxygen tension after endotracheal suctioning. *Heart and Lung* 14:11–17.

Goodnough, S.K.C. 1988. Reducing tracheal injury and aspiration. *Dimensions of Critical Care Nursing* 7:324–331.

Hanley, M.V., and Tyler, M.L. 1987. Ineffective airway clearance related to airway infection. *Nursing Clinics of North America* 22:135–150.

Hanley, V., Rudd, T., and Butler, J. 1978. What happens to intratracheal instillations? *American Review of Respiratory Diseases* 117:124–127.

Hardie, D., and Kirchhoff, K. 1989. A comparison of the open versus closed system suction catheter. *Heart and Lung* 18:305.

Harken, S. 1975. A routine for safe, effective endotracheal suctioning. *American Surgeon* 41:398–404.

Heffner, J.E. 1990. Airway management in the critically ill patient. *Critical Care Clinics* 6:533–550.

Heffner, J.E., Miller, S., and Sahn, S.A. 1986a. Tracheostomy in the intensive care unit. Part I. *Chest* 90:269–274.

Heffner, J.E., Miller, S., and Sahn, S.A. 1986b. Tracheostomy in the intensive care unit. Part II. *Chest* 90:430–436.

Hess, D., and Easter, G. 1986. Delivery 100% oxygen with a ventilator. A study of lag time. *Respiratory Therapy* 31:17–21, 39.

Hipenbecker, D., and Guthrie, M. 1981. The effects of negative pressure generated during suctioning on lung volumes and pulmonary compliance. *American Review of Respiratory Diseases* 123:120–122.

Hirsch, J., Tokayer, J., and Robinson, M. 1975. Effect of dry air and subsequent humidification on tracheal mucous velocity in dogs. *Journal of Applied Physiology* 39:242–246.

Hoffman, L.A. 1987. Ineffective airway clearance related to neuromuscular dysfunction. *Nursing Clinics of North America* 22:151–166.

Hoffman, L.A., and Maszkiewicz, R.C. 1987. Airway management. *American Journal of Nursing* 87:40–53.

Hravnak, M. 1984. Ventilator tubing stabilization for the tracheostomized patient. *Critical Care Nurse* 4(5):20–21.

Hunsinger, D., Lisnerski, K., Maurizi, J., and Phillips, M. 1980. *Respiratory technology procedure and equipment manual.* Reston, Va.: Reston Publishing Co.

Janson-Bjerklie, S. 1983. Defense mechanisms protecting the healthy lung. *Heart and Lung* 12:643–649.

Jones, G. 1989. *Effectiveness of two suction methods.* Unpublished master's thesis, University of Iowa, College of Nursing, Iowa City.

Kastanos, N., Miro, R.E., Perez, A.M., Mir, A.X., and Agusti-Vidal, A. 1983. Laryngotracheal injury due to endotracheal intubation: Incidence, evolution and predisposing factors. A prospective long-term study. *Clinical Care Medicine* 11:362–367.

Kim, M.J., and Larson, J.L. 1987. Ineffective airway clearance and ineffective breathing patterns: Theoretical and research base for nursing diagnosis. *Nursing Clinics of North America* 22:125–134.

King. E.G. 1988. Respiratory failure in the critically ill. In W. Sibbald (ed.), *Synopsis of critical care* (3d ed.). Baltimore: Williams & Wilkins.

Kirilloff, L. H., Owens, G.R., Rogers, R.M., and Mazzocco, M.C. 1985. Does chest physical therapy work? *Chest* 88:436–444.

Klainer, A., Turndorf, H., Wu, W.H., Maewal, H., and Allener, P. 1975. Surface alterations due to endotracheal intubation. *American Journal of Medicine.* 58:674–681.

Knipper, J.S. 1986. Minimizing the complications of tracheal suctioning. *Focus on Critical Care* 13(4):23–26.

Kronberg, F.G., and Goodwin, W.J., Jr. 1985. Sinusitis in intensive care unit patients. *Laryngoscope* 95:936–942.

Kuzenski, B. 1978. Effect of negative pressure on tracheobronchial trauma. *Nursing Research* 27:260–263.

Landa, J.F., Kwoka, M.A., Chapman, G.A., Brito, M., and Sackner, M. 1980. Effects of suctioning on mucociliary transport. *Chest* 77:202–207.

Lane, G.H. 1990. Pulmonary therapeutic management. In L.A. Thelan, J.K. Davie, and L.D. Urden (eds.). *Textbook of critical care nursing: Diagnosis and management* (pp. 444–471). St. Louis: C.V. Mosby.

Langrehr, E.A., Washburn, S.C., and Guthrie, M.P. 1981. Oxygen insufflation during endotracheal suctioning. *Heart and Lung,* 10:1028–1036.

Lareau, S., and Larson, J.L. 1987. Ineffective breathing pattern related to airflow limitation. *Nursing Clinics of North America* 22:179–191.

Lucke, K. 1982. A comparison of two methods of preoxygenation and hyperinflation associated with tracheal suction. *American Review of Respiratory Diseases* 125:141–145.

McCauley, M., and VonRueden, K.T. 1988. Noninvasive monitoring of the mechanically ventilated patient. *Critical Care Nursing Quarterly* 11(3):36–49.

Magovern, G.J., Shively, J.G., and Fecht, D. 1972. The clinical and experimental evaluation of a controlled-pressure intratracheal cuff. *Journal of Cardiovascular Surgery.* 64:747–750.

McHugh, J.M. 1985. Airway management. In S. Millar, L.K. Sampson, and M. Soukup (eds.), *AACN procedural manual for critical care* (pp. 203–239). Philadelphia: W.B. Saunders.

Mackenzie, C.F. 1983. Compromises in the choice of orotracheal or nasotracheal intubation and tracheostomy. *Heart and Lung* 12:485–492.

Malen, J., and Bochuck, J. 1989. Advances in pulmonary care: The immunocompromised. *Critical Care Nursing Clinics of North America* 1:713–717.

Marsh, H.M., Gillespie, D.J., and Baumgartner, A.E. 1989. Timing of tracheostomy in the critically ill patient. *Chest* 96:190–193.

Mathis, D.B., and Wendley, J.R. 1974. The effects of cuffed endotracheal tubes on the tracheal wall. *British Journal of Anaesthesia* 46:849–852.

Naigow, D., and Powaser, M. 1977. The effect of different endotracheal suction procedures on arterial blood gases in a controlled experimental model. *Heart and Lung* 6:808–816.

Nelson, D.M. 1989. *Defining activities for the validation of respiratory nursing interventions.* Unpublished master's thesis, University of Iowa, College of Nursing, Iowa City.

Noll, M., Hix, C., and Scott, G. 1990. Closed tracheal suction systems: Effectiveness and nursing implications. *AACN Clinical Issues* 1:318–328.

Nordin, U. 1977. The trachea and cuff-induced tracheal injury. *Acta Otolaryngology Supplement* 345:1–74.

Norton, L., and Conforti, C. 1985. The effects of body position on oxygenation. *Heart and Lung* 14:45–52.

Oldenburg, F.A., Dolovich, M.B., Montgomery, J.M., and Newhouse, M.T. 1979. Effects of postural drainage, exercise and cough on mucous clearance in chronic bronchitis. *American Review of Respiratory Diseases* 120:739–745.

Openbrier, D.R., and Covey, M. 1987. Ineffective breathing pattern related to malnutrition. *Nursing Clinics of North America.* 22:225–247.

O'Reilly, M.J., Reddick, E.J., Black, W., Carter, P.L., Erhardt, J., Fill, W., Maughn, D., Sado, A., and Klatt, G.R. 1984. Sepsis from sinusitis in nasotracheally intubated patients. A diagnostic dilemma. *American Journal of Surgery* 147:601–604.

Pardowsky, B.J., and Guthrie, M.M. 1983. Negative airway pressure during endotracheal suctioning. *American Review of Respiratory Diseases* 127:147–151.

Persons, C. 1987. *Critical care procedures and protocols: A nursing process approach.* Philadelphia: J.B. Lippincott.

Pierce, J., and Piazza, D. 1987. Difference in postsuctioning arterial blood oxygen concentration values using two postoxygenation methods. *Heart and Lung* 16:34–38.

Plum, F., and Dunning, M.F. 1956. Techniques for minimizing trauma to the tracheobronchial tree after tracheostomy. *New England Journal of Medicine* 254:193–200.

Plummer, A.L., and Gracey, D.R. 1989. Consensus conference on artificial airways in patients receiving mechanical ventilation. *Chest* 96:178–180.

Polacek, L., and Guthrie, M.M. 1981. The effect of suction catheter size and suction flow rate on negative airway pressure and its relationship to the fall in arterial oxygen tension. *American Review of Respiratory Diseases* 123:120–122.

Pressuer, B.A. 1985. The efficiency of commercially available manual resuscitation bags. *Focus on Critical Care* 12:59–61.

Preusser, B., Stone, K., Gonyon, D., Winningham, M.L., Groch, K.F., and Karl, J.E. 1988. Effects of two methods of preoxygenation on mean arterial pressure, cardiac output, peak airway pressure, and postsuctioning hypoxemia. *Heart and Lung* 17:290–299.

Pryor, S., Webber, B., Hodson, M., and Batten, J. 1979. Evaluation of the forced expiration technique as an adjunct to postural drainage in treatment of cystic fibrosis. *British Medical Journal* 2:417–418.

Rashkin, M.C., and Davis, T. 1986. Acute complications of endotracheal intubation. *Chest* 89:165–167.

Riegel, B., and Forshee, T. 1985. A review of the literature on preoxygenation for endotracheal suctioning. *Heart and Lung* 14:507–518.

Rindfleisch, S., and Tyler, M. 1983. Duration of suctioning: An important variable. *Respiratory Care* 28:457–459.

Ritz, R., Scott, L.R., Coyle, M.B., and Pierson, D.J. 1986. Contamination of a multiple-use suction catheter in a closed-circuit system compared to contamination of a disposal, single-use suction catheter. *Respiratory Care* 31:1086–1091.

Rogge, J., Bunde, L., and Baun, M. 1989. Effectiveness of oxygen concentrations of less than 100% before and after endotracheal suction in patients with chronic obstructive pulmonary disease. *Heart and Lung* 18:64–71.

Rosen, M., and Hillard, E.K. 1962. The effects of negative pressure during tracheal suction. *Anesthesia Analgesia* 41:322–325.

Routh, G., Hanning, C.D., and Ledingham, I. 1979. Pressure on the tracheal mucosa from cuffed tubes. *British Medical Journal* 282:1425–1428.

Ruby, E., Baun, M., Stone, K., and Turner, B. 1986. The relationship between endotracheal suctioning and changes in intracranial pressure. A review of the literature. *Heart and Lung.* 15:488–494.

Sackner, M.A., Hirsch, J., and Epstein, S. 1975. Effect of cuffed endotracheal tubes on tracheal mucous velocity. *Chest* 68:774–777.

Sackner, M.A., Landa, J.F., Greeneltch, N., and Robinson, M.J. 1973. Pathogenesis and prevention of tracheobronchial damage with suction procedures. *Chest* 64:284–290.

Shekleton, M.E., and Nield, M. 1987. Ineffective airway clearance related to artificial airway. *Nursing Clinics of North America* 22:167–177.

Skelley, V., Deeren, S., and Powaser, M. 1980. The effectiveness of two preoxygenation methods to prevent endotracheal suction-induced hypoxemia. *Heart and Lung* 9:316–323.

Smith, A.E. 1983, January. Endotracheal suctioning. "Are we harming our patients?" *Critical Care Update.* 29–31.

Snowberger, P. 1986. Decreasing tracheal damage due to excessive cuff pressures. *Dimensions of Critical Care Nursing* 5:136–142.

Stauffer, J.L., Olson, D.E., and Petty, T.L. 1981. Complications and consequences of endotracheal intubation and tracheostomy. A prospective study of 150 critically ill adult patients. *American Journal of Medicine* 70:65–68.

Stauffer, J.L., and Silvestri, R.C. 1982. Complications of endotracheal intubation, tracheostomy, and artificial airways. *Respiratory Care* 27:417–433.

Stone, K. 1989. Endotracheal suctioning in the critically ill. *Critical Care Nursing Currents* 7(2):5–8.

Stone, K., Preusser, B., Groch, K., and Karl, J. 1988. The effect of lung hyperinflation on cardiopulmonary hemodynamics and postsuctioning hypoxemia. *Heart and Lung* 17:309.

Stone, K., and Turner, B. 1988. Endotracheal suctioning. *Annual Review of Nursing Research* 7:27–49.

Stone, K., Vorst, E., Lanham, B., and Zahn, S. 1989. Effects of lung hyperinflation on mean arterial pressure and postsuctioning hypoxemia. *Heart and Lung* 18:377–385.

Sutton, P., Parker, R., Webber, B., Newman, S., Garland, N., Lopez-Vidriero, M., Pavia, D., and Clark, S.W. 1983. Assessment of forced expiration technique, postural drainage and directed coughing in chest physiotherapy. *European Journal of Respiratory Disease* 64:62–68.

Szaflarski, N.L., and Cohen, N.H. 1989. Use of pulse oximetry in critically ill adults. *Heart and Lung* 18:444–452.

Taggart, J., Dorinsky, N., and Sheahan, J. 1988. Airway pressures during closed system suctioning. *Heart and Lung* 17:536–542.

Techlin, J.S. 1979, March. Positioning, percussing and vibrating patients for effective bronchial drainage. *Nursing 79*, 64–71.

Traver, G. 1985. Ineffective airway clearance: Physiology and clinical application. *Dimensions in Critical Care Nursing* 4:198–208.

Traver, G.A., and Flodquist-Priestley, G. 1986. Management problems in unilateral lung disease with emphasis on differential lung ventilation. *Critical Care Nurse* 6(4):40–50.

Update: Universal precautions for prevention of transmission of human immunodeficiency virus, hepatitis B virus, and other bloodborne pathogens in health-care settings. 1988. *Morbidity and Mortality Weekly Report* 37(24):377–382.

Via-Reque, E., and Rattenburg, C. 1981. Prolonged oro- or nasotracheal intubation. *Critical Care Medicine* 9:37–42.

Walsh, J.M., Vanderwarf, C., Hoscheit, D., and Fahey, P.J. 1989. Unsuspected hemodynamic alterations during endotracheal suctioning. *Chest* 95:162–165.

Wanner, A. 1986. Mucociliary clearance in the trachea. *Clinical Chest Medicine* 7:247–258.

Wanner, A. 1977. Clinical aspects of mucociliary transport. *American Review of Respiratory Diseases* 116:73–125.

Yelderman, M., and New, W. 1983. Evaluation of pulse oximetry. *Anesthesiology* 59:349–352.

York, K. 1985. Clinical validation of two respiratory nursing diagnoses and their defining characteristics. *Nursing Clinics of North America* 20:657–667.

40

VENTILATORY SUPPORT

JANE S. KNIPPER
MICHELE A. ALPEN

Ventilation is the movement of air between the atmosphere and the alveoli. The proper functioning of this process relies on the respiratory system and its interactions with the neurological and cardiovascular systems. Failure of one or more of these systems may result in ventilatory failure and impending death if an artificial means of ventilation is not instituted.

The focus of this chapter is the intervention of Ventilatory Support, defined as the care and management of patients who require a mechanical ventilator to assist with respiratory gas exchange requirements. The use of machines to provide artificial ventilation was described as early as the sixteenth century; however, consistently successful techniques were not developed until the 1920s (Shapiro 1984), and the routine use of ventilators was not incorporated into clinical practice until the 1950s, when this intervention was required to sustain the life of polio victims (Hubmayr, Abel, and Rehder 1990).

DESCRIPTION OF THE INTERVENTION

Ventilatory Support is an intervention that is physician initiated; however, successful implementation requires the combined effort of physicians, nurses, and respiratory therapy technicians. The nurse coordinates the efforts of the team in carrying out all components of the intervention: initiation of mechanical ventilation, management of the equipment, monitoring patient response and management of complications, and weaning from mechanical ventilatory support.

Initiation of Mechanical Ventilation

The members of the health care team determine when ventilatory support is indicated based on the status of the patient's oxygenation, ventilation, and respiratory mechanics. Specific criteria for institution of mechanical ventilation are listed in Table 40–1. When the decision has been made to institute mechanical ventilation, the nurse prepares the ventilator or contacts the respiratory therapy department if these services are available. The nurse prepares the patient by obtaining the necessary equipment for endotracheal intubation, discussing the need for

The authors acknowledge Dr. Gloria Bulechek, assistant professor, the University of Iowa College of Nursing, and Margo Halm, MA, RN, CCRN, Clinical Nurse Specialist II, University of Iowa Hospital and Clinics for their review of this chapter.

TABLE 40–1. CRITERIA FOR INITIATION OF MECHANICAL VENTILATORY SUPPORT

Oxygenation
$PaO_2 \leq 60$ mm Hg on $\geq .5$ FiO_2

Ventilation
$PaCO_2 \geq 50$–60 mm Hg (or ≥ 10 mm Hg above patient's normal $PaCO_2$)
pH < 7.20

Respiratory mechanics
Apnea
Sustained respiratory rate >35 breaths/minute
Vital capacity <10–15 mL/kg body weight

Sources: Luce et al. (1984); Shapiro (1984).
Note: PaO_2, arterial oxygen tension; FiO_2, fraction of inspired oxygen; $PaCO_2$, arterial carbon dioxide tension; pH, hydrogen ion concentration.

ventilation, and providing reassurance that the machine will breathe for the patient. The patient must be alerted to the alarms that will sound and be assured that a nurse is always close by to deal with the alarms and be certain that the machine is functioning correctly. The nurse explains to the patient and family that he or she will not be able to talk following intubation. Alternative communication techniques, such as lip reading, writing notes, hand signals, electronic spellers, and using picture boards, will have to be experimented with in order to learn which is the easiest and best means of communication for the patient.

Management of Equipment

A decision must be made regarding which type of mechanical ventilator is best to achieve the goals of improving oxygenation and ventilation while decreasing the patient's work of breathing (Luce, Pierson, and Hudson 1981). There are two types of ventilators, each with its own specific purpose, and both function by very different principles. Negative pressure ventilation operates externally, without the use of an artificial airway; positive pressure ventilation requires airway intubation. The latter type of ventilator is most often found in the acute-care setting. Table 40–2 compares the two types of ventilators and their indications for use.

An understanding of the physiological effects of mechanical ventilation as it compares to spontaneous ventilation can assist the nurse in understanding not only

TABLE 40–2. TYPES OF VENTILATORS

TYPE	PRINCIPLE OF OPERATION	INDICATION FOR USE	EXAMPLE
Negative pressure ventilator	Inspiration: Externally applied apparatus creates negative pressure, expanding the thoracic cage, allowing air to flow into lungs	Patients with neuromuscular disease with mild respiratory failure	Iron lung Cuirass Pulmowrap
	Expiration: Passive by lung recoil		
Positive pressure ventilator	Inspiration: An inspiratory flow of gas is forced into airways under pressure	Patients with severe acute or chronic respiratory failure	Bourns Bear V Servo 900
	Expiration: Passive by lung recoil		

TABLE 40–3. POSITIVE PRESSURE VENTILATORS

TYPE	MECHANICS	LIMITATIONS
Pressure cycled	Inspiratory flow of gas delivered to airway until preset pressure reached	Inability to guarantee delivery of exact volumes of gas and precise oxygen concentrations Inability to ventilate noncompliant lung
Time cycled	Inspiratory gas flow occurs over a preset length of time	Volume of gas and pressures delivered to lung may vary greatly with changes in airway resistance
Volume cycled pressure limited	Inspiratory gas flow occurs until a preset volume is reached or until the pressure limit is reached, ensuring delivery of precise volumes of gas and oxygen concentrations	Potential delivery of excessive pressures to lung

the benefits of this intervention but the adverse effects as well. During spontaneous respiration, a negative intrathoracic pressure is created, which initiates the flow of gas from the atmosphere into the lungs. As alveolar pressure becomes more positive, inspiration is inhibited, and the elastic recoil properties of the lung force gas out of the airway. The decreased intrathoracic pressure on inspiration enhances venous return to the thorax, resulting in more blood available to be pumped to the body tissues. Positive pressure ventilation creates the opposite effect of spontaneous respiration. As air is forced into the lung on inspiration, positive pressure is attained. This state reduces venous return to the heart, which leads to a decreased blood supply available to the tissues and increases pooling in peripheral vessels. However, the delivery of larger than usual volumes of gas to the lung allows for the expansion of otherwise collapsed or underventilated alveoli. This improves the exchange of oxygen and carbon dioxide at the alveolar-capillary level.

There are several types of positive pressure ventilators available. The types of ventilators are described according to the method they use to terminate inspiration and are summarized in Table 40–3. A positive pressure ventilator functions in one of many different modes of operation. The decision of which mode will best meet a patient's ventilatory requirements ultimately lies with the physician. However, there is often a discussion among the members of the health care team as to the benefits and limitations of particular modes. The nurse must be informed on the various modes of ventilation and the desired outcomes of each in order to perform astute assessments and continual surveillance of the adequacy of overall alveolar ventilation. The nurse must also be alert to the patient's tolerance of a particular mode and to the presence of any adverse effects related to mechanical ventilation.

The technology of mechanical ventilation is rapidly growing. Many new, nontraditional modes of ventilation are being investigated. Table 40–4 discusses common modes of ventilation and their clinical indications. (For more detailed information on traditional and nontraditional modes of ventilation, see Kersten 1989 and Weilitz 1989.)

Monitoring of Patient Response and Management of Complications

Nursing care for patients requiring ventilatory support is multifaceted. At the most basic level, the nurse cares for a patient and a ventilatory support device.

TABLE 40-4. MODES OF VENTILATION

MODE	FUNCTION	CLINICAL INDICATION	SURVEILLANCE CRITERIA
Control mode	Machine provides all inspiratory power by delivering set number of breaths per minute at specific volume	No spontaneous respiratory effect	Monitor for presence of any spontaneous respiratory effort
Assist control (A/C)	Machine initiates inspiration at set rate and volume; if senses patient effort, machine assists at set volume	Respiratory muscle fatigue Patient comfort	Monitor for tachypnea to prevent hyperventilation
Intermittent mandatory ventilation (IMV)	Patient breathes spontaneously, but machine breath is delivered at predetermined interval	Allows patient to adjust $PaCO_2$ Respiratory muscle fatigue (if machine rate is adequate) Weaning	Monitor for asynchrony between patient and ventilator Assess for tachypnea (increases work of breathing)
Synchronized intermittent mandatory ventilation (SIMV)	Patient breathes spontaneously, but machine provides a breath intermittently	When benefits of spontaneous ventilation are desired Allows patient to adjust $PaCO_2$ Weaning	Monitor for tachypnea (increases work of breathing)
Positive end-expiratory pressure (PEEP)	Positive pressure delivered and maintained in the airway; used with any inspiratory mode previously listed	Hypoxemia resistant to oxygen therapy and not responding to inspiratory mode above Avoidance of oxygen toxicity Atelectasis Decreased pulmonary shunting and improved matching of ventilation and perfusion	Monitor airway pressures Monitor for complications (barotrauma, decreased cardiac output)
Continuous positive airway pressure (CPAP)	Positive pressure delivered and maintained in the airway; used without an inspiratory mode	To achieve optimal airway inflation	Monitor for adequate spontaneous respiratory rate Monitor work of breathing
Pressure support ventilation (PSV)	Augmentation of spontaneous breathing by delivery of a predetermined constant positive pressure throughout most of inspiration; used with another mode of ventilation (usually IMV/SIMV)	To decrease the work of spontaneous breathing	Monitor airway pressures

Continuous monitoring of this patient-device system is vital to ensure proper functioning, achieve ventilatory goals, and promote early detection of complications. Monitoring of ventilatory support begins with the development of an individualized plan of care with input from the patient, family, and health care team. Systematic monitoring is key in the care of these patients. Nurses gather and interpret data from a variety of systems: thorax (lung sounds, respiratory rate, chest expansion, ventilator settings), hemodynamic (heart rate, blood pressure, temperature, hemodynamic monitoring indexes), nutritional status (type of feed-

TABLE 40–5.   VENTILATOR SETTINGS

FiO_2	Set at lowest setting to achieve a PaO_2 of >60 mm Hg (Shapiro 1984)
	Set at 1.0 in emergency situations until adequate oxygenation is achieved (Luce et al. 1984)
Tidal volume (V_T) (normal: 5–7 mL/kg)	Set at 10–15 mL/kg of ideal body weight to prevent atelectasis
Respiratory rate	Somewhat dependent on mode of ventilation; 10–14 breaths/minute

Sources: Luce et al. (1984); Kersten, (1989).
Note: These settings should achieve desired arterial blood gas values.

ings, intake, and output), and psychological (patient's level of anxiety and general overall mental status). Diagnostic testing, such as pulmonary function tests, ventilation and perfusion scans, and laboratory values, especially arterial blood gases, complete blood count, electrolytes, and sputum cultures, are essential components of nursing assessment for the patient receiving Ventilatory Support. The data gathered from this comprehensive assessment are used to determine further nursing action.

To assess ventilator function, the nurse verifies that the parameters or settings ordered by the physician are in use and achieving the goals established for the patient. These parameters include the fractionated inspired oxygen concentration (FiO_2; the tidal volume (V_T), which is the volume of gas inspired or expired in a respiratory cycle; respiratory rate delivered by the machine; and the mode of ventilation. Key factors related to FiO_2, V_T, and respiratory rate are supplied in Table 40–5. Ongoing monitoring of respiratory muscle function is important to determine if the mode of ventilation is increasing the work of breathing for the patient. Increased work of breathing is most often associated with the intermittent mandatory ventilation (IMV) and synchronized intermittent mandatory ventilation (SIMV) modes (Kanak, Fahey, and Vanderwarf 1985).

In addition to these four settings, the nurse must note the patient's peak inspiratory airway pressure, paying particular attention to trends showing increasing airway pressure, which may signal the need for tracheal suctioning, impending barotrauma, or decreasing lung elasticity (Kersten 1989).

Most ventilators currently in use have sophisticated alarm systems to alert the health care team to potential problems. The nurse and respiratory therapist should determine that all alarm parameters are individualized to each patient and ensure that alarms remain activated. The nurse must provide constant surveillance of the patient-ventilator system, troubleshooting alarms and assessing for signs and symptoms of complications that may occur as a result of mechanical ventilatory support. These complications are listed in Table 40–6.

The establishment of a regular schedule is of importance with the intervention of Ventilatory Support. Regular muscle reconditioning can be established through weaning activities and getting the patient out of bed, being cautious to ensure adequate periods of rest. Efforts to enhance the intensive care unit environment should also be undertaken. Assistance to families in relating to their loved one is often needed. Regular visiting by family members should be encouraged. They should be told the patient's schedule and the importance of keeping the patient's spirit up. They can keep the patient up to date on family happenings and world news through activities such as personalizing the bedside by placing pictures, cards, religious symbols, and other items of importance to the patient.

TABLE 40–6. COMPLICATIONS OF MECHANICAL VENTILATION

POTENTIAL COMPLICATION	RELATED TO
Decreased venous return to the heart	High intrathoracic pressures (especially prolonged PEEP)
Barotrauma	High intrapulmonary pressures
Oxygen toxicity	Prolonged periods of high oxygen administration
Positive fluid balance	Release of antidiuretic hormone and change in renal perfusion Overhydration by humidification
Gastric distention and ileus	Ischemia secondary to altered mesenteric blood flow from high intrathoracic pressures
Gastrointestinal bleeding	Increased gastric acid secretion secondary to hypoxia and/or hypercapnia
Jaundice	Concurrent disease or portal perfusion changes secondary to decreased cardiac output
Pulmonary infection	Presence of artificial airway and bypassing of normal filtering system Break in aseptic suctioning technique Possible aspiration of gastric contents Cross-contamination
Malnutrition	Absence of nutritional support or hypercatabolic state Decreased appetite
Respiratory muscle fatigue	Increased work of breathing
Acid-base disturbance	Inappropriate ventilatory settings, especially V_T and respiratory rate Malfunctioning ventilator
Airway obstruction	Thick secretions Bronchospasm Improper positioning of artificial airway
Arrhythmias	Hypoxemia and acid-base disturbance
Atelectasis	Obstruction from retained secretions

Sources: Kersten (1989); Montenegro (1984).

Weaning

Weaning is the transition from full or partial ventilatory support to spontaneous unassisted breathing. For some patients, this may mean immediate extubation following general anesthesia; in other individuals, it may entail months of respiratory muscle reconditioning with multiple weaning attempts and setbacks. Some patients and their families may need counseling to arrive at suitable alternatives if weaning cannot be achieved. In this situation, the various options may include a do-not-resuscitate (DNR) status, terminal wean, long-term acute-care hospitalization, and/or home-going ventilation (Lundberg and Noll 1990). One fact is certain: over the years weaning has been a source of frustration for the entire health care team, particularly when faced with the difficult-to-wean patient.

Criteria for Weaning

Weaning criteria have been well documented in the literature and are listed in Table 40–7. These objective measures provide guidelines when considering

TABLE 40-7. OBJECTIVE CRITERIA
FOR WEANING

Oxygenation
  $PaO_2 > 60$ mm Hg on $FiO_2 \leq .4-.5$
  PEEP < 5 cm H_2O

Ventilation
  Minute ventilation $v_E < 10$ L/min
  $v_T > 5$ mL/kg body weight
  $PaCO_2$ within usual range for patient

Respiratory mechanics
  Spontaneous respiratory rate $< 30-35$ breaths/minute

  Maximal inspiratory force ≤ -20 cm H_2O

Sources: Geisman (1989); Witta (1990).

which patients will tolerate weaning and who will not. Subjective questions that should also be considered are:

1. Is the patient getting better?
2. Is the reason for mechanical ventilation on its way to being resolved?
3. Is the patient clinically stable?
4. Can the patient cough, deep breathe, and swallow effectively?
5. What is the patient's work of breathing (WOB)?
6. What are the characteristics of the patient's secretions?
7. Is the patient awake, cooperative, and alert (King 1988; Norton and Neureuter 1989; Scoggin, 1980)?

Clinical problems identified by these objective and subjective criteria must be systematically addressed, and plans should be developed to resolve them before weaning attempts are initiated.

Differences exist between routine weaning and weaning from prolonged ventilation. The definition of routine weaning typically involves the patient who has been ventilated for fewer than 7 days and required mechanical ventilation for a reversible process, such as cardiac surgery or drug overdose (Morganroth and Grum 1988). Utilizing the basic criteria for weaning, the majority of mechanically ventilated patients will successfully wean. However, the 9% to 10% of patients considered difficult to wean may never meet these criteria and yet be successfully weaned (Nett, Morganroth, and Petty 1984).

Morganroth, Morganroth, Nett, and Petty (1984) conducted a restrospective evaluation of patients ($N = 11$) who required prolonged ventilation for over 30 days. None of these patients met conventional criteria on either successful or unsuccessful weaning episodes, yet 9 of the 11 were eventually weaned via the T-piece method. The authors developed a tool based on ventilatory and patient data, factoring in such variables as level of mobility, emotional status, level of consciousness, secretion quality and quantity, triggered respiratory rate, and infection. This study underscored the importance of considering subjective as well as objective patient data when determining a patient's ability to wean. This is particularly true in the case of patients with chronic obstructive pulmonary disease, congestive heart failure, and other debilitating diseases. Four etiologies must be considered when patients fail to wean from ventilatory support: respiratory muscle weakness, inadequate respiratory drive, inability of the lung to carry out gas exchange, and failure of the cardiovascular system (Morganroth and Grum 1988).

Weaning Modes

Traditional weaning modes include SIMV, CPAP, and T piece. (SIMV and CPAP are discussed in Table 40–4.) T-piece weaning involves removing the patient from the ventilator, connecting the endotracheal tube or tracheostomy tube to a blow-by tubing, and allowing the patient to breathe spontaneously. Usually after a predetermined period of time, the patient is placed back on the ventilator to rest. Ideally the T-piece trials will become progressively longer until the patient no longer needs the ventilator.

Several important aspects must be kept in mind when utilizing T-piece trials. The patient must be able to breathe spontaneously, maintain a PaO_2 of 60 mm Hg to 70 mm Hg and appropriate $Paco_2$ on the ventilator, and require 5 cm H_2O positive end-expiratory pressure or less to be considered a candidate for this technique. Prior to the trial, position the patient, schedule all procedures and activities at a different time, and ensure a clear airway by suctioning the patient if indicated. Once the trial begins, the nurse must monitor the patient continuously, noting any signs of respiratory muscle fatigue, and observing the end of the T-piece tubing for a continuous flow of humidified oxygen. If continuous flow is not present or if the stream starts and stops with the patient's respiratory cycle, the flow of oxygen must be increased. This adjustment will ensure that the patient is receiving the optimum percentage of oxygen and not the percentage mixed with room air. A patient who develops respiratory fatigue should be placed back on an A/C or IMV mode to ensure little or no spontaneous effort is required. A high mandatory rate should be set on the ventilator to accomplish this goal. Shapiro (1984) suggested it may take 48 hours for a patient to regain strength following severe respiratory muscle fatigue.

Debate over the best weaning modes has existed for many years. Techniques fade in and out of popularity, but to date no experimental research shows any method to be superior to another (Hess 1988). New techniques introduced include pressure support ventilation and mandatory minute ventilation. As these new modes make their way into clinical practice, nurses must keep in mind the basic principles of the ventilatory modes in order to coach the patient to successful weaning. Johanson, Wells, Hoffmeister, and Dungca (1988) and Kersten (1989) provide additional discussion of weaning protocols.

RELATED RESEARCH

Research related to mechanical ventilation is lacking in the nursing literature. Investigations cited previously in this chapter have primarily been gleaned from the medical literature. Medical research has examined the usefulness of various types of ventilators, clinical indications of specific modes of ventilation, and the clinical response to those modes. There have been numerous studies evaluating the newer modes of ventilation, some of which remain experimental. Weaning has been the focus of many studies as well, focused on the usefulness of various modes in achieving successful discontinuation of ventilatory support.

The American Association of Critical-Care Nurses utilized the Delphi technique to survey nurse experts on the research priorities for critical care nursing. The results, published by Lewandowski and Kositsky in 1983, ranked problems associated with mechanical ventilation among the top 10 research priorities. The majority of nursing research to date has investigated activities focused at airway management of the patient receiving mechanical ventilatory support. (These findings are discussed in Chapter 39.) Use of relaxation therapy and examination of the psychological issues surrounding the patient on ventilatory support have appeared in the nursing literature.

In 1988, Acosta published a case study describing the successful use of biofeedback and progressive relaxation during T-piece weaning of an anxious patient. Heart rate, respiratory rate, and oxygen saturations were measured before, during, and after each session. Use of these techniques resulted in a lowering of heart and respiratory rates and an increase in oxygen saturations following each session. The patient was progressively able to tolerate longer T-piece trials and eventually went on to be successfully weaned. Although use of relaxation techniques require specialized training, nurses could implement these in their daily practice. Research evaluating the response to these techniques in larger patient populations could then follow.

Two studies examined psychological issues surrounding the patient on ventilatory support (Gries and Fernsler, 1988; Riggion, Singer, Hartman, and Sneider 1982). Both studies identified communication as a primary problem. Gries and Fernsler (1988) suggested that nurses deal with the communication difficulty by providing repeated explanations until patients demonstrate understanding. The majority of subjects in this study indicated that the overall experience of mechanical ventilatory support was a negative one, a finding with important implications for nursing that suggests that research is needed to examine how the negative aspects can be minimized. The most frequently cited stressors were related to the discomfort associated with the endotracheal tube and suctioning. Patient responses such as "the most inhumane treatment I ever had" indicate the need for further research to investigate means of decreasing the stress related to mechanical ventilatory support.

NURSING DIAGNOSES

The decision to begin Ventilatory Support entails one or all three of the primary respiratory diagnoses: Impaired Gas Exchange, Ineffective Airway Clearance, and Ineffective Breathing Pattern. Because of the restrictions and demands placed by a life support system such as a ventilator, these patients are at risk for numerous other nursing diagnoses. Table 40 – 8 identifies nursing diagnoses commonly seen in patients requiring ventilatory support.

Several diagnoses encompass the psychosocial or behavioral realm of nursing and can be a major determinant in the success or failure of ventilatory support.

TABLE 40 – 8. NURSING DIAGNOSES APPLICABLE TO PATIENTS REQUIRING MECHANICAL VENTILATION

PHYSIOLOGICAL	PSYCHOSOCIAL
Impaired Gas Exchange	Anxiety
Ineffective Airway Clearance	Impaired Verbal Communication
Ineffective Breathing Pattern	Knowledge Deficit
Altered Nutrition: Less Than Body Requirements	Hopelessness
Potential for Infection	Powerlessness
Altered Comfort	
Decreased Tissue Perfusion	
Altered Level of Consciousness	

Most of these diagnoses can be managed independently by the nurse, yet by enlisting the expertise of mental health colleagues, patient outcomes will be maximized (Roberts 1988). The remaining physiological diagnoses fall into a domain where collaboration between nursing and medicine is necessary. Consultaion with other health team members, such as respiratory therapists and dietitians may also be required.

CASE STUDIES

Case Study 1

Mrs. P is a 70-year-old married white female who has been experiencing atypical chest pain over the past 6 years. She denies any alcohol or tobacco use and engages in water exercises two times per week. After a positive exercise treadmill on February 20, she underwent a cardiac catheterization. The results showed her left ventricular ejection fraction to be 60% and the presence of three-vessel coronary artery disease. The lesions ranged from 75% to 90% stenosis. Bypass surgery was thought to be the best option, so on March 22 she underwent coronary artery bypass surgery. When Mrs. P returned to the surgical intensive care unit at 1300, she had in place a 7.5 French oral endotracheal tube and was connected to a Bourns Bear V ventilator. Initial cardiac indexes and arterial blood gases were obtained (Table 40–9). Mrs. P was awake and following commands within 3 hours postoperatively, mediastinal tube drainage was within parameters, and epinephrine and nipride infusions quickly weaned off. By 2300 after a trial of CPAP, Mrs. P was extubated. The next morning at 0500 she was placed on 4 L oxygen per nasal cannula with oxygen saturations of 97% and by late morning was transferred to the monitored step-down unit.

Case Study 2

Mrs. A is an 81-year-old female admitted to the medical intensive care unit with a medical diagnosis of Guillain-Barré syndrome. For the past 8 days, she has been experiencing diffuse myalgias that have progressed to an inability to ambulate, increased dysphagia, and now respiratory fatigue. On the morning of admission, Mrs. A was on a 3 L oxygen per nasal cannula with arterial blood gases (ABGs) as follows: pH, 7.31; pCO_2, 40; pCO_2, 94. By 1600 that afternoon, it was necessary to provide Mrs. A with ventilatory support. This was

TABLE 40–9. MRS. P: THE DAY OF CARDIAC SURGERY

PARAMETER	TIME SEQUENCE							
	1300	1332	1355	1431	2130	2210	2300	2350
pH	7.47			7.42	7.38	7.34		7.40
pCO_2	33			32	38	37		39
pO_2	284			99	89	82		112
HCO_3	24			20	21	19		24
Base excess	1			−3	−4	−5		0
Mode	SIMV	SIMV	SIMV	SIMV	SIMV	CPAP	Face mask	Face mask
Rate	10/min	10	10	10	4			
Tidal volume	700cc	700	700	700	700			
FiO_2	1.0	.8	.6	.4	.4	.4	.4	.4
PEEP	0	0	0	0	0	0	0	0
O_2 Sat.	100%	100%	100%	99%	97%	98%	97%	100%
Cardiac output	4.70				5.97	4.7		
Cardiac index	2.47				3.16	2.49		
Systemic vascular resistance	1412				1005	1429		

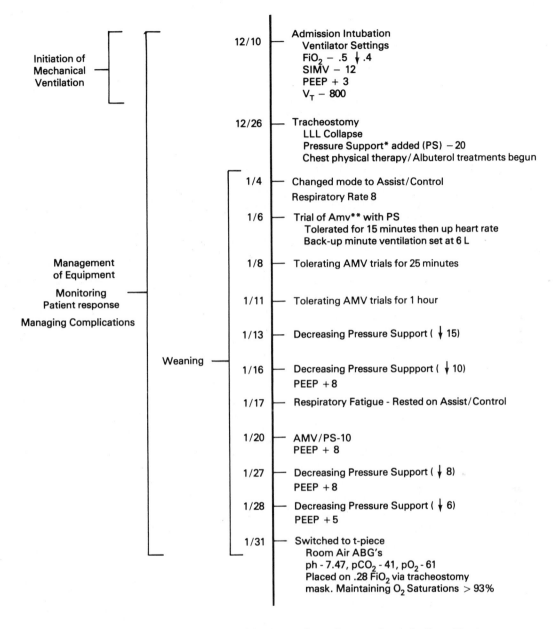

Initiation of Mechanical Ventilation	12/10	Admission Intubation
		   Ventilator Settings
		   FiO_2 − .5 ↓ .4
		   SIMV − 12
		   PEEP + 3
		   V_T − 800

	12/26	Tracheostomy
		   LLL Collapse
		   Pressure Support* added (PS) − 20
		   Chest physical therapy / Albuterol treatments begun

Management of Equipment	1/4	Changed mode to Assist/Control Respiratory Rate 8

Monitoring Patient response	1/6	Trial of Amv** with PS
		   Tolerated for 15 minutes then up heart rate
		   Back-up minute ventilation set at 6 L

Managing Complications	1/8	Tolerating AMV trials for 25 minutes
	1/11	Tolerating AMV trials for 1 hour
	1/13	Decreasing Pressure Support (↓ 15)
Weaning	1/16	Decreasing Pressure Suppport (↓ 10) PEEP + 8
	1/17	Respiratory Fatigue - Rested on Assist/Control
	1/20	AMV/PS-10 PEEP + 8
	1/27	Decreasing Pressure Support (↓ 8) PEEP + 8
	1/28	Decreasing Pressure Support (↓ 6) PEEP + 5

	1/31	Switched to t-piece
		   Room Air ABG's
		   ph - 7.47, pCO_2 - 41, pO_2 - 61
		   Placed on .28 FiO_2 via tracheostomy
		   mask. Maintaining O_2 Saturations > 93%

*Pressure support mode: Used in conjunction with other modes to decrease the work of breathing by maintaining a predetermined positive pressure throughout the majority of inspiration.
**Augmented minute ventilation: Ensures that the patient receives a preset constant minute ventilation (V_E) regardless of the patient's spontaneous V_T or RR.

FIGURE 40 – 1. Weaning Progression of Mrs. A.

accomplished by endotracheal intubation and placement on a Bourns Bear V. The next day, Mrs. A underwent plasmaphoresis and during the exchange developed hypotension and hemodynamic instability, requiring a dopamine infusion. She subsequently suffered a non–Q wave myocardial infarction. Mrs. A continued to decline neurologically to eventual quadriparesis and the inability to blink her eyes. A 5-day course of immunoglobulins did result in some improvement but only in eye movement. Two and a half weeks following admission, Mrs. A received a tracheostomy, at which time chest films also revealed a left-lower-lobe collapse and the need for aggressive pulmonary care and mucolytic aerosol treatments.

Approximately a month had passed before Mrs. A began experiencing full range of motion of her eyes and some extremity movement. She relied completely on the intensive care unit (ICU) nurses for ventilatory support, nutritional maintenance, skin care, pain control, passive range of motion, and emotional support. Once she was able to blink her eyes, a yes-no communication signal was established. When she was able to move her head, a soft-push call light was placed by the side of her face at all times.

Weaning from ventilatory support began with the return of motor movement. The primary nurse, physician, and daughter met with Mrs. A to discuss the goals and plans for weaning and identified the possible difficulties. A psychiatric nurse specialist was consulted to help Mrs. A with relaxation therapy and her feelings of depression and hopelessness.

Within three and a half weeks, Mrs. A was off the ventilator and transferred to a pulmonary step-down unit. Figure 40–1 highlights the major stages of Mrs. A's ICU stay and her progression through the components of Ventilatory Support. Monitoring of Mrs. A's oxygenation was accomplished primarily by close surveillance and trending of oxygen saturations using a pulse oximeter attached to her ear. Occasional arterial blood gases were drawn when major ventilator changes occurred or when she was experiencing respiratory distress. Mrs. A spent several more weeks in the hospital receiving aggressive pulmonary care and physical therapy. She currently is in a rehabilitation center closer to home and her daughter.

SUMMARY

Ventilatory Support is a complex intervention requiring the coordination of a multidisciplinary health care team. The team functions collaboratively in initiating ventilatory support, managing the equipment, monitoring patient response and managing complications, and finally weaning from the mechanical ventilator. The greatest implications for nursing center around monitoring the patient's response to the ventilator. Through careful monitoring of patients requiring Ventilatory Support, we will ensure progression toward goal achievement, minimize the number of complications, and maintain the patient's psychological well-being.

REFERENCES

Acosta, F. 1988. Biofeedback and progressive relaxation in weaning the anxious patient from the ventilator: A brief report. *Heart and Lung* 17(3):299–301.

Geisman, L.K. 1989. Advances in weaning from mechanical ventilation. *Critical Care Nursing Clinics of North America* 1(4):697–705.

Gries, M.L., and Fernsler, J. 1988. Patient perceptions of the mechanical ventilation experience. *Focus on Critical Care* 15(2):52–59.

Hess, D. 1988. Controversies in respiratory critical care. *Critical Care Nursing Quarterly* 11(3):62–78.

Hubmayr, R., Abel, M., and Rehder, K. 1990. Physiologic approach to mechanical ventilation. *Critical Care Medicine* 18(1):103–113.

Johanson, B.C., Wells, S.J., Hoffmeister, D., and Dungca, C.U. 1988. *Standards for critical care* (3d ed.) (pp. 41–49). St. Louis: C.V. Mosby Co.

Kanak, R., Fahey, P.J., and Vanderwarf, C. 1985. Oxygen cost of breathing: Changes dependent on mode of ventilation. *Chest* 87(1):126–127.

Kersten, L. 1989. *Comprehensive respiratory nursing.* Philadelphia: W.B. Saunders Company.

King, E.G. 1988. Respiratory failure in the critically ill. In W. Sibbald (ed.), *Synopsis of critical care* (3d ed.) (pp. 53–65). Baltimore: Williams & Wilkins.

Lewandowski, L.A., and Kositsky, A.M. 1983. Research priorities for critical care nursing: A study by the American Association of Critical-Care Nurses. *Heart and Lung* 12(1):35–44.

Loughran, S. 1987. High frequency ventilation: Application of nursing diagnosis. *Dimensions of Critical Care Nursing* 6(6):328–334.

Luce, J., Pierson, D., and Hudson, L. 1981. Intermittent mandatory ventilation. *Chest* 79(6):678–685.

Luce, J., Tyler, M., and Pierson, D. 1984. *Intensive respiratory care.* Philadelphia: W.B. Saunders Company.

Lundberg, J.A., and Noll, M.L. 1990. The long-term acute care hospital: A new option for ventilator-dependent individuals. *AACN Clinical Issues in Critical Care Nursing* 1(2):280–288.

MacIntyre, N. 1986. Respiratory function during pressure support ventilation. *Chest* 89(5):677–683.

Montenegro, H.D. 1984. Complications of mechanical ventilation. *Respiratory Therapy* 14(5):20–27.

Morganroth, M.L., and Grum, C.M. 1988. Weaning from mechanical ventilation. *Journal of Intensive Care Medicine* 3(2):109–120.

Morganroth, M.L., Morganroth, J.L., Nett, L.M., and Petty, T.L. 1984. Criteria for weaning from prolonged mechanical ventilation. *Archives of Internal Medicine* 144(5):1012–1016.

Nett, L.M., Morganroth, M., and Petty, T.L. 1984. Weaning from mechanical ventilation: A perspective and review of techniques. In R.C. Bone (ed.), *Critical care: A comprehensive approach* (pp. 171–188). Parkridge, Ill.: American College of Chest Physicians.

Norton, L.C., and Neureuter, A. 1989. Weaning the long-term ventilator-dependent patient: Common problems and management. *Critical Care Nurse* 9(1):42–44, 46, 48–52.

Riggion, R.E., Singer, R.D., Hartman, K., and Sneider, R. 1982. Psychological issues in the care of the critically ill respirator patient: Differential perceptions of patients, relatives, and staff. *Psychological Reports* 51:363–369.

Roberts, S.L. 1988. Physiologic nursing diagnoses are necessary and appropriate for critical care. *Focus on Critical Care* 15(5):42–49.

Scoggin, C.H. 1980. Weaning respiratory patients from mechanical support. *Journal of Respiratory Diseases* 1:13–23.

Shapiro, B. 1984. *Respiratory critical care: State of the art Volume 6* (February). Respiratory Care Seminar. Chicago, Ill.

Thelan, L.A., Davie, J.K., and Urden, L.D. 1990. *Textbook of critical care nursing: Diagnosis and management* (pp. 444–471). St. Louis: C.V. Mosby Co.

Weilitz, P. 1989. New modes of mechanical ventilation. *Critical Care Nursing Clinics of North America* 1(4):689–695.

Weisman, I., Rinaldo, J., Rogers, R., and Sanders, M. 1983. State of the art—intermittent mandatory ventilation. *American Review of Respiratory Disease* 127(5):641–647.

Willatts, S. 1985. Alternative modes of ventilation. Part I. Disadvantages of controlled mechanical ventilation: Intermittent mandatory ventilation. *Intensive Care Medicine* 11(2):51–55.

Witta, K. 1990. New techniques for weaning difficult patients from mechanical ventilation. *AACN Clinical Issues in Critical Care Nursing* 1(2):260–266.

41

HEMODYNAMIC REGULATION

MARLA PRIZANT-WESTON
KATHLEEN CASTIGLIA

The human body supplies nutrients and removes wastes from the cells through a complicated network called the circulatory system. This system consists of three components: the heart, the intravascular volume, and the vascular structures. Hemodynamics is the interrelationship of these components in maintaining the delivery and elimination of physiologic substances to and from the tissues. Hemodynamic stability is dependent on a proportionate equilibrium of the pumping action of the heart, the quantity of intravascular volume, and resistance to flow offered by the vascular structures.

Hemodynamic Regulation, the adjustment of the components of the circulatory system to enhance the delivery of physiologic substances to and from the tissues, is indicated when a disequilibrium exists in the pumping action of the heart, the quantity of intravascular volume, and the peripheral resistance to blood flow. Hemodynamic Regulation restores the equilibrium by enhancing the pumping action of the heart, altering the quantity, quality, or distribution of intravascular volume, and altering peripheral resistance to blood flow.

To maximize patient outcome, Hemodynamic Regulation must be directed toward the component in the circulatory system in which disequilibrium has occurred. Selection of the appropriate nursing activities can be done only if the nurse has a comprehensive understanding of hemodynamics, as well as the impact of altering any of the components of the circulatory system.

INTERRELATIONSHIP OF THE HEART, VASCULAR STRUCTURES, AND INTRAVASCULAR VOLUME

The Pumping Action of the Heart

The ventricles of the heart provide the main force for propelling intravascular volume through the circulatory system (Guyton 1986). The pumping action of the heart is dependent on the rhythmic electrical stimulation of the heart coupled with an organized contraction. As blood enters the ventricles of the heart, the myocardial fibers stretch. With stimulation to contract, the muscle fibers shorten, generating a pressure that causes a displacement of volume from within the chamber (Weber and Janicki 1979). The volume of blood expelled during one contraction is referred to as stroke volume. Stroke volume is determined by myocardial contractility, preload, and afterload. Cardiac output (CO), the volume of blood ejected from the heart in 1 minute, reflects the transport of substances to and from the

544

tissues (Guyton 1986). CO is determined by multiplying stroke volume by heart rate.

Contractility, an inherent mechanism of the myocardium, enables the heart to increase the extent and force of shortening of the actin-myosin fibers. An increase in contractility produces an increase in the velocity and degree of contraction, resulting in increased stroke volume and CO. Contractility is influenced by the ionic environment, oxygen availability, beta-receptor stimulation, and amount of functioning myocardium.

The myocardium does not contract without the presence of oxygen. Because myocardial extraction of oxygen is near maximum even at rest, myocardial oxygenation can be improved only by reducing demand or increasing supply (Riegel 1985). Myocardial oxygen consumption can be estimated by calculating pressure-rate product (PRP). PRP equals heart rate multiplied by systolic blood pressure. Although PRP does not reflect myocardial contractility or tension states, it has been shown to correlate well with myocardial oxygen consumption during rest and exercise (Alteri 1984; Quaglietti, Stotts, and Lovejoy 1988).

Preload is the volume of blood in the ventricles before contraction (ventricular end-diastolic volume), which establishes the stretch and resting muscle length of the myocardial fiber. Within physiologic limits, increasing preload increases ventricular fiber stretch, resulting in a more forceful contraction (Frank-Starling law). Over- or understretching fibers results in a weakened contraction.

Preload can be increased with volume, which causes stretching of myocardial fibers; a weakened or noncompliant myocardium that fails to eject sufficient volume; or peripheral vasoconstriction, which increases venous return and resistance to ventricular ejection. Preload is primarily a function of venous return; however, other determinants of preload are ventricular compliance and ventricular filling time. Systemic venous return influences right ventricular preload, whereas left ventricular preload is determined by return from the pulmonary venous circulation. Left ventricular preload can be reduced with decreased right ventricular preload, when right ventricular contractility is impaired, or when pulmonary blood flow is obstructed.

Afterload is defined as the resistance that the heart must pump against. Afterload is determined primarily by the diameter of the blood vessels and, to a lesser extent, blood viscosity and the length of the vessels. As afterload increases, the ventricle must generate increased ventricular wall tension to overcome arterial resistance. Thus, increases in afterload result in an increase in the work of the heart and a marked increase in myocardial requirements. In hypovolemia and cardiogenic shock, afterload increases as a compensatory attempt to increase venous return and salvage cardiac output.

Afterload for the left ventricle is determined by the diameter of arterioles in the systemic circulation. Right ventricular afterload is determined by pulmonary circuit resistance and is increased with pulmonary vascular constriction from hypoxia. Afterload of either side of the heart can be increased by an occlusion of a vessel in the corresponding circuit.

Heart rate and rhythm also influence cardiac output. Heart rate is controlled by metabolic demands and autonomic nervous system stimulation. With a rise in metabolic demand, heart rate increases, thereby increasing cardiac output. Parasympathetic stimulation slows heart rate, which may reduce cardiac output and tissue perfusion. Normally the heart rate can increase to approximately 180 beats per minute through sympathetic stimulation. As stroke volume decreases, for whatever reason, sympathetic stimulation increases heart rate as a compensatory mechanism to maintain cardiac output. However tachycardias of rates greater than

120 beats per minute and premature beats can adversely affect cardiac output by reducing diastolic filling time and preventing effective preload. Diastolic filling can also be adversely affected by atrial arrhythmias. Normally atrial contraction contributes up to 30% of ventricular filling volume. When atrial contraction is absent, ventricular preload is reduced and cardiac output may fall. Because coronary arteries fill during diastole, reducing diastolic time also decreases coronary artery perfusion, potentially decreasing oxygen delivery to the myocardium.

Quantity, Quality, and Distribution of Intravascular Volume

More than half of intravascular volume is composed of plasma. Plasma is 93% water with a small amount of colloids. The remainder of intravascular volume is formed elements such as red blood cells, white blood cells, and platelets. The hemodynamically significant components of intravascular volume are water, colloids, and red blood cells. While all components of intravascular fluid contribute to volume, water contributes to the hydrostatic pressure gradient, colloids create the osmotic pressure gradient, and red blood cells provide for oxygen-carrying capacity. Interstitial-intracellular fluid stability is maintained by a stable capillary membrane and the gradient between hydrostatic and colloid pressures.

Decreased intravascular volume can occur when fluid leaks through the capillary wall and enters the interstitial space. Edema, defined as excess interstitial fluid in the tissues, can occur with increased hydrostatic pressure, increased capillary permeability, decreased colloidal osmotic pressure (from decreased plasma protein concentration), and lymphatic obstruction (Guyton 1986). The imbalance of the pressure gradients, present in edema, inhibits the transport of substances to and from the tissues.

The storage and redistribution of intravascular volume is primarily controlled by the venous system. Sixty percent to 80% of intravascular volume is held in the venous system, providing a ready volume for use during physiological times of demand. The venous system volume functions as a hemodynamic reserve, meaning that venous intravascular volume does not directly contribute to blood pressure or other hemodynamic parameters.

The redistribution of intravascular volume is influenced by venous tone, skeletal muscle compression, intrathoracic pressures, and intra-abdominal pressures. Venoconstriction and venodilation redistribute the volume between the heart and the periphery. For example, in the initial stages of volume depletion, vasoconstriction occurs, thereby redistributing intravascular volume to the central organs to maintain hemodynamic stability.

In the upright position, the return of intravascular volume to the heart (venous return) must overcome the resistance posed by the force of gravity. Many veins, most commonly found in the legs, are equipped with valves to overcome the effects of gravity and to ensure blood flow only in the direction of the heart. In the upright position, venous return from the legs depends almost entirely on the pumping action of skeletal leg muscles compressing venous walls.

Venous return to the heart is increased during the slightly negative intrathoracic pressure at the beginning of normal inspiration. When this negative pressure is lost or when intrathoracic pressure is positive, venous return decreases. Prolonged inspiration during a Valsalva maneuver elevates intrathoracic pressures, which impedes venous return. With exhalation at the end of a Valsalva, intrathoracic pressure dramatically decreases, resulting in a significant surge of volume into the heart and, potentially, reflex bradycardia (Hickey 1986). Venous return can also be decreased when intra-abdominal pressures increase. A venous obstruction impedes blood flow, resulting in an engorgement of vessels with blood, raising venous pressure and causing edema.

Peripheral Resistance to Flow

Peripheral resistance to flow refers to the impediment to the flow of intravascular volume through the arterial and venous vessels. Resistance to flow is chiefly affected by the diameter of blood vessels and, to a lesser extent, blood vessel length and blood viscosity. The arterioles and venules are innervated by sympathetic system fibers, which allow for changes in vessel diameter. Because of their predominantly muscular construction, the arterioles constrict more dramatically and to a smaller diameter than venules, thereby constituting the majority of peripheral resistance to flow. Additionally, the terminal portions of the arterioles regulate blood flow by changing diameter with local changes in temperature, pH, oxygen, or metabolite levels. Normally local tissue perfusion is enhanced by vasodilation and reduced with vasoconstriction. Systemic vasodilation decreases preload and afterload, affecting cardiac output. Vasoconstriction increases afterload by narrowing vessel diameter and increases preload by displacing peripheral intravascular volume into the heart.

Arterial or venous interruption of flow increases peripheral resistance by narrowing or occluding the diameter of the vessel. Four pathological states cause interruption to flow in arterial and venous vessels: edema, inflammation, acute occlusion by a clot, and structural changes within the vessel. Structural changes include plaque buildup, which reduces arterial flow (chronic arterial insufficiency), and incompetent valves, resulting in venous stasis (chronic venous insufficiency).

Blood vessel length is not clinically significant to hemodynamic regulation since it does not normally change. However, blood viscosity, determined almost entirely by the concentration of red blood cells, can be altered clinically. Reducing an elevated blood viscosity decreases peripheral resistance to flow.

NURSING DIAGNOSES

Hemodynamic regulation is indicated for patients with nursing diagnoses having defining characteristics related to disruption of the interrelationship of the components of the circulatory system. Table 41–1 indicates variables to assess. Nursing diagnoses involving alterations in the pumping action of the heart; the quantity, quality, or distribution of intravascular volume; or peripheral resistance to flow include:

Decreased Cardiac Output
Fluid Volume Excess
Fluid Volume Deficit
Altered Tissue Perfusion (Peripheral)

Decreased Cardiac Output results from one or a combination of the following: decreased contractility, increased preload, decreased preload, increased afterload, decreased afterload, increased heart rate or arrhythmias, and/or decreased heart rate. Fluid volume alterations occur with an excessive increase or decrease in fluid volume intake, retention, or excretion or with a shift in distribution between interstitial and intracellular spaces. Altered Tissue Perfusion (Peripheral) results from an interruption in flow through the vascular circuit. If, through the assessment, the nurse can define the etiology or contributing factor(s) for the nursing

TABLE 41-1. PHYSICAL EXAMINATION OF THE CIRCULATORY SYSTEM

CIRCULATORY SYSTEM COMPONENT	ASSESSMENT VARIABLES
Heart action	Blood pressure, heart rate, respiratory rate, breath sounds, heart sounds, peripheral pulses, capillary filling, skin turgor and temperature, peripheral edema, urine output, level of consciousness, cardiac output, cardiac index, mixed venous oxygen saturation (SvO_2)
Contractility	Left ventricular stroke work index, right ventricular stroke work index
Preload	Jugular venous distention, hepatojugular reflex, peripheral edema, breath sounds, heart sounds, CVP, PAWP, PAD, LAP
Afterload	Peripheral pulses, capillary filling, skin temperature and color, SVR, PVR
Heart rate/rhythm	Apical/radial pulse, heart rate, electrocardiogram
Intravascular volume	Weight, intake and output, heart rate, blood pressure, postural vital signs, respiratory rate, breath sounds, heart sounds, peripheral pulses, capillary filling, skin turgor, peripheral edema, urine output, urine specific gravity, CVP, PAWP, PAD, LAP
Peripheral perfusion	Peripheral pulses, capillary filling, skin temperature and color, skin condition and integrity, hair distribution, peripheral edema, presence/absence of pain

Note: CVP = central venous pressure; PAWP = pulmonary capillary wedge pressure; PAD = pulmonary artery diastolic pressure; LAP = left atrial pressure; SVR = systemic vascular resistance; PVR = peripheral vascular resistance.

diagnosis, Hemodynamic Regulation can be aimed directly at the source of the problem.

ADMINISTERING THE INTERVENTION

When administering Hemodynamic Regulation, it is imperative that the nurse accurately determines the primary cause of the hemodynamic instability. Otherwise an inappropriate set of nursing actions may be selected, which may result in a detrimental patient outcome. Therefore, the intervention has been structured into three components: the nurse needs to select the appropriate component based on the nursing diagnosis, etiology or contributing factor, and the goals for treatment.

Cardiac Output

Nursing activities to enhance the pumping action of the heart are classified as optimizing the ionic environment, administering and titrating medications, optimizing preload and afterload, managing mechanical devices, and altering heart rate and rhythm. Optimizing the ionic environment includes reducing oxygen demand, increasing oxygen supply, and correcting acid-base and electrolyte abnormalities.

Nursing care is planned to minimize myocardial oxygen demand. Promoting rest by decreasing environmental stimuli, assisting or performing self-care activities, and pacing patient activities reduces myocardial oxygen demand. For example, bed baths and tub baths may be preferable to a shower for patients with recent acute hemodynamic system events. In subjects 3-days to 5-days postinfarction, showering increased oxygen consumption as demonstrated by a higher pressure-rate product (PRP) and greater number of ST segment changes than bed baths or tub baths (Johnston, Watt, and Fletcher 1981). No significant physiological differences were found for the three types of bathing in subjects 5-days to 17-days postinfarction (Winslow, Lane, and Gaffney 1985).

Patients recovering from an acute myocardial infarction consumed significantly less oxygen during bathing than control subjects (Winslow, Lane, and Gaffney 1985). This was attributed to acutely ill patients' naturally pacing their activities by moving slowly and deliberately to conserve energy. Nevertheless, rest periods should be provided after activities of daily living whether or not the patient reports a need for rest. Although subjects in one study reported a readiness to continue with additional activity immediately, their PRP did not return to baseline levels for some time after activities of daily living. Ninety percent of the subjects took up to 30.5 minutes to return to baseline after showering, 10 minutes after walking, and 7 minutes after climbing stairs (Alteri 1984).

For most patients, activity does not need to be limited following meals. Although PRP rises above fasting level approximately 30 minutes to 60 minutes after beginning a meal, the response is considerably lower than those seen with other daily activities, such as bathing. The duration and magnitude of this response is greater after a large meal than for small meals (Bagatell and Heymsfield 1984), so patients with postprandial angina may benefit from both smaller meal sizes and limiting activities after meals.

No significant difference was found in PRP for uncomplicated postinfarction patients when placed in supine, semi-Fowler's, dangling, and chair positions (Quaglietti, Stotts, and Lovejoy 1988). Prakash, Parmley, Dikshit, Forrester, and Swan (1973) found insignificant hemodynamic alterations associated with moving from a supine to a semierect position, concluding, "The patient's preference for comfort [in positioning] is a reasonable guide to nursing" (p. 7).

Although complete bed rest may be indicated at times to reduce oxygen demand, the nurse should use caution when prescribing this action. Prolonged bed rest has been associated with losses of blood and plasma volume, increases in heart rate of up to 15 beats per minute, and reduced stroke volume and cardiac output during exercise. Also, orthostatic intolerance begins after as little as 6 hours of bed rest (Winslow, Lane, and Gaffney 1985). Therefore, the nurse should gradually progress a patient's activity after periods of bed rest.

The nurse must evaluate the patient's tolerance to any activity. Activity that is poorly tolerated by individuals results in increased heart rate, blood pressure, and myocardial oxygen demand (Riegel 1988). Any activity that results in the patient's experiencing angina, fatigue, shortness of breath, dizziness, unsteady gait, tachycardia greater than 120 beats per minute, ST segment depression of greater than 1.5 mm, drop in systolic blood pressure, and/or significant arrhythmias must be terminated (Alteri 1984).

Oxygen administration is often initiated by nurse's request or with standing protocols (Riegel 1988). Supplemental oxygen increases oxygen availability to the myocardium, particularly in hypoxic patients. Myocardial oxygen supply is also increased by restoring coronary artery perfusion. For example, the coronary vasodilating effects of nitroglycerin make it a common therapy for a patient with chest pain due to myocardial ischemia. In patients with myocardial ischemia of less than 4-hours to 6-hours duration, thrombolytic therapy offers the possibility of reperfusing the myocardium and thereby restoring myocardial oxygen delivery. The nurse is "important in both identifying appropriate candidates for thrombolytic therapy and facilitating early administration" (Kline 1987, p. 784). In addition, the nurse prevents or minimizes bleeding by obtaining intravenous access prior to thrombolytic administration, maintaining patency of access sites, applying pressure to puncture sites, and instructing and assisting the patient to avoid activities that may cause bleeding (such as shaving or vigorous toothbrushing).

Another area where a nurse can optimize the ionic environment is in identifying

TABLE 41-2. ACTIONS OF COMMONLY USED INOTROPIC AND VASOACTIVE MEDICATIONS

MEDICATION	INOTROPIC	CHRONOTROPIC	VASOCONSTRICTION	ARTERIAL DILATION	VENOUS DILATION
Epinephrine	++	++	++	+	+
Norepinephrine	++	++	++	0	0
Isoproterenol	++	++	0	++	++
Dopamine 2.0–5.0[a]	++	0	0	++[b]	0
Dopamine > 10.0[a]	++	+	++	0	0
Dobutamine	++	0/+	0	+	+
Amrinone	++	0	0	+	+
Digoxin	+	−	0	0	0
Inderal	−	−	0	0	0
Nitroprusside	0	0	0	++	++
Nitroglycerin < 2.0[a]	0	0	0	+	++
Nitroglycerin > 2.0[a]	0	0	0	++	++
Hydralazine	0	0	0	++	0
Nifedipine	0/−	0/−	0	++	++
Captopril	0	0	0	+	+
Prostaglandin E1	0	0	0	++	++

Note: +positive effect, ++greatly positive effect, 0 no effect, −negative effect
[a] Dosages are in mcg/kg/min.
[b] Vasodilation of renal and mesenteric arteries.

and correcting electrolyte and acid-base abnormalities. Correcting acidosis improves contractility, as does normalizing potassium, calcium, magnesium, and sodium levels.

Within defined parameters, the nurse independently titrates inotropic and vasoactive agents, alone and in combination, to improve the pumping action of the heart. Thus, the nurse must be familiar with the purpose, actions, and limitations of pharmacologic agents utilized to improve hemodynamics. Table 41–2 summarizes the primary actions of commonly used medications.

Inotropic medications increase the strength of myocardial contraction; however, positive inotropes also increase the work of the heart, particularly if they increase heart rate. Vasodilators reduce afterload, decreasing the work of the left ventricle. Also, vasodilators decrease preload, allowing for a stronger contraction when the ventricle is overstretched by volume. Thus, combining inotropes with vasodilators enhances the pumping action of the heart by increasing the force of contraction while decreasing peripheral resistance to flow. Vasoconstrictors increase contractility by increasing preload when a patient has adequate intravascular volume but is pathologically vasodilated.

Because preload and afterload influence the strength and work of contraction, optimizing preload and afterload improves the pumping action of the heart.

If conventional pharmacology fails to restore adequate heart pumping, mechanical devices may be utilized. Mechanical devices to assist or replace the failing myocardium include the intra-aortic balloon pump, the ventricular assist device, and the total artificial heart. Intra-aortic balloon pumping enhances the pumping action of the heart by mechanically reducing left ventricular afterload. The nurse is responsible for timing balloon deflation and inflation to maximize afterload reduction and coronary artery perfusion, respectively. When the intra-aortic balloon is timed to deflate just prior to systole, aortic pressure is greatly reduced. In this manner, left ventricular afterload is dropped, allowing for reduced ventricular workload and oxygen demand. Intra-aortic balloon inflation during diastole provides for increased coronary artery perfusion, thereby increasing oxygen delivery to the myocardium.

Ventricular assist devices provide a means for partially or totally supporting cardiac output and resting the ventricles, whereas total artificial hearts completely replace heart functioning. Nursing responsibilities when caring for a patient with a ventricular assist device or total artificial heart include adjusting flow rates and manipulating preload.

Although increasing contractility is a more common method of enhancing heart action, contractility may be decreased as an attempt to reduce the work of the heart, particularly in a patient who has had an acute myocardial infarction. Contractility is decreased by administering negative inotropic agents such as beta-blocking and calcium channel-blocking agents.

The final area for acting to enhance the effectiveness of the heart's pumping is through altering or maintaining an effective heart rate and rhythm. Traditionally nurses have withheld caffeinated beverages from patients with cardiac disorders. However, small doses of caffeine (1 cup of coffee) do not appear to affect heart rate, blood pressure, or the incidence of arrhythmias, even in patients with cardiac disorders (Schneider 1987).

Because tachycardias are associated with decreased diastolic filling time and increased myocardial oxygen demand, nursing activities are aimed at preventing or minimizing conditions associated with rapid heart rates. If tachycardia is a compensatory response to pathology, nursing activities are directed at correcting the underlying condition. For example, tachycardia in the febrile patient is best alleviated by nursing activities that restore the patient to a normothermic state. When decompensating tachycardias or arrhythmias occur, nurses are often responsible for determining activities based on identification of the rhythm (Breu and Dracup 1982). For patients with arrhythmias, medication administration, pacemaker therapy, or defibrillation may be provided by a nurse using written protocols.

Intravascular Volume

Amount and type of fluid replacement is dependent on the assessment of estimated loss and hemodynamic response. Oral fluids can completely or partially replace fluid loss. By offering oral fluids that appeal to the patient, the nurse may effectively restore intravascular volume and preserve hemodynamic stability.

Frequently hemodynamic regulation for patients with decreased preload or fluid volume deficit involves volume replacement, with either crystalloids or colloids. When hypovolemia is due to blood loss, the appropriate treatment is to replace the volume with blood products. In addition, actions should be aimed at controlling the bleeding, whether through direct pressure, elevation of a bleeding limb, pharmacologic agents (such as Pitressin), or surgical intervention (Holloway 1988; Kuhn et al. 1990).

Although much controversy remains regarding the appropriate selection of fluids for resuscitation, crystalloids are primarily used to replace isotonic fluid loss, whereas colloids are most often used when third spacing has led to hypovolemia. When administering fluid volume replacement, the nurse must remember that crystalloids replace both intravascular and extravascular fluid volume, whereas colloids increase colloid osmotic pressure and remain in the intravascular space longer than crystalloids. Because crystalloids move freely between the intravascular and interstitial compartments, the volume of replacement solution required may be as much as four times the actual volume loss (Rice 1984; Weil and Rackow

1984). Edema and dilution of plasma proteins (including hemoglobin) may ensue. In patients with increased capillary permeability, colloids leak into the interstitial space and locally increase osmotic pressure (Rice 1984).

When a patient is suffering from extreme fluid volume deficit, an intravenous access must be secured that allows for rapid fluid administration. A short, large-bore catheter (2 inch, 14 or 16 gauge) offers the least resistance to fluid flow (Rice 1984). Administering fluids under pressure using a blood pump or pressurized bag also increases the rate of fluid administration (Rice 1984).

Positioning the patient flat with legs elevated 20 degrees to 30 degrees is the preferred treatment for increasing preload through displacing peripheral blood to the central organs (Wilcox and Vandam 1988). The Trendelenburg position was once considered a logical maneuver to shift venous blood from the periphery to the heart and, consequently, increase venous return and cardiac output in hypovolemic patients. However, studies have demonstrated that mean arterial blood pressure did not change significantly in normotensive and hypotensive patients placed in this position (Sibbald, Paterson, Holliday, and Baskerville 1979; Wilcox and Vandam 1988). Hypotensive patients placed in the Trendelenburg position actually showed a decrease in cardiac index, probably related to an increase in systemic vascular resistance, whereas normotensive patients demonstrated significant increases in central venous pressure, pulmonary capillary wedge pressure, and cardiac index and significant decreases in systemic vascular resistance (Sibbald et al. 1979).

Pneumatic antishock garments (PASGs) are widely used for prehospital control of shock associated with hypovolemia or spinal cord injury. PASGs function in improving end-diastolic volume, stroke volume, and cardiac output by increasing preload and increasing peripheral resistance to flow. Approximately 4 mL/kg autotransfusion has been shown to occur with the use of PASGs in animal models of hypovolemic shock (Kaback, Sanders and Meislin 1984). However, PASGs have been shown to elevate blood pressure primarily by reducing the diameter of blood vessels (Kaback, Sanders, and Meislin 1984). Inflation of PASGs increases peripheral resistance, sacrificing perfusion to the lower half of the body to increase blood pressure and flow to the central organs. Inflating the calf and leg bladders simultaneously and then inflating the abdominal bladder of the PASG allows for the optimal increase in end-diastolic volume, stroke volume, and cardiac output (Jennings, Seaworth, Howell, Tripp, and Goodyear 1986). Deflating the PASG must be done only after hemodynamic stability has been restored to avert a precipitous drop in blood pressure.

Increases in intrathoracic pressure can decrease preload. The nurse is instrumental in recognizing when increases in positive end-expiratory pressure in a mechanically ventilated patient are compromising cardiac output by decreasing venous return. Patients with cardiovascular disorders should be taught to avoid the Valsalva maneuver. Patients under age 45 years can be expected to have more extreme hemodynamic changes during the Valsalva maneuver. In addition, patients in more upright sitting positions have larger drops in systolic blood pressure during the Valsalva maneuver than patients in a flat or side-lying position (Metzger and Therrien 1990). Use of stool softeners coupled with instruction on breathing through the mouth when straining, turning, or moving up in bed can eliminate the Valsalva maneuver in most bedridden patients. When patients cannot avoid the Valsalva maneuver—for example, during suctioning—the nurse can minimize hemodynamic changes by positioning the patient in a flat or side-lying position.

The nurse should limit fluid volume intake for patients with increased preload. Fluid intake is limited by setting up a fluid restriction schedule with patient input and by administering medications in their most concentrated form. When increased preload is accompanied by acute respiratory distress, placing patients in a sitting position with their legs dependent increases pooling of blood in the extremities, reducing preload and pulmonary congestion.

Vasodilators and diuretics are used to decrease preload and circulating volume. Venous system vasodilators are used to displace intravascular volume to the venous vascular bed, thereby decreasing preload. Diuretic therapy has been associated with an early fall in stroke volume and cardiac output, directly related to the decrease in intravascular volume. This effect is counteracted by a rapid rise in systemic vascular resistance, which maintains mean arterial blood pressure. However, when used for long-term therapy for hypertension, the hemodynamic actions of diuretics differ from the acute effects in that systemic vascular resistance returns from the initial elevation to, or even below, baseline levels (Struyker-Boudier, Smits, Kleinjans, and van Essen 1983).

For patients with altered peripheral tissue perfusion, redistributing volume from the lower extremities decreases venous stasis. If venous pooling is anticipated, compression stockings should be applied. If venous pooling does occur, the extremity should be elevated. Exercising, whether active or passive, enhances the pumping action of the muscles, thereby increasing venous return and reducing venous stasis.

Peripheral Flow

Hemodynamic Regulation for patients with increased peripheral resistance to flow is directed toward reducing blood viscosity and dilating vessels. Blood viscosity can be reduced using hemodilution, which is done by increasing fluid intake, by administering crystalloid solutions, or by phlebotomy. Twenty-minute whole body massage therapy was reported in one study to reduce blood viscosity by increasing perfusion and hemodilution of intravascular volume (Ernst, Matrai, Magyarosy, Liebermeister, Eck, and Breu 1987).

Before vasodilating a patient, the nurse should assess for fluid volume deficit by evaluating if the increase in peripheral resistance to flow represents the normal physiological response to hypovolemia. If afterload reduction is utilized when the patient is experiencing fluid volume deficit, cardiac output can be precipitously affected. If tachycardia or hypotension are observed as afterload is reduced, the nurse should suspect the need to increase preload.

Warming a cold, vasoconstricted patient may reduce peripheral resistance to flow. However, the nurse must use caution when warming a patient. A normothermic patient may report feeling cold due to compensatory vasoconstriction. A nurse should only warm hypothermic patients in whom vasoconstriction is causing an increase in afterload that is deleteriously affecting hemodynamics. Numerous techniques are available for increasing a patient's body temperature: warming the patient's room, applying blankets to the patient's torso and/or extremities, covering the patient's head, and using room-temperature or warmed intravenous fluids and blood products (Phillips and Skov 1988). Nonwarmed thermal blankets were as effective as warmed thermal blankets and electric heating blankets in raising body temperature to normal in postoperative cardiovascular surgery patients (Oliver and Fuessel 1990). To warm overweight patients, the patient's torso and extremities are completely covered because these patients take longer to rewarm than patients at normal body weight (Oliver and Fuessel 1990).

Pharmacologic agents that vasodilate peripheral vessels are used to reduce left ventricular afterload and the resistance to flow (Table 41–2). When patients are administered vasodilators, their vessel diameter increases, reducing systemic vascular resistance and displacing intravascular volume to the periphery. Both events contribute to a reduction in ventricular filling pressure. Vigorous fluid administration is often necessary in conjunction with vasodilators to maintain preload. During vasodilator therapy, hypotension, reflex tachycardia, and/or chest pain (because coronary blood flow is reduced) may indicate inadequate preload or excessive afterload reduction. Some vasodilators may be administered to improve end-organ perfusion. For example, low-dose dopamine is used to increase renal perfusion by dilating the renal arteries.

Enhancing peripheral flow in patients with altered tissue perfusion is done by body positioning, decreasing blood viscosity, medication administration, and vasodilation. Positioning an extremity dependently enhances arterial flow. Conversely, elevation increases venous flow from the extremity. Decreasing blood viscosity through methods already described improves flow to the periphery. Frequently, heparin or thrombolytic agents are used for vessel thrombosis. Vasodilation, through the application of warmth and the administration of vasodilating medications, can also be used to increase peripheral tissue perfusion. Vasoconstricting substances, such as caffeine and nicotine, should be avoided when peripheral tissue perfusion is compromised.

For pathologically vasodilated patients, systemic pressure can be maintained with vasoconstricting medications (Table 41 – 2). Activities for treating hyperthermic patients are based on the origin of the fever: antipyretics for febrile illness and external cooling measures when antipyretics are contraindicated or when the fever is inordinately high, unresponsive to antipyretics, or due to external heat exposure (Enright and Hill 1989). External cooling measures include removing clothes and bed covers, cooling the room temperature, applying ice packs to the groin and axilla, tepid sponging, and applying a mechanical cooling blanket.

CASE STUDY

RF is a 60-year-old male who was admitted to a surgical unit after removal of a sigmoid tumor. His cardiovascular medical history included a small lateral myocardial infarction (MI) at age 58. Since having his MI, he had quit smoking but remained overweight and sedentary. Postoperative assessments included the following information:

	ADMISSION	FOURTH HOUR	FIFTH HOUR
Blood pressure	152/86	144/84	112/72
Heart rate	80	92	112
Heart rhythm	Regular	Regular	Irregular
Respiratory rate	18	22	28
Consciousness	Drowsy	Awake	Restless
Breath sounds	Clear	Crackles in bases	Crackles lower half
Heart sounds	S1, S2	S1, S2	S1, S2, S3
Jugular venous distention (45°)	3 cm	4 cm	6 cm
Peripheral pulses	2+/=	2+/=	1+/=
Peripheral edema	Absent	Absent	Absent
Urine output (cc/hr)	35	25	20
Intake (cc/hr)	150	150	150
Specific gravity	1.024	1.028	1.028

The nursing diagnosis was Decreased Cardiac Output related to increased preload and decreased contractility. The desired patient goal, to enhance heart action, was to be determined by the following criteria:

1. Absence of crackles, dyspnea, orthopnea, S_3
2. Return of blood pressure, heart rate, respiratory rate to baseline
3. Urine output of ≥ 1.0 mL/kg/hr
4. Peripheral pulses $2+/=$, jugular venous distention of 3 cm or less at a 45° angle.

The nurse administered the intervention of Hemodynamic Regulation by following the protocol to decrease preload and increase contractility. Fluid intake was limited by slowing the intravenous rate. The patient was placed in a sitting position by elevating the head of the bed and lowering the feet, a position of comfort that reduced preload. After consultation with the physician, the nurse administered low-flow oxygen and diuretics. The outcome criteria were met within the hour.

TABLE 41–3. INTERVENTION PROTOCOL FOR HEMODYNAMIC REGULATION

CARDIAC OUTPUT: GOAL—ENHANCE HEART ACTION

Increase contractility	Decrease contractility	Increase preload	Decrease preload
Optimize oxygen to myocardium	Administer negative inotropic agents	Increase fluid volume	Decrease fluid volume
promote rest		Decrease intrathoracic	Increase contractility
pace activities		or intraabdominal	Decrease afterload
position of comfort		pressure	
administer low-flow oxygen		Maintain diastolic filling time	
Correct acid-base balance		Increase afterload	
Correct electrolyte balance			
Administer and titrate inotropic agents			
Optimize preload and afterload			
Manage mechanical devices			

Increase afterload	Decrease afterload	Maintain heart rate and diastolic filling time
Cool hyperthermic patient	Ensure adequate preload	Follow protocol/standard
Administer and titrate vasoconstrictors	Hemodilute blood administer fluids	for emergency interventions
Increase preload	massage whole body	Administer antidysrhythmic agents
Place and inflate PASG	Warm	Insure adequate pacemaker functioning
	Administer and titrate vasodilators	

INTRAVASCULAR VOLUME:
Goal—Alter Intravascular Volume

PERIPHERAL FLOW:
Goal—Enhance Peripheral Flow

Increase fluid volume	Decrease fluid volume	Improve arterial flow	Improve venous flow
Replace fluid	Limit fluid intake	Place extremity in a dependent position	Decrease venous stasis
encourage oral fluids	Place in sitting position	Increase hydration	apply compression stockings
administer crystalloids or colloids intravenously	Administer diuretics	Warm	elevate extremity
administer blood products	Administer and titrate vasodilators	Avoid vasoconstricting agents	exercise extremity
Position flat with legs elevated			
Place and inflate PASG			

Note: PASG = pneumatic antishock garment

SUMMARY

The appropriate set of nursing activities to administer Hemodynamic Regulation must be based on the etiology of or contributing factors to the alteration in hemodynamics. Table 41–3 summarizes the actions to carry out the three components of Hemodynamic Regulation according to the appropriate goal.

REFERENCES

Alteri, C.A. 1984. The patient with myocardial infarction: Rest prescriptions for activities of daily living. *Heart and Lung* 13:355–360.

Bagatell, C.J., and Heymsfield, S.B. 1984. Effect of meal size on myocardial oxygen requirements: Implications for postmyocardial infarction diet. *American Journal of Clinical Nutrition* 39:421–426.

Breu, C., and Dracup, K. 1982. Survey of critical care nursing practice. Part III. Responsibilities of intensive care unit staff. *Heart and Lung* 11:157–161.

Enright, T., and Hill, M.G. 1989. Treatment of fever. *Focus on Critical Care* 16(2):96–102.

Ernst, E., Matrai, A., Magyarosy, I., Liebermeister, R.G., Eck, M., and Breu, M.C. 1987. Massages cause changes in blood fluidity. *Physiotherapy* 73:43–45.

Guyton, A.C. 1986. *Textbook of medical physiology* (7th ed.). Philadelphia: W.B. Saunders Company.

Hickey, J. 1986. *The clinical practice of neurological and neurosurgical nursing.* Philadelphia: Lippincott.

Holloway, N.M. 1988. *Nursing the critically ill adult* (3d ed.). Menlo Park, Calif.: Addison-Wesley.

Jennings, T.J., Seaworth, J.F., Howell, L.L., Tripp, L.D., and Goodyear, C.D. 1986. The effects of various antishock trouser inflation sequences on hemodynamics in normovolemic subjects. *Annals of Emergency Medicine* 15:1193–1197.

Johnston, B.L., Watt, E.W., and Fletcher, G.F. 1981. Oxygen consumption and hemodynamic and electrocardiographic responses to bathing in recent post-myocardial infarction patients. *Heart and Lung* 10:666–671.

Kaback, K.R., Sanders, A.B., and Meislin, H.W. 1984. MAST suit update. *Journal of American Medical Association* 252:2598–2603.

Kline, E.M. 1987. Recombinant tissue-type plasminogen activator in acute myocardial infarction: Role of the critical care nurse. *Heart and Lung* 16:779–786.

Kuhn, R.C., et al. (eds.). 1990. *Outcome standards for nursing care of the critically ill.* Laguna Niguel, Calif.: American Association of Critical-Care Nurses.

Metzger, B.L., and Therrien, B. 1990. Effect of position on cardiovascular response during the Valsalva maneuver. *Nursing Research* 39:198–202.

Oliver, S.K., and Fuessel, E. 1990. Control of postoperative hypothermia in cardiovascular surgery patients. *Critical Care Nurse Quarterly* 12(4):63–68.

Palmar, P.N. 1982. Advanced hemodynamic assessment. *Dimensions of Critical Care Nursing* 1:139–144.

Phillips, R., and Skov, P. 1988. Rewarming and cardiac surgery: A review. *Heart and Lung* 17:511–520.

Prakash, R., Parmley, W.W., Dikshit, K., Forrester, J., and Swan, H.J. 1973. Hemodynamic effects of postural changes in patients with acute myocardial infarction. *Chest* 64:7–9.

Quaglietti, S.E., Slotts, N.A., and Lovejoy, N.C. 1988. The effect of selected positions on rate pressure product of the postmyocardial infarction patient. *Journal of Cardiovascular Nursing* 2(4):77–85.

Rice, V. 1984. Shock management: Part I. Fluid volume replacement. *Critical Care Nurse* 4(6):69–82.

Riegel, B. 1985. The role of nursing in limiting myocardial infarct size. *Heart and Lung* 14:247–254.

Riegel, B. 1988. Acute myocardial infarction: Nursing interventions to optimize oxygen supply and demand. In L.S. Kern (ed.), *Cardiac critical care nursing* (pp. 59–90). Rockville, Md.: Aspen.

Schneider, J.R. 1987. Effects of caffeine ingestion on heart rate, blood pressure, myocardial oxygen consumption, and cardiac rhythm in acute myocardial infarction patients. *Heart and Lung* 16:167–174.

Sibbald, W.J., Paterson, N.A., Holliday, R.L., and Baskerville, J. 1979. The Trendelenburg position: Hemodynamic effects in hypotensive and normotensive patients. *Critical Care Medicine* 7:218–224.

Struyker-Boudier, H.A., Smits, J.F., Kleinjans, J.C., and van Essen, H. 1983. Hemodynamic actions of diuretic agents. *Clinical and Experimental Hypertension* 5:209–223.

Urban, N. 1990. Hemodynamic clinical profiles. *AACN Clinical Issues in Critical Care Nursing* 1:119–130.

Weber, K.T., and Janicki, J.S. 1979. The heart as a muscle-pump system and the concept of heart failure. *American Heart Journal* 98:371–384.

Weil, M.H., and Rackow, E.C. 1984. A guide to volume repletion. *Emergency Medicine* 16(8):100–110.

Wilcox, S., and Vandam, L.D. 1988. Alas, poor Trendelenburg and his position! A critique of its uses and effectiveness. *Anesthesia and Analgesia* 67:574–578.

Winslow, E.H., Lane, L.D., and Gaffney, F.A. 1985. Oxygen uptake and cardiovascular response in control adults and acute myocardial infarction patients during bathing. *Nursing Research* 34:164–169.

42

SECONDARY BRAIN INJURY REDUCTION

PAMELA H. MITCHELL
LAURIE L. ACKERMAN

Conscious thought, memory, personality, movement, and sensation are but a few of the functions originating from and controlled by the brain. It is the source of the uniquely human functions that separate humans from other mammals. Brain function is protected in any situation that threatens the integrity of the brain or its component functions.

A variety of systemic or localized disorders can result in altered brain function. Often these changes result from cerebral insufficiency by diminishing overall cerebral circulation, decreasing perfusion of specific brain tissues, or directly compromising the physical integrity of brain cells. The primary health goal of therapy is to protect patients from secondary brain injury. Nursing has a central role in achieving this goal through the application of the intervention. Secondary Brain Injury Reduction, is defined as protecting the patient's brain from further neurological insult resulting from compressive or ischemic damage.

ACUTE BRAIN INSUFFICIENCY AND SECONDARY INJURY

Examples of the many sources of acute brain injury include focal contusion or compression from head trauma, cerebral vascular embolism or occlusion, intracerebral hemorrhage from a cerebral aneurysm or hypertension, widespread axonal shearing from trauma, or anoxia following prolonged cardiac arrest. Regardless of the source of the acute injury, a set of cellular responses is set into motion. Cellular perfusion is reduced by tissue compression, reduction of blood flow, or loss of metabolic substrate (oxygen and glucose, for example). Vasoactive neurotransmitters are released in an attempt to dilate intracerebral vessels and thus restore perfusion. These neurotransmitters initiate cerebral vasodilation with a subsequent hyperemic state, often called brain swelling. Brain swelling (or hyperemia) is to be distinguished from brain edema, which is excess water within brain cells themselves. Brain edema may follow hyperemia if cell membranes are injured, if systemic injury alters serum osmolar equilibrium, or if the internal cellular metabolic machinery is damaged (Klatzo 1985; Miller 1985). In either case (brain swelling or brain edema), the intracranial volumes of blood and brain may expand sufficiently to increase intracranial pressure (ICP). Normal intracranial pressure is approximately 0 mm Hg to 10 mm Hg in adults, children, and neonates, with values exceeding 10 mm Hg to 15 mm Hg considered elevated (Miller 1977,

558

1985). Sustained increases in baseline ICP (greater than 15 mm Hg to 20 mm Hg) are termed intracranial hypertension. The degree to which the intracranial compartment is able to compensate for additional volumes of blood, brain, or cerebrospinal fluid has been considered the adaptive capacity of the intracranial system and is measured in terms of intracranial compliance or elastance (Miller 1977; Mitchell 1986).

While intracranial hypertension may occur as a sequela to the primary brain damage, secondary insults such as hypoxia, hypotension, or sustained large cerebrospinal fluid pulsations can increase damage and are assumed to influence both survival and its quality (Eisenberg, Bary, Aldrich, Saydjari, Turner, Fourlkes, Jane, Marmarov, Marshall, and Young 1990; Eisenberg, Cayard, Papanicolaou, 1983; Miller 1977; Pettarossi, DiRocco, Manicinelli, Calderalli and Vedard 1978; Pfenniger, Reith, Breitig, Gunert, and Ahnefeld 1989). Available cerebral oxygen may be reduced by systemic hypoxia, even with constant cerebral perfusion pressure. In contrast, hypotension promotes tissue injury by decreasing cerebral perfusion pressure and, thus, cerebral blood flow.

SECONDARY BRAIN INJURY REDUCTION AND NURSING DIAGNOSIS

The terminology relating to care of the neuroscience patient in the NANDA taxonomy is inadequate. The most relevant diagnosis from the NANDA taxonomy in relation to secondary brain injury reduction is Altered (Cerebral) Tissue Perfusion. A variety of other NANDA diagnoses relate to portions of secondary brain injury reduction by targeting individual components that are dealt with in treating the primary problem:

Altered Thought Processes
Ineffective Breathing Pattern
Fluid Volume Deficit
Potential Fluid Volume Deficit
Impaired Gas Exchange
Impaired Physical Mobility
Potential for Infection
Self Care Deficit
Sensory/Perceptual Alterations

Several other diagnoses relating to care of the patient at risk for secondary brain injury have been identified by the American Nurses' Association Council on Medical-Surgical Nursing Practice and the American Association of Neuroscience Nurses in their 1985 document on neuroscience nursing practice: high risk of secondary brain injury and altered level of responsiveness. Another potential diagnosis, Decreased Intracranial Adaptive Capacity, has been proposed (Mitchell 1986b; Rauch, Mitchell, and Tyler 1990).

DESCRIPTION OF THE INTERVENTION

Three primary nursing care components are involved in Secondary Brain Injury Reduction: ongoing monitoring of the patient's physiological status, promotion of cerebral perfusion, and decreasing or controlling stimuli in the patient's environment.

Monitoring

Ongoing monitoring of the patient at risk for secondary brain injury should include ongoing clinical examination of the neurological, respiratory, and cardiovascular systems (Henneman 1989). Ideally, the patient's intracranial and cerebral perfusion pressure are monitored. Monitoring would also include watching for signs and symptoms of brain herniation syndromes.

Neurologial Monitoring

McGuffin (1983) states that the neurological examination is the "single most important parameter in deciding the management of the cerebral trauma patient" (p. 192). In fact, "subtle changes, if acted upon promptly, can mean the difference between a good or poor recovery or even between survival and death" (Marshall, Marshall, Vos, and Chestnut 1990, p. 90).

There are good physiological reasons for this. The Monro-Kellie hypothesis identifies the skull as a rigid compartment with essentially constant volumes of brain tissue, cerebrospinal fluid, and blood. Any increase in volume in one of these components must be offset by a reciprocal decrease in the volume of another component, or the intracranial pressure will rise. A patient whose adaptive capacity of the system is exhausted eventually will manifest symptoms of neurological change. If the change is detected early, it is often possible to prevent further deterioration to the point of brain herniation syndromes. (Brain herniation is the movement of brain tissue from one compartment to another. It occurs with growth of mass lesions, such as tumor or hematoma, or with rapid increases in ICP. Herniation of cerebral hemisphere tissue onto the brain stem is often fatal.)

It is well accepted in the nursing and medical literature that the patient's level of consciousness is one of the first parameters to show appreciable change when neurological deterioration begins to occur (Becker, Miller, Ward, Greenberg, Young, and Sakalas 1977; Jess 1987; Mauss and Mitchell 1976). The concept of consciousness incorporates the physiological components of arousal the state of wakefulness — and content processing — the interpretation of the internal and external environment and stimuli (Crigger and Strickland 1985; Plum and Posner 1980; Wong, Wong, and Dempster 1984). Some degree of arousal is required for content processing to take place.

The Glascow Coma Scale, initially developed to promote consistent, objective assessment of head injury patients, is often utilized as an initial screening type of monitoring tool in critical care units. Scoring is based on best response in three areas of behavioral response: eye opening, verbal, and motor responses (Teasdale and Jennett 1974). It measures arousal as a function of eye opening and content processing as a function of response to orientation questions and ability to understand and perform requests for motor movement. There are problems associated with the use of this and other standardized tools in that they often do not provide enough information for the nurse to visualize patient performance fully at a given time so as to be of value for later comparison. Descriptive terminology used to describe level of consciousness (*stupor, obtundation, lethargy*) varies greatly in meaning from source to source and is of minimal value in actual practice. Arousal may perhaps be best described as the stimulus required to attract and keep the patient's attention. This is best documented as a stimulus-response statement — for example, "opens eyes to voice" or "decerebrates upper extremities to nail bed pressure" — and use of descriptive terminology should be avoided.

Cognition is best monitored as a product of response in terms of memory,

TABLE 42-1.   CRANIAL NERVE ASSESSMENT

NUMBER	NAME	TEST
I	Olfactory	Sense of smell
II	Optic	Visual acuity Visual fields
III	Oculomotor	Pupillary constriction Extraocular movements (moves eye down and laterally, up and medially, up and laterally, and nasally) Eyelid elevation
IV	Trochlear	Extraocular movements (moves eye down and medially)
V	Trigeminal	Facial sensation Corneal reflex Jaw movement
VI	Abducens	Extraocular movements (moves eye laterally)
VII	Facial	Facial symmetry Taste (anterior two-thirds of tongue) Corneal reflex Eyelid closure
VIII	Auditory	Hearing Balance/equilibrium
IX	Glossopharyngeal	Taste (posterior one-third of tongue) Throat and pharnyx sensation Gag reflex Swallowing
X	Vagus	Gag reflex Swallowing Voice quality Vital signs (parasympathetic innervation)
XI	Spinal accessory	Shoulder shrugs Strength of head turn
XII	Hypoglossal	Tongue movement Swallowing

thought processes, ability to follow commands, and mood/affect. It is important that the overall content and behaviors of the interchange with the patient are evaluated for appropriateness to the situational context, since significant deficit can be present in patients classically oriented to time, place, and person. Changes in language abilities are often concomitantly observed and monitored during this portion of the examination. These could include the presence of aphasias, echolalia, perseveration, or a variety of other disorders.

Cranial nerve functioning incorporates testing of the functions of the 12 cranial nerves exiting from the brain stem. These nerves incorporate both motor and sensory components and are generally associated with such functions as visual scope and acuity, pupillary size and reactivity, gaze characteristics, facial movement and sensation, and hearing and balance, as well as the corneal, oculocephalic, oculovestibular, cough, gag, and swallowing reflexes. Table 42-1 illustrates activities to monitor cranial nerve function.

Motor and sensory testing is a function of the cerebral hemispheres and spinal nerves associated with various segmental functions. Common activities tested in conscious patients include grip and leg strength and assessment of the patient for a

TABLE 42-2. TYPES OF MOTOR RESPONSES

Follows commands	Able to comply with simple requests (gripping, holding up fingers)
Localizes	Organized, purposeful attempt to remove a noxious stimulus
Withdrawal	Reflexive response in which the extremity being examined withdraws or pulls away from the source of the stimulus
Decortication (abnormal flexion)	Flexion of the arms at the wrist and elbows with shoulder adduction; lower extremities exhibit extension of the legs with plantar flexion
Decerebration (abnormal extension)	Extension, adduction, and internal rotation of the arms; legs may be rigidly extended, and arching of the back with backward flexion of the head and feet may also be seen
Flaccid	No muscle tone or response to stimuli

pronator drift. Examination of the patient with an altered level of consciousness often requires monitoring of focal monitor movements in which a stimulus such as nail bed pressure or a sternal rub is applied, and the response in each extremity is individually noted. Table 42-2 lists types of movement that may be seen in response to stimulus application. It is useful to note these responses in a stimulus utilized–patient response format. Patient posture and gait should also be monitored because they reflect muscle tone and cerebellar function.

Respiratory Monitoring

It has been well documented and established that it is possible to recognize and potentially localize evolving cerebral insult on the basis of respiratory rate and pattern. Cheyne-Stokes respirations, central neurogenic hyperventilation, and apneustic, cluster, and ataxic breathing patterns are several examples (Gifford and Plaut 1975; Hickey 1986; Plum and Posner 1980). These patterns are reproduced in Figure 42-1.

Changes in rate, rhythm, and depth of respiration should be noted because they can affect cerebral perfusion. It is important to distinguish between changes in these parameters due to cerebral origin as opposed to primary respiratory or metabolic changes. Monitoring and analysis of arterial blood gases, O_2 saturation, end-tidal CO_2, and pulmonary artery pressures in conjunction with the clinical examination of the patient, including chest expansion and breath sounds, are necessary activities in accomplishing this.

If mechanical ventilation is necessary, the nurse also monitors parameters relevant to this activity. In general, positive end-expiratory pressure is used cautiously due to potential increased ICP pursuant to its use. Some investigators have found that head elevation minimizes ICP change; others have not. In some instances, administration of prn sedative medications or paralyzing agents as ordered by the physician may be necessary to maximize respiratory function needed for optimal cerebral recovery.

Cardiovascular Monitoring

Portions of the hypothalamus and the vasomotor center of the medulla are responsible for regulating blood pressure and may be disrupted in certain types of intracranial pathology. Hypotension is rarely due to cerebral injury (Hickey 1986), and patients displaying such symptoms should be evaluated for shock or other

Type	Respiratory Pattern	Neuroanatomical Lesion
Cheyne-Stokes respiration		Usually bilateral in cerebral hemispheres Cerebellar sometimes Midbrain Upper pons
Central neurogenic hyperventilation		Low midbrain Upper pons
Apneustic breathing		Mid pons Low pons
Cluster breathing		Low pons High medulla
Ataxic breathing		Medulla

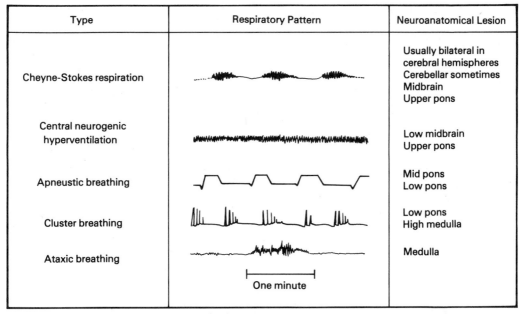

One minute

Source: Gifford, R.R., Plaut, M.R.: Abnormal respiratory patterns in the comatose patient caused by intracranial dysfunction. Journal of Neurosurgical Nursing, 7(1):58, July 1975

FIGURE 42–1. Abnormal Respiratory Patterns

hemorrhagic injuries, particularly in the presence of a tachycardia. Hypotension with bradycardia is commonly seen following cervical cord injury due to disruption of the sympathetic nervous system below the level of injury.

In some cases, ongoing monitoring of arterial blood pressures (ABP), central venous pressures (CVP), or pulmonary artery wedge (PAW) pressures is required. These parameters are often monitored when utilizing hypervolemic hemodilution or other forms of volume expansion therapy to ensure cerebral perfusion (Stewart-Amidei 1989). The nurse administers colloid or crystalloid in conjunction with the physician's orders to maintain the patient's ABP, PAW, or CVP within a certain therapeutic range. Continuous infusion of vasoactive drugs such as sodium nitroprusside, dopamine, epinephrine, or dobutamine may be required to raise or lower the systolic blood pressure (SBP) to keep it within a specified therapeutic range.

Monitoring of the electrocardiogram (ECG) may also be required. Major ECG changes associated with acute intracranial disease may include A-V block or dissociation, premature ventricular contractions, large, upright T waves with a prolonged QT interval, Q waves with ST depression, supraventricular tachycardias, atrial flutter-fibrillation, sinus bradycardia, nodal rhythms, and cardiac arrest. These types of changes are frequently seen in patients with aneurysmal subarchnoid hemorrhage or severe acute head injury (Adams 1984; Hickey 1986; Plum and Posner 1980).

The pulse is evaluated in respect to rate, rhythm, and quality. Bradycardia is of note because of its relationship to the Cushing response. This response, incorporating bradycardia, elevated systolic blood pressure, and widened pulse pressure, is a compensatory mechanism attempting to maintain cerebral blood flow in the pressure of rising intracranial pressure. These symptoms indicate that brain herniation is imminent and are so late that reversal of herniation is often not possible.

TABLE 42-3. COMPARISON OF MONITORING DEVICES: ADVANTAGES
AND DISADVANTAGES

MONITORING DEVICE	ADVANTAGES	DISADVANTAGES
Intraventricular catheter (IVC)	Accurate measurement of ICP Allows drainage/sampling of CSF Allows installation of contrast media Provides reliable evaluating volume/pressure responses	Provides additional site for potential infection Most invasive method for monitoring ICP <> Must be balanced and recalibrated frequently Catheter can become occluded by blood or tissue
Subarachnoid bolt/screw	Allows sampling of CSF Lower infection rates than with the IVC Quickly and easily placed	Tendency for dampened waveforms Less accurate at high ICP pressures May become occluded by tissue or blood Must be balanced and recalibrated frequently (i.e., q 4 hours and whenever the patient is repositioned)
Subdural, extradural catheter/sensor	Least invasive Easily and quickly placed	Increasing baseline drift over time; therefore, accuracy and reliability are questionable Does not provide for CSF sampling
Fiberoptic probe/catheter	Can be placed in subdural or subarachnoid space, ventricle, or into brain tissue Easily transported Requires zeroing only once (during insertion) Baseline drift to 1 mm Hg/day No irrigation—less risk of infection Less waveform artifact No need to adjust transducer to patient position	Does not provide for CSF sampling Cannot be recalibrated once it is placed Breakage of the fiberoptic cable

Source: Gilliam Intracranial hypertension: advances in intracranial pressure monitoring. Critical Care Nursing Clinics of North America, Vol. 2(1), p. 25.

Intracranial Pressure (ICP) Monitoring

Rises in ICP can also occur in the absence of neurological examination findings. (Gilliam 1990). For this reason, an ICP monitoring device can assist in identifying the problem and guiding medical and nursing actions or therapy.

Several types of ICP monitoring devices are available: fluid-transduced systems such as an intraventricular catheter (ventriculostomy), subarachnoid screw and bolt, and the subdural or extradural catheter/sensor or fiberoptically transduced probes and catheters. These monitoring devices are compared in Table 42-3.

Nurses are responsible for several activities that ensure accuracy of the monitoring device. Fluid-transduced systems require frequent recalibration, inspection for bubbles in the transducer tubing, and leveling to ensure accurate readings. The transducer of the system is generally leveled to the external auditory canal to approximate the location of the lateral ventricle at the foramen of Monro.

Other nursing responsibilities include documentation and interpretation of intracranial pressure recordings and waveform tracings. Historically, waveform interpretation was difficult, since trending over time was required for identification of the A, B, and C waves described in the literature. Recently the analysis of the component portions of the ICP pulse wave that occur in real time has gained attention (Cardosa, Rowan, and Galbraith 1983; Germon 1988). More research is needed to investigate the clinical significance of these waveforms.

The actual mean ICP values must be evaluated in the light of the patient's clinical status. ICP readings of greater than 20 mm Hg are uniformly recognized as indicative of intracranial hypertension and are generally treated with direct or standing medical orders for hyperventilation, osmotic or loop active diuretics, and CSF drainage via ventriculostomy or lumbar drainage system, as well as various other nursing actions discussed in the next section.

Infection is a serious complication that can result in ventriculitis, meningitis, or death (Hickman and Muwaswes 1990). In general, devices that pierce the dura, utilize external drainage system components, or are in place for more than 5 days are associated with a greater risk of infection. (Franges and Beiderman 1988; Mayhall, Archer, Lamb, Spadora, Baggett, Ward, and Narayan 1984; Narayan, Kishore, Becker, Ward, Enes, Greenberg, DaSilva, Lipper, Choi, Mayhall, Lutz, and Young 1982). Administration of prophylactic antibiotics, tunneling approaches in catheter insertion, and not changing the system have been associated with lower infection rates (Friedman and Vries 1980; Kanter, Winer, Patti, and Robson 1985; Mayhall et al. 1984).

No standard group of activities is appropriate for all patients in need of monitoring. The nurse must incorporate information from the medical history, current illness, including diagnosis, and type and timing of medical, surgical, or nursing activities in deciding on components of the initial neurological examination. Performance of this examination is measured against each succeeding examination. These data are then reintegrated with information regarding various therapies, with the nurse continuing to make choices about what components are monitored and how frequently. This component of the intervention consists of the choices made regarding type and frequency of activities to monitor, as well as the synthesis and analysis of the information obtained (Ackerman 1991).

Cerebral Perfusion Promotion

The brain has high metabolic energy requirements and thus requires a constant supply of glucose and oxygen to perform its necessary cell functions. The brain does not have the ability to store these substrates and requires 750 mL, or 20% of the body's resting cardiac output, each minute to extract these nutrients (Marshall et al. 1990). Cessation of blood flow to the brain results in the CNS's using up the available oxygen and glucose in a matter of seconds. It is therefore essential that blood flow to the brain be monitored and maintained in order to prevent deleterious changes in cell functioning.

Cerebral Gas Exchange and Acid Base Balance

A cornerstone of intracranial hypertension treatment is controlled hyperventilation (Marshall et al. 1990). The $PaCO_2$ is reduced to 27 mm Hg to 30 mm Hg, thereby constricting cerebral blood vessels and reducing intracranial pressure by decreasing volume in the vascular compartment. More severe reduction of the $PaCO_2$ may induce ischemia by loss of adequate cerebral blood flow (CBF) or loss of autoregulation (the brain's ability to direct regional blood flow on a needs basis). Since it is not possible to measure CBF at the bedside, the cerebral perfusion pressure (CPP) is the parameter utilized. CPP is calculated by subtracting the intracranial pressure from the mean arterial pressure (MAP − ICP = CPP). When the CPP falls below 60 mm Hg, there is danger of irreversible ischemia and further secondary damage (Walleck 1986).

Hyperventilation generally results in respiratory alkalosis, with pH of up to 7.55 being acceptable. A pH of greater than 7.55 may result in shifting of the oxygen-hemoglobin curve to the right, resulting in potential tissue hypoxia secondary to failure of the hemoglobin to release the oxygen to the tissue. Sources vary, but generally the PaO_2 should be kept above 70 mm Hg to 80 mm Hg (Marshall et al. 1990; Mitchell 1989). Frequent interpretation of arterial blood gases and end-tidal CO_2 from capnometer readings is utilized by the nurse in maintaining $PaCO_2$ in the proper therapeutic range.

Airway Management and Suctioning

Nursing activities include use of airway adjuncts, such as nasopharnyngeal and oral airways, and positioning techniques to maintain the airway. Pulse oximetry may be utilized for ongoing monitoring of O_2 saturation and early identification of desaturation episodes (Andrus 1991; Marshall et al. 1990).

Frequently the neurological patient is at high risk for pneumonia and other respiratory complications secondary to immobility and ineffective airway clearance. A strong association between suctioning episodes and rises in ICP has been established (Boortz-Marx 1985; Hendrickson 1987; Mitchell and Mauss 1978; Parson and Shogun 1984; Rudy, Baun, Stone, and Turner 1986; Shalit and Umansky 1977; Snyder 1983; Tsementzis and Loizou 1982). In order to prevent deleterious changes in ICP, the need for suctioning should be evaluated prior to each suctioning episode. Research is underway to define the most effective presuctioning ventilation protocol. Current practice recommends that the patient be well ventilated with 100% oxygen prior to and following each suction pass to avoid hypoxia, and individual suctioning passes should be limited to no longer than 15 seconds (Andrus 1991; Johanson, Wells, Hoffmeister, and Dungca 1985; Marshall et al. 1991). Additionally, if a monitor is in place, ICP should be monitored during suctioning. If dramatic rises in ICP are noted, the suctioning should be terminated. Lidocaine may be given to suppress the cough reflex, or other pharmocologic agents may be required to sedate the patient prior to suctioning (Donegan and Bedford 1980).

Positioning

The literature regarding positioning patients with acute brain injury has been almost entirely devoted to examining the effects of various body positions on ICP in an attempt to determine whether various body positions cause potentially harmful rises in ICP (Boortz-Marx 1985; Goldberg, Joshi, Moscoso, and Castillo 1983; Hulme and Cooper 1976; Kenning, Toutant, and Saunders 1981; Lee 1989; Lipe and Mitchell 1980; Magnaes 1976; March, Mitchell, Grady, and Winn 1990; Mitchell, Amos, Astley, Johnson, Habermann-Little, Van Inwegan-Scott, and Tyler 1986; Mitchell and Mauss 1978; Mitchell, Ozuna, and Lipe 1981; Nornes and Magnaes 1971; Parson and Wilson 1984; Ropper, O'Rourke, and Kennedy 1982; Rosner and Coley 1986; Shalit and Umansky 1977; Snyder 1983). Implicitly, these studies are examining the demand on the intracranial adaptive system induced by changing position. They have small samples (4 to 30 subjects) and most commonly report only grouped data. Only ICP was measured in the older studies, making it impossible to know the effect of the positioning on cerebral perfusion. Studies that did include individual data have shown considerable individual variability in response to being passively turned and to what has been considered the standard therapeutic head-up position.

Neck flexion and head rotation have shown consistently harmful changes and should be avoided. Neutral head and neck alignment should be maintained whenever possible. Manual holding of the head in neutral position while turning the patient should also be performed because the findings suggest that lateral neck flexion alone may account for the ICP changes (Mitchell et al. 1986). Prone positioning of the patient is also contraindicated (Nornes and Magnaes 1971). Changes in ICP and CPP in response to turning have been highly individualized; therefore, the turning prescription needs to be based on the individual's response to a trial of any position.

While elevation of the head to 15 degrees to 30 degrees has been the standard protocol for patients with head injury and other sources of increased ICP, current research is challenging this position. It had been believed that head elevation reduced ICP by optimizing venous outflow and reducing intracranial CSF volume, but the action was not always therapeutic since ICP was not uniformly reduced. Cerebral perfusion is decreased with head elevation, and CPP may actually be reduced to clinically dangerous levels. Further research on this topic is needed since there are few studies examining changes in CPP with head position and therefore no prescriptive information to guide practice. Currently, head position should be modified to achieve optimal neurological status and ICP and CPP readings, with an exception for patients with identified perfusion problems (such as vasospasm) whose optimal head position will probably be minimally elevated or supine for the purpose of enhancing blood delivery.

Fluid Balance

The use of fluid restriction and osmotic or loop-active diuretics is advocated in treating intracranial hypertension. Osmotic agents remove fluid from cerebral tissue via an osmotic gradient, while loop-active diuretics such as furosemide or acetazolamide reduce total body fluid volume and may inhibit cerebrospinal fluid production up to 70% (Andrus 1991; Hickey 1986; Littleton 1988; McCabe 1973; Walleck 1989). Potential difficulties are inherent in the use of these therapies. "Rebound" swelling after therapy is discontinued, hyperosmolarity, and renal dysfunction have been noted with use of osmolar diuretics, and electrolyte imbalance or hypovolemia resulting in decreased perfusion to the brain and other body tissues can result when any of these therapies is used (Walleck 1989). The nurse must monitor the patient's vital signs, intake and output, and serum and urine laboratory values for abnormalities or evidence of hypovolemia. It is particularly important to monitor the serum osmolarity since patients with values greater than 320 mOsm may require fluid replacement therapy (Marshall et al. 1990). Central venous pressure or pulmonary artery wedge pressures may also need to be utilized in obtaining an accurate picture of fluid status.

Minimizing Metabolic Demands

A variety of situations can increase the metabolic needs of the brain, resulting in increased waste product accumulation and potential for further cerebral compromise. Hyperthermia increases ICP by elevating the brain's metabolic rate 7% for every Fahrenheit degree increase in body temperature above 100° F (Andrus

1991; Boortz-Marx 1985; Walleck 1986). Body temperature should be monitored, and antipyretic therapy such as aspirin, acetaminophen, cooling blankets, and frequent sponge baths may be indicated (Andrus 1991).

Seizure activity can also increase the brain's metabolic demands, which may in turn alter autoregulation. Tonic-clonic seizure activity may elevate intrathoracic pressure, resulting in decreased venous outflow (Simon 1985). Administration of antiepileptic medication, monitoring drug levels, and observing the patient for seizure activity is indicated. Utilization of an airway management device, administration of supplemental oxygen, and prompt notification of medical staff for potential pharmacologic intervention are necessary.

Barbiturate coma may be instituted to treat intracranial hypertension that has not responded to conventional treatment, such as hyperventilation, dehydration, or surgical decompression. Expected outcomes from use of barbiturate therapy include cerebral vasoconstriction, decreased metabolism, reduced ICP, and preservation of ischemic cerebral cells from irreversible damage by improving and stabilizing the blood supply in the cerebral arterial system (Hickey 1986). Pentobarbital and thiopental are commonly used agents in barbiturate coma induction and maintenance. The patient generally requires ICP monitoring since there is no neurological examination to follow as the patient is "paralyzed" during the therapy. Mechanical ventilation is required. The nurse must monitor the ICP and other vital sign parameters carefully. Frequently, hypotension occurs during induction into barbiturate coma. Erratic dose response to the barbiturate may require ongoing titration of the drug to achieve appropriate blood levels or continuous electroencephalogram (EEG) monitoring to achieve burst suppression of the EEG according to parameters.

Narcotic Sedation

Narcotic sedation may be utilized in an attempt to control agitation, cerebral metabolic rate, and ICP (Walleck 1989). This is used with care because it may depress respiratory activity, resulting in increased $PaCO_2$ from hypoventilation.

Environmental Stimuli Control

In critically ill patients, a variety of "normal" stimuli may be perceived by the injured individual as a noxious stimulus with potentially deleterious effects on ICP and neurological functioning. It is vitally important that nurses caring for these patients have a good understanding of the effects of routine care activities on the individual's ICP and neurological status. Two categories of environmental stimuli encountered in routine patient care are the sequencing of care delivery and sensory stimulation.

Sequencing of Care

Sequencing of care refers to the deliberate design of a series of nursing care activities to include either a planned period of rest or a specified sequence of activities. Presumably an activity that results in a large and relatively sustained increase in ICP creates a new, elevated baseline that could be sustained or further elevated by an otherwise neutral care activity.

The clinical literature recommends temporal spacing between necessary known noxious stimuli, such as endotracheal suctioning and neck rotation, and normally nonnoxious stimuli or use of medical protocols to lower baseline ICP prior to these noxious care activities (Hickey 1986; Kinney, Packa, and Dunbar 1988; Marshall et al. 1990). There is limited evidence for this therapy in terms of clinical studies supporting these recommendations. Only two studies (Bruya 1981; Hugo 1987) have been conducted comparing ICP in patients treated with planned rest periods compared with those with no planned rest periods. The numerous methodological problems in the studies reviewed make it difficult to interpret the findings. The best action continues to be ongoing monitoring of the patient's neurological examination and ICP readings in response to care activities and allowing the examination or ICP findings to return to baseline before initiating another potentially noxious stimulus.

Sensory Stimulation

Deliberate, multimodal sensory input consists of programmatically stimulating the visual, auditory, olfactory, tactile, kinesthetic, and gustatory senses in a standardized fashion. This is intended to improve cognitive function in brain-injured patients and is usually not introduced until the patient is physiologically stable. The stimuli may be introduced in planned, time-limited sessions (45 minutes twice daily) and is continued for the duration of "coma" (Kater 1989). These sessions are reported to have increased cognitive functioning levels at 3 months and a shorter mean duration of coma as compared to controls (Kater 1989; Mitchell, Bradley, Welch, and Britton 1990).

Incidental sensory stimulation encompasses stimulation as it occurs either incidental to ongoing care giving or on a systematic basis to determine if there are physiologically detrimental effects. The effects on ICF of touch, conversation, and family presence have been reported.

There are numerous studies on the effects of touch singly (Mitchell et al. 1985; Pollack and Goldstein 1981; Walleck 1983) and in combination with conversation (Mitchell et al. 1986; Osband, Blackburn, Zuill, Casey, Fahey, and Mitchell 1989; Pollack and Goldstein 1981). Walleck (1983) found a significant decrease in ICP with stroking of the face or hand of head trauma patients, although a later study (Mitchell, Johnson, and Habermann-Little 1985) reported no difference. Considerable variability in response was reported when touching and talking occurred together. The direction of response was a function of the stability of the baseline preceding the episode of touching and talking. When the baseline was stable, little change in ICP occurred with touching and talking. When the baseline was unstable, the conditional probability of the baseline's becoming more stable (and ICP decreasing) was 30%, with the increased stability being 96% sensitive to touch. These findings suggest a therapeutic effect for touching and talking (Mitchell, Johnson, and Habermann-Little 1985). This activity should be individualized to patient response; another study reports ICP increases with stimulation in preterm infants (Osband et al. 1989).

There are anecdotal and descriptive reports of both increases and decreases in ICP associated with bedside conversations (Boortz-Marx 1985; Bruya 1981; Hugo 1985; Mitchell and Mauss 1978; Snyder 1983). Only one experimental study of the effect on conversation on ICP was found (Johnson, Omery, & Nikas 1989). While the overall study was not clinically significant, presentation of individual data once again shows some individuals for whom there were large and sustained increases in ICP during conversation. The authors suggest individual evaluation of patient response to bedside conversation. Family presence (Prins 1989) was studied in relation to ICP changes. Visits were not associated with a particular detrimental or therapeutic effect and should be evaluated individually.

CASE STUDY

Ms. Smith is a 34-year-old white female admitted to University Hospitals with sudden onset of the "worst headache of her life," neck stiffness, and a decreased level of consciousness. A computerized tomography (CT) scan and four-vessel angiogram were performed and revealed subarachnoid hemorrhage from an anterior communicating artery aneurysm. Ms. Smith was taken emergently to the operating room for a right frontotemporal craniotomy and aneurysm clipping. Following surgery, she was extubated and placed in the surgical intensive care unit for monitoring.

Nursing diagnoses for Ms. Smith at this time included potential for Altered (Cerebral) Tissue Perfusion; high risk of secondary brain injury secondary to postoperative swelling or vasospasm; Altered Thought Processes; and altered level of responsiveness.

Ms. Smith's neurological examination at 0800 was remarkable for a slight flattening of the left nasolabial fold, indicating a mild seventh cranial nerve dysfunction, and she was not oriented to place or time, although she could state her home address and name. She was also intermittently agitated, which was treated with PRN narcotic sedation. The remainder of her neurologic examination was normal, with briskly reactive pupils, intact cranial nerve function except for the left seventh, strong grips and leg movements, and absence of a pronator drift. Blood pressure was 152/92, pulse 110, respirations 28, and CVP 8 mm Hg, and the ECG showed a sinus tachycardia without ectopy. A nipride drip was titrated to keep the systolic blood pressure between 140 mm Hg and 160 mm Hg, and the HOB was positioned at 15 degrees to promote cerebral perfusion and venous drainage. She was receiving 5% dextrose in ½ strength normal saline with 20 mEq potassium chloride at 125 cc per hour for fluids and O_2 at 40% face mask, and blood gases were within normal limits. Breath sounds were clear, and O_2 saturation was 97%. The craniotomy dressing was dry and intact, and a Hemovac drain had minimal dark red drainage. Urine output was 200 cc for the previous hour, and the serum potassium was 3.7. The remainder of the physical examination was unremarkable.

Ms. Smith was examined again at 0825 by the staff physician and the nurse with the findings consistent with the 0800 examination. New orders were given to keep her CVP over 10 mm Hg as part of hypervolemic therapy to prevent cerebral vasospasm, and a 500 cc plasmanate bolus was begun. At 0847 Ms. Smith's heart rate dropped into the low 70s, and the monitor showed a junctional rhythm with frequent PVCs and T wave inversion. After consultation with one of Ms. Smith's physicians, a 20 mEq bolus of KCl over 1 hour was begun and a 12-lead ECG ordered. At 0851 Ms. Smith attempted to sit up and stated, "My head hurts." The nurse noted her systolic pressure had risen to the 180s, and widening of the pulse pressure was noted. Recognizing that this was consistent with a Cushing response, the nurse rechecked the neurological examination and paged the physician.

Ms. Smith now had pupils that were 6 mm on the right, 4 mm on the left, and no light reaction or corneal reflex in the right eye. She had no verbalization, did not follow commands, and moved all extremities nonpurposefully to noxious stimuli. Respirations were 24 and shallow. The nurse began hyperventilating Ms. Smith with 100% O_2 at a rate of 30 breaths per minute. At 0905 a 500 cc mannitol bolus was initiated per physician's order. At 0910 pupils were 7/5 and bilaterally nonreactive with absent corneals, and there was minimal flexion to noxious stimuli. A small amount of bright red drainage was now visible on the head dressing on the operative side. Ms. Smith was emergently intubated by the physician, continued to be hyperventilated, and was taken to CT scan, which revealed an epidural hematoma and compression of brain tissue consistent with impending transtentorial herniation. She was taken directly from CT to the operating room for removal of the hematoma.

Because of planned monitoring and quick nursing action, this patient received appropriate medical, diagnostic, and surgical care within minutes of deterioration. After discharge from University Hospitals, Ms. Smith spent several weeks in therapy at a rehabilitation center and is now living at home with minimal supervision as she continues to recover.

SUMMARY

The 1990s were officially recognized as the Decade of the Brain when House Joint Resolution 174 was signed by President George Bush on July 25, 1989. A "call went out to acknowledge the devastation of neurologic disease" (Stewart-Amidei 1990). Intracranial events, including head trauma, stroke, and tumor, continue to strike down large numbers of people. Nurses caring for patients with intracranial disease or trauma have a tremendous responsibility in preventing or minimizing secondary brain injury in order to return the injured individual to a functional role in society. The nursing actions comprising the intervention Secondary Brain Injury Reduction are a vitally important component of the care of any patient with an intracranial disease or event. Ongoing implementation of these actions is imperative since change can occur quickly, leading to potentially catastrophic events such as those outlined in the case study. It is by the ongoing monitoring, early identification of changes, and quick initiation of nursing actions encompassed in Secondary Brain Injury Reduction that nurses will continue to enhance the potential for recovery for all patients with intracranial events.

REFERENCES

Ackerman, L.L. 1991. *Development and validation of selected interventions for neuroscience nursing.* Unpublished master's thesis, University of Iowa, Iowa City.

Ackerman, L.L. In press. Interventions related to neurologic care. *Nursing Clinics of North America.*

Adams, H.P., Jr. 1984. Clinical manifestations and diagnosis of subarachnoid hemorrhage. *Seminars in Neurology* 4(3):304–314.

American Nurses' Association Council on Medical-Surgical Nursing and American Association of Neuroscience Nurses. 1985. *Neuroscience nursing practice: Process and outcome for selected diagnosis.* Kansas City, Mo.: American Nurses' Association.

Andrus, C. 1991. Intracranial pressure: Dynamics and nursing management. *Journal of Neuroscience Nursing* 23(2):85–92.

Arrling, J.K., Thompson, N.M., and Minor, M.E. 1990. Neuropsychological outcome in children with gunshot wounds to the brain. *Journal of Neuroscience Nursing* 19(4):211–215.

Becker, D.P., Miller, J.D., Ward, J.D., Greenberg, R.P., Young, H.F., and Sakalas, R.S. 1977. The outcome from severe head injury with early diagnosis and intensive management. *Journal of Neurosurgery* 47(4):491–502.

Boortz-Marx, R. 1985. Factors affecting intracranial pressure: A descriptive study. *Journal of Neurosurgical Nursing* 17:89–94.

Bruya, M.A. 1981. Planned periods of rest in the intensive care unit: Nursing care activities and intracranial pressure. *Journal of Neurosurgical Nursing* 13:184–194.

Cardosa, E.R., Rowan, J.O., and Galbraith, S. 1983. Analysis of cerebrospinal fluid pulse wave in intracranial pressure. *Journal of Neurosurgery* 59:817–821.

Crigger, N.J., and Strickland, C.C. 1985. Selecting a nursing diagnosis for changes in consciousness. *Dimensions of Critical Care Nursing* 4(3):156–163.

Donegan, M.F., and Bedford, R.F. 1980. Intravenously administered lidocaine prevents intracranial hypertension during endotracheal suctioning. *Anesthesiology* 52:516–518.

Eisenberg, H.M., Cayard, C.A., Papanicolaou, R.L., Franklin, D., Jani, J., Grossman, R., Tabaddor, K., Becker, L.F., and Kunitz, S. 1983. The effects of three potentially preventable complications on outcome after severe closed head injury. In S. Ishi, H. Nugui, and M. Brock (eds.), *Intracranial pressure V* (pp. 549–553). Berlin: Springer-Verlag.

Eisenberg, H.M., Bary, H.E., Aldrich, D.F., Saydjari, D., Turner B., Fourlkes, M.A., Jane, J.A., Marmarou, A., Marshall, L.F., and Young, H.F. 1990. Initial CT findings in 753 patients with severe head injury. *Journal of Neurosurgery* 73:688–698.

Franges, E.Z., and Beiderman, M.E. 1988. Infections related to intracranial pressure monitoring. *Journal of Neuroscience Nursing* 20(2):94–103.

Friedman, W.A., and Vries, J.K. 1980. Percutaneous tunnel ventriculostomy. *Journal of Neurosurgery* 53(5):662–665.

Germon, K. 1988. Interpretation of ICP pulse waves to determine cerebral compliance. *Journal of Neuroscience Nursing* 20:344–349.

Gifford, R.R.M., and Plaut, M.R. 1975. Abnormal respiratory patterns in the comatose patient caused by intracranial dysfunction. *Journal of Neurosurgery Nursing* 7:57–61.

Gilliam, E.W. 1990. Intracranial hypertension: Advances in intracranial pressure monitoring. *Critical Care Nursing Clinics of North America* 2(1):21–27.

Goldberg, R.N., Joshi, A., Moscoso, P., and Castillo, T. 1983. The effect of head position on intracranial pressure in the neonate. *Critical Care Medicine* 11:428–430.

Hendrickson, S.L. 1987. Intracranial pressure changes and family presence. *Journal of Neuroscience Nursing* 19:14–17.

Henneman, E.A. 1989. Clinical assessment and neurodiagnostics. *Critical Care Nursing Clinics of North America* 1(1):131–142.

Hickey, J. 1986. *The clinical practice of neurological and neurosurgical nursing* (2d ed.). Philadelphia: Lippincott.

Hickman, K.M., and Muwaswes, M. 1990. Intracranial pressure monitoring: A review of risk factors associated with infection. *Heart and Lung* 19(1):84–90.

Hugo, M. 1987. Alleviating the effects of care on the intracranial pressure (ICP) of head-injured patients by manipulating nursing care activities. *Intensive Care Nursing:* 3(2):78–82.

Hulme, A., and Cooper, R. 1976. The effects of head position and jugular vein compression on intracranial pressure. In J. Beks, et al. (eds.), *Intracranial pressure III* (pp. 259–263). Berlin: Springer-Verlag.

Jess, L.W. 1987. Assessing your patient for increased ICP. *Nursing 87* 17(6):34–41.

Johanson, B.C., Wells, S.J., Hoffmeister, D., and Dungca, C.U. 1985. *Standards for Critical Care* (3d ed.). St. Louis: CV Mosby.

Johnson, S., Omery, A., and Nikas, D. 1989. Effects of conversation on intracranial pressure in comatose patients. *Heart and Lung* 18:56–63.

Kantor, R.K., Weiner, L.B., Patti, A.M., and Robson, L.K. 1985. Infectious complications and duration of intracranial pressure monitoring. *Critical Care Medicine* 13(10):837–839.

Kater, K.M. 1989. Response of head-injured patients to sensory stimulation. *Western Journal of Nursing Research* 11(1):20–33.

Kenning, J.A., Toutant, S.M., and Saunders, R.L. 1981. Upright positioning in the management of intracranial hypertension. *Surgical Neurology* 15:148–152.

Kinney, M., Packa, D., and Dunbar, S. (eds.). 1988. *AACN clinical reference for critical care nursing* (2d ed.). New York: McGraw-Hill.

Klatzo, I. 1985. Brain oedema following brain ischaemia and the influence of therapy. *British Journal of Anaesthesia* 57:18–22.

Lee, S.T. 1989. Intracranial pressure changes during positioning of patients with severe head injury. *Heart and Lung* 18:411–414.

Lipe, H.P., and Mitchell, P.H. 1980. Positioning the patient with intracranial hypertension: How turning and head rotation affect the internal jugular vein. *Heart and Lung* 9:1031–1037.

Littleton, M.T. 1988. Pathophysiology and assessment of sepsis and septic shock. *Critical Care Nursing Quarterly* 11(1):30–47.

McCabe, W.R. 1973. Serum complement levels in bacteremia due to gram-negative organisms. *New England Journal of Medicine* 288:21–73.

Magnaes, B. 1976. Body position and cerebrospinal fluid pressure. Part I: Clinical studies on the effect of rapid postural changes. *Journal of Neurosurgery* 44:687–697.

McGuffin, J.F. 1983. Basic cerebral trauma care. *Journal of Neurosurgical Nursing* 15(4):183–190.

March, K., Mitchell, P., Grady, S., and Winn, R. 1990. Effect of backrest position on intracranial and cerebral perfusion pressures. *Journal of Neuroscience Nursing* 22:375–381.

Marshall, S.B., Marshall, L.F., Vos, H.R., and Chestnut, R.M. 1990. *Neuroscience critical care: Pathophysiology and patient management.* Philadelphia: WB Saunders.

Mauss, N.K., and Mitchell P.H. 1976. Increased intracranial pressure: An update. *Heart and Lung* 5(6):919–926.

Mayhall, G., Archer, N., Lamb, V.A., Spadora, A.C., Baggett, J.W., Ward, J.D., and Narayan, R.K. 1984. Ventriculostomy related infection: A prospective epidemiologic study. *New England Journal of Medicine* 310(9):553–559.

Miller, J.D. 1977. Significance of intracranial hypertension severe head injury. *Journal of Neurosurgery* 47:503–517.

Miller, J.D. 1985. Head injuries and brain ischaemia. *British Journal of Anaesthesia* 57:120–130.

Miller, J.D., Sweet, R.C., Narayan, R., and Becker, D.P. 1978. Early insults to the injured brain. *Journal of the American Medical Association* 240:439–442.

Mitchell, M. 1989. *Neuroscience nursing: A nursing diagnosis approach.* Baltimore: Williams & Wilkins.

Mitchell, P.H. 1986. Intracranial hypertension: Influence of nursing care activities. *Nursing Clinics of North America* 21(4):563–576.

Mitchell, P.H. 1986. Decreased adaptive capacity, intracranial: A proposal for a nursing diagnosis. *Journal of Neuroscience Nursing* 18:170–175.

Mitchell, P.H., Amos, D., Astley, C., Johnson, F.B., Habermann Little, B., Van Inwegen-Scott, D., and

Tyler, D. 1986. Nursing and ICP: Studies of two clinical problems. In JD Miller et al. (eds.), *Intracranial pressure VI* (pp. 701–703).

Mitchell, P.H., Johnson, F.B., and Habermann-Little, B.H. 1985. Promoting physiologic stability: Touch and ICP. *Communicating Nursing Research* 18:93. (abstract)

Mitchell, P.H., Johnson, F.B., Habermann-Little, B.H., VanInwegen-Scott, D., and Tyler, D. 1985. Critically ill children: The importance of touch in a high technology environment. *Nursing Administration Quarterly* 9(4):38–46.

Mitchell, P.H., and Mauss, N.K. 1978. The relationship of patient and nurse activity to intracranial pressure variations. *Nursing Research* 27:4–10.

Mitchell, P.H., Ozuna, J., and Lipe, H.P. 1981. Moving the patient in bed: Effects of turning and range of motion on intracranial pressure. *Nursing Research* 30:212–218.

Mitchell, S.W., Bradley, V.A., Welch, J.L., and Britton, P.G. 1990. Coma arousal procedure: A therapeutic intervention in the treatment of head injury. *Brain Injury* 4:273–279.

Narayan, R.K., Kishore, P.R.S., Becker, D., Ward, J.D., Enas, G.G., Greenberg, R.P., DaSilva, A.D., Lipper, M.H., Choi, S.C., Mayhall, C.G., Lutz, H.A., and Young, H.F. 1982. Intracranial pressure: To monitor or not to monitor. *Journal of Neurosurgery* 56(5):650–659.

Nornes, H., and Magnaes, B. 1971. Supratentorial epidural pressure recorded during posterior fosse surgery. *Journal of Neurosurgery* 35:541–549.

Osband, B.A. (Foerder), Blackburn, S., Zuill, R., Casey, L., Fahey, D., and Mitchell, P. 1989. Intracranial pressure in preterm infants: Effects of nursing and parental care. In J.T. Hoff and A. Betz (eds.), *Intracranial pressure VII* (pp. 511–513). Berlin: Springer-Verlag.

Parson, L.C., and Shogun, J.S.L. 1984. The effects of the endotracheal tube suctioning/manual hyperventiliation procedures on patients with severe closed head injuries. *Heart and Lung* 13(4):372–380.

Parson, L.C., and Wilson, M.M. 1984. Cerebrovascular status of severe closed head injury patient following passive position changes. *Nursing Research* 33:68–75.

Pettarossi, V.E., DiRocco, C., Mancinelli, R., Calderelli, M., and Vedard, F. 1978. Communicating hydrocephalus induced by mechanically increasing the amplitude of the intraventricular cerebrospinal fluid pulse pressure: Rationale and method. *Experimental Neurology* 59:30–39.

Pfenninger, E.G., Reith, A., Breitig, D., Grunert, A., and Ahnefeld, F.W. 1989. Early changes of intracranial pressure, perfusion pressure and blood flow after severe head injury. *Journal of Neurosurgery* 70:774–779.

Plum, F., and Posner, J. 1980. *The diagnosis of stupor and coma* (3d ed.). Philadelphia: FA Davis Company.

Pollack, L.D., and Goldstein, G.W. 1981. Lowering of intracranial pressure in Reye's syndrome by sensory stimulation (letter). *New England Journal of Medicine* 304:732.

Prins, M.M. 1989. The effect of family visits on intracranial pressure. *Western Journal of Nursing Research* 11(3):281–297.

Rauch, M.E., Mitchell, P.H., and Tyler, M.L. 1990. Validation of risk factors for the nursing diagnosis of decreased intracranial adaptive capacity. *Journal of Neuroscience Nursing* 22:173–178.

Ropper, A.H., O'Rourke, D., and Kennedy, S.K. 1982. Head position, intracranial pressure, and compliance. *Neurology* 32:1288–1291.

Rosner, M., and Coley, I. 1986. Cerebral perfusion pressure, intracranial pressure and head elevation. *Journal of Neurosurgery* 60:636–641.

Rudy, E., Baun, M., Stone, K., and Turner, B. 1986. The relationship between endotrachial suctioning and changes in intracranial pressure: A review of the literature. *Heart and Lung* 15:488–494.

Shalit, N.M., and Umansky, G.W. 1977. Effect of routine bedside procedures on intracranial pressure. *Israeli Journal of Medical Science* 13:881–886.

Simon, R.H. 1985. Management of critical head injuries. *Emergency Care Quarterly* 1(1):40–47.

Snyder, M. 1983. Relation of nursing activities to increases in intracranial pressure. *Journal of Advanced Nursing* 8:273–279.

Stewart-Amidei, C. 1989. Hypervolemic hemodilution: A new approach to subarachnoid hemorrhage. *Heart and Lung* 18(6):590–598.

Stewart-Amidei, C. 1990. Decade of the brain (editorial). *Journal of Neuroscience Nursing* 22(4):205.

Teasdale, G., and Jennett, B. 1974. Assessment of coma and impaired consciousness: A practical scale. *Lancet* 2:81–84.

Tsementzis, P.H., and Loizou, L.A. 1982. The effect of routine nursing care procedures on the ICP in severe head injuries. *Acta Neurochirurgica* 65(3):153–166.

Walleck, C. 1983. The effects of purposeful touch on intracranial pressure (abstract). *Heart and Lung* 12:428–429.

Walleck, C.A. 1986. Pharmacological control of cerebral metabolism. In J. Lundgren (ed.), *Acute neuroscience nursing: Concepts and care* (pp. 55–56). Boston: Jones & Bartlett Publishers.

Walleck, C.A. 1989. Controversies in the management of the head-injured patient. *Critical Care Nursing Clinics of North America* 1(1):67–74.

Wong, J., Wong, S., and Dempster, I.K. 1984. Care of the unconscious patient: A problem oriented approach. *Journal of Neurosurgical Nursing* 16(3):145–50.

43

SHOCK MANAGEMENT

MEG GULANICK
CAROL RUBACK

Recent advances in medicine have necessitated the expansion of the nurse's role in delivery of patient care. Nowhere is this demonstrated more clearly than in the challenging care of a patient in impending or actual shock. Although complication and mortality rates remain persistently high for patients in shock, especially those in cardiogenic shock, chances for a successful outcome are contingent on early recognition and prompt, aggressive therapy. Nurse monitoring of sometimes subtle changes in the patient's hemodynamic status, followed by immediate and appropriate intervention in the presence or absence of the physician, can improve patients' chances of survival.

The acute-care nurse caring for the shock patient must have an armamentarium of knowledge and skills: sound understanding of the pathophysiology of shock and its potential complications, the ability to assess multiple parameters simultaneously, understanding of current treatment modalities and their rationale, and the ability to provide rapid emergency care calmly and deliberately. Shock Management entails a variety of nursing actions — independent as well as collaborative. There are four essential concepts the nurse utilizes in assisting the patient to maintain integrity in this process of survival: providing surveillance, maintaining tissue perfusion, maintaining vital organ function, and providing emotional support.

TYPES OF SHOCK

The circulatory system is made up of the chambers of the heart and the blood vessels. To function properly, there must be adequate blood to fill this system (blood volume), the heart muscle must pump efficiently to keep the blood circulating, and the blood vessels must dilate or constrict appropriately to channel the blood to all vital tissues. If there is significant failure anywhere within this system and perfusion to one vital organ is reduced, a myocardial infarction, stroke, or renal failure may occur. If perfusion to several vital organs is compromised, shock occurs (Bordicks 1980).

Shock as a clinical entity represents inadequate tissue perfusion, resulting in metabolic changes at the cellular level. The subsequent metabolic derangements are most crucial in the cells of the vital organs: the brain, the heart, and the kidneys (Guyton 1981; Wilson 1976). Shock can be classified in several different ways. For our purposes, shock is classified according to its cause: cardiogenic, hypovolemic, or distributive (Lanros 1988; Weil, von Planta, and Rackow 1988).

In cardiogenic shock (CGS), cardiac dysfunction (inability of the heart to pump blood efficiently) is the primary problem. It can result from mechanical, structural, or electrical problems with the heart (Weeks 1986). It is a self-perpetuating condition because the early compensatory mechanism of increased arterial vasoconstriction later becomes a liability for the failing pump. To compensate for the increased afterload, the heart must pump harder, which requires additional coronary artery blood flow. But since the shock has reduced coronary blood flow, the myocardium now becomes even more ischemic, causing further ventricular dysfunction and ischemia (Bordicks 1980).

Hypovolemic shock is caused by a decrease in the circulating blood volume. Usually this is due to a reduction in the intravascular volume relative to the vascular capacity. It is associated with a blood volume deficit of at least 15% to 25% (Wilson 1976; American College of Surgeons 1988). Distributive shock is due to excessive dilation of the blood vessels, resulting in pooling of blood in the peripheral vessels. This category encompasses three types of shock: septic, anaphylactic, and neurogenic.

Whatever the initiating cause of the shock state, the ultimate defect involved is the inadequacy of cardiac output to perfuse vital organs. This results in a chain reaction, beginning with impaired tissue perfusion, anaerobic metabolism, and metabolic acidosis, which leads to increased capillary permeability, cell membrane deterioration, cell death, and organ failure. The body has homeostatic mechanisms to meet this crisis. Initially, as the sympathetic system is stimulated, the heart's rate and force of contraction increase in an attempt to correct the drop in blood pressure and cardiac output. The peripheral blood vessels constrict in order to redistribute blood in priority tissue areas. Both effects may be immediately useful; however, they increase oxygen demands on the heart itself, which may interfere with its normal functioning (Weil, von Planta, and Rackow 1988).

NURSING DIAGNOSES AND TREATMENT GOALS

Regardless of the primary cause of the shock, the patient is at risk for several nursing diagnoses: Fluid Volume Deficit, Decreased Cardiac Output, and Alterated Tissue Perfusion. As the shock state progresses, disturbances in ventilatory status, such as Impaired Gas Exchange or Ineffective Breathing Pattern, may be diagnosed. Other diagnoses commonly seen include Altered Level of Consciousness, and in septic shock, Potential for Infection and Hyperthermia.

The immediate goal in treating shock is to improve tissue perfusion in an effort to maintain vital organ function (Rice 1981). This is best accomplished by determining the underlying cause of the shock state and treating it specifically with appropriate fluids, pharmacologic agents, and adjunctive therapy. The nurse has a crucial role in providing ongoing evaluation of patients' specific responses to these collaborative treatments. There are numerous other independent nursing actions essential in managing shock.

DESCRIPTION OF THE INTERVENTION

Provide Surveillance

The classic description of the shock patient — hypotensive, oliguric, rapid weak pulse, cold clammy skin, restless, and anxious — is easy to recognize. By the time most patients reach this stage, their chances for a successful recovery are limited. Therefore, the nurse needs to be skilled at assessing the earlier signs of shock — those subtle trends and changes that signal potential problems with tissue perfusion. The assessment tools available are clinical findings, laboratory data, and hemodynamic monitoring.

Since the patient is changing constantly, the nurse in attendance at the bedside has a primary role in ongoing surveillance (Cohen 1982). Knowing what to look for, when, and how are basic characteristics of surveillance. Ongoing assessment involves not only observation of the relevant parameters but also the complex process of integrating the information in a meaningful way so as to be useful in guiding nursing actions. There are several specific parameters for surveillance in shock.

Skin Temperature and Color

One of the most immediate, simple, and extremely useful assessments the nurse makes is that of peripheral skin temperature and color. The nurse should check the nail beds for blanching, since a quick return of color suggests adequate tissue oxygen perfusion. In cardiogenic and hypovolemic shock, the profound vasoconstriction that occurs causes the skin to be pale, cool, and diaphoretic. These changes reflect inadequate tissue oxygenation. Cyanosis is a late sign in the shock state. Persistently cold, clammy skin despite fluid and pharmacologic treatment signals the nurse to the need for reevaluation of therapy. In contrast, early septic shock due to generalized vasodilation commonly finds the patient to be warm, pink, and dry, as well as to have an increase in urine output.

Body temperature should be assessed with a rectal probe, not by oral or axillary methods. Most patients in shock are cool to touch secondary to the vasoconstrictive responses. This clinical picture is changed for patients in the early stages of septic shock, for their skin is usually warm and dry.

Mentation

Changes in sensorium or level of consciousness are early manifestations of impending shock. This response is characterized by restlessness, anxiety, and confusion. Serial assessments are critical so the earliest changes or signs of deterioration can be identified.

Blood Pressure

Blood pressure measurements are used frequently to assess the status of the circulating blood volume. However, the measurements can be misleading. For example, in early septic shock, the blood pressure is relatively normal secondary to peripheral shunting. And in cardiogenic or hypovolemic shock, the alpha-stimulating effects of the sympathetic nervous system (vasoconstriction) may produce a near-normal blood pressure. Therefore, arterial hypotension may or may not be an early manifestation of shock.

Nurses need to realize that blood pressure by the ausculatory method usually produces values significantly lower than the central aortic pressure (Robenson-Piano, Holm, and Powers 1987). This "error" or difference is even greater if the patient is peripherally vasoconstricted from physiologic compensatory mechanisms or by vasopressor drug treatment. Therefore, it can be risky for nurses to rely on cuff pressures to guide titration of inotropic and vasopressor drug treatment. While increasing drug dosages to achieve a cuff pressure of 100 mm Hg, the central pressure may increase to much more than 100 mm Hg. For some patients, such as those in cardiogenic shock, a systolic pressure greater than 100 mm Hg puts increased demands on the heart, further compromising the cardiac output.

Because of the unreliability of the cuff, direct intra-arterial monitoring of pressures should be instituted as soon as possible. Once monitoring is initiated, the nurse needs to monitor the patient for the potential hazards associated with such hemodynamic monitoring: infection, bleeding, and air embolism.

Several important measurements can be derived from an accurate blood pressure reading. The mean arterial pressure provides information about the overall perfusion pressure to the tissues and organs. The pulse pressure (the difference between systolic and diastolic pressures) provides an estimate of the heart's stroke volume or pumping ability. Pulse pressure generally narrows in shock since the systolic pressure falls more rapidly than the diastolic pressure. In fact, diastolic pressure initially increases secondary to vasoconstriction. The body generally needs a systolic pressure of 80 mm Hg to 90 mm Hg for optimal perfusion. A fall below 80 mm Hg generally indicates inadequate coronary blood flow.

The nurse needs to be cognizant of the patient's normal blood pressure so that future changes can be assessed more accurately. The patient must be assessed simultaneously for mentation changes and signs of oliguria. If these signs are not present and a slight reduction in baseline pressure is being well tolerated, then the low readings should not be aggressively treated. Similarly, in patients who were previously hypertensive, a fall of 30 mm Hg or more systolic accompanied by clinical signs of impaired tissue perfusion may require treatment. Since the patient in shock is changing constantly, the nurse must be alert for the earliest changes that may signal danger.

Pulses

The pulse rate of hypotensive patients is usually rapid — an adaptive mechanism to optimize cardiac output. However, significant and persistent tachycardia reduces the filling time of the heart and increases myocardial oxygen demands — both of which can lead to reduced cardiac output and subsequent inadequate tissue perfusion if left unchecked.

The nurse must evaluate both central and peripheral pulses regularly to detect critical changes in the patient's hemodynamic status. Palpation of the central pulses (femoral, carotid) provides valuable information about stroke volume and arterial pressure. Weak, thready pulses require treatment. Assessment of peripheral pulses provides data on the amount of vasoconstriction, which indicates impaired peripheral perfusion. The need for early detection of subtle changes is vitally important.

The pulses need to be monitored for at least 30 seconds to determine the presence of arrhythmias, and the patient should be placed on continuous electrocardiographic (ECG) monitoring as soon as possible. Tachycardia or bradycardia and frequent ectopic beats can compromise cardiac output further and must be treated promptly according to medical orders or protocols (Standards and Guidelines 1986).

The nurse also should take routine 12-lead ECGs to monitor for signs of myocardial ischemia (ST-T wave changes) or frank infarction patterns (Q waves) occurring from reduced coronary blood flow.

Invasive Hemodynamic Monitoring

Hemodynamic monitoring is essential for accurately assessing the filling pressures of the heart (preload) in critically ill patients (Davis and Silverman 1984). Central venous pressure (CVP) catheters inserted into the vena cava or right atrium provide information on the circulating fluid volume and thus on the ability of the right side of the heart to handle fluid challenges. Low CVP readings indicate hypovolemia. However, CVP pressures are not accurate indicators of left ventricular filling pressures. Although fluid challenges may be required to assess the cardiovascular response to increased fluid volume, it can be risky giving intravenous (IV) fluid therapy without first assessing the left side of the heart.

Flow-directed balloon-tipped (Swan-Ganz) catheters, which can be positioned in the pulmonary artery, can be easily inserted at the bedside. The nurse needs to anticipate their use and be prepared to assist promptly with their insertion (Woods 1976). These catheters monitor pulmonary artery end diastolic pressures, as well as pulmonary capillary wedge pressures (PCWP). In the absence of mitral valve disease, these measurements provide the most accurate evaluation of the preload of the left ventricle. In healthy individuals, the normal range is 4 mm Hg to 12 mm Hg. Lower values indicate hypovolemia; higher values around 30 mm Hg indicate pulmonary congestion and left ventricular impairment. However, for acutely ill patients, especially those with significant left ventricular impairment, a higher filling pressure, or wedge pressure of at least 18 mm Hg to 20 mm Hg, is usually required for maintaining an optimal cardiac output (Dossey 1984; Forrester, Diamond, Chatterjee, and Swan 1976; Weeks 1986).

Swan-Ganz catheters also provide indirect determination of cardiac output, information useful when evaluating response to therapeutic measures.

Urine Output

The shock state is associated with reduced renal blood flow and the subsequent decrease in urine formation. Inadequate renal perfusion is reflected in oliguria (less than 30 cc urine per hour). If it is uncompensated, renal damage will occur. Even when vital signs return to normal, it is important for the nurse to continue monitoring urine output, since continuing oliguria is a feature of impending renal shutdown.

It is imperative that the nurse insert a Foley catheter early so that hourly trends in urine output can be monitored. Laboratory studies of urine specific gravity and osmolality are indicated, as well as serum tests of blood urea nitrogen (BUN) and creatinine for evaluation of renal status.

Respirations

In general, the body responds to tissue hypoxia with both rapid and shallow respirations. In the presence of tachypnea, the nurse must auscultate for crackles and wheezes and monitor arterial blood gases.

Arterial Blood Gases

Measurement of arterial blood gases provides needed information about the adequacy of both gas exchange and acid-base balance. The nurse must be knowledgeable of normal parameters and report immediately any significant deviations. Hypoxemia (low O_2) can contribute to cardiac arrhythmias. Metabolic acidosis (low pH) is expected due to anaerobic metabolism and lactic acid production. Metabolic or lactic acidosis impairs the contractility of the heart and inactivates most vasoactive drugs (Standards and guidelines 1986). Respiratory acidosis (low pH secondary to elevated CO_2) decreases the availability of oxygen to the tissues and needs to be treated with improved ventilatory methods. The pH must be maintained within the 7.35 to 7.45 range. Metabolic alkalosis (high pH) is a problem too, occurring usually from overzealous treatment with sodium bicarbonate or from use of citrated bank blood. Bicarbonate levels should be held within 15 mEq/L to 18 mEq/L.

Most acid-base imbalances correct spontaneously once tissue perfusion is restored and adequate ventilation is maintained. If the acidosis is severe and persistent, sodium bicarbonate can be administered. The nurse nevertheless should use caution when administering sodium bicarbonate, which can lead to alkalosis when tissue perfusion improves.

Maintain Tissue Perfusion

The basic defect in shock from any cause is a decrease in tissue perfusion; therefore, many of the nursing actions used to treat shock are the same despite different etiologies.

Position

The nurse places the patient into a position that will facilitate both perfusion to vital organs and ventilation. The ideal position is supine. This position provides adequate blood flow to the brain and promotes venous return from the brain to the heart. If the patient is hypovolemic, the nurse may elevate the patient's legs slightly in order to mobilize fluids. However, the patient should not be placed in the Trendelenburg position; although blood flow to the brain will be increased, venous return of blood to the heart will be impeded. This causes the blood to pool in the brain, resulting in tissue hypoxia. Additionally, the Trendelenburg position can interfere with ventilation because gravity will push the abdominal organs upward against the diaphragm. For the patient experiencing respiratory distress, the nurse can elevate the head of the bed slightly to facilitate ventilation. Turning the patient frequently prevents pooling of secretions and also improves ventilation. The nurse must determine the priority needs of the patient: ventilation or perfusion.

Ventilation and Oxygenation

Shock results in hypoperfusion of cells and resultant tissue hypoxia. The nurse intervenes promptly to optimize the patient's state of oxygenation, positioning as described, suctioning to remove secretions, and inserting a nasogastric tube into the patient's stomach to prevent aspiration of stomach contents.

Once the airway has been established, supplemental oxygen must be administered. The patient in shock has an increased need for oxygen to offset the hypoperfusion and increased metabolic state. If previous actions are not effective, the patient may require tracheal intubation and mechanical ventilation to maintain oxygenation. Nursing management of such patients is discussed in Chapter 40.

Volume Replacement

The patient in hypovolemic shock needs fluid replacement immediately, and restoring blood volume is the priority. The physician determines the appropriate fluid for replacement based on the source of fluid loss and the patient's clinical condition. Two large-bore intravenous catheters should be inserted and a balanced solution such as Ringer's lactate rapidly infused. Normal saline and dextrose solution should never be given to the hypovolemic patient, as they are hypotonic solutions and may lead to water intoxication (Bordicks 1980; Lanros 1988; Thompson 1977). Colloid volume expanders such as albumin, dextran, and hetastarch are effective hypertonic solutions. They may be useful in patients with normal or excessive total body water but with intravascular dehydration. These fluids increase the osmolality of intravascular fluid, drawing interstitial fluid into the vascular space. As a result, the circulating blood volume is expanded.

The volume replacement of choice in the hemorrhagic patient with a hematocrit level of less than 35% is blood and blood components. Type-specific crossmatched packed red blood cells (PRBC) are preferred. Universal-donor, blood type O can be given emergently and is relatively safe (Lanros 1988). PRBC are preferred over whole blood in both type-specific and universal donor transfusion because they reduce the risk of transfer of donor antibodies.

Warming the blood prior to transfusion of large amounts of blood is generally recommended (Lanros 1988). Multiple transfusions of unwarmed blood are associated with cardiac arrhythmias.

Packed red blood cells do not contain the normal clotting factors; when multiple transfusions are given, the patient's own clotting factors are diluted. Properly crossmatched fresh frozen plasma and packed platelets should be given to patients receiving more than 10 units of packed red blood cells to prevent coagulopathy (Lanros 1988; Wilson 1976).

It is essential for the nurse to have an understanding of the character of the prescribed fluid therapy and its effects in order to evaluate the patient's response to treatment. The nurse carefully records the type and amount of fluid and the effect on the patient.

Once blood volume replacement has been initiated, the source of the bleeding or fluid loss should be found and stopped. If no obvious bleeding points are found, occult bleeding must be considered, especially with patients with pelvic and femur fractures and those having undergone invasion of a major vessel for any reason (e.g., cardiac catheterization procedure).

Medication Therapy

Several types of drugs are used to treat shock. The nurse assumes responsibility for titrating the administration of these powerful medications to regulate vital signs within established parameters.

Inotropic Agents

In the normovolemic patient in shock, the physician may order an inotropic agent such as dobutamine, amrinone, or low-dose dopamine to optimize cardiac output and hence, oxygen delivery (Shoemaker, Kram, and Appel 1990) (Table 43–1). They are one of the main therapies for patients in cardiogenic shock associated with reduced myocardial contractility. The acute-care nurse should use caution when administering these agents to patients with minimal cardiac reserve

TABLE 43 – 1. EFFECTS OF INOTROPIC AGENTS

Dobutamine: Has a positive inotropic effect that increases stroke volume and cardiac output. Reduces afterload by decreasing peripheral vasoconstriction, also resulting in higher cardiac output.

Dopamine: In low- and medium-range doses, has a positive inotropic and chronotropic effect on the heart, which improves stroke volume and cardiac output. Low-dose dopamine also enhances renal blood flow, thus improving renal output. Dopamine, however, greatly increases myocardial demand for oxygen. High doses of dopamine can cause peripheral vasoconstriction and can be arrhythmiogenic.

Amrinone: Similar effects as dobutamine but with a different mechanism of action; therefore, some patients may respond better to amrinone than to dopamine. It has both a positive inotropic and peripheral vasodilation effect to improve cardiac output.

Note: Drugs may be used in combination for enhanced effect.

or coronary artery disease since these medications increase the myocardial oxygen demand (Underhill, Woods, Froelicher, and Halpenney 1990).

Additionally, the use of these agents can be disastrous in hypovolemic patients since they cause vasodilation, which can lead to dangerous hypotension. This reaction can be prevented and even reversed with administration of fluid.

Diuretics

Diuretics may be helpful in maintaining renal function once blood volume deficits are corrected. Diuretics also are used to remove excess extravascular fluid associated with heart failure in cardiogenic shock.

Vasopressors

The patient should receive vasopressors only as a last resort (Lanros 1988; Shoemaker, Kram, and Appel 1990; Thompson 1977; Wilson 1976). When the patient is in shock, compensatory neurohormonal mechanisms are maximally activated to produce vasoconstriction, which maintains blood pressure, and to shunt blood away from nonessential tissues to the heart, brain, and working muscle. As this maldistribution of blood flow continues and tissues become anoxic, the shock state worsens and becomes irreversible. The use of vasopressors hastens and worsens this process. Exceptions to the precaution of vasopressors include patients with compromised coronary or cerebral blood flow secondary to atherosclerosis (Lanros 1988; Shoemaker, Kram, and Appel 1990; Thompson 1977). These individuals may benefit from the increased perfusion pressure produced by a vasopressor.

Vasodilators

Vasodilators increase cardiac output by decreasing the resistance (afterload) to ejection of blood from the left ventricle. They may be beneficial in the treatment of shock by improving the delivery of oxygen to anoxic tissues. For patients in cardiogenic shock, the use of vasodilators in conjunction with inotropic agents will enhance the pumping ability of the heart. Vasodilators must be used cautiously in hypotensive patients, however, and any hypovolemia should be corrected before administration.

The nurse has a critical role in maintaining parameters at prescribed levels. According to protocols and based on her assessments and judgment, the nurse may titrate inotropic, vasodilator, and/or diuretic medications along with fluid challenges to maintain the fragile balance between over- and underhydration.

Antiarrhythmics

Although cardiac arrhythmias are not usually the precipitating cause of shock, they can severely aggravate an already existing low output state. Therefore, the nurse needs to intervene appropriately according to unit protocol.

Antibiotics

For septic patients, antibiotics must be initiated to treat the infection, usually caused by the release of gram-negative bacilli into the blood. The nurse collects specimens for culturing and drug sensitivities and monitors the patient for drug reactions. The nurse should, if indicated, anticipate the removal of the source of infection, either surgically or at the bedside.

Additional Medication

Benadryl and epinephrine are used in the treatment of anaphylactic shock to counteract the massive effects of histamine and bradykinin release, resulting in bronchospasm and dilation of peripheral blood vessels.

Corticosteroids in physiological doses, such as hydrocortisone 100 mg, are beneficial as replacement therapy in patients with clinical or subclinical adrenal insufficiency. Their use in pharmacological doses (large doses) remains controversial (Lanros 1988). The beneficial effect that corticosteroids produce is related to their membrane stabilizing ability (Thompson 1977).

Counterpulsation

Counterpulsation, through the use of an intra-aortic balloon pump, is another therapeutic modality used in cardiogenic shock to enhance the heart as a pump. The use of an intra-aortic balloon pump is confined to critical care units because of the high degree of technical monitoring and skill required (McHenry and Schultz 1986).

Regulate Vital Body Functions

Temperature

Typically in shock, the body's compensatory mechanisms are fully activated, causing peripheral vasoconstriction and resultant cool skin. However, the nurse should never apply external heat to such a patient. Applying heat causes vasodilation, which leads to a decrease in the blood pressure. Additionally, an elevation of body temperature of 1°C increases the body metabolism by 7%. Any increase in metabolism increases the need for oxygen and the production of carbon dioxide, worsening the state of shock. However, in situations where the patient is shivering (the body's way of increasing internal temperature by muscle contractions), the nurse *should* apply heat. External heat such as a lightweight blanket will not increase the metabolic rate as much as shivering. In the septic febrile patient, the nurse administers antipyretics to maintain normothermia and prevent the hypermetabolism caused by fever.

Nutrition

The nurse acts to ensure that the patient's nutritional needs are met. The patient in shock requires supplemental nutrition because of the hypermetabolism and increased catabolism that occur. However, the patient will not be able to consume or digest food normally. The preferred route of supplemental nutrition in all cases of shock is enteral rather than parenteral (Kuhn 1990). Enteral nutrition maintains the structure and function of the gastrointestinal tract and prevents the translocation of gastrointestinal flora, which can lead to septicemia. Another advantage of enteral alimentation is the avoidance of the risk of infection associated with the intravenous catheter necessary for parenteral nutrition. If the patient cannot take nutrients orally, a nasoduodenal feeding tube can be placed for short-term or a jejunostomy tube for long-term use (Kuhn 1990). If the gastrointestinal tract cannot be used, parenteral nutrition may be necessary. The patient should begin to receive supplemental nutrition via either route within 36 hours of admission.

Provide Emotional Support

The priority in caring for the patient in actual or impending shock must be directed first toward prompt recognition and diagnostic investigation of inadequacies in vital organ perfusion and then to implementation of appropriate therapeutic modalities. The acute-care nurse must also understand how critical it is to focus on the whole patient: to render "emergency care" to the patient's emotional and spiritual needs, as well as to those of significant others. This can be accomplished in several ways. Nurses need to display intelligent nursing action in a calm, confident manner so both patients and family feel secure in the care rendered during this stressful time. If the patient is alert, the nurse needs to explain the purpose for the myriad tubes, monitors, and machines that may suddenly be attached to the patient. Finally, the patient must be assured that the close continuous monitoring being provided ensures prompt action. When specific procedures are undertaken (tracheal intubation, invasive monitoring, etc.), the nurse must discuss the rationale for these procedures as appropriate. Health professionals should avoid unnecessary technical conversations about equipment and therapeutics when near patients so as not to increase patients' apprehension.

Emotional needs can be addressed by identifying and utilizing support systems available to the patient (family, significant other, clergy, psychiatric liaison staff). When the patient is hemodynamically stable, staff should encourage selective visiting by family members and significant others, which may assist the patient in coping with this stressful situation.

Nurses also need to be cognizant of the special needs of family members, such as honest and frequent information about the patient's status and prognosis, mechanisms by which they can contact physicians and nurses, and reassurances that their family member is receiving optimal care (Hickey 1990).

The four components of the intervention Shock Management have been summarized in a protocol, which appears in Table 43–2.

CASE STUDY

Mr. H is a 70-year-old man recovering on the cardiac stepdown unit from an acute anterior myocardial infarction that occurred 4 days ago. He suddenly complains of chest pressure and shortness of breath. The nurse notes that he is pale, and his skin is cool and damp. His blood pressure is 94/76 mm Hg (normal for him is 140/70); his pulse is weak at 120 min and irregular. The ECG monitor shows premature ventricular beats and ST segment elevation in the anterior V leads. His breathing is rapid at 32 breaths per minute; new crackles are heard upon auscultation. The nurse administers supplemental oxygen at 4 L/min, positions him supine with the head of the bed slightly elevated, and calls for assistance. Next, the nurse inserts a large-bore intravenous catheter

TABLE 43–2. NURSING PROTOCOL FOR MANAGEMENT OF ACUTE SHOCK

Provide surveillance
Perform ongoing assessments
    Skin color, temperature, moisture
    Mental status
    Hemodynamic parameters (BP, HR, CVP, PAP, PCWP)
    Heart rhythm, ECG changes
    Respiratory rate, rhythm
    Nutritional status
    Presence of frank or occult blood
Monitor lab results: Hgb/crit; serum and urine electrolytes and osmolality, BUN, creatinine
Insert Foley catheter; monitor intake and output
Monitor ABGs and acid-base balance
Monitor response to treatment
Keep physician informed of change in status

Maintain tissue perfusion
Place patient in optimal position, usually supine; turn and reposition every 2 hours; suction as needed
Initiate oxygen therapy as prescribed
Maintain hemodynamics within prescribed parameters
Initiate and maintain aggressive fluid therapy as ordered
For hypovolemic shock with low hematocrit, keep crossmatched blood available
Initiate and titrate drug therapy as ordered or by protocol (inotropes, vasodilators, vasopressors,
    etc.); for septic shock, initiate antibiotics as ordered
Treat arrhythmias according to protocol or order
Anticipate and assist with adjunct therapies within prescribed protocol (mechanical ventilation,
    counterpulsation, etc.)

Maintain vital body function
Regulate body temperature
Give enteral or parenteral feedings as ordered

Provide emotional support
Ensure continuity of care
Deliver competent care in a calm, professional manner
Initiate patient/family education as appropriate
Facilitate involvement of the patient's significant support system

---

and infuses fluids at a keep-open rate in anticipation of medication administration.

The nurse correctly identifies Mr. H's problem as myocardial ischemia, causing pump failure and impending cardiogenic shock, a situation requiring immediate action. The nurse intervenes in the early stages of shock by positioning Mr. H for optimal tissue perfusion and ventilation, administering supplemental oxygen to enhance oxygen delivery to the peripheral tissues and myocardium, and initiating IV fluids.

Next, the nurse mobilizes the health care team; the decision is made to transfer Mr. H to the coronary care unit for further management. In this setting, Mr. H continues to complain of chest pain. His blood pressure is now 90/60, and a 12-lead ECG confirms extension of his myocardial infarction. He is given the prescribed analgesic. Mr. H is anxious and concerned. The critical care nurse maintains a calm, professional manner and explains the need for specialized equipment and procedures. She tries to relieve Mr. H's anxiety as much as possible, for anxiety will cause further catecholamine release and vasoconstriction, which would increase his cardiac demands. The nurse hangs a continuous dobutamine infusion to optimize cardiac output and inserts a Foley catheter to monitor his urine output. Low-dose dopamine is started to improve renal perfusion. The critical care nurse assists with insertion of a Swan-Ganz catheter, used to evaluate the filling pressures in the heart. On its insertion, Mr. H's pressures are markedly elevated (PCWP = 26 mm Hg). The nurse titrates his dose of dobutamine upward, and amrinone is added in an effort to increase his cardiac output further. IV Lasix is given to promote diuresis of excessive pulmonary extravascular fluid. Mr. H responds to these measures with lower pulmonary artery and capillary wedge pressures and an increase in his urinary output. Despite optimal pharmacological therapy, however, Mr. H remains hypotensive with cool extremities and continues to complain of chest pain. The cardiologist elects to insert an intra-aortic balloon. Once the nurse connects it to the pump, Mr. H's chest pain is relieved, and his vital signs stabilize. Because Mr. H's condition has improved, the nurse starts to titrate the inotropic agents downward so that the myocardial oxygen demand will be reduced.

In collaboration with the physician and other members of the health team, the nurses in this situation used both assessment skills and expert judgment in correctly identifying critical actions needed to treat Mr. H. Their prompt, aggressive treatment improved Mr. H's chance of survival.

CONCLUSION

Shock is a devastating syndrome with dire consequences. This condition may be reversible if an accurate diagnosis is made early and aggressive shock management is implemented immediately. Because of their constant presence at the bedside, acute-care nurses play a prominent role in providing surveillance, alerting the health team members when indicated, and initiating further Shock Management modalities as needed. At the same time, these nurses attend to the psychosocial needs of both the critically ill patient and significant others. Shock Management presents a true challenge to the professional nurse.

REFERENCES

American College of Surgeons Committee on Trauma. 1988. *Advanced trauma life support (ATLS) student manual.* Chicago: American College of Surgeons.

Bordicks, K. 1980. *Patterns of shock: Implications for nursing care* (2d ed). New York: Macmillan.

Cohen, S. 1982. Nursing care of patients in shock (Programmed instruction): Part 3: Evaluating the patient. *American Journal of Nursing* 82:1723–1746.

Davis, S., and Silverman, B. 1984. Hemodynamic monitoring. In C. Guzzetta and B. Dossey (eds.), *Cardiovascular nursing: Mindbody tapestry.* St. Louis: C.V. Mosby.

Dossey, B. 1984. The person in cardiogenic shock. In C. Guzetta and B. Dossey (eds.), *Cardiovascular nursing: Mindbody tapestry.* St. Louis: C.V. Mosby.

Forrester, J., Diamond, G., Chatterjee, K., and Swan, H. 1976. Medical therapy of acute myocardial infarction by application of hemodynamic subsets (part 1 of 2). *New England Journal of Medicine* 295:1356–1362.

Forrester, J., Diamond, G., Chatterjee, K., and Swan, H. 1976. Medical therapy of acute myocardial infarction by application of hemodynamic subsets (part 2 of 2). *New England Journal of Medicine* 295:1404–1413.

Guyton, A. (ed). 1981. *The textbook of medical physiology.* Philadelphia: W.B. Saunders.

Hickey, M. 1990. What are the needs of families of critically ill patients? A review of the literature since 1976. *Heart and lung* 19:401–415.

Kuhn, N. 1990. Nutritional support for the shock patient. Review article. *Critical Care Nursing Clinics of North America* 2:201–220.

Lanros, N. 1988. *Assessment and intervention in emergency nursing* (3d ed.). Norwalk, Conn.: Appleton & Lange.

McHenry, L., and Schultz, M. 1986. Cardiac assist devices. In L. Weeks (ed.), *Advanced cardiovascular nursing.* Boston: Blackwell Scientific Publications.

Rice, V. 1981. Shock: A clinical syndrome. Part IV: Nursing intervention. *Critical Care Nurse* 1:34–43.

Robenson-Piano, M., Holm, K., and Powers, M. 1987. An examination of the differences that occur between direct and indirect blood pressure measurement. *Heart and Lung* 16:285–294.

Shoemaker, W., Kram, H., and Appel, P. 1990. Therapy of shock based on pathophysiology, monitoring, and outcome prediction. *Critical Care Medicine* 18:S19–S25.

Standards and guidelines for cardiopulmonary resuscitation (CPR) and emergency cardiac care (ECC). 1986. *Journal of the American Medical Association* 255:2841–3044.

Thompson, W.L. 1977. The patient in shock (A clinical discussion from the proceedings of a symposium). Kalamazoo: Upjohn Co.

Underhill, S., Woods, S., Froelicher, E.S., and Halpenney, C.J. 1990. *Cardiovascular medications for cardiac nursing.* Philadelphia: J.B. Lippincott.

Weeks, Lin (ed.). 1986. Heart failure. In L. Weeks (ed.), *Advanced cardiovascular nursing.* Boston: Blackwell Scientific Publications.

Weil, M., von Planta, M., and Rackow, E. 1988. Acute circulatory failure (shock). In E. Braunwald (ed.), *Heart disease.* Philadelphia: W.B. Saunders, 1988.

Wilson, R. (ed.). 1976. *Principles and techniques of critical care.* Kalamazoo: Upjohn Co.

Woods, S. 1976. Monitoring pulmonary artery pressures. *American Journal of Nursing* 76:1765–1771.

DIALYSIS THERAPY

MARGERY O. FEARING
LAURA K. HART

Dialysis Therapy is a treatment prescribed for patients diagnosed with renal failure. The process of dialysis, whereby solutes and fluids are removed from a solution by use of diffusion and osmosis, was demonstrated as early as 1914. Technical advances and clinical research undertaken from 1940 to the mid-1960s successfully demonstrated that a person diagnosed as having renal failure did not automatically receive a death sentence. Instead, hemodialysis and peritoneal dialysis could be utilized as therapies to sustain the life of a person for months and even years (Fearing 1967; Hoffert 1989).

Both hemodialysis and peritoneal dialysis therapy require that essential nursing care center on actions that address the following: preparing patients for treatments, management of technology, and monitoring the treatment and possible complications. The chronicity of this treatment requires life-style adjustments by patients and their families. Therefore, it is important to maintain a collaborative role with not only the patient and family but with a circle of health team members —the physician, social worker, dietitian, and technicians—so that plans of care can be developed (Fearing 1973; Lancaster 1986; Richard 1986). This chapter focuses on the care for patients undergoing hemodialysis and peritoneal dialysis therapy.

CLIENT GROUPS

Every year 1 in 10,000 persons in the United States experiences end-stage renal disease and chronic glomerulonephritis, nephrosclerosis, chronic reflux nephropathy, diabetes, and polycystic kidney. The incidence of renal disease is four and a half times higher in the black population (Brunner, Wing, Dykes, Brynger, Fassbinder, and Selwood 1989).

Acute renal failure is a relatively common syndrome. Although the incidence in the general population is not known, one study found 5% of patients on a medical surgical unit in a general hospital had episodes of acute renal failure. Approximately 60% of these cases related to surgery or trauma. Half of the cases of acute renal failure appear to be iatrogenic (Grantham 1982). Acute renal failure is usually the result of a toxic, acute inflammatory or ischemic process. The origin of the causative condition may be prerenal, intrarenal (parenchymal), or postrenal (Anderson and Schrier 1985).

Chronic renal failure is not a specific disease, so its etiology is often obscure. The term refers to any situation that causes a permanent renal dysfunction sufficient to cause significant chemical abnormalities. As renal function decreases, clinical disease develops from the retention of substances normally excreted by the kidneys, the loss of substances normally retained by the kidneys, and compensatory responses to lost function. When chronic renal failure is severe enough to cause uremia, the condition is referred to as end-stage kidney or end-stage renal disease (ESRD).

Uremia is a clinical syndrome of systemic disorders that involves multiple organs precipitated by advanced renal failure. The uremic syndrome becomes clinically apparent after 90% of the functioning nephron population is lost, and it quickly leads to death unless dialysis is utilized or a kidney transplant is received. It is generally thought that the pathogenesis of uremia occurs due to the retention of toxic metabolite products called the uremic toxins; however, no one toxin has been identified as the basic factor causing uremia. The accumulation of nitrogenous metabolites constitutes only one facet of this complex condition to which malnutrition, anemia, acidosis, water and electrolyte imbalance, hypertension, and circulatory insufficiency may contribute (Robbins, Catran, and Kumar 1984; Vanholder, Schoots, and Ringoir 1989).

Patients with renal failure can be treated by dialysis until a reversible condition is corrected or as a lifelong treatment. Currently about 80,000 persons in the United States with ESRD are being treated with dialysis. About 20% of this population are receiving their dialysis treatments at home (Brunner et al. 1989). Dialysis is usually initiated when the glomerular filtration rate (GFR) falls below 5 mL/min, the blood urea nitrogen is above 99 mg/100mL, creatinine is greater than 10 mg/100 mL, and the patient is experiencing progressive uremic symptoms such as nausea, vomiting, anorexia, lethargy, pruritis, and fatigue. The presence of pericarditis, progressive peripheral neuropathy, severe acidosis, and severe electrolyte and fluid imbalances also indicate the need for dialysis (Brenner, Dworkin, and Ichikawa 1986; Delano 1989).

RELATED NURSING DIAGNOSES

Dialysis therapy is initiated to correct the priority problems of fluid, electrolyte, and acid-base imbalance subsequent to renal failure (Hart, Reese, and Fearing 1981). The 1986 NANDA nursing diagnoses associated with these problems include: Fluid Volume Excess, Altered Cardiac Perfusion, Ineffective Breathing Pattern, and Sensory/Perceptual Alterations (All senses). Other possible diagnoses currently not listed by NANDA could include Altered Nutrition; Potential for More Than Body Requirements, Acid-Base Disturbance, and Electrolyte Disturbance.

Additional problems related to unavoidable dependency imposed by this treatment modality include body image disturbance, social isolation, reduced productivity, and psychological immobility. The nursing diagnoses associated with these problems are Body Image Disturbance, Powerlessness, Social Isolation, and Diversional Activity Deficit related to changes in life-style.

Body Image Disturbance often surfaces because of loss of body function, changes in physical appearance, reduced energy, and an inability to fulfill expected social roles. Signs and symptoms that present with this diagnosis are denial of limitations or life changes, not accepting self-care responsibilities, noncompliance, increased dependency, and feelings of uselessness, anger, depression, and hostility. The patient's reduced ability to perform activities of daily living or to meet social responsibilities, reduced financial income, extensiveness of treatment regimen, and social isolation may contribute to the inference of a diagnosis of Powerlessness. The signs and symptoms that present with this diagnosis are noncompliance, depression, withdrawal, apathy, anxiety, and acting out. The patient's activity intolerance, fatigue, reduced social role, and anxiety and the regimen's time commitment support the inference of the diagnosis of Social Isolation. Patients with this diagnosis may have reduced social interaction and activity, reduced decision-making ability, and feelings of anger, anxiety, depression, loneliness, and abandonment. Depression, fatigue, lengthy treatments, and loss of ability to perform work, social, and leisure activities support the inference of a diagnosis of Diversional Activity Deficit related to change in life-style. Patients with this diagnosis may appear distinterested and withdrawn and express feelings of boredom, monotony, uselessness, restlessness, depression, inactivity, anger, and hostility.

The kidney function deficit, even with the treatment of dialysis, continues to produce problems with fatigue (anemia), infection (depressed T cell–mediated functions), and pruritis (increased toxins). Compliance, constipation, and sexual dysfunction can also be problems in this patient population. The nursing diagnoses related to these problems include Fatigue or Activity Intolerance, Potential for Infection, Impaired Skin Integrity, Noncompliance, Constipation, and Sexual Dysfunction related to impotence and physiologic limitations.

HEMODIALYSIS PROTOCOL

Access

Hemodialysis requires access to the bloodstream so the patient's blood can be diverted to the extracorporeal circuit within the dialyzer. It is in fact the patient's lifeline, so all nursing activities are directed at maintaining its patency. Access for hemodialysis is of two types: those used on a temporary basis and those used for long-term therapy. Temporary accesses include catheterization of the subclavian and femoral vein and occasionally an arterioventricular (A-V) shunt (Scribner shunt). Temporary access is used for patients who have acute renal failure or are long-term patients awaiting a more permanent access. The femoral catheter is relatively safe and simple to insert but awkward to connect to the dialyzer. Also, because it is difficult to maintain asepsis at the femoral vein, the catheter is usually used only 1 day or 2 days to reduce the risk of infection or venous thrombosis. Subclavian catheterization is more convenient for dialysis connections, and the catheter can be left in place for several treatments. The use of these sites allows the peripheral veins to be reserved for a more permanent access. Insertion of a subclavian catheter requires X-ray confirmation that it is properly placed and that a pneumothorax has not occurred during placement. Patency is maintained by instilling 1000 units of heparin in 1 mL of normal saline solution in the catheter (a heparin lock) between treatments. If the patient has adequate peripheral vessels, an A-V or Scribner shunt (a silastic/Teflon apparatus) can be used. This access provides a direct, external line from an artery back to a vein, making the two blood pathways immediately available. The major disadvantages of the external shunt are the risk of infection, clotting, and possible disconnection (Bell and Veitch 1990).

A fistula provides more permanent vascular access. Usually a side-by-side or an end-to-end fistula between a radial artery and cephalic vein at the wrist is created. The superficial veins become arteriolized and can be repeatedly cannulated with large-bore, 14-gauge to 16-gauge needles. This allows 200 mL/min to 400 mL/

min of blood to be diverted through the arterial needle when a blood pump is used. A fistula may take up to 3 weeks to 4 weeks to develop but has the advantage that no foreign bodies are present and the exit sites are sealed, reducing the risk of infection. Also, no external appliance is present, and clotting is unusual. However, repeated venipunctures and extravasation of blood can result in scarring and fibrosis along the vessel.

Prosthetic grafts are also used to form fistulas. The risk of clot formation in these grafts increases during periods of prolonged hypovolemia and hypotension (Bell and Veitch 1990).

When a temporary femoral access is used, it is usually removed after dialysis and pressure is applied to the site for 5 minutes or longer to stop internal and external bleeding. The site should be monitored for at least 1 hour postdialysis for signs of bleeding. When a subclavian cannula is used, dialysis should not be done until its position has been validated by X ray. The dressing should be kept clean and dry. A Luer lock infusion set should always be used for intravenous infusions. If the cannula slips out, no matter what distance, it should not be pushed back in. The doctor should be called to change the cannula. All clots and residual heparin should be aspirated from the cannula before dialysis, and then it should be flushed with heparinized normal saline. Smooth, guarded clamps should be used to avoid puncturing the silastic tube. When shunts are used, the prepump arterial negative pressure should not exceed -50 mm Hg because the intima of the arterial wall can be damaged. Only a person trained in the technique should declot shunts.

When the access needle is inserted into a fistula, the needle should be inserted bevel down to reduce coring, postdialysis bleeding time, and the need to rotate the needle to improve flow. Puncture sites should be rotated and allowed to heal before reusing.

Procedure

To begin dialysis, the patient's arterial vascular access is entered to allow the blood to flow through blood tubing into the dialyzer. The cleansed blood exits the dialyzer through blood tubing and is returned to the patient's bloodstream by the venous access. A blood pump circulates the blood at 250 mL/minute to 400 mL/min. The blood circuit is a closed system and has three monitors. An arterial pressure monitor indicates if improper arterial access has occurred or if there is poor blood flow in the patient's access. These conditions will be reflected in a low reading. A high arterial reading may indicate clotting, tubing kinks, or that a clamp has inadvertently been left on the blood tubing. The venous monitor gives readings that signal any obstruction causing a cessation of flow to the patient. The third monitor signals the presence of air within the blood circuit. An alarm from any of the three monitors stops the blood pump and applies a clamp to the venous return tubing until the problem is corrected.

Since the blood is in an extracorporeal circuit, in contact with a foreign substance (the dialyzer), it is necessary to use an anticoagulant to prevent clotting. A bolus of heparin (usually 1000 units to 5000 units) is injected at the start of the procedure with either intermittent doses or continuous infusion by an infusion pump. Clotting time is monitored and the heparin dose adjusted. The goal is to prevent clotting within the dialyzer yet not cause the patient to bleed. A 25% increase above the baseline clotting time is usually sufficient for this purpose (Swartz 1990).

The dialysate for hemodialysis is a solution containing electrolytes in amounts that approximate normal extracellular fluid. Although this composition is prescribed by the physician, nurses are responsible for analyzing the laboratory results to determine the effectiveness of the solution. This solution can be tailored to suit the patient's individual need but usually contains sodium 140 mEq/L, potassium 0 mEq/L to 2 mEq/L, calcium 2.5 mEq/L to 3.5 mEq/L, magnesium 1.0 mEq/L, chloride 104 mEq/L, and acetate 38 mEq/L or bicarbonate 35 mEq/L (Stewart 1989). The water used to prepare dialysate must be free of electrolytes, microorganisms, and foreign material. The use of filters, ion exchangers, and reverse osmosis can be used to purify the water. The water treatment used depends on the location from which the water is obtained and the constituents present in the water. Whichever method is used, the content of the water needs to be known so adjustments can be made when mixing the dialysis solution (Keshaviah 1990).

The dialysate is delivered to the dialyzer most commonly by a proportioning single-pass delivery system. Some dialyzing facilities still use batch or partial recirculating single-pass dialysate systems, but the single-pass proportioning system is preferred. In the proportioning single-pass system, treated water and dialysis concentrate are constantly mixed by a proportioning pump, usually in the ratio of 1 part concentrate to 34 parts water. The solution is pumped past the membrane and carried directly to the drain. Just as the blood circuit is monitored, so too is the dialysate circuit monitored at three points. A temperature regulator is utilized to maintain a temperature of 36°C to 40°C. Overheated dialysate could cause hemolysis of the blood. If the temperature is lower than 35°C, the patient shivers and is uncomfortable. A second monitor checks the conductivity of the solution. It will indicate if there is a problem with the proportioning pump (that it is infusing too little or too much concentrate to yield the correct composition). A third monitor notes the presence of hemoglobin in the dialysate circuit. A tear in the dialysis membrane will allow the blood to escape into the dialysate solution. When any of these alarms is activated, the dialysate pump shuts off (Keshaviah 1990).

Nursing action to prevent or correct complications arising from a disruption in the external blood circuit must be properly addressed. If a blood leak occurs during dialysis, the dialysate hoses should be disconnected and the blood returned to the patient. If a break in the blood tubing occurs, the open ends are cleansed and reconnected. If air has entered the system, as much blood as possible is returned to the patient, and dialysis is restarted using a new circuit. If dialyzer clotting occurs, dialysis is discontinued without returning the blood. If fever and chills occur, dialysis should be stopped and the patient's blood cultured. If air does reach the patient, the blood pump should be stopped, the patient placed on the left side in the Trendelenburg position, and the physician notified immediately (Levin, Kupin, Zasuwa, and Venkat 1990).

Deciding on the type of dialyzer, length of treatment, and place of treatment is a collaborative effort based on the patient's individual needs. Dialyzers consist of a support structure for the blood compartment separated from the dialysate compartment by a semipermeable membrane. Currently dialyzers are of two types: parallel plate or hollow fiber. Selection of the type to use depends on the dialysis prescription and preference of the nephrologist (Corea, Ohanian, Anderson, and Holloway 1990). Consideration is given to the surface area of the membrane, priming volume, ultrafiltration capabilities, and clearance rates of blood urea nitrogen, creatinine, and phosphate (Hoenich, Woffindin, and Ward 1989).

The use of hemodialysis for an acute renal failure patient is determined on a daily basis by the patient's condition. The type of dialyzer, the content of the dialysate, and the heparinization should be tailored to the individual's needs. The patient who needs hemodialysis on a regular long-term basis will usually need to run each treatment 3 hours to 4 hours three times a week, in either a hospital or at home. A center-based program is used for patients who lack facilities for home treatment or are considered medically unsuited to treatment at home. The patient comes to the center three times a week at the time slot assigned for treatment. This schedule can be rather inflexible due to the number of patient treatments that have to be fitted into a center-based program. Recently high-efficiency treatments (high-flux dialysis) have been used to reduce treatment time. High-efficiency dialysis delivers the treatment in less than 3 hours three times per week, has blood flow rates of greater than 300 mL/min, urea clearances greater than 210 mL/min, and an index greater than three obtained by dividing urea clearance by patient body weight. When high-efficiency treatments are kept within these parameters, intra-treatment complications are no greater than with standard acetate hemodialysis. However, comparative morbidity and mortality have not been validated (Collins and Keshaviah 1990).

When home dialysis is selected, the patient and helper are taught the procedure until they are capable of conducting a safe and therapeutic dialysis. This can take as little as 3 weeks or as long as 6 months. The average time is about 6 weeks to 8 weeks. A 24-hour answering service is maintained between the home-treated patient and the teaching facility. Return clinic visits are scheduled at 2-month to 3-month intervals to monitor for medical, social, and psychological problems. Whichever modality is used, efforts should be made to help the patient achieve a schedule that minimizes interference with the patient's work and leisure activities supporting the rehabilitation of the patient.

Complications

Knowing the potential complications and selecting appropriate corrective action will ensure the patient receives safe, therapeutic treatment. The effects of hemodialysis on blood pressure can be formidable due to the electrolyte and fluid alterations that occur during treatment. Hypotension, hypertension, edema, muscle cramps, chest pain, and cardiac arrhythmias can occur. Dialysis disequilibrium can occur in patients just starting hemodialysis if dialysis is rapid over an extended period. The patient will manifest signs of headache, rising blood pressure, nausea, occasional blurred vision, and even seizures. This appears related to a rapid change of the urea and electrolyte concentrations and pH in the peripheral blood during dialysis that are not reflected in the central nervous system tissue because of the blood-brain barrier. The use of a gentler approach with slower flow rates or more frequent, shorter periods of dialysis can prevent this problem (Blagg 1989). The risk of bleeding—intracranially, intramuscularly, and in the gastrointestinal tract—is everpresent because of the required anticoagulant used during dialysis. The platelet dysfunction common to uremia coupled with heparinization during dialysis can also lead to severe menstrual bleeding in women.

Hypotension, resulting from excessive fluid removal, is common during dialysis. Yawning and feeling hot may precede the actual drop in blood pressure, with nausea and vomiting following. Either a decrease in ultrafiltration pressure or an infusion of normal saline may eliminate this problem. The patient's weight and lying and standing blood pressure should be measured before and after dialysis to monitor fluid loss (Blagg 1989).

If the monitoring devices of the dialysate circuit malfunction and a salt-free solution is delivered, blood hemolysis, hyperkalemia, and death would occur if immediate adjustments are not made. A hyperconcentrated solution would cause hypernatremia with subsequent hypertension and then later hypotension. If this were not corrected within 15 minutes to 20 minutes, the patient would suffer irreversible brain damage (Sullivan and Chami 1981). Air embolism, bacteremia, and septicemia are also possible should the monitoring devices fail (Levin et al. 1990).

Many of the problems of chronic renal failure persist. Chief among them is the presence of anemia. If the patient experiences severe dsypnea, chest pain, or tachycardia, blood transfusions may be administered. However, the conservative approach using iron or androgens along with r-HuEPO (erythropoietin) is usually favored (Eschbach and Adamson 1988; Eschbach 1989). When peripheral neuropathies persist, the length of dialysis may need to be increased. Persistence of hypertension leading to cardiac problems can occur. This, due to acceleration of atherosclerosis, is the greatest cause of morbidity and mortality in patients on long-term dialysis (Heyka and Paganini 1989).

The serum calcium of patients on dialysis should stay between 8.5 mg/100mL and 10.0 mg/100mL and the phosphate level between 3.0 mg/100 and 5.0 mg/100. While hypercalcemia may occur, it is more common to have insufficient control of phosphate. Intractable pruritis and metastatic calcifications may be the clinical manifestation of an elevated phosphate-calcium product. Renal osteodystrophy with diffuse bone pain and spontaneous fractures are possible long-term complications of poor calcium and phosphorus control. Calcium and vitamin D_3 supplements may be used to maintain calcium levels. Intestinal phosphate binders are administered to maintain the phosphate level. These must be used with caution because of potential aluminum toxicity. If a calcium phosphate balance problem persists, a subtotal parathyroidectomy may be necesssary (Llach and Coburn 1989).

The risk of hepatitis has been modulated with the use of Heptavax. However, patients on dialysis who require frequent transfusions are at risk, and precautions should be taken. Regular monitoring for the hepatitis virus in patients and staff should be done. In some dialysis units, monitoring for the acquired immunodeficiency syndrome is routine (Crosnior, Degos, and Jungers 1989; Rao 1989).

Psychosocial problems are generally influenced by the amount of support the patient has in addition to past experiences with meeting and adjusting to crises. Adaptation to dialysis takes varying lengths of time. A honeymoon phase occurs in the early weeks and months after dialysis initiation when the patient feels relieved to be rid of some of the unpleasant symptoms of uremia. After this, a period of depression may set in when the realization occurs that this treatment is lifelong. Patients confronted with this treatment are forced to relinquish much of their autonomy, independent judgment, and control over their body. A patient's capacity to establish a trusting relationship with the personnel of the dialysis team and to delegate much of his or her control to others will influence the emotional reaction to the treatment. Ultimately the patient either successfully adapts or continues to experience a great deal of anxiety and depression (Wolcott 1990). The nurse can help the patient throughout this period by offering support, explaining treatments and expected outcomes, providing constant reinforcement, and teaching. In addition, a major responsibility of the nurse caring for dialysis patients is to teach the patients and family about the purpose, side effects, and proper administration of necessary medications. Some medications interfere with dialysis by increasing side effects, such as hypotension, and other medications may be removed from the blood by dialysis. Time of drug ingestion may need to relate to the time of the dialysis treatment.

PERITONEAL DIALYSIS PROTOCOL

Access

Preparing the patient for placement of the catheter and teaching him or her about its care is the first step in caring for the patient receiving peritoneal dialysis. Access for peritoneal dialysis can be temporary or permanent. A temporary peritoneal catheter consists of a metal stylet inside a semirigid catheter 3 mm in diameter and 25 cm to 30 cm in length. The metal stylet protrudes from the end, providing a sharp tip for penetrating the abdominal wall. The catheter is perforated at its distal portion to allow the dialysate to flow into and out of the abdominal cavity. Since the number of dialysis treatments can be unpredictable, a permanent-type catheter is often used to eliminate the need for repeated punctures of the abdominal wall. Permanent peritoneal catheters come in many configurations. Almost all are constructed of silastic, making them soft and pliable. The cuffs on the catheter (one or two) are placed within the bulk of the abdominal muscle to maintain mechanical fixation and create a barrier against bacterial invasion. Radiopaque material in the catheter helps visualize catheter placement (Nolph 1986).

The catheter can be inserted at the bedside, using local anesthesia, if asepsis can be maintained. The catheter is usually placed below and lateral to the navel in a location that will not interfere with clothing at the beltline or impede sexual activity. Once the catheter is placed, it may be used for small volume exchanges if the patient remains in bed. If immediate dialysis is unnecessary, the catheter insertion site is allowed to heal for 10 days to 14 days while the catheter is irrigated weekly with a heparinized saline solution. The solution is usually 5000 units of heparin in 250 cc of normal saline. During the first weeks of dialysis, heparin 500 units/L is often used to prevent clotting in the catheter. If immediate dialysis is required, intermittent peritoneal dialysis is used every other day for approximately 2 weeks. Thereafter, the patient is placed on the prescribed dialysis schedule. The dialysate exchange volume is kept under 1 L during the first weeks to keep leakage to a minimum and to enhance healing around the cuffs (Ash et al. 1990).

Procedure

The nursing activities during peritoneal dialysis include adherence to the prescribed procedure and monitoring the patient's response. The prevention of complications is also required. The dialysate solution is delivered to the abdominal cavity through the catheter in varied intervals, usually every 1 hour to 2 hours for intermittent peritoneal dialysis or every 4 hours to 6 hours for continuous therapy. The peritoneal membrane has a larger pore size than the manufactured membrane used in hemodialysis. This allows higher molecular weight substances, such as vitamin B_{12} and insulin, to traverse from the capillaries within the peritoneal membrane to the dialysate solution bathing the membrane. Clearance of urea is 20 mL/min to 30 mL/min and creatinine is 15 mL/min to 20 mL/min. Hemodialysis clearance rates are about five to six times higher. The slower clearance rates of peritoneal dialysis require longer periods of time to obtain results comparable to those of hemodialysis. Factors that affect the peritoneal clearance rate are the dwell time (how long the solution stays within the abdominal cavity), the dialysate composition, the temperature, flow rate, and the intra-abdominal condition of the patient. The optimal amount of dwell time for solute removal is 10 minutes. Peritoneal clearance is higher when a dialysate is 37°C. The higher is the concentration gradient between blood and dialysate, the greater is the volume of solute removed. A high concentration gradient can be maintained by using large volumes of dialysate or inducing rapid exchanges. A dialysate volume above 40 cc/kg of body weight or a flow rate above 4 L/hr is impractical. The best peritoneal clearances are usually obtained with a 2 L exchange volume at a rate of 1.5 exchanges to 2 exchanges per hour. This obtains a flow rate of 3 L to 4 L per hour. A hypertonic dialysate containing a 4.25 g/dL of dextrose also increases peritoneal clearance. This is thought to occur because of the large volume of fluid that is removed seems to drag other constituents with the water. The addition of a vasodilator, such as nitroprusside, to the dialysate can enhance the clearances by as much as 20% (Nolph 1989).

While intermittent peritoneal dialysis is still used, the current usual schedules of conducting peritoneal dialysis are continuous ambulatory peritoneal dialysis (CAPD) and continuous cyclic peritoneal dialysis (CCPD). In intermittent peritoneal dialysis, 2 L of dialysate solution are infused into the peritoneal cavity and allowed to equilibrate for 10 minutes to 20 minutes and then drained out by gravity. The exchanges are repeated until the desired clinical and biochemical improvements occur. This method can be used for patients who have acute or chronic renal failure. Continuous ambulatory peritoneal dialysis keeps dialysate in the peritoneal cavity 24 hours, 7 days a week. The solution in the cavity is replaced by fresh dialysate three or four times a day. The continuous cyclic peritoneal dialysis is a slight modification of the CAPD technique. The patient uses an automatic cycler to exchange 6 L to 8 L of dialysate during the night over a 10-hour period. Two liters of solution are left in the peritoneal cavity during the day to be removed the next evening (Diaz-Buxo 1990; Mion 1989).

The composition of the dialysate fluid used in peritoneal dialysis is similar to that used during hemodialysis except that it is generally potassium free for patients undergoing maintenance dialysis. This is because the peritoneal membrane clears potassium very slowly and the patient is usually hyperkalemic. Potassium is added to the dialysate if the patient is receiving digitalis or is undergoing frequent exchanges (every 1 hour to 2 hours) for an extended period of time, such as over a 24-hour period, to prevent myocardial irritability of a potentially fatal arrhythmia. The amount added is usually 2 mEq to 3 mEq of KCl/L. Lactate is added to the dialysate at the concentration of 35 mEq/L and is metabolically converted to bicarbonate.

The level of dextrose concentration in the dialysate solution is determined by the weight desired, the lying and standing blood pressure, and the presence of edema or congestion. Diarrhea, vomiting, or other fluid losses or fluid increases must also be considered. The following guidelines are used for deciding on the type of dextrose solution (Diaz-Buxo 1990):

Patient's weight is greater than 0.5 kg below ideal weight: Use 0.5%.
Patient's weight is at ideal weight (0.5% kg): Use 1.5%.
Patient's weight is between 0.5 kg and 1 kg above ideal weight: Use 2.5%.
Patient's weight is greater than 1 kg above ideal weight: Use 4.25%.

The peritoneal membrane is porous enough to allow some protein, approximately 30 g/week to 100 g/week, to escape from the blood into the dialysate solution. To compensate for this loss dietary protein should be about 1.2 g/kg to 1.5 g/kg of body weight per day (Sullivan and Chami 1981).

Indications for the Use of Peritoneal Dialysis

When a patient is considering dialysis, a nurse can discuss factors that indicate the use of peritoneal dialysis:

1. The possibility of home dialysis.
2. An older patient with a complicating cardiovascular disease.
3. A child with small body size and poor vascular access.
4. A diabetic with ESRD.
5. Uncontrollable hypotension during dialysis.
6. Malignant hypertension with renal failure.
7. Severe anemia requiring multiple blood transfusions.
8. Pretransplant maintenance dialysis.
9. Acute renal failure.

Poor peritoneal clearance is an absolute contraindication for peritoneal dialysis. Relative contraindications include the following:

1. Backache with vertebral disease.
2. Abdominal hernias.
3. Presence of colostomy, ileostomy, recurrent diverticular disease, or a similar condition.
4. Concurrent immunosuppressive treatment.
5. Chronic obstructive lung disease.
6. Poorly motivated and/or depressed patients (Khanna and Oreopoulos 1983; Mion 1989).

Complications

Problems associated with peritoneal dialysis can occur at any time. Anticipating these complications will prepare the nurse for correct action. Complications that can accompany catheter placement include perforation of the bladder, bowels, and possibly the aorta. This happens more commonly when the rigid catheter with the stylet is used; it rarely happens with the use of the silastic catheters. Occasionally the catheter becomes dislodged, with the cuff migrating out through the skin exit site. Exit site infections with localized cellulitis or a subcutaneous tunnel abcess extending into the deep cuff area can occur. Also, fluid may leak through the catheter tunnel and out of the skin exit site when large volume exchanges or ambulation occur too soon after catheter insertion.

The catheter may become covered by omentum and migrate to the upper abdomen. The omental covering will obstruct the flow. A change of position or the use of cathartics, creating vigorous bowel movement, may help relieve the obstruction. Fibrin clots may form and cause permanent catheter obstruction, requiring replacement. The use of heparin, urokinase, and continuous flushing helps reduce this problem. A bloody outflow often occurs shortly after catheter placement but usually clears spontaneously. Leakage around the catheter is not uncommon immediately following catheter insertion. This can usually be corrected by temporarily stopping dialysis and reducing the exchange volume used.

Patients may report pain in the rectal or suprapubic area during the first 5 weeks to 6 weeks after catheter implantation. Abdominal pain may occur if the patient is using a dialysate with the higher dextrose concentrations. Overfilling with dialysate will distend the abdomen, creating discomfort or pain. When this happens, the fluid should be drained immediately (Diaz-Buxo 1990).

Possible medical complications include abdominal hernia resulting from the continuously raised intra-abdominal pressure exerted by the presence of dialysate in the abdominal cavity. Females may develop rectoceles or cystoceles with or without uterine prolapse. The raised pressure may aggravate previous conditions of hiatal hernia and hemorrhoids. If the patient has a vertebral disease, the weight may exaggerate lordosis and aggravate back pain.

Circulation to the lower extremities is compromised by this increased abdominal pressure with partial occlusion of the ileal femoral vessels. This may produce hypotension and ischemic complications and accelerate atherosclerosis. These patients have increased problems with their cardiovascular and cerebrovascular systems such as angina, arrhythmias, acute myocardial infarction, transient ischemic attacks, and strokes (Diaz-Buxo 1990).

Peritonitis is one of the most dangerous complications of peritoneal dialysis. It is manifested clinically by abdominal pain, a cloudy effluent, rebound abdominal tenderness, and sometimes fever, vomiting, and ileus. About 25% to 30% of these patients become extremely ill. The presence of enteric organisms in the effluent suggests a bowel leak; however, occasionally organisms may cross the enteric wall when abnormal bowel motility occurs, as with diverticulosis or chronic constipation. Aseptic peritonitis may occur caused by chemical plasticizers and/or endotoxins and coincidental administration of antibiotics. Peritonitis is initially treated by a number of very rapid exchanges. Heparin and antibiotics are then added to the dialysate, and the exchanges are done every 3 hours to 6 hours. Since peritonitis increases protein loss, serum albumin may fall during infections. If the peritonitis treatment is going to work, a favorable response should occur within 24 hours to 48 hours after treatment initiation. The therapy is continued until two consecutive daily cultures are negative. Heparin and antibiotics are added to the dialysate, and oral antibiotics are usually administered for a period of 3 weeks after the episode. Strict aseptic technique when handling any of the connections and inserting needles into fluid containers is the key to the prevention of this complication. Removal of the catheter is necessary when the infection persists for more than 4 days to 5 days in spite of the use of appropriate antibiotics, if fungal, tuberculosis, or fecal peritonitis is present or if there is severe skin exit or subcutaneous tunnel infection. If fecal contamination occurs, a laparotomy to seal off the leaky bowel may be necessary (Walshe and Morse 1990).

Since CAPD is a form of continuous dialysis, wide fluctuations between hemodialysis treatments do not occur. Anemia is less severe, and transfusion requirements are lower. The mechanism of this improvement is unknown, but it might result from the more consistent removal of the toxic substances that suppress the bone marrow's response to erythropoietin. The constant low-grade loss of blood seen with hemodialysis also does not occur. After 1 month to 2 months, CAPD patients become sodium depleted, and hypertension becomes easier to manage. These patients often become normotensive within 2 months of treatment initiation.

The psychological impact of long-term peritoneal dialysis relates to a changed body image. In addition to the placement of the external appliance (the catheter and bag), it is not unusual for patients of CAPD to gain more than 5 kg during the first year of treatment. Use of hypertonic exchanges and high caloric intake effect this weight gain. In addition, glucose tolerance may be impaired secondary to pancreatic exhaustion in CAPD. The feeling of fatigue is a side effect of their state of hyponatemia, and depression may ensue because of the demanding regimen requiring the completion of the dialysis procedure four to five times per day, 7 days a week.

Following catheter implantation, patients learn to tolerate 2 L of dialysate in their abdomen and learn how to identify and deal with mechanical problems with the catheter. They need to become aware of the importance of meticulous aspesis with every bag change to prevent complications. It will usually take approximately

2½ weeks to 3½ weeks for patients to learn how to carry out the dialysis procedure. They must learn aseptic techniques and other procedures and be able to manipulate either the bags or cycler machine before they can be discharged from the hospital.

If a leakage at the exit site occurs and the dressings become wet, the dressings should be changed completely rather than reinforced. Outflow is often dependent on position and may improve when repositioning allows gravity to have a greater effect. An accurate record of fluid balance should be kept. Dialysis should not be continued if a cumulative positive balance of more then 2000 mL occurs. Weight and blood pressure should be checked at least every 3 hours during prolonged dialysis treatments, as may be done for acute failure (Mion 1989).

After discharge, home visits and clinic appointments provide opportunity to evaluate the patient's techniques and do additional teaching as needed. The patients should be taught the signs and symptoms of infection and encouraged to report the signs of peritonitis promptly.

DISCHARGE PLANS

Teaching plans are individualized to address the patient's prescription needs. Planning should begin as early as possible to allow time to deal with problems such as impaired learning ability, emotional problems, lack of adequate funds, physical limitations, and transportation difficulties. The home situation needs to be reviewed to determine if adjustments are required before the patient is discharged. For example, when the patient receives home hemodialysis, the patient's water system needs to be adequate. All patients will need adequate storage space for supplies and adequate funds to support the therapy and a mode of transportation.

Since dialysis is a government-funded program, it is important that the patients become aware of the financial assistance available through Medicare. Usually the most knowledgeable person about this program is the renal social worker. If the patient needs to return to the treatment center frequently, transportation must be arranged. The family, volunteers, and civic or church organizations might be used to help ensure that the patient receives treatment in a timely fashion. All patients return to the hospital or clinic at some periodic interval for evaluation of their status and adjustment of treatment regimen. Patients who need the services of a home health care nurse should make arrangements before discharge. Including the patient and significant others as partners in the care and planning for dialysis therapy has consistently proved to be an essential and successful long-term nursing approach for thousands of persons who have received dialysis therapy (Cummings 1989).

CASE STUDIES

Case 1

This 71-year-old married male's ESRD is secondary to polycystic kidney disease. Diverticulitis terminated CAPD treatment. Currently in-center, 4-hour hemodialysis is used three times per week with a Gambro AK-10. The dialysate contains 2 mEq/L of potassium, 3.5 mEq/L of calcium, plus bicarbonate. The flow rate is 350 mL/min. Access is a right brachial fistula. Current diet is 2500 Kcal/day, 90 g protein, 3 g Na, 80 mEq potassium, low phosphorus, low cholesterol, and fluid restriction to 1000 cc/day. Nutritional status is good, with albumin staying about 3.5 g/dL. Current medications are calcium carbonate 650 mg 4 times a day, DHT 0.4 mg every day, Deca-Durabolin 200 mg intramuscular every other week, Stuart Prenatal Tablets 1 + 1 1 every day, hypertonic saline (23.5%) 10 cc intravenous as needed for cramps, and Ecotrin 1 every day. Pneumovax and Heptavax immunizations have been used.

The patient condition is unstable with mild congestive heart failure when weight gain exceeds 4 kg to 6 kg. Hypotension occurs postdialysis when weight gains exceed 4 kg. During the past decade, the patient's medical history includes a right nephrectomy, arteriosclerotic cardiovascular disease with a myocardial infarction and left hemisphere cerebrovascular accident, a tracheostomy for sleep apnea, a right brachial artery aneurysm rupture due to needle trauma, and osteopenia with spinal compression.

His immediate family consists of a wife and three adult children living in the home area. He is semiretired, owning a feed and grain business with other family members. Current health care coverage through Medicare and private insurance is adequate. He is ineligible for any state or local program so the family must pay extra costs, such as travel expenses. The wife transports the patient to his center treatments. Compliance with dietary, medication, and activity prescriptions has been good.

His primary problems currently relate to altered fluid and electrolyte balance, cardiac output, respiratory status, mobility, and energy level. The associated nursing diagnoses are Fluid Volume Excess, Altered Nutrition: Potential for More Than Body Requirements, Altered Cardiac Perfusion, Ineffective Breathing Pattern, Potential for Trauma, Activity Intolerance, and Fatigue. Nursing activities, in addition to following prescribed dialysis parameters, include reinforcing the need for fluid restriction and maintaining a dry weight goal of 97 kg and monitoring lung sounds, episodes of coughing, bone pain, and electrolyte, hemoglobin, and hemotocrit levels.

Case 2

This 53-year-old married male's ESRD is secondary to focal segmental glomerulosclerosis. He receives home hemodialysis on a Travenol SPS 450 for 4 hours three times a week. The dialysate contains 1 mEq/L of potassium, 3.5 mEq/L of calcium, and 200 mg of dextrose. The flow rate is 300 mL/min with the access an AV fistula, right arm. Current diet is 2700 Kcal, 95 g protein, 4 g Na, 80 mEq potassium, low phosphorus, and 1500 cc fluid restriction per day. Current nutritional status is adequate, with normal serum albumin levels. He has periodic problems with hyperphosphatemia. Current medications are calcium carbonate 650 mg three times a day, DHT 0.2 mg every day, Deca-Durabolin 200 mg intramuscular every 2 weeks, AluCaps three times a day, Verapamil 240 SR every day, Synthroid 0.15 mg every day, and Stuart Prenatal Tablets one per day. Pneumovax and Heptavax immunizations have been used.

Although the patient's condition is stable, he is hypertensive and has hypothyroidism, anemia, and hyperphosphatemia. The patient's immediate family consists of his wife and an adult son and daughter. The son resides in their home. The wife is his dialysis partner and after some initial anxiety has adjusted to and is doing well with the home treatment. The patient has a trucking business and plans to continue working for at least 3 more years until the daughter finishes her schooling. Current health care coverage is provided through Medicare and private insurance. Transportation to the clinic is provided by the patient or family. He occasionally misses a treatment due to his truck driving activities. Social activities are often limited.

His primary problems relate to altered fluid and electrolyte balance, reduced social activities, and limited energy reserves. The associated nursing diagnoses are Fluid Volume Excess, Altered Nutrition: Potential for More Than Body Requirements, Diversional Activity Deficit, Fatigue, and Activity Intolerance: Potential. Current nursing activities include reinforcing dietary teaching, encouraging social outings and vacations to give a break to his routine, helping the patient set priorities regarding energy use, and monitoring electrolyte, hemoglobin and hematocrit levels.

SUMMARY

The nursing intervention of Dialysis Therapy consists of preparing patients for treatments, managing the technology, monitoring the treatment and possible complications, and collaborating with the patient, family, and health team members in developing a plan of care.

REFERENCES

Anderson, R., and Schrier, R. 1985. Acute renal failure. In R.G. Petersdorf, R.E. Adams, E. Braunwald, K. Isselbacker, J.B. Martin, and J.D. Wilson (eds.), *Harrison's principles of internal medicine* (10th ed.). New York: McGraw-Hill.

Ash, S.R., Carr, D.J., and Diaz-Buxo, J.A. 1990. In A.R. Nissesson, R.N. Fine, and D.E. Gentile (eds.), *Clinical dialysis* (2d ed.). Norwalk, Conn.: Appleton & Lange.

Bell, P.R.F., and Veitch, P.S. The development of hemodialysis and peritoneal dialysis. In A.R. Nissesson, R.N. Fine, and D.E. Gentile (eds.), *Clinical dialysis* (2d ed.). Norwalk, Conn.: Appleton & Lange.

Blagg, C.R. 1989. Acute complications associated with hemodialysis. In J.F. Maher (ed.), *Replacement of renal function by dialysis*. (3d ed.). Boston: Kluwer Academic Publishers.

Brenner, B.M., Dworkin, L.D., and Ichikawa, I. 1986. Glomerular filtration. In B.M. Brenner and F.C. Rector, Jr. (eds.), *The kidney* (vol. 1) (3d ed.). Philadelphia: W.B. Saunders Co.

Brunner, F.P., Wing, A.J., Dykes, S.R., Brynger, H.O.A., Fassbinder, W., and Selwood, N.H. 1989. International review of renal replacement therapy: Strategies and results. In J.F. Maher (ed.), Replacement of renal function by dialysis (3d ed.). Boston: Kluwer Academic Publishers.

Cheung, A.K. 1990. Membrane biocompatibility. In A.R. Nissesson, R.N. Fine, and D.E. Gentile (eds.), *Clinical dialysis* (2d ed.). Norwalk, Conn.: Appleton & Lange.

Collins, A.J., and Keshaviah, P.K. 1990. High-efficiency therapies for clinical dialysis. In A.R. Nissesson, R.N. Fine, and D.E. Gentile (eds.), *Clinical dialysis* (2d ed.). Norwalk, Conn.: Appleton & Lange.

Corea, A.L., Ohanian, N., Anderson, M., and Holloway, M. 1990. The hemodialysis procedure. In A.R. Nissesson, R.N. Fine, and D.E. Gentile (eds.), *Clinical dialysis* (2d ed.). Norwalk, Conn.: Appleton & Lange.

Crosnior, J., Degos, F., and Jungers, P. 1989. Dialysis associated hepatitis. In J.F. Maher (ed.), *Replacement of renal function by dialysis* (3d ed.). Boston: Kluwer Academic Publishers.

Cummings, N.B. 1989. Social, ethical and legal issues involved in chronic maintenance dialysis. In J.F. Maher (ed.), *Replacement of renal function by dialysis* (3d ed.). Boston: Kluwer Academic Publishers.

Delano, B.G. 1989. Regular dialysis treatment. In J.F. Maher (ed.), *Replacement of renal function by dialysis* (3d ed.). Boston: Kluwer Academic Publishers.

Diaz-Buxo, J.A. 1990. Clinical use of peritoneal dialysis. In A.R. Nissesson, R.N. Fine, and D.E. Gentile (eds.), *Clinical dialysis* (2d ed.). Norwalk, Conn.: Appleton & Lange.

Eschbach, J.W. 1989. The anemia of chronic renal failure: Pathophysiology and the effects of recombinant erythropoietin. *Kidney International* 35:134–148.

Eschbach, J.W., and Adamson, J.W. 1988. Correction of the anemia of hemodialysis (HD) in patients with recombinant human erythropoietin (rHuEPO): Results of a multicenter study. *Kidney International* 33:189–192.

Fearing, M.O. 1967. *Nursing implications for patients on chronic hemodialysis*. American Nurses Association Clinical Conferences. New York: Appleton-Century Crofts.

Fearing, M.O. 1973. Standards of clinical practice of nephrology patients. *Journal of Renal Technology: Dialysis and transplant* 2:41–44.

Grantham, J. 1982. Acute renal failure. In J.B. Wyngaarden and L.H. Smith (eds.), *Cecil textbook of medicine* (16th ed.). Philadelphia: W.B. Saunders Co.

Hart, L.K., Reese, J.L., and Fearing, M.O. 1981. *Concepts common to acute illness: Identification and management.* St. Louis: C.V. Mosby Co.

Heyka, R.J., and Paganini, E.P. 1989. Blood pressure control in chronic dialysis patients. In J.F. Maher (ed.), *Replacement of renal function by dialysis* (3d ed.). Boston: Kluwer Academic Publishers.

Hoenich, N.A., Woffindin, C., and Ward, M.K. 1989. Dialysers. In J.F. Maher (ed.), *Replacement of renal function by dialysis* (3d ed.). Boston: Kluwer Academic Publishers.

Hoffert, N. 1989. Nephrology nursing 1915–1970: A historical study of integration of technology and care. *American Nephrology Nurses' Association Journal* 3:169–178.

Keshaviah, P.R. 1990. Equipment for hemodialysis. In A.R. Nissesson, R. N. Fine, and D.E. Gentile (eds.), *Clinical dialysis* (2d ed.). Norwalk, Conn.: Appleton & Lange.

Khanna, R, and Oreopoulos, D.G. 1983. Peritoneal dialysis. In D.Z. Levine (ed.), *Care of the renal patient*. Philadelphia: W.B. Saunders Co.

Lancaster, L.E. 1987. *Core curriculum for nephrology nursing*. Pitman, N.J.: American Nephrology Nurses' Association.

Levin, N.W., Kupin, W.L., Zasuwa, G., and Venkat, L.L. 1990. In A.R. Nissesson, R.N. Fine, and D.E. Gentile (eds.), *Clinical dialysis* (2d ed.). Norwalk, Conn.: Appleton & Lange.

Llach, F., and Coburn, J.W. 1989. Renal osteodystrophy and maintenance dialysis. In J.F. Maher (ed.), *Replacement of renal function by dialysis* (3d ed.). Boston: Kluwer Academic Publishers.

Mion, C.M. 1989. Practical use of peritoneal dialysis. In J.F. Maher (ed.), *Replacement of renal function by dialysis* (3d ed.). Boston: Kluwer Academic Publishers.

Nolph, K.D. 1986. Peritoneal dialysis. In B.M. Brenner and F.C. Rector, Jr. (eds.), *The kidney*. Philadelphia: W.B. Saunders Co.

Nolph, K.D. 1989. Peritoneal anatomy and transport physiology. In J.F. Maher (ed.), *Replacement of renal function by dialysis* (3d ed.). Boston: Kluwer Academic Publishers.

Rao, T.K.S. 1989. Dialysis in the acquired immunodeficiency syndrome. In J.F. Maher (ed.), *Replacement of renal function of dialysis* (3d ed.). Boston: Kluwer Academic Publishers.

Richard, C.J. 1986. *Comprehensive nephrology nursing*. Boston: Little, Brown.

Robbins, S.L., Catran, R., and Kumar, V. 1984. *Pathologic basis of disease* (3d ed.). Philadelphia: W.B. Saunders Co.

Stewart, W.K. 1989. The composition of dialysis fluid. In J.F. Maher (ed.). *Replacement of renal function by dialysis* (3d ed.). Boston: Kluwer Academic Publishers.

Sullivan, J.F., and Chami, J. 1981. Dialysis treatment. In J.S. Cheigh, K.H. Stenzel, and A.L. Rubin (eds.), *Manual of clinical nephrology: Developments in nephrology* (vol. 1). Boston: Martinus Nijhoff.

Swartz, R.D. 1990. Anticoagulation in patients on hemodialysis. In A.R. Nissesson, R.N. Fine, and D.E. Gentile (eds.), *Clinical dialysis* (2d ed.). Norwalk, Conn.: Appleton & Lange.

Vanholder, R., Schoots, A., and Ringoir, S. 1989. Uremic toxicity. In J.F. Maher (ed.), *Replacement of renal function by dialysis* (3d ed.). Boston: Kluwer Academic Publishers.

Walshe, J.J., and Morse, G.D. 1990. Infectious complications of peritoneal dialysis patients. In A.R. Nissesson, R.N. Fine, and D.E. Gentile (eds.), *Clinical dialysis* (2d ed.). Norwalk, Conn.: Appleton & Lange.

Wolcott, D.L. 1990. Psychosocial adaption of dialysis patients. In A.R. Nissesson, R.N. Fine, and D.E. Gentile (eds.), *Clinical dialysis* (2d. ed.). Norwalk, Conn.: Appleton & Lange.

FUTURE DIRECTIONS

GLORIA M. BULECHEK
JOANNE C. McCLOSKEY

The first edition of this book was a new effort to define nursing interventions at a conceptual level. It examined 26 independent nursing interventions, those initiated by a nursing diagnosis. Most of the treatments were psychosocial in nature. This book, the second edition, has been expanded to cover 44 interventions. The definition of a nursing intervention in this edition encompasses both nurse-initiated and physician-initiated treatments. Sections on Self-Care Assistance and Life Support have been developed for this edition. This has resulted in the inclusion of more pathophysiological treatments, including Feeding, Positioning, Intermittent Catheterization, Airway Management, and Shock Management. All of the interventions are listed in alphabetical order in Table 1 with their related nursing diagnoses as identified by the chapter authors. Some of the linkages of interventions with diagnoses are based on research, but most are based on the authors' judgments and clinical experiences.

Examination of Table 1 leads to several observations. First, the number of diagnoses related to each intervention ranges from 3 to 19. At the top end, Environmental Structuring has 19; Support Groups has 18; related nursing diagnoses; and Reminiscence Therapy has 17 diagnoses; Patient Teaching has 15; Surveillance has 13; and Counseling has more than 11. Are these intervention labels too global? It does not seem that a definitive therapy should treat 19 diagnoses. Maybe more specific intervention labels are needed for clinical practice—or maybe future research will establish that the interventions do not work for all the suggested diagnoses.

Second, the chapter authors suggested 24 diagnostic labels that are not on the current NANDA list. Several physiological nursing diagnoses have been suggested by the authors of the chapters on Bowel Management, Dry Skin Care, Dialysis Therapy, and Secondary Brain Injury. In addition, more diagnoses are needed for urinary incontinence. Although the NANDA taxonomy contains five labels for this phenomenon the authors of the chapter on Intermittent Catheterization suggested two more. Nurses are operating incontinence clinics and conducting detailed assessments to make the differential diagnosis and establish treatments tailored to the specific diagnosis.

The multiple diagnosis and intervention labels in the area of incontinence illustrate the level of specificity needed to direct clinical practice. Other areas also need this level of specificity. For example, Structured Preoperative Teaching, an intervention with a well-established research base, lacks a precise diagnostic label. The diagnosis label Knowledge Deficit (Specify) seems too general to direct this well-established nursing treatment. Other authors have expressed concern about the

Text continued on page 608

TABLE 1. NURSING INTERVENTIONS AND RELATED NURSING DIAGNOSES

NURSING INTERVENTIONS	NURSING DIAGNOSES
Airway Management	Impaired Gas Exchange Ineffective Airway Clearance Ineffective Breathing Pattern
Art Therapy[a]	Altered Family Processes Diversional Activity Deficit Fear Dysfunctional Grieving Impaired Verbal Communication Ineffective Individual Coping Potential for Violence Powerlessness Rape-Trauma Syndrome Self Esteem Disturbance Social Isolation Spiritual Distress
Bowel Management	Bowel Incontinence Colonic Constipation Constipation Diarrhea *Fecal Impaction *Idiopathic Bowel Incontinence Perceived Constipation *Stool Retention
Cognitive Reappraisal	Altered Health Maintenance Altered Thought Processes Fear Ineffective Individual Coping Powerlessness
Concrete Objective Information	Fear *Potential for Ineffective Individual Coping
Confusion Management	Altered Thought Processes *Impaired Communication Potential for Injury Potential for Violence Sensory/Perceptual Alterations
Counseling[a]	Altered Parenting Altered Sexuality Patterns Anxiety Body Image Disturbance Decisional Conflict Fear Anticipatory Grieving Dysfunctional Grieving Ineffective Individual Coping Noncompliance Self-Esteem Disturbance
Crisis Intervention	Anxiety Dysfunctional Grieving Fear Impaired Adjustment Ineffective Family Coping: Disabling Ineffective Individual Coping Knowledge Deficit Potential for Violence Powerlessness Rape-Trauma Syndrome Social Isolation Spiritual Distress

Table continued on following page

TABLE 1. NURSING INTERVENTIONS AND RELATED
NURSING DIAGNOSES *Continued*

NURSING INTERVENTIONS	NURSING DIAGNOSES
Dialysis Therapy[a]	*Acid/Base Disturbance Altered Nutrition: Potential for More Than Body Requirements *Electrolyte Disturbance Fluid Volume Excess
Discharge Planning	[Altered Health Maintenance Knowledge Deficit Impaired Home Maintenance Management Self Care Deficit (Specify) Social Isolation *Translocation Syndrome]
Dry Skin Care	*Impaired Skin Integrity: Dry Skin
Environmental Structuring	Activity Intolerance Altered Thought Processes Diversional Activity Deficit Hyperthermia Hypothermia Impaired Home Maintenance Management Impaired Skin Integrity Impaired Physical Mobility Impaired Verbal Communication Pain Potential Altered Body Temperature Potential for Infection Potential for Injury Powerlessness Self-Care Deficit (Specify) Sensory/Perceptual Alterations Social Isolation Sleep Pattern Disturbance
Exercise Program	Altered Health Maintenance Altered Nutrition: More Than Body Requirements Constipation Decreased Cardiac Output Health Seeking Behaviors Impaired Physical Mobility Sleep Pattern Disturbance
Family Therapy	[Altered Family Processes Family Coping: Potential for Growth Ineffective Family Coping: Compromised Ineffective Family Coping: Disabling Ineffective Individual Coping]
Feeding	Altered Nutrition: Less Than Body Requirements Altered Thought Processes Feeding Self-Care Deficit Impaired Physical Mobility Impaired Swallowing Sensory/Perceptual Alterations
Fluid Therapy	Altered Nutrition: Less Than Body Requirements Altered Urinary Elimination Decreased Cardiac Output Fluid Volume Deficit Fluid Volume Excess Impaired Gas Exchange Ineffective Breathing Pattern *Potential for Injury: Cerebral Edema

TABLE 1. NURSING INTERVENTIONS AND RELATED
NURSING DIAGNOSES *Continued*

NURSING INTERVENTIONS	NURSING DIAGNOSES
Group Psychotherapy	Body Image Disturbance *Impaired Interpersonal Relationships Impaired Social Interaction Ineffective Individual Coping Self Esteem Disturbance
Hemodynamic Regulation	Altered Tissue Perfusion (Peripheral) Decreased Cardiac Output Fluid Volume Deficit Fluid Volume Excess
Hygiene Assistance[a]	Bathing/Hygiene Self-Care Deficit
Infection Control	Potential for Infection *Potential for Infection: Nosocomial
Intermittent Catheterization	*Iatrogenic Incontinence *Overflow Incontinence Reflex Incontinence Urge Incontinence
Medication Management	Altered Health Maintenance Knowledge Deficit Noncompliance *Potential for Poisoning: Drug Toxicity
Mutual Goal Setting	Health Seeking Behaviors Noncompliance Self Esteem Disturbance Social Isolation
Pain Control	Chronic Pain Pain
Patient Contracting	Altered Parenting Ineffective Individual Coping Knowledge Deficit Noncompliance Self-Care Deficit (Specify)
Patient Teaching	Altered Parenting Altered Protection Altered Role Performance Decisional Conflict Family Coping: Potential for Growth Health Seeking Behaviors Impaired Home Maintenance Management Impaired Social Interaction Ineffective Breastfeeding Ineffective Family Coping: Compromised Ineffective Individual Coping Knowledge Deficit Noncompliance Self-Care Deficit (Specify) Sexual Dysfunction
Positioning	Impaired Physical Mobility *Potential for Injury: Physiological
Presence	Anticipatory Grieving Anxiety Fear Impaired Verbal Communication Ineffective Individual Coping Potential for Injury Powerlessness Social Isolation Spiritual Distress

Table continued on following page

TABLE 1. NURSING INTERVENTIONS AND RELATED NURSING DIAGNOSES Continued

NURSING INTERVENTIONS	NURSING DIAGNOSES
Pressure Reduction	Chronic Pain Impaired Skin Integrity Pain Potential Impaired Skin Integrity
Relaxation Training	Activity Intolerance Anxiety Fear Impaired Physical Mobility Ineffective Breathing Pattern Ineffective Individual Coping Pain Powerlessness Sleep Disturbance
Reminiscence Therapy[a]	Altered Growth and Development Anxiety Diversional Activity Deficit Decisional Conflict Defensive Coping Fear Anticipatory Grieving Dysfunctional Grieving Health Seeking Behaviors Hopelessness Impaired Adjustment Impaired Social Interaction Ineffective Denial Powerlessness Self Esteem Disturbance Social Isolation Spiritual Distress
Secondary Brain Injury Reduction	*Altered Level of Responsiveness *Decreased Intracranial Adaptive Capacity Altered Tissue Perfusion (Cerebral) Altered Thought Processes Ineffective Breathing Pattern Fluid Volume Deficit Impaired Gas Exchange Impaired Physical Mobility Potential for Infection *Potential for Secondary Brain Injury Self Care Deficit (Specify) Sensory/Perceptual Alterations
Shock Management	*Altered Level of Consciousness Altered Tissue Perfusion Decreased Cardiac Output Fluid Volume Deficit Hyperthermia Impaired Gas Exchange Ineffective Breathing Pattern *Potential for Infection
Sleep Promotion	*Sleep Deprivation Sleep Pattern Disturbance
Smoking Cessation	Activity Intolerance Altered Health Maintenance Health Seeking Behaviors Ineffective Airway Clearance

TABLE 1.   NURSING INTERVENTIONS AND RELATED
NURSING DIAGNOSES *Continued*

NURSING INTERVENTIONS	NURSING DIAGNOSES
Structured Preoperative Teaching	Knowledge Deficit (Specify) Anxiety Fear Ineffective Individual Coping Ineffective Family Coping Potential Activity Intolerance
Support Groups	Altered Family Processes Altered Parenting Altered Protection Anxiety Diversional Activity Deficit Fear Anticipatory Grieving Dysfunctional Grieving Hopelessness Impaired Adjustment Ineffective Individual Coping Knowledge Deficit Noncompliance Potential for Injury Potential for Violence Powerlessness Self Esteem Disturbance Social Isolation Spiritual Distress
Surveillance	Altered Thought Processes Decreased Cardiac Output Diarrhea Fluid Volume Deficit Impaired Adjustment Impaired Gas Exchange Impaired Swallowing Ineffective Airway Clearance Ineffective Breathing Pattern Potential Altered Body Temperature Potential for Suffocation Potential for Violence
Terminal Care	Altered Nutrition: Less Than Body Requirements Altered Oral Mucous Membrane Altered Thought Processes Constipation Fatigue Anticipatory Grieving Impaired Skin Integrity Pain Spiritual Distress
Therapeutic Touch	Anticipatory Grieving Anxiety Fear Ineffective Individual Coping Impaired Physical Mobility Pain Powerlessness Sleep Pattern Disturbance
Truth Telling	Anticipatory Grieving Body Image Disturbance Impaired Adjustment Knowledge Deficit Spiritual Distress

Table continued on following page

TABLE 1. NURSING INTERVENTIONS AND RELATED
NURSING DIAGNOSES Continued

NURSING INTERVENTIONS	NURSING DIAGNOSES
Values Clarification	Decisional Conflict *Inadequate Decision Making *Spiritual Despair Spiritual Distress
Ventilatory Support[a]	Impaired Gas Exchange Ineffective Airway Clearance Ineffective Breathing Pattern
Weight Management	Activity Intolerance Altered Health Maintenance Altered Nutrition: More Than Body Requirements Impaired Physical Mobility Ineffective Individual Coping Knowledge Deficit (Exercise) Knowledge Deficit (Nutrition) Powerlessness Self-Esteem Disturbance Social Isolation

Notes: An asterisk before the label means that the diagnosis is not on the NANDA list. The diagnoses in brackets were supplied by the editors for this table; they do not appear in the pertinent chapter.
[a] See the chapter for others.

global nature of the Knowledge Deficit label. It needs to be made more precise to direct the many types of patient teaching that nurses do. The intervention Patient Teaching also needs more specific intervention labels to identify the type of teaching activity required. What is needed is enough specificity to be useful to clinicians without losing the conceptual focus. The new suggested diagnosis labels should be developed for submission to the NANDA review committee. The guidelines for submission are available in NANDA publications.

Third, there is much research and development work ahead of the profession. Several types of work related to interventions are needed. More work on concept development is needed to refine some labels. When the operational definitions are examined, several labels appear similar. Is Presence the same as empathy, caring, or reassurance? What is the distinction between Support Groups and Group Psychotherapy? Research utilizing experimental designs is needed to test the effectiveness of the interventions for the nursing diagnoses suggested in Table 1. Clinical trials comparing the benefits of two or more interventions for a specific diagnosis should be done.

A current goal of the Agency for Health Care Policy and Research and the American Nurses' Association (ANA) is to produce practice guidelines—statements that link diagnoses, treatments, and outcomes. The intent is to assist practitioners and consumers in making decisions about health care. Practice guidelines are based on several sources of knowledge. The gold standard is knowledge derived from clinical trials; the next best is other types of empirical evidence; and the least acceptable is clinical judgment. Several guidelines are in process by the federal agency. ANA is deliberating about the approach to use in producing guidelines within the professional associations. These efforts require standardized language to describe diagnoses, interventions, and outcomes, and empirical work from which the knowledge to link diagnoses, interventions, and outcomes can be derived.

Nursing has only begun to develop and test its standardized language. We believe this book is a valuable contribution to the needed work. The chapter authors have made enormous strides in defining and describing the essential nursing treatments. Vast amounts of literature have been synthesized and combined with the authors' experiences to articulate the intervention concepts and provide direction for clinical practice. We commend the chapter authors for contributing to the continuing evolution of nursing knowledge.

INDEX

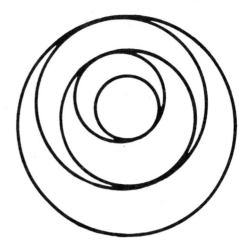